GERIATRIC DIABETES

GERIATRIC DIABETES

Edited by

Medha N. Munshi
Joslin Diabetes Center
Beth Israel Deaconess Medical Center
Boston, Massachusetts, USA

Lewis A. Lipsitz
Beth Israel Deaconess Medical Center
Hebrew SeniorLife Institute for Aging Research
Boston, Massachusetts, USA

informa
healthcare

New York   London

Informa Healthcare USA, Inc.
52 Vanderbilt Avenue
New York, NY 10017

International Standard Book Number-10: 0-8493-7065-5 (hb.: alk. paper)
International Standard Book Number-13: 978-0-8493-7065-6 (hb.: alk. paper)

Library of Congress Cataloging-in-Publication Data

Geriatric diabetes/[edited by] Medha N. Munshi, Lewis A. Lipsitz.
    p. ; cm.
  Includes bibliographical references and index.
  ISBN-13: 978-0-8493-7065-6 (hb.: alk. paper)
  ISBN-10: 0-8493-7065-5 (hb.: alk. paper) 1. Geriatrics. 2. Diabetes. 3. Older people--Health and hygiene. I. Munshi, Medha N. II. Lipsitz, Lewis A.
  [DNLM: 1. Diabetes Mellitus--therapy. 2. Aged. 3. Diabetes Complications.
4. Diabetes Mellitus--diagnosis. WK 815 G369 2007]

RC952.G4779 2007
618.97'6462--dc22   2007009436

Visit the Informa Web site at
www.informa.com

and the Informa Healthcare Web site at
www.informahealthcare.com

We wish to dedicate this book to our families.
Who I am as a person was guided by my parents Vila and Anil Mehta,
my sister Madhavi and my brother Milind.
Who I have become personally and professionally is due to my husband
Nikhil and sons Vidit and Manit.
No words can express my gratitude!

Medha Munshi

My commitment to the health and wellbeing of older people is inspired by my parents,
Jeanne and Paul Lipsitz, and my Mother-in-Law, Marion Preston.
My ability to pursue this commitment is due to the love and support of my wife,
Louise, and my sons Matthew, and Ethan.

Lewis Lipsitz

Preface

The good physician treats the disease; The great physician treats the patient who has the disease.

—Sir William Osler

The world population is rapidly aging, and the prevalence of diabetes is reaching epidemic proportions. Diabetes in older populations poses unique challenges that have not been fully addressed in medical textbooks or educational programs for health care professionals. Diabetes is not the same disease in the elderly as it is in the young. Its pathophysiology, diagnostic criteria, pharmacologic management, dietary recommendations, and lifestyle impact are quite different. In addition, older adults are not a homogeneous population. Community-dwelling adults, individuals in assisted living facilities, and nursing home residents all have unique functional characteristics and needs. Before developing a management plan the physical, social, emotional, and cognitive status of an older adult must be considered. Specific barriers to their ability to perform self-management must be taken into account. Moreover, the goals of care may differ in elderly patients, emphasizing quality rather than quantity of life.

At present there are few evidence-based recommendations to guide the care of elderly patients with diabetes, largely because there are very few prospective studies that include adequate numbers of representative elderly subjects. When the same criteria and strategies used in young adults are applied to the elderly without considering their special circumstances, there is increased risk of non-adherence, complications of treatment such as hypoglycemia or falls, and diabetic complications.

The unique feature of this book is its primary focus on diabetes in older adults and the challenges encountered in caring for these patients. The chapters in this book illustrate how diabetes presents differently in older adults, how it affects other diverse systems of the body, and how it should be diagnosed and treated with attention to its protean manifestations and related comorbidities. There is a detailed discussion of physical, social, emotional, and cognitive problems that affect older adults with diabetes, and the effects of these problems on their disease and their ability to perform self-management. In addition, the authors have presented strategies to modify the management plan to overcome these barriers and thereby improve diabetes control without compromising quality of life.

Optimal diabetes care has much in common with geriatric medicine, since it requires multidisciplinary teamwork, attention to comorbidity, knowledge of pharmacology, and a variety of social, psychological, nutritional, economic, and environmental interventions. It is our hope that this book provides enough practical information about all of these aspects to help clinicians provide excellent care for their elderly patients with diabetes.

The editors would like to thank the Joslin Diabetes Center and Beth Israel Deaconess Medical Center for supporting our mission and providing us with the opportunity to care for many elderly patients with diabetes. We also thank our distinguished colleagues who have contributed the chapters of this book. Finally, we wish to acknowledge the John A. Hartford Foundation's Center of Excellence in Geriatric Medicine and the Donald W. Reynolds Program to Strengthen Training in Geriatric Medicine at Harvard Medical School, for supporting our efforts to educate physicians about the care of elderly patients.

Medha N. Munshi
Lewis A. Lipsitz

Contents

Contributors

Martin J. Abrahamson   Joslin Diabetes Center, Department of Medicine, Harvard Medical School, Boston, Massachusetts, U.S.A.

Lloyd Paul Aiello   Beetham Eye Institute, Joslin Diabetes Center and Department of Ophthalmology, Harvard Medical School, Boston, Massachusetts, U.S.A.

Sunil Asnani   Department of Medicine, Section of Endocrinology, UMDNJ-Robert Wood Johnson Medical School, Jersey Shore University Medical Center, Neptune, New Jersey, U.S.A.

Caroline S. Blaum   University of Michigan Medical School, Ann Arbor, Michigan, U.S.A.

Suzanne F. Bradley   Geriatric Research Education and Clinical Center, Veterans Affairs Ann Arbor Healthcare Center, and Divisions of Geriatric Medicine and Infectious Diseases, Department of Internal Medicine, University of Michigan Medical School, Ann Arbor, Michigan, U.S.A.

Christina Bratcher   Department of Medicine, Section of Endocrinology and Metabolism, Tulane University Health Sciences Center, New Orleans, Louisiana, U.S.A.

Mark R. Burge   Department of Medicine, Endocrinology Division, University of New Mexico Health Sciences Center, Albuquerque, New Mexico, U.S.A.

Jerry D. Cavallerano   Beetham Eye Institute, Joslin Diabetes Center and Department of Ophthalmology, Harvard Medical School, Boston, Massachusetts, U.S.A.

Ronni Chernoff   Geriatric Research Education and Clinical Center, Central Arkansas Veterans Healthcare System, Department of Geriatrics, Arkansas Geriatric Education Center and Reynolds Institute on Aging, University of Arkansas for Medical Sciences, Little Rock, Arkansas, U.S.A.

Marshall H. Chin   Section of General Internal Medicine, The University of Chicago, Chicago, Illinois, U.S.A.

Virginia K. Cummings   Division of Gerontology, Beth Israel Deaconess Medical Center, Boston, Massachusetts, U.S.A.

Robin M. Daly   School of Exercise and Nutrition Sciences, Deakin University, Melbourne, Victoria, Australia

Jatin K. Dave   Division of Aging, Brigham and Women's Hospital, Harvard Medical School, Boston, Massachusetts, U.S.A.

Catherine E. DuBeau   Section of Geriatrics, The University of Chicago, Chicago, Illinois, U.S.A.

David W. Dunstan   Department of Epidemiology and Clinical Research, NOT Geriatric Research Education and Clinical Center, Melbourne, Victoria, Australia

Hermes Florez   Divisions of Endocrinology and Geriatric Medicine, University of Miami Miller School of Medicine and Geriatric Research, Education, and Clinical Center, Miami Veterans Affairs Medical Center, Miami, Florida, U.S.A.

Vivian A. Fonseca   Department of Medicine, Section of Endocrinology and Metabolism, Tulane University Health Sciences Center, New Orleans, Louisiana, U.S.A.

Jason L. Gaglia   Joslin Diabetes Center, Department of Medicine, Harvard Medical School, Boston, Massachusetts, U.S.A.

Leslie Gamache   Department of Medicine, Endocrinology Division, University of New Mexico Health Sciences Center, Albuquerque, New Mexico, U.S.A.

J. Michael Gaziano   Division of Aging, Brigham and Women's Hospital, Harvard Medical School, Boston, Massachusetts, U.S.A.

Sudeep S. Gill   Departments of Medicine and Community Health and Epidemiology, Queen's University, Kingston, and Institute for Clinical Evaluative Sciences, Toronto, Ontario, Canada

Rola N. Hamam   Beetham Eye Institute, Joslin Diabetes Center and Department of Ophthalmology, Harvard Medical School, Boston, Massachusetts, U.S.A.

Elbert S. Huang   Department of Medicine, The University of Chicago, Chicago, Illinois, U.S.A.

Hsu-Ko Kuo   Department of Geriatrics and Gerontology and Department of Internal Medicine, National Taiwan University Hospital, Taipei, Taiwan

Suzanne G. Leveille   Department of Medicine, Beth Israel Deaconess Medical Center, Harvard Medical School, Boston, Massachusetts, U.S.A.

Lorraine L. Lipscombe   Department of Medicine, University of Toronto, and Institute for Clinical Evaluative Sciences, Toronto, Ontario, Canada

Lewis A. Lipsitz   Hebrew SeniorLife Institute for Aging Research, Beth Israel Deaconess Medical Center, Harvard Medical School, Boston, Massachusetts, U.S.A.

Thomas E. Lyons   Division of Podiatry, Beth Israel Deaconess Medical Center, Harvard Medical School, Boston, Massachusetts, U.S.A.

Jennifer B. Marks   Divisions of Endocrinology, Diabetes, and Metabolism, University of Miami Miller School of Medicine, and Miami Veterans Affairs Medical Center, Miami, Florida, U.S.A.

Graydon S. Meneilly   Department of Medicine, Vancouver Hospital and the University of British Columbia, Vancouver, British Columbia, Canada

Medha N. Munshi   Joslin Diabetes Center, Beth Israel Deaconess Medical Center, Boston, Massachusetts, U.S.A.

Peter Novak   Department of Neurology, Boston University Medical Center, Boston, Massachusetts, U.S.A.

Vera Novak   Division of Gerontology, Department of Medicine, Beth Israel Deaconess Medical Center, Harvard Medical School, Boston, Massachusetts, U.S.A.

Hemanth Pai   Department of Medicine, Endocrinology Division, University of New Mexico Health Sciences Center, Albuquerque, New Mexico, U.S.A.

Seema Parikh   Division of Gerontology, Department of Medicine, Beth Israel Deaconess Medical Center, Harvard Medical School, Boston, Massachusetts, U.S.A.

Monica E. Peek   Section of General Internal Medicine, The University of Chicago, Chicago, Illinois, U.S.A.

Frank B. Pomposelli   Division of Vascular and Endovascular Surgery, Beth Israel Deaconess Medical Center, Harvard Medical School, Boston, Massachusetts, U.S.A.

Attila Priplata   Hebrew SeniorLife Institute for Aging Research, Beth Israel Deaconess Medical Center, Harvard Medical School, Boston, Massachusetts, U.S.A.

Paula A. Rochon   Departments of Medicine and Health Policy, Management and Evaluation, University of Toronto, and Institute for Clinical Evaluative Sciences, Toronto, Ontario, Canada

James L. Rosenzweig   Joslin Diabetes Center, Harvard Medical School, Boston, Massachusetts, U.S.A.

Deborah K. Schlossman   Beetham Eye Institute, Joslin Diabetes Center and Department of Ophthalmology, Harvard Medical School, Boston, Massachusetts, U.S.A.

Richard E. Scranton   Division of Aging, Brigham and Women's Hospital, Harvard Medical School, Boston, Massachusetts, U.S.A.

Alissa Segal   College of Pharmacy, University of New Mexico Health Sciences Center, Albuquerque, New Mexico, U.S.A.

Gautam V. Shrikhande   Department of Surgery, Beth Israel Deaconess Medical Center, Harvard Medical School, Boston, Massachusetts, U.S.A.

Kristi D. Silver   Division of Endocrinology, Department of Medicine, Diabetes, and Nutrition, University of Maryland, Baltimore, Maryland, U.S.A.

Alan J. Sinclair   Bedfordshire and Hertfordshire Postgraduate Medical School, University of Bedfordshire, Luton, U.K.

Lilya Sitnikov   Section of Behavioral and Mental Health Research, Joslin Diabetes Center, Boston, Massachusetts, U.S.A.

Kenneth J. Snow   Section of Adult Diabetes, Joslin Diabetes Center, and Department of Clinical Medicine, Harvard Medical School, Boston, Massachusetts, U.S.A.

Robert C. Stanton   Renal Section, Joslin Diabetes Center, Harvard Medical School, Boston, Massachusetts, U.S.A.

William M. Sullivan   Joslin Diabetes Center, Beth Israel Deaconess Medical Center, and Department of Medicine, Harvard Medical School, Boston, Massachusetts, U.S.A.

Tina K. Thethi   Department of Medicine, Section of Endocrinology and Metabolism, Tulane University Health Sciences Center, New Orleans, Louisiana, U.S.A.

Aristidis Veves   Joslin-Beth Israel Deaconess Foot Center and Microcirculation Laboratory, Harvard Medical School, Boston, Massachusetts, U.S.A.

Stefano Volpato   Department of Clinical and Experimental Medicine, Section of Internal Medicine, Gerontology, and Geriatrics, University of Ferrara, Ferrara, Italy

Jeremy D. Walston   Department of Medicine, Johns Hopkins University, Baltimore, Maryland, U.S.A.

Katie Weinger   Section of Behavioral and Mental Health Research, Joslin Diabetes Center and Department of Psychiatry, Harvard Medical School, Boston, Massachusetts, U.S.A.

Mark E. Williams   Renal Section, Joslin Diabetes Center, Harvard Medical School, Boston, Massachusetts, U.S.A.

1 | Descriptive Epidemiology of Diabetes

Caroline S. Blaum
University of Michigan Medical School, Ann Arbor, Michigan, U.S.A.

INTRODUCTION

Diabetes is one of the most common chronic diseases affecting older persons, and diabetes prevalence is increasing among older Americans as well as among all other age groups. Over 95% of people with diabetes have type 2 diabetes. In 2004, the Centers for Disease Control (CDC) estimated that nearly 17% of the population of the United States aged 65 to 74 had diabetes, with a slightly lower prevalence among those 75 years and older (1). Over the past 20 years, the prevalence of diagnosed diabetes has increased even when different diagnostic criteria and practices are considered.

In the United States, people aged 65 and older now comprise nearly 40% of all people with diabetes. As the current CDC incidence data shows, because of the population aging and increasing rates of obesity among middle-aged adults (2), older adults will make up the majority of people with diabetes in the United States and in other developed countries in the coming decades. For example, in 2004, the incidence of diabetes among people aged 65 to 79 was over five times as high as the incidence among people under 45 years of age (14.9 per 1000 population vs. 2.9 per 1000) (3). Among people aged 65 to 79, incidence increased 43% (from 10.4 to 14.9 per 1000) from 1997 to 2004; among people aged 45 to 64, incidence increased 34% (from 8.5 to 11.4 per 1000 population) during that time period. Figures are not available for those older than 79, but the incidence is thought to decrease in the oldest age groups.

The CDC also estimates that up to one-third of adults with diabetes mellitus are unaware of their condition, presumably because diabetes is often asymptomatic for several years (4). Despite the early asymptomatic period, diabetes mellitus is a serious condition associated with significant morbidity and a shortened survival. Older persons with diabetes experience a mortality rate nearly twice that of persons without this disease; mortality is increased even more in the presence of coronary artery disease (5,6). In addition, older adults experience disproportionately high number of clinical complications and comorbidities associated with diabetes. These complications include atherosclerosis, neuropathies, loss of vision, and renal insufficiency. The rates of myocardial infarction, stroke, and renal failure are increased approximately twofold (7). Diabetes is the major cause of blindness in people up to the age of 65, and the risk of blindness is increased approximately 40% in older persons with diabetes. Diabetes is also the major reason for end-stage renal disease and dialysis in people who are 60 and older (4).

Research is accumulating about important clinical consequences of diabetes that are common in older adults and have serious implications for health status and quality of life. In older patients, poorly controlled hyperglycemia can lead to physical decline and symptoms such as fatigue, weight loss, and muscle weakness (7). Observational studies have documented that older adults with diabetes are at higher risk than those without diabetes for geriatric conditions (conditions that are prevalent in older adults, which are not associated with any single disease and are associated with disability and decreased quality of life) (8) including incontinence (9), falls (10), frailty (11), cognitive impairment (12), and depressive symptoms (13). Older patients with diabetes also have a higher prevalence of functional impairment and disability than older adults without diabetes. Mobility disability is about two to three times more likely, and activities of daily living (ADL) disability about 1.5 times more likely, in older adults with diabetes compared to those without (14). CDC data shows that, in 2003, the prevalence of mobility limitations among people aged 75 and older with diabetes was 78%, nearly twice that of younger people with diabetes (4).

The fastest growing segment of the older population in the United States includes people aged 80 and older. This group has the highest disability rates, resulting in an increased need for personal assistance and caregiver attention. These trends result in a substantial number of functionally disabled elders, either in the community or in nursing homes, who have diabetes, and their numbers will increase. Up to 15% of nursing home patients have diabetes, and these patients have higher levels of comorbid diseases, diabetes complications, and disability than nursing home patients without diabetes (15). This issue is discussed in detail in Chapter 27.

The epidemic of type 2 diabetes is experienced by other developed countries, as well as the United States. In addition, as modernization occurs throughout Asia and Latin America, the incidence and prevalence of diabetes are increasing worldwide (16). Diabetes is becoming a common chronic disease in developing countries as life expectancy increases and modernization leads to more adoption of Western work and eating habits. The World Health Organization estimates that at least 171 million people worldwide have diabetes. This figure is likely to more than double by 2030 to reach 366 million (17,18).

Diabetes is increasing worldwide for several reasons. In developed countries, better treatment, particularly the decrease in mortality from atherosclerotic heart disease, leads to increased survival of people with diabetes. Although not all sociodemographic groups benefit equally, the net result is that more people survive with diabetes into older age. However, the increasing incidence of diabetes worldwide is related to changes in diet and activity level associated with modernization and globalization. An increasing amount of processed food is available and work patterns lead to a sedentary lifestyle, increasing the numbers of people who are overweight and obese-risk factors for type 2 diabetes (19).

Diabetes is a difficult public health problem because of its pathophysiological characteristics: its few symptoms are easily treated early in the disease, but as it progresses, the associated vascular disease and neurological and other complications lead to excess morbidity and mortality. Also, effective diabetes management depends on patient self-management and diet and physical activity changes, which are difficult for many people to accomplish. As the developed countries already know, and the developing world is rapidly discovering, diabetes is a major strain on health-care resources and adversely affects population health.

Recently in the United States, concern has been growing over the increasing incidence of type 2 diabetes in childhood and among teenagers, attributed to inactivity and increasing obesity levels in childhood (20). Early appearance of type 2 diabetes appears to be a growing problem, particularly among minority groups in the United States, including Hispanic Americans, African Americans, and Native Americans.

PATHOPHYSIOLOGICAL CONSIDERATIONS

The vast majority of older adults with diabetes, about 95%, have type 2 diabetes, formally called non insulin dependent diabetes (NIDDM), which involves a complex interaction of genetic factors, diet, and activity level. Risk factors linked with the modern lifestyle, including inactivity and obesity, are associated with insulin resistance, lipid disorders, hypertension, and vascular disease. In the setting of β-cell dysfunction, whether genetic or acquired, hyperglycemia develops and magnifies the associated disorders. However, some older adults with diabetes mellitus do have other forms of diabetes, not as well described. Fewer than 5% have type 1 diabetes, related to autoimmune mechanisms. Other rarer and mainly genetic forms of diabetes are characterized clinically by dysfunctions in signaling and/or insulin utilization, or β-cell abnormalities. Clinically, most physicians caring for older patients with diabetes will have a few patients who are thin and insulin sensitive, and in whom it is difficult to achieve glycemic control. Epidemiological studies of older adults with diabetes have documented a small group of thin, older people with diabetes who may not have high insulin levels, or other characteristics such as hypertension and hyperlipidemia associated with type 2 diabetes and the metabolic syndrome (21).

As people age with diabetes, or develop type 2 diabetes after years of having insulin resistance and cardiovascular risk factors, physiological changes common to both aging and diabetes may interact to further decrease physiological reserve. Type 2 diabetes and obesity are associated with inflammatory dysregulation, which may also be associated with aging and lead to clinical sequelae such as sarcopenia (decreased muscle mass) (22). Changes in body composition that occur with aging, such as increased visceral fat leading to insulin resistance, may also contribute to alternations in carbohydrate metabolism in aging (23). Aging is associated with decreased physiological reserve in multiple organ systems (renal, cardiovascular, neurological), which may interact with end-organ damage due to diabetes, resulting in increased vulnerability to physiological stressors.

HEALTH BURDEN OF OLDER PEOPLE WITH DIABETES: DISTAL OUTCOMES

Despite its worrisome recent increase in children and young adults, type 2 diabetes still is mainly a disease of middle-aged and older adults. As a chronic disease, diabetes lasts for many years, allowing people with diabetes to accumulate complications and comorbidities over time, which add to several prediabetes risks and unrelated comorbidities. Eventually, these complications and comorbidities lead to physical limitations, disability, and increased mortality.

Figure 1 illustrates the multiple effects of diabetes on health. Although it depicts type 2 diabetes, many of these pathways would exist in any type of diabetes. Most diabetes management efforts and research are directed at the pathway from diabetes to its atherosclerotic and microvascular complications. Over the past 10 years, however, it has become clearer that risk factors for diabetes related to insulin resistance (24), obesity, and inactivity are themselves risk factors for atherosclerotic diseases. As diabetes has come to be recognized as a major disease of older adults, including people in their late 70s and 80s, and many people in nursing homes, the more distal complications of diabetes have also begun to be recognized. Although many of the impairments and distal outcomes illustrated in Figure 1 are due to vascular complications of diabetes, other pathways involving glycated proteins and inflammatory disruption may be involved (*dotted lines*).

Diabetes is associated with risks of atherosclerotic disease, microvscular complications, related and unrelated comorbidities, multiple impairments, and distal outcomes. Clinically, that means that older adults with diabetes have tremendous clinical complexity, multiple comorbidities (multimorbidity), and, often, geriatric conditions and disabilities. Therefore, the key characteristic of older adults with diabetes is heterogeneity (8,25). Most have type 2 diabetes, but some do not. Many are functional and relatively healthy; many are not. Some have few risks and comorbidities; many have multiple comorbid conditions and complications.

Compare, for example, three 75-year-old women with diabetes. One may have developed type 2 diabetes last year, has mild hypertension requiring one medication, and has no hint of diabetes complications or hyperlipidemia, speed walks 10 miles/wk, volunteers extensively and travels widely. Another developed type 2 diabetes about 15 years ago, is obese and fairly sedentary, has hyperlipidemia, hypertension, coronary artery disease, depression, peripheral neuropathy, and mild chronic kidney disease, takes 10 prescription medications, feels unsteady, and has had one fall, but still volunteers at church, drives, cares for her husband with Alzheimer's, handles the finances, and visits her children and grandchildren often. Another has had diabetes for over 15 years, has dry gangrene of toes, coronary artery disease, hypertension, atrial fibrillation, a minor stoke with left arm weakness, and depression, walks minimally with a walker, requires assistance with ADLs, is incontinent of urine, and cannot remember her medications. Clearly, for these three older women with diabetes, the goals of diabetes

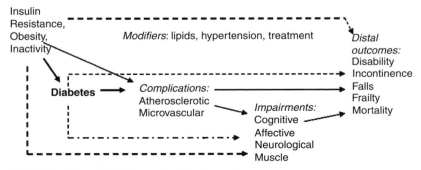

FIGURE 1 Effects of diabetes on health outcomes.

management are different. Clinicians who care for older adults with diabetes can easily recall patients similar to and different from these three women.

The tremendous heterogeneity of older adults with diabetes may be one way in which older adults with diabetes differ from middle-aged people with diabetes. However, there is little epidemiological information on differences between older and middle-aged adults with diabetes. Although older adults have more functional limitations and disability associated with their diabetes, the strength of the association of disability and diabetes is the same among middle-aged and older adults (26). Comorbidity increases with age, and older adults with diabetes have a higher comorbidity burden than middle-aged people with diabetes. The duration of diabetes increases with age. CDC data shows that, among people with diabetes, aged 65 to 79, the median diabetes duration was 9.1 years, while among those aged 45 to 64, the median diabetes duration was 5.3 years (1). Geriatric conditions such as cognitive impairment, falls, incontinence, and frailty are known to increase with age; so older diabetes patients are more likely to have co-occurring geriatric conditions, and diabetes itself may increase the risk of geriatric conditions.

Clinically, older diabetes patients are less likely to have classic symptoms of hyperglycemia such as polyuria and polydipsia, but may have others, including worsened incontinence, declining mental status, increased falls, more infections, or weight loss. Some older adults with poorly controlled diabetes may have no specific symptoms at all or may demonstrate only a nonspecific slow decline (7). Older adults are more likely to experience hypoglycemia with tightly controlled diabetes, but hypoglycemia requiring medical assistance is relatively uncommon (27). The longer duration of diabetes among older people places them at higher risk of autonomic dysfunction, hypoglycemia unawareness, or metabolic hormonal dysregulation, leading to a higher risk of complications of hypoglycemia (28). In some people, however, hypoglycemia can be traced to associated comorbidities and geriatric conditions such as mild cognitive impairment leading to medication error or irregular food intake due to difficulty with cooking or shopping. Among older adults with diabetes, there are some who are vulnerable and frail, with conditions such as advanced dementia, multiple dependencies in ADL, or shortened life expectancy; diabetes management for that group should have different goals. On the other hand, it is critical to remember that some older adults with diabetes are healthy and highly functional and can expect to live for many more years. Many older diabetes patients should not be deprived of high-quality diabetes care on the basis of age.

Clinicians and researchers have suggested several ways to capture the heterogeneity among older adults with diabetes to better inform management goals. Perhaps the most common suggestion involves the estimation of life expectancy (8,25). Because many diabetes management interventions are directed toward preventing or mitigating vascular complications rather than improving symptomatology, they take several years to achieve this goal. If a person's life expectancy is short, the interventions would not be reasonable, although, clearly, inventions to improve symptoms would continue to be indicated. Another approach suggests that considering functional status would be helpful (9). If patients are unable to comply with diabetes management recommendations, it may not be reasonable to attempt aggressive management. Regardless of how such a summarization is done, it is clear that many older adults with diabetes are healthy and functional and should have diabetes management similar to middle-aged adults. However, some older diabetes patients have multiple disabilities and diseases and would not benefit or could be harmed by aggressive diabetes management (29). Goal-setting in older adults is discussed elsewhere in this book. Of course, many patients are between these extremes and have individual preferences and capabilities regarding their diabetes management.

CARE DELIVERY FOR DIABETES

The key characteristics of older adults with diabetes—heterogeneity, multimorbidity, and physiological complexity—have major implications for management of diabetes. As the population ages and obesity rates rise among middle-aged people, more people will be aging with diabetes in the coming years and the complexity of management of diabetes will increase.

Several trends have intersected to influence current diabetes management. First, there is an imperative for better control of vascular disease risks associated with diabetes that is generated by increasing obesity, decreasing activity levels, and high prevalences of prediabetes syndromes and diabetes. Second, we have a relatively good understanding of the causal relationship of diabetes to atherosclerotic and microvascular complications, poor quality of life, and increased costs of care. Third, although less discussed, clinicians and researchers are beginning to realize that diabetes is related to additional, distal, negative health outcomes, illustrated in Figure 1, which also demean quality of life and increase health-care and personal care costs. Finally, high-quality randomized controlled trials (RCTs) have proven that some diabetes management interventions (blood pressure and cholesterol control) decrease macrovascular diabetes complications (in some populations and under some conditions) and some interventions (glycemic control, blood pressure control, eye and foot exams, urine protein monitoring, angiotensin converting enzyme inhibitor/angiotensin receptor blocker) can prevent or decrease microvascular complications (8,30). All these factors have led to the current interest codifying high-quality diabetes management by developing and using diabetes clinical quality indicators to measure the quality of primary care delivery to patients with diabetes (31–33).

Diabetes clinical performance quality indicators are derived from research-based evidence of intermediate outcomes that decrease complications of diabetes or are process measures related to this evidence (i.e., if you do not measure the A1C, you cannot intervene if it is too high, so the quality indicator is the measurement of A1C). Unfortunately, older adults are poorly represented in the classic RCTs that are the basis of current diabetes management. In the United Kingdom Prospective Diabetes Study (UKPDS), for example, the mean age was about 54 (slightly different in different reported substudies) (34) and the participants were people with newly diagnosed diabetes. Most studies that relate level of glycemic and blood pressure control to vascular outcomes involved participants with mean ages in the late 50s and 60s (8,30). The Heart Protection Study is one of the few that randomized people with diabetes, aged up to 80 (35). In general, applying management recommendations on the basis of trials carried out in people aged 70 and under, who were able to participate in an RCT, to complex patients in their late 70s and older, requires extrapolation that may or may not be appropriate. A critical area for geriatric clinical and outcome research is to determine the appropriateness of diabetes management goals derived mainly in late middle-aged populations, to older populations (36). As a rough guide, it would seem reasonable that for people 75 and younger, or for those older adults with diabetes of any age who are functional and healthy, the extrapolation is appropriate. However, for patients with diabetes in their late 70s and older, for patients with comorbidities, disability, and geriatric conditions, and for the over 15% of nursing home residents with diabetes, it remains unclear as to how the quality of care can be assessed. Recent methodological work points out that those most at risk of vascular complications or worsening vascular complications experience the most benefit from diabetes management interventions (37). However, older adults with diabetes who have clinical vascular disease and multimorbidity and have high risk of worsening diabetes complications are often also at risk of adverse affects from management interventions (27), may lack the capacity or desire for a complex self-management regimen, or may have a decreased life expectancy (25). Further research on the feasibility and benefits of different diabetes management interventions in the heterogeneous older population is needed.

Regardless of patient age, diabetes is the most complicated disease managed in primary care with a progressive, multiyear course. Care delivery is complex and time consuming and requires a high-quality medical information system and decision support in order to track interventions (38). In addition, successful diabetes management depends on patient self-management, making patient education and self-management support critical (39). However, education and self-management support can be difficult for a busy physician to handle appropriately. These roles are rendered even more complex as it becomes necessary to understand whether an individual older adult with diabetes has the capacity or desire to comply with complex diabetes self-management recommendations, along with all their other chronic disease self-management needs, and how much caregiver involvement is necessary. Taken together, the optimal management of diabetes in older adults is best facilitated by using a team, with diabetes educators, nurses, and social workers who can work with a patient and caregiver over time to support self-management and connect the patient to community-based services, if needed. Most primary care practices are not yet organized to handle chronic disease in this way. For primary care practices that are part of large health systems, such as academic practices or large physician groups, gradual reorganization toward care delivery models that use strategies to support both provider management decisions and patient self-management may improve diabetes care (and care of other chronic diseases) for patients of any age (40,41).

DIABETES AND PUBLIC POLICY

Care for diabetes is expensive, and most of the expense is due to management of diabetic complications: atherosclerotic disease, retinal disease, and renal failure. The chronic medical management of diabetes—control of hypertension, cholesterol and hyperglycemia, and screening for complications—is suboptimal among adults of all ages with diabetes (32). There is no clear evidence that older adults with diabetes achieve diabetes management goals less often than middle-aged people with diabetes, although low-income elders may be at risk for poor diabetes care quality (42). There is evidence, however, that ethnic disparities exist in diabetes management and achievement of treatment goals (43,44), although this may be mitigated by managed care (45). This issue is discussed in detail in Chapter 26. African Americans and Hispanics, due to socioeconomic considerations or location, may have less access to medical care and insurance coverage.

Much of the health-care bill for diabetes patients is paid for by the taxpayers through Medicare and Medicaid. This financial imperative, as well as the public health goal to decrease morbidity and mortality due to chronic diseases and the significant evidence base for diabetes management interventions, has led to interest in the use of health policy to improve diabetes care. Policy interventions, through legislation and regulation at the state and federal level and through larger insurers, are being directed toward health-care insurers such as Managed Care Organizations (MCOs), group practices, individual physicians, and even patients. Some incentivization schemes involve indirect financial incentives to improve diabetes care. For example, MCOs can be ranked according to the scores of their beneficiary population on clinical quality performance indicators for diabetes. A large employer might encourage employees to choose MCOs with good scores during insurance enrollment by using advertising or favorable pricing. Large group practices can similarly report performance on diabetes clinical quality performance indicators to insurance companies or employer groups in hopes of favorable contracts or advertising. Individual physician profiling for performance on diabetes quality indicators can be used for educational purposes, maintenance of certification, or quality assurance.

Over the past few years, the idea of paying hospitals, large group practices, or individual physicians based on the quality of care provided has intrigued payers—the government, insurance companies, and large employers (46). Although value-based purchasing is being tested widely throughout the clinical arena, the ambulatory care of diabetes is a primary target of many value-based purchasing models. Diabetes is targeted because of its prevalence, its effects on health and costs, and the strong research evidence that medical interventions can change the natural history of diabetes by preventing vascular complications, and, by implication, improving population health, and decreasing costs.

As diabetes clinical quality performance monitoring becomes incorporated into the accountability and payment mix for physician groups and physicians, there remain several technical problems to resolve. For example, in the fee for service system, it is not clear how to allocate patients, who generally see several physicians, to any particular physician. Nor is it clear which of the many physicians seen by an older adult with diabetes should be the physician held accountable for particular quality measures. More important than these issues, however, are concerns about the "evidence base" and the patient. For example, if patient is unable or unwilling to comply with evidence-based care, is the physician "incentivized" to discharge the patient from the practice? For many older adults with diabetes, the evidence base, which is the foundation of the entire system, may be flawed because older patients with multiple diseases were not included in relevant studies. Older patients are more likely to suffer adverse reactions to evidence-based medications, may have different opinions about quality of life, or may have limited life expectancy.

Currently, there are no agreed-upon clinical criteria to exclude a patient from "usual" diabetes quality measures, other than shortened life-span, and age itself (older than 75 is sometimes an exclusion). Life span is difficult to estimate for most patients, which decreases utility of that criterion. On the other hand, many people with diabetes who are 75 and older are healthy, functional, and able to handle diabetes self-management; so age criteria are also not satisfactory. It remains unclear how to target older patients for appropriate diabetes management or how to measure quality of care among different groups of older adults with diabetes.

The complexity and heterogeneity of older adults with diabetes requires the development of an individualized care plan for diabetes and high-quality care addressing diabetes complications and comorbidities, distal outcomes, and geriatric conditions. Currently, there are no defined clinical quality performance indicators, which measure complex care quality. Rather, current physician "accountability" and quality programs provide incentives for providers to focus their attention on those patients who, for whatever reasons, are successful in reaching desired goals of diabetes care, (e.g., A1C < 7.0%, blood pressure < 130/80, low density lipoprotein < 100 mg/dL) (30) and to decrease attention paid to the quality of care of patients who are more complex and may not, for a variety of reasons, achieve these goals. To improve the quality of life and health status of many older adults with diabetes, however, it is important that we learn how to measure diabetes care quality for patients with multiple comorbidities who are medically and socially complex and often vulnerable and, who in fact, require the highest-quality care.

SUMMARY

Diabetes is a common disease among older adults, which will become even more common as diabetes increases in prevalence and the older population grows in number. Older adults with diabetes experience, disproportionately, all the vascular complications of diabetes. In addition, older adults with diabetes may have multiple other diabetes associated impairments including cognitive impairment, incontinence, falls, and disability. Older adults with diabetes are heterogeneous in their health status. Many are extremely healthy; others are disabled with multiple comorbidities; many others are in between these two extremes. The complexity and heterogeneity of older adults with diabetes require the development of an individualized care plan for diabetes and high-quality care addressing diabetes complications and comorbidities, distal outcomes, and geriatric conditions.

Randomized clinical trials have shown that several clinical interventions in diabetes care can decrease vascular complications. Although many of the relevant studies have not included people 75 and older, it is likely that most of these evidence-based diabetes care interventions are appropriate for many older adults with diabetes. However, for complex older patients with diabetes, who often have multiple comorbidities, geriatric syndromes, and personal care needs, individualized and coordinated care is necessary. As physicians are held accountable for the quality of care provided to people with diabetes, it is important to define quality of care for the most complex and vulnerable older adults with diabetes.

REFERENCES

1. Centers for Disease Control and Prevention. Crude and Age-Adjusted Prevalence of Diagnosed Diabetes per 100 Population, United States, 1980–2004. http://www.cdc.gov/DIABETES/statistics/prev/national/figage.htm.
2. Centers for Disease Control and Prevention. Overweight and Obesity: Obesity Trends: U.S. Obesity Trends 1985–2004. http://www.cdc.gov/nccdphp/dnpa/obesity/trend/maps/index.htm.
3. Centers for Disease Control and Prevention. Crude and Age-Adjusted Incidence of Diagnosed Diabetes per 1000 Population Aged 18–79 Years, United States, 1997–2004, 2005. http://www.cdc.gov/diabetes/statistics/incidence/fig 2.htm
4. Centers for Disease Control and Prevention. National diabetes fact sheet: general information and national estimates on diabetes in the United States, 2005. www.cdc.gov/DIABETES/pubs/pdf/ndfs_2005.pdf.
5. Gu K, Cowie CC, Harris MI. Mortality in adults with and without diabetes in a national cohort of the U.S. population, 1971–1993. Diabetes Care 1998; 21(7):1138–1145.
6. Hu FB, Stampfer MJ, Solomon CG, et al. The impact of diabetes mellitus on mortality from all causes and coronary heart disease in women: 20 years of follow-up. Arch Intern Med 2001; 161(14):1717–1723.
7. Blaum CS, Halter JB. Treatment of older adults with diabetes. In: Kahn CR, King GL, Moses AC, Weir GC, Jacobson AM, Smith RJ, eds. Joslin's Diabetes Mellitus. 14th ed. Phildelphia: Lippincott, Williams and Wilkins, 2005:737–746.

8. Brown AF, Mangione CM, Saliba D, Sarkisian CA. Guidelines for improving the care of the older person with diabetes mellitus. J Am Geriatr Soc 2003; 51(suppl 5 Guidelines):S265–S280.

9. Blaum CS, Ofstedal MB, Langa KM, Wray LA. Functional status and health outcomes in older Americans with diabetes mellitus. J Am Geriatr Soc 2003; 51(6):745–753.

10. Volpato S, Leveille SG, Blaum C, Fried LP, Guralnik JM. Risk factors for falls in older disabled women with diabetes: the women's health and aging study. J Gerontol A Biol Sci Med Sci 2005; 60(12): 1539–1545.

11. Fried LP, Tangen CM, Walston J, et al. Frailty in older adults: evidence for a phenotype. J Gerontol A Biol Sci Med Sci 2001; 56(3):M146–M156.

12. Strachan MW, Deary IJ, Ewing FM, Frier BM. Is type II diabetes associated with an increased risk of cognitive dysfunction? A critical review of published studies. Diabetes Care 1997; 20(3):438–445.

13. Anderson RJ, Freedland KE, Clouse RE, Lustman PJ. The prevalence of comorbid depression in adults with diabetes: a meta-analysis. Diabetes Care 2001; 24(6):1069–1078.

14. Songer TJ. Disability in diabetes. In: Harris MI, Cowie CC, Stern MP, Boyko EJ, Reiber G, Bennet PH, eds. Diabetes in America. Vol. NIH Pub. No. 95-1468. 2nd ed. Bethesda, MD: National Institute of Diabetes and Digestive and Kidney Diseases, 1995:259–283.

15. Mayfield J, Deb P, Potter D. Diabetes and long term care. In: National Diabetes Data Group, ed. Diabetes in America. 2nd ed. National Institutes of Health, 1995:571–590.

16. Zimmet P, Shaw J. Diabetes—A worldwide problem. In: Kahn CR, King GL, Moses AC, Weir GC, Jacobson AM, Smith RJ, eds. Joslin's Diabetes Mellitus. 14th ed. Philadelphia: Lippincott, Williams and Wilkins, 2005.

17. World Health Organization. Country and regional data. http://www.who.int/diabetes/facts/world_figures/en/print.html. Accessed 6/5/2006, 2006.

18. World Health Organization. Controlling the global obesity epidemic. http://www.who.int/nutrition/topics/obesity/en/index.html.

19. World Health Organization. Obesity and Overweight. http://www.who.int/mediacentre/factsheets/fs311/en/index.html

20. Liese AD, D'Agostino RB Jr, Hamman RF, et al. The burden of diabetes mellitus among US youth: prevalence estimates from the SEARCH for Diabetes in Youth Study. Pediatrics 2006; 118(4): 1510–1518.

21. Haffner SM, D'Agostino R Jr, Mykkanen L, et al. Insulin sensitivity in subjects with type 2 diabetes. Relationship to cardiovascular risk factors: the Insulin Resistance Atherosclerosis Study. Diabetes Care 1999; 22(4):562–568.

22. Park SW, Goodpaster BH, Strotmeyer ES, et al. Decreased muscle strength and quality in older adults with type 2 diabetes: the health, aging, and body composition study. Diabetes 2006; 55(6):1813–1818.

23. Walston J, McBurnie MA, Newman A, et al. Frailty and activation of the inflammation and coagulation systems with and without clinical comorbidities. Arch Intern Med 2002; 162:2333–2341.

24. Semenkovich CF. Insulin resistance and atherosclerosis. J Clin Invest 2006; 116(7):1813–1822.

25. Durso SC. Using clinical guidelines designed for older adults with diabetes mellitus and complex health status. JAMA 2006; 295(16):1935–1940.

26. Wray LA, Ofstedal MB, Langa KM, Blaum CS. The effect of diabetes on disability in middle-aged and older adults. J Gerontol A Biol Sci Med Sci 2005; 60(9):1206–1211.

27. Shorr RI, Ray WA, Daugherty JR, Griffin MR. Incidence and risk factors for serious hypoglycemia in older persons using insulin or sulfonylureas. Arch Intern Med 1997; 157(15):1681–1686.

28. Cryer PE, Davis SN, Shamoon H. Hypoglycemia in diabetes. Diabetes Care 2003; 26(6):1902–1912.

29. Vijan S, Stevens DL, Herman WH, Funnell MM, Standiford CJ. Screening, prevention, counseling, and treatment for the complications of type II diabetes mellitus. Putting evidence into practice. J Gen Intern Med 1997; 12(9):567–580.

30. American Diabetes Association. Standards of medical care in diabetes. Diabetes Care 2006; 29:S4–S42.

31. Kerr EA, Gerzoff RB, Krein SL, et al. Diabetes care quality in the Veterans Affairs Health Care System and commercial managed care: the TRIAD study. Ann Intern Med 2004; 141(4):272–281.

32. Saaddine JB, Cadwell B, Gregg EW, et al. Improvements in diabetes processes of care and intermediate outcomes: United States, 1988–2002. Ann Intern Med 2006; 144(7):465–474.

33. Hayward RA, Hofer TP, Kerr EA, Krein SL. Quality improvement initiatives: issues in moving from diabetes guidelines to policy. Diabetes Care 2004; 27(suppl 2):B54–B60.

34. UK Prospective Diabetes Study Group. Intensive blood-glucose control with sulphonylureas or insulin compared with conventional treatment and risk of complications in patients with type 2 diabetes. Lancet 1998; 352:837–852.

35. Heart Protection Study Collaborative Group (writing committee: Collins R, Armitage J, Parish S, Sleight P, Peto R). MRC/BHF Heart Protection Study of cholesterol-lowering with simvastatin in 5963 people with diabetes: randomised placebo-controlled trial. Lancet 2003; 361:2005–2016.

36. Blaum CS. Management of diabetes mellitus in older adults: are national guidelines appropriate? J Am Geriatr Soc 2002; 50(3):581–583.

37. Hayward RA, Kent DM, Vijan S, Hofer TP. Reporting clinical trial results to inform providers, payers, and consumers. Health Aff (Millwood) 2005; 24(6):1571–1581.

38. O'Connor PJ. Electronic medical records and diabetes care improvement: are we waiting for Godot? Diabetes Care 2003; 26(3):942–943.
39. Gary TL, Genkinger JM, Guallar E, Peyrot M, Brancati FL. Meta-analysis of randomized educational and behavioral interventions in type 2 diabetes. Diabetes Educ 2003; 29(3):488–501.
40. Bodenheimer T, Wagner EH, Grumbach K. Improving primary care for patients with chronic illness: the chronic care model, Part 2. JAMA 2002; 288(15):1909–1914.
41. Bodenheimer T, Wagner EH, Grumbach K. Improving primary care for patients with chronic illness. JAMA 2002; 288(14):1775–1779.
42. McCall DT, Sauaia A, Hamman RF, Reusch JE, Barton P. Are low-income elderly patients at risk for poor diabetes care? Diabetes Care 2004; 27(5):1060–1065.
43. de Rekeneire N, Rooks RN, Simonsick EM, et al. Racial differences in glycemic control in a well-functioning older diabetic population: findings from the health, aging, and body composition study. Diabetes Care 2003; 26(7):1986–1992.
44. Heisler M, Smith DM, Hayward RA, Krein SL, Kerr EA. Racial disparities in diabetes care processes, outcomes, and treatment intensity. Med Care 2003; 41(11):1221–1232.
45. Brown AF, Gregg EW, Stevens MR, et al. Race, ethnicity, socioeconomic position, and quality of care for adults with diabetes enrolled in managed care: the Translating Research Into Action for Diabetes (TRIAD) study. Diabetes Care 2005; 28(12):2864–2870.
46. Institute of Medicine. Rewarding Provider Performance: Aligning Incentives in Medicare. Washington DC: National Academies Press, 2006.

2 The Genetics of Diabetes and Its Complications in Older Adults

Jeremy D. Walston
Department of Medicine, Johns Hopkins University, Baltimore, Maryland, U.S.A.

Kristi D. Silver
Division of Endocrinology, Department of Medicine, Diabetes, and Nutrition, University of Maryland, Baltimore, Maryland, U.S.A.

INTRODUCTION

Population studies demonstrate that up to 25% of the U.S. population over the age of 65 years has diabetes, making it one of the most common genetic diseases in the United States (1). In addition, it is a major contributing factor to many chronic medical conditions and to the development of disability in older adults (2,3). The prevalence of diabetes increases with age, with the vast majority of cases of diabetes in older adults consisting of type 2 diabetes mellitus (T2DM) (1). While progress toward the understanding of the environmental, physiological, and molecular and genetic basis of diabetes in older adults has been made over the past several years, substantial gaps in knowledge remain, in part because of the complex and heterogeneous nature of diabetes (4,5). Type 1 DM (T1DM) usually develops in childhood or early adulthood and is due to the autoimmune destruction of insulin-secreting beta cells in the pancreas. Although T1DM is found in older adults, it is uncommon for older adults to develop new onset T1DM. The etiology of T2DM in older adults is more complex, with increased insulin resistance and impaired insulin secretion being the key predisposing features of this disorder (1). In fact, T2DM appears to be a complex of multiple metabolic alterations that in sum ultimately contribute to the development of hyperglycemia and the diagnosis of diabetes (4). Aging-related changes in body composition and activation of inflammatory pathways with related declines in lean body mass and increased fat mass profoundly influence these metabolic processes (6). In addition, age-related environmental factors including declines in activity, chronic medical conditions, and pharmaceutical interventions likely alter insulin sensitivity in older adults as well. Given that the vast majority of cases of diabetes that impact older adults are T2DM, the main focus of this chapter will be on genes that contribute to T2DM and related endophenotypes as well as epigenetic mechanisms that influence the development of this disease in older adults. Gene variants that may influence diabetic complications and the utility of some diabetes therapies will also be covered, as will the clinical relevance of this type of research.

DIABETES IS A HEREDITABLE TRAIT

Genetic variants underlie most, if not all, of the physiological abnormalities that influence the development of T2DM (4). Evidence for this comes from several sources. First, monozygotic twin studies show concordance rates at nearly 1.0, and dizygotic twins concordance rates between 0.3 and 0.4 (7–9). Second, having a sibling or a parent with T2DM increases the chance of developing T2DM between three-, and four-fold (10). Finally, large population studies have demonstrated substantial differences in diabetes prevalence between ethnic and racial groups of the same age and country of origin, suggesting that genetic differences may play an important role in determining these differences (1). Although several specific single gene variants that contribute to a rare subtype of T2DM called maturity onset diabetes of the young have been identified in the past decade, no other single gene variants have been demonstrated to have a strong and predictable influence on the development of more common types of T2DM (4). This finding is likely due to the fact that there are multiple molecular pathways influencing the development of the DM phenotype, and that the more common forms of T2DM that impact older adults are likely influenced by a pool of susceptibility genes in many of these pathways (4).

GENES OR PATHWAYS THAT MAY INFLUENCE DIABETES IN OLDER ADULTS

Using both candidate gene and whole genome approaches hundreds of gene variants thought to influence the development of T2DM via alterations in metabolic pathways have been identified. Several of these genes that have consistently (but not necessarily always) been shown to have a modest effect on diabetes or a related endophenotype such as insulin resistance or lower metabolic rate (4,11). Other highly studied gene variants have inconsistently been associated with diabetes. Most of these genes impact more than one diabetes endophenotype (i.e., heritable traits that influence the end phenotype of diabetes mellitus) as well as T2DM itself. Some of these endophenotypes include insulin resistance, insulin secretion, satiety/hunger sensing, body composition, and energy expenditure (Fig. 1). A few select genes and gene variants that may contribute to T2DM in older adults as well as categories of age-related physiological changes that have been demonstrated to have some genetic effect on the development of diabetes or diabetes-related traits are described in the following section.

   Adiponectin is a circulating protein that has both anti-inflammatory and insulin sensitizing properties (12). Levels of adiponectin are inversely related to T2DM, obesity, characteristics of the metabolic syndrome including hypertension and dyslipidemia, and cardiovascular disease. This protein contains C1Q and collagen domains and is encoded by the *APM1* gene located on chromosome 3q27. Single nucleotide polymorphisms (SNPs) in exon 2 (SNP 45 T/G) and intron 2 (SNP 276 G/T) have been associated with lower adiponectin levels in Japanese, Amish, French and Polish (13) Caucasians, insulin resistance in Italian and German (14) Caucasians, and T2DM in French and Polish Caucasians and Japanese. These same SNPs were also predictive of conversion from impaired glucose tolerance (IGT) to T2DM in subjects participating in the STOP-NIDDM trial, with SNP 45 GG and GT genotypes associated with a 1.8-fold higher risk of developing T2DM compared with the TT genotype (OR = 1.84, 95% CI = 1.12–3.00, P = 0.015) (12). Subjects with both the SNP 45 G allele and SNP 276 T allele had a 4.5-fold increased risk of progressing to T2DM (95% CI = 1.78–11.3, P = 0.0001) (12). Other adiponectin gene SNPs that have been associated with either adiponectin levels or T2DM include Ilc164Thn (Japanese) (15), 5'-11391 6/4 (French Caucasians) and 11377 C/G (French Caucasians) and 5' G/A -11391 C/G 11377 (French Caucasians) (16).

β-CELL ADENOSINE TRIPHOSPHATE–SENSITIVE POTASSIUM CHANNEL

The β-cell adenosine triphosphate (ATP)-sensitive potassium channel plays a critical role in insulin secretion. The channel is composed of two subunits: the sulfonylurea receptor-1 (SUR1), a member of the ATP binding cassette transporter family of proteins, and an inward rectifying potassium channel (Kir6.2) which are encoded by the *ABCC8* and *KCNJ11* genes on chromosome 11p15.1 about 4.5 kb apart. SUR1 is a 13-membrane-spanning protein with two

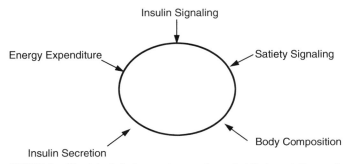

FIGURE 1 Physiologic factors under genetic control that may influence the development of type 2 diabetes mellitus in older adults.

nucleotide-binding folds that bind ATP. Binding sites for sulfonylurea and meglitinides are most likely located at the amino terminus of the protein. Kir6.2 has two membrane spanning domains and homodimerizes to form the potassium channel. Molecular scanning of the *Kir6.2* gene has identified several missense mutations, with the Glu23Lys mutation being the most studied (17). In most studies of Caucasians, the Glu23Lys variant is significantly associated with T2DM. For example, the Glu23Lys variant was significantly associated with T2DM in French Caucasians (allele frequency 0.27 vs. 0.14, $P = 0.015$) (18) and in UK Caucasians [OR for Lys23 heterozygotes = 1.23 (95% CI = 1.12–1.36), $P = 0.000015$; and for Lys23 homozygotes = 1.65 (95% CI = 1.34–2.02), $P = 0.000002$] (19). A meta-analysis of four Caucasian populations [French, United Kingdom (two populations), Danish] (T2DM $n = 521$, control $n = 367$) demonstrated an association of the Lys23 variant with T2DM ($P = 0.0016$; corrected for multiple comparisons $P < 0.01$) (18). Another meta-analysis of the Glu23Lys variant by van Dam et al. in over 7000 Caucasian subjects found a 1.12-fold increase in the likelihood of glucose intolerance for subjects heterozygous for Glu23Lys (95% CI = 1.01–1.23, $P = 0.03$) and 1.44-fold increase in the likelihood of glucose intolerance for Lys23 homozygosity (95% CI = 1.17–1.78, $P = 0.0007$) (20). In several other studies, Kir6.2 variants have not been directly associated with T2DM; however, the variants have been associated with traits related to diabetes including decreased insulin secretion in glucose tolerant controls (21). Despite these findings, it is not clear if the association is due to the Glu23Lys variant, since it is in strong linkage disequilibrium with *SUR1* gene Ala 1369Ser variant, thus making it difficult to determine which variant is responsible for the association.

Several polymorphisms have been identified in the *SUR-1* gene including exon 18 (AC**C**→AC**T**, Thr759Thr) and in the intron 5′ of exon 16 (t→c change located at position -3 of the exon 16 splice acceptor site) [numbering of SUR1 exons is done according to Hansen et al. (22)], which are associated with T2DM in two Caucasian populations of European descent (Utah Mormons and UK) (23). However, not all studies have found a similar association, including the above-mentioned meta-analysis by van Dam et al. (20). In the Finnish Diabetes Prevention Study, the 1273 AGA allele of the *SUR1* gene was associated with a two-fold risk of progression from IGT to T2DM. The 1273 AGA allele is part of a high-risk haplotype that includes promoter variants G-28886A, G-1561A, and A-1273G. Subjects with the high risk SUR1 haplotype and the Kir6.2 Lys23 allele were at a six-fold increased risk for converting to T2DM compared with those without any of the at-risk genotypes (OR = 5.68, 95% CI = 1.75–18.32, $P = 0.004$) (24).

β-3-Adrenergic Receptor Trp64Arg

Using the classical candidate gene approach, investigators discovered a Trp64Arg variant in the gene that codes for a seven trans membrane receptor that likely contributes to the regulation of beta-3-adrenergic receptor adrenergic function in visceral fat, muscle, and islet cells. Early population studies showed associations between the Arg variant and accelerated onset of T2DM in Pima Indians and in Finnish Caucasians (25,26). Subsequent studies in dozens of populations showed mixed results in the study of the relationship of the variant allele to insulin resistance, obesity, and T2DM (27). Physiological studies demonstrated that those homozygous for the Arg variant secreted lower levels of insulin during an IV glucose tolerance test and that they had a lower resting metabolic rate than those who were homozygous for the common Trp allele (28,29). Subsequent molecular studies also demonstrated that islet cells transfected with the Arg/Arg receptor secreted less insulin after stimulation with a beta adrenergic agonist (30). This evidence suggests that the Arg variant impacts both insulin secretion and insulin resistance, perhaps through alteration of metabolic rate. It also provides a good example of how genes may play a modifying role rather than a direct role in the development of diabetes in older adults.

Calpain 10

Calpain 10 is the first gene for T2DM identified by genome wide scan and positional cloning. The gene for calpain 10 is located at chromosome 2q37.3 and consists of 15 exons and at least eight isoforms (a–h). It is a member of a family of cytoplasmic cysteine proteases that are activated by calcium and is expressed diffusely in tissues including liver, muscle, adipocytes, and pancreatic islets. All of these tissues are important in the metabolic processes involved with either insulin sensitivity or insulin secretion.

The initial positional cloning effort that was performed in Mexican Americans from Starr County Texas, identified SNP UCSNP 43 (G/A) in intron 3 that was associated with T2DM (31). Further studies demonstrated that a common haplotype (112/121) including UCSNP43 (G/A), UCSNP19 (two to three repeats of a 32 bp sequence in intron 6), and UCSNP63 (C/T in intron 13) was more strongly associated with T2DM than the UCSNP43 alone (OR = 3.02, 95% CI = 1.37–6.64). The group also performed association studies of this haplotype in Caucasian Finns from Botnia and Caucasians from Germany and found in the combined group a similar association with T2DM (OR = 3.16, 95% CI = 1.19–8.40) (31).

Subsequent studies have shown mixed results, with some demonstrating association (32,33) [Finish/Botnia (34) and African Americans (35)] and others demonstrating no association [Japanese (36), South Indians (37), Samoans (38), Mexican Americans (39) and OjiCree (46)].

In 2004, Song et al. performed a meta-analysis (47) of 26 studies that demonstrated no effect of the UCSNP43 on T2DM when analyzed under a dominant or additive model; however, when analyzed under a recessive model, there was a 19% higher risk of T2DM in those homozygous for the G allele than in those homozygous or heterozygous for the A allele (OR = 1.19, 95% CI = 1.07–1.33). In a recent pooled analysis and meta-analysis for the UCSNP43, -19, and -63, individually and as haplotypes in 3237 subjects with T2DM and 2935 controls with European ancestry, the UCSNP43 G allele showed a modest, but significant, association with T2DM (OR = 1.11, 95% CI = 1.02–1.20, $P = 0.01$) (48). Two haplotypes increased the risk of T2DM (121/121, OR = 1.20, 95% CI = 1.03–1.41, $P = 0.002$ and 112/121, OR = 1.26, 95% CI = 1.01–1.59, $P = 0.04$) and one haplotype decreased the risk of T2DM (111/221, OR = 0.86, 95% CI = 0.75–0.99). When only the population case–control samples were analyzed (pooled and meta-analysis) the association with T2DM increased.

In other populations, UCSNP44 (T/C), which is 11 base pairs from the UCSNP43, but not in linkage disequilibrium with this SNP, has been associated with T2DM (39,45). A meta-analysis by Weedon et al. (49) that included over 3000 British, Chinese (50), Japanese (36,43), Finish/Botnia (33), South Indian (37), and Mexican American (31) subjects from 10 case–control studies and additional 4213 Caucasian, Japanese and Mexican subjects genotyped for the study gave an OR of 1.17 (95% CI = 1.07–1.29, $P = 0.007$) for an increased risk of the SNP44 C allele and the development of T2DM.

While it is not yet known how these calpain variants increase the development of T2DM, calpain has been shown to have a role in glucose metabolism that could potentially lead to diabetes. In calpain 10 transgenic mice, enhanced ryanodine induced apoptosis occurs in pancreatic β cell (51). Nonspecific calpain inhibitors enhanced insulin secretion in short-term culture; however, these inhibitors suppressed glucose metabolism in 48-hour cultures (52,53). Calpain 10 may affect fusion of insulin granules to the cell membrane via SNAP 25 (54). These studies suggest a role for Calpain 10 in insulin secretion. Thus, mutations in the gene could lead to decreased insulin secretion.

HEPATOCYTE NUCLEAR FACTOR 4α

The hepatocyte nuclear factor 4 alpha (HNF4α) is a β cell transcription factor that regulates expression of genes involved with glucose metabolism and insulin secretion. The HNF4α gene localizes to chromosome 20q13, a region that has been linked to T2DM in a number of genome wide linkage studies (55–58). There are several isoforms for the gene as a result of alternate splicing and transcription from two different promoters. The predominant transcription start site in pancreatic β cells is the P2 promoter.

In a study of Ashkenazi Jews, Love-Gregory et al. identified a SNP in the P2 promoter (rs1884614) that was significantly associated with T2DM (26.9% cases vs. 20.3% controls, $P = 0.00078$, OR = 1.45) (dm 4/04 p1134). Through further studies, this group identified a >10 kb haplotype block that is associated with T2DM and accounted for a linkage signal on chromosome 20q. In an independent association analysis of T2DM in the Finland–United States Investigation of NIDDM (FUSION) Genetics cohort, Silander et al. identified a SNP (rs2144908) which was located 1.3 kb downstream of the P2 promoter that was also associated with T2DM (OR = 1.33, 95% CI = 1.06–1.65, P = 0.011) (59). Each of these SNPs was tested in the other population and the associations confirmed. Similar associations with either individual SNPs or haplotypes have been found in the Japanese (60), Pima Indians (61), and Caucasian (62,63) populations though not in all populations (64,65).

PEROXISOME PROLIFERATOR-ACTIVATED RECEPTOR-GAMMA

Peroxisome proliferator-activated receptor-gamma (PPAR-γ) is a nuclear receptor that has been implicated in the regulation of adipocyte differentiation as well as insulin sensitivity and lipid metabolism. The PPAR-γ2 isoform is expressed almost exclusively in adipose tissue (66,67). It is encoded on chromosome 3p25. A proline to alanine substitution at codon 12 (Pro12Ala PPAR-γ2) was identified in the γ2 specific isoform of PPAR-γ (68) and is common in diverse populations with the highest allele frequency in Caucasians (0.10–0.19) and the lowest in African Americans (0.02) (69). Functional evaluation of the proline to alanine substitution by Deeb et al. (70) demonstrated that PPAR-γ Ala12 allele had lower affinity for the PPAR-γ response element than PPAR-γ2 Pro12 allele. In vitro studies show decreased activation of the PPAR-γ2 Ala12 variant by PPAR-γ agonist rosiglitazone compared with the Pro12 allele (70,71). In most studies (72–76), but not all [German (80), Italian (81), and French Caucasian (82)], the Ala12 variant is associated with a decreased prevalence of T2DM. A meta-analysis by Altshuler et al. revealed a significantly higher risk for T2DM in subjects carrying the Pro12 allele (relative risk = 1.25, P = 0.002) (83). Because the prevalence of the Pro allele is high, the population attributable risk of the variant is large.

There is greater consistency among studies of the effects of the Pro12Ala PPARγ2 variant on endophenotypes, including insulin sensitivity and body mass index (BMI), than T2DM. Several studies have shown that nondiabetic subjects with the Ala12 allele are significantly more insulin sensitive and have lower fasting insulin levels (84–86). In a large cohort of African Americans, subjects with the Ala12 PPARγ2 allele had significantly lower fasting insulin levels and insulin to glucose ratio, indicating increased insulin sensitivity. Using euglycemic hyperinsulinemic clamps, Jacob et al. (87) showed that German Caucasian subjects with the PPARγ2 Ala variant had significantly greater glucose uptake and lipolysis index, indicating greater insulin sensitivity. However, the association with greater insulin sensitivity has not been confirmed in all populations [in another Japanese cohort (88), Italians (81), or Koreans (72)].

Several studies have also shown an association between Ala12 carriers and increased BMI (73,74). Differences in the direction and magnitude of associations with BMI and insulin sensitivity may be due, in part, to interaction of the Pro12Ala variant with dietary fat intake (75) and/or with obesity itself (76,77). For example, in a weight loss study, postmenopausal Caucasian women with the Ala12 allele lost similar amounts of weight as those homozygous for the Pro12 allele (77). However, those with the Ala12 allele became significantly more insulin sensitive after weight loss and regained the weight more rapidly after the weight loss intervention ended. In summary, the PPAR-γ2 Ala12 variant appears to be protective against the development of insulin resistance and susceptibility to T2DM, and at the same time, increases susceptibility to obesity and/or weight gain. PPAR-γ2 may thus be considered a "thrifty gene" (78).

TRANSCRIPTION FACTOR 7–LIKE 2

Transcription factor 7–like 2 (TCF7L2) is a member of the family of high mobility group box containing transcription factors. The *TCF7L2* gene may alter levels of glucagon-like peptide 1 secreted by enteroendocrine cells via WNT signaling (79). The *TCF7L2* gene is located at 10q25.2 and is made up of 14 exons with five alternate splicing sites. Grant et al. identified a microsatellite marker (DG10S478) in intron 3 of the *TCF7L2* gene that is associated with T2DM in Icelandic individuals from the DeCODE study (P = 2.1 × 10^{-9}) (89). This association with T2DM was replicated in Danish female (P = 4.8 × 10^{-3}) and European American (P = 3.3 × 10^{-9}) cohorts. Nearby SNPs include rs122553372, rs7903146, rs122553372, rs7903146, and rs7901695. Of these

SNPs, rs122553372 (T allele) and rs7903146 (T allele) had strong associations with T2DM and increased relative risk of T2DM by 1.52 ($P = 2.5 \times 10^{-16}$) and 1.54 ($P = 2.1 \times 10^{-17}$), respectively (89). Subsequent studies in French Caucasians (90), European Caucasians (91), Indian Asians (91), Dutch Caucasians (92), and Amish Caucasians (93) have confirmed the initial findings. In addition to increasing the risk of T2DM, variants in TCF7L2 also increased the risk of subjects participating in the Diabetes Prevention Program of Progressing from IGT to T2DM [rs7903145 TT vs. CC (hazard ratio = 1.55, 95% CI = 1.20–2.01, $P < 0.001$)]. The TT genotype was also associated with decreased insulin secretion. Similar effects on progression to T2DM and decreased insulin secretion were found for rs1255372. In Caucasian subjects from Baltimore ($n = 48$), in whom intravenous glucose tolerance tests were performed, an association between rs7901695 and rs7903146 and insulin sensitivity ($P = 0.003$ and $P = 0.005$, respectively) and disposition index ($P = 0.04$ and $P = 0.007$, respectively) was identified, suggesting that the variants in TCF7L2 likely influence both insulin secretion and insulin sensitivity.

OTHER T2DM CANDIDATE GENES

The genes discussed in detail above give only the briefest overview of the many gene variants thought to have some influence over the development of diabetes in older adults. Dozens of other genes have been evaluated in multiple genetic studies of varied design. Some of these genes are listed in Table 1. Many of the identified associations have been inconsistent, or the biological basis of how the variants influence the phenotype is poorly understood. Although strong proof that these genes are influential in the development of diabetes-related phenotypes does not currently exist, many of these variants may prove to play modest roles in other study populations or in more rigorous study designs (Table 1).

OTHER PATHWAYS THAT MAY INFLUENCE THE DEVELOPMENT OF DIABETES IN OLDER ADULTS

In addition to these diabetes-related endophenotypes, aging-related physiologic changes, including activation of inflammatory and oxidative stress pathways, declines in mitochondrial function, and epigenetic changes are also under genetic control and can influence the development of diabetes and related endophenotypes.

GENES INFLUENCING INFLAMMATION

Multiple recent population studies of older adults have shown that increased serum markers of inflammatory pathway activation such as interleukin (IL)-6 and C reactive protein increase the risk for adverse health outcomes in older adults (165,166). Some of these same markers are also thought to play a role in the development of T2DM via activation of insulin resistance pathways (167,168). Most of the inflammatory cytokines, including IL-6, tumor necrosis factor-α (TNF-α), and IL-1, are known to be heritable traits with heritability estimates up to 50% (169,170). Given this heritability, and the potential influence of these cytokines on the development of insulin resistance and diabetes, several investigators have explored the relationship between inflammatory cytokine gene variants and T2DM. Studies of variants in IL-6 and IL-1 cluster genes have demonstrated significant association between specific gene variants and T2DM. For example, a study of North Indians revealed a strong association between a haplotype consisting of IL-1β-511C and IL-1 RN*2 variants was associated with high risk of developing T2DM (171). Other studies demonstrate that a very common polymorphism in the IL-6 promoter (-174 C) modulates insulin resistance (172), although a recent well-performed meta-analysis does not demonstrate a relationship between this allele and the development of T2DM (173). While variants in inflammatory genes may influence or modify diabetes or traits related to diabetes, especially as individuals age and develop medical illnesses that may trigger inflammatory pathways, it is unlikely that variants in inflammatory related genes alone will be major contributors to the diabetes phenotype.

TABLE 1 Selected Polymorphisms in Candidate Genes for Type 2 Diabetes

Candidate gene (genbank name)	Position	Variant[a]	Reference
Neuro D1	7q32	Ala45Thr, Arg111Leu	94,95
Carboxypeptidase E (*CPE*)	4q32.3	-53G/T, -144G/A, Val219Val (G/A nt 657)	96
(*CD38*)	4p15	Arg140Trp	97
(*CTLA4*)	2q33	Ala17Thr	98
Frataxin (*FRDA*)	9q13-q21	GAA triplet repeats	99–101
Gastric inhibitory polypeptide receptor (*GIPR*)	19q13.3	Gly198Cys, Glu354Gln, Ala207Val	102,103
Glucagon receptor (*GCGR*)	17q25	Gly40Ser	104–106
Glucagon-like peptide-1 receptor (*GLP1R*)	6p21	Polymorphic repeats GLP-1R-CA1 $[(GT)_n TAT(GT)_n CT(GT)_n]$ (intron 3), GLP-1CA3 $[(GT)_n]$ (3′UTR)	107,108
Glucose transporter-2 (*GLUT-2*)	3q26.1-q26.2	Thr110Ile, Val197Ile, Val101Ile, Gly519Glu	109–111
Glucose transporter-4 (*GLUT-4*)	17p13	Ile383Val	112–114
Glycogen synthase (*GYS1*)	19q13.3	A2 Allele, Met416Val, Gln71His	116–118
Hexokinase II (*HK2*)	2p13	Gln142His	119,120
Insulin (*INS*)	11p15.5	8 bp insertion at position −315, VNTR in 5′UT	121,122
Intestinal fatty acid binding protein-2 (*FABP2*)	4q28-q31	Thr54Ala	123–130
Inward rectifying potassium channel (*Kir6.2*) (*KCNJ11*)	11p15.1	Glu23Lys, Leu270Val	17–19,131,132
Islet amyloid polypeptide (*IAPP*)	12p12.3	Ser20Gly	133–136
Islet-1 (*Isl-1*)	5q11.1	Gln310Stop,-47 A/G	137,138
Lamin A/C (*LMNA*)	1q21.2-q21.3	His566His (C/T nt 3408)	139
Paired box gene 4 (*PAX4*)	7q32	Pro321His, Pro334Ala	95
Phosphatidylinositiol 3-kinase (*PI3K*)	17p13.1	Met326ILe	140,141
Plasma cell differentiation antigen (*PC-1*)	6q22	Lys121Gln	142,143
Presenilin 2 (*PSEN2*)	1q31-q42	Met239Val	144
Prohormone convertase 1 (*PCSK1*)	5q15-21	Arg53Gln, Gln638Glu	145,146
Prohormone convertase 2 (*PCSK2*)	20p11.2	A1 allele	147
Protein phosphatase type 1 (*PPP1R3*)	7q31.1	Asp905Tyr, Arg883Ser, 3′ UTR 5-bp insertion/deletion	148–153
Ras associated with diabetes (*RAD*)	16q22	Polymorphic repeat (GTT)n (ATT)n	104,154
Resistin (*RSTN*)	19p13.2	3′ UTR G/A 1326, C/T -167, C/G −394, C/T 157 (intron 2), G/A 299 (intron 2)	155–157
Sarco(endo)plasmic reticulum *Ca(2+)* transport ATPase 3 (*SERCA3*) (*ATP2A3*)	17p13	Gln108His, Val648Met, Arg674Cys	158
Sulfonylurea receptor-1 (*SUR1*) (*ABCC8*)	11p15.1	Thr759Thr (C/T nt 2277), -3 t/c 5′ of exon 16 splice acceptor site	22–24,159,160
Vitamin D–binding protein (*GC*)	4q12	Asp416Glu, Thr420Lys	161
Vitamin D receptor (*VDR*)	12q12-q14	ΔMet1-Ala3, ApaI (intron 8), Taq 1 (3′ UTR)	162–164

[a]Variants are numbered according to provided references.

GENES INFLUENCING MITOCHONDRIAL FUNCTION AND OXIDATIVE STRESS

Mitochondria are the powerhouse of the cell, and as such are crucial in the generation of ATP, the biosynthesis of heme and steroids, and calcium and iron homeostasis. As part of these processes, the free radicals, superoxide and hydrogen peroxide, are produced, which can alter gene expression, activate inflammatory pathways, and damage protein, lipid, and DNA (174). Mitochondria have their own genome that is inherited directly from the mother. Interest in mitochondrial gene based etiologies of T2DM comes in part from the discovery of maternally inherited diabetes and sensorineural deafness (MIDD), which presents in mid-life (175). An A to G substitution at position 3234 in the leucine to RNA gene is the most common genetic variant associated with MIDD. The variant likely leads to increased oxidative stress and mitochondria damage from ROS as well as reduce ATP production due to direct cellular respiration (176). Ultimately, this leads to altered insulin secretion and the development of diabetes (177). Although MIDD is relatively rare, there is some evidence that other mutations in the mt DNA may contribute to some cases of diabetes later in life. For example, a recent North Indian population study consisting of two cohorts demonstrated an increased odds ratio of developing diabetes with 10398A and 16189C, two specific mt DNA variants (178). Other alleles, including a 16189 mtDNA variant, are higher in those with T2DM when compared with those without the variant. In addition, this influence is stronger with higher BMI (179). These and other studies suggest that mt DNA variants may contribute to the development of diabetes through alterations in both insulin secretion and insulin resistance.

EPIGENETIC FACTORS

Recent advances in the understanding of epigenetic control have demonstrated at least three "extra DNA" mechanisms by which gene transcription is controlled. These mechanisms, including DNA methylation, histone modification, and RNA silencing, are crucial for normal growth and development of all organisms (180). These mechanisms, which change with age and environmental exposure, may explain some of the late life variation in gene expression which is thought to contribute to the increased rates of chronic disease observed in older adults (181,182). Although no direct links between epigenetic control alterations and the development of diabetes have been discovered, there is emerging evidence that epigenetic control of NF-kappaB signaling is crucial to inflammatory gene expression (183). In addition, many of the noncoding polymorphic variants identified in linkage studies of T2DM may only be relevant to age-related changes in methylation (4). Future studies of the age-related changes in epigenetic control of specific disease candidate genes or in genome wide epigenetic controls may reveal important links between epigenetic regulation and the development of diabetes in older adults (184).

GENES RELATED TO DM COMPLICATIONS

Diabetic complications of retinopathy, nephropathy, neuropathy, and atherosclerosis are in general related to vascular disease. These complications are driven in large part by chronic hyperglycemia (185). Recent evidence suggests that there may also be genetic predictors of these complications, and a number of studies have now shown that specific gene variants correlate with increased rates of complications (186–191). For example, review of over 80 publications on genes impacting retinopathy suggest that aldose receptor, vascular endothelial growth factor, intercellular adhesion molecule 1, β-3-adrenergic receptor, and $\alpha 2 \beta 1$ integrin all may have gene variants that contribute to the development of diabetic retinopathy (187). Other genes of interest include *IGF-1*, which is associated with an odds ratio of 1.8 for developing retinopathy in those with diabetes and the variant IGF-1 allele compared with those with diabetes and the more common allele (188). Linkage analysis to ascertain important chromosomal regions for diabetic nephropathy (DN) identified susceptibility loci on chromosome 10 and chromosome 3 (189–191), although no firm candidate genes or polymorphisms within chromosomal loci have been confirmed to date (186). Numerous SNPs in candidate genes have been studied in DN with some positive associations and some negative associations, including angiotensin I–converting enzyme (ACE), apolipoprotein E, heparin sulfate, aldose reductase, insulin, and angiotensinogen, among others (186). These mixed results, much like those of candidate gene studies of the T2DM phenotype, suggest that there are multiple genes likely play a modest role in the development of diabetes complications of diabetes, especially when combined with chronically elevated glucose levels.

CLINICAL RELEVANCE

The clinical relevance of genes associated with chronic diseases has long been debated, especially given the fact that much of the diabetes that is observed in older adults is attributable to overnutrition and underactivity (4,5). However, critical clinical information can be obtained from the identification of gene variants that influence the development of diabetes. Knowledge of molecular pathways that impact glucose levels through altered body composition, appetite regulation, insulin resistance, insulin secretion, and inflammatory activation can provide evidence critical to the development of targeted interventions. For example, understanding the role of incretins and GLP1 in insulin seretion has led to the development of drugs sitagliptin [to treat T2DM] that work in this pathway (better example). In the growing field of pharmacogenomics, knowledge of patients' genotype for genes targeted by specific medications may, in the future predict which medications will be effective in controlling blood sugars or preventing complications. For example, polymorphisms in the ACE gene predicts who will respond to treatment with ACE inhibitors, a drug which lows the progression of DN (186). Gene and epigenetic variation discovered in diabetes research may also further our understanding of age-related metabolic changes that impact function and multiple systems beyond glucose metabolism. Finally, the knowledge of meaningful genotypes will help identify those younger individuals who are at the highest risk of developing diabetes or diabetic complications. With this knowledge, more targeted educational and intervention protocols could be initiated before disease and complications develop in these most vulnerable individuals.

SUMMARY

T2DM is among the most common genetic diseases impacting older adults. Multiple genes in many metabolic pathways have been identified that associate with the development of diabetes or at least one or more of the physiological characteristics that underlie diabetes. For typical T2DM no one gene variant is sufficient to trigger T2DM in all individuals. For most people, multiple gene variants with modest affects combine with environmental factors and aging lead to the development of T2DM. As individuals age, and gene expression patterns, activity levels, and diets change, some of these gene variants may become more relevant and some less. In addition, it is likely that various combinations of gene variants combined with activity and dietary factors will ultimately affect how and when the phenotype is expressed, and how severe it will be. Future genetic studies utilizing whole genome scanning technology may provide clues as to which combinations of gene variants are most important for the ultimate development of the phenotype. In addition, understanding age-related changes in epigenetic control may be critical in further genetic discovery. This knowledge will help to identify the most influential metabolic pathways in the development of diabetes in older adults, provide targets for interventions, and help to identify age-related changes in physiological systems that influence chronic disease and the development of disability.

REFERENCES

1. Engelgau MM, Geiss LS, Saaddine JB, et al. The evolving diabetes burden in the United States. Ann Intern Med 2004; 140(11):945–950.
2. Okoro CA, Denny CH, Greenlund KJ, et al. Risk factors for heart disease and stroke among diabetic persons, by disability status. J Diabetes Complicat 2005; 19(4):201–206.
3. Wray LA, Ofstedal MB, Langa KM, Blaum CS. The effect of diabetes on disability in middle-aged and older adults. J Gerontol A Biol Sci Med Sci 2005; 60(9):1206–1211.
4. Das SK, Elbein SC. The genetic basis of type 2 diabetes. Cellscience 2006; 2(4):100–131.
5. Sabra M, Silver KD, Shuldiner AR. Candidate genes for type 2 diabetes. In: LeRoth D, Olefsky JM, Taylor SI, eds. In: Diabetes Mellitus: A Fundamental and Clinical Text. Philadelphia: Lippincott, 2004:1003–1012.
6. Zamboni M, Mazzali G, Zoico E, et al. Health consequences of obesity in the elderly: a review of four unresolved questions. Int J Obes (Lond) 2005; 29(9):1011–1029.
7. Barnett AH, Eff C, Leslie RD, Pyke DA. Diabetes in identical twins. A study of 200 pairs. Diabetologia 1981; 20(2):87–93.
8. Poulsen P, Kyvik KO, Vaag A, Beck-Nielsen H. Heritability of type II (non-insulin-dependent) diabetes mellitus and abnormal glucose tolerance—a population-based twin study. Diabetologia 1999; 42(2):139–145.
9. Newman B, Selby JV, King MC, Slemenda C, Fabsitz R, Friedman GD. Concordance for type 2 (non-insulin-dependent) diabetes mellitus in male twins. Diabetologia 1987; 30(10):763–768.
10. Meigs JB, Cupples LA, Wilson PW. Parental transmission of type 2 diabetes: the Framingham Offspring Study. Diabetes 2000; 49(12):2201–2207.

11. Huang QY, Cheng MR, Ji SL. Linkage and association studies of the susceptibility genes for type 2 diabetes. Yi Chuan Xue Bao 2006; 33(7):573–589.

12. Zacharova J, Chiasson JL, Laakso M. The common polymorphisms [single nucleotide polymorphism (SNP) +45 and SNP +276] of the adiponectin gene predict the conversion from impaired glucose tolerance to type 2 diabetes: the STOP-NIDDM trial. Diabetes 2005; 54(3):893–899.

13. Kretowski A, Gugala K, Okruszko A, Wawrusiewicz-Kurylonek N, Gorska M. Single nucleotide polymorphisms in exon 3 of the adiponectin gene in subjects with type 2 diabetes mellitus. Rocz Akad Med Bialymst 2005; 50:148–150.

14. Stumvoll M, Tschritter O, Fritsche A, et al. Association of the T-G polymorphism in adiponectin (exon 2) with obesity and insulin sensitivity: interaction with family history of type 2 diabetes. Diabetes 2002; 51(1):37–41.

15. Kondo H, Shimomura I, Matsukawa Y, et al. Association of adiponectin mutation with type 2 diabetes: a candidate gene for the insulin resistance syndrome. Diabetes 2002; 51(7):2325–2328.

16. Vasseur F, Helbecque N, Lobbens S, et al. Hypoadiponectinaemia and high risk of type 2 diabetes are associated with adiponectin-encoding (ACDC) gene promoter variants in morbid obesity: evidence for a role of ACDC in diabesity. Diabetologia 2005; 48(5):892–899.

17. Sakura H, Wat N, Horton V, Millns H, Turner RC, Ashcroft FM. Sequence variations in the human Kir6.2 gene, a subunit of the β-cell ATP-sensitive K-channel: no association with NIDDM in while Caucasian subjects or evidence of abnormal function when expressed in vitro. Diabetologia 1996; 39:1233–1236.

18. Hani EH, Boutin P, Durand E, et al. Missense mutations in the pancreatic islet β cell inwardly rectifying K+ channel gene (KIR6.2/BIR): a meta-analysis suggests a role in the polygenic basis of Type II diabetes mellitus in Caucasians. Diabetologia 1998; 41(12):1511–1515.

19. Gloyn AL, Weedon MN, Owen KR, et al. Large-scale association studies of variants in genes encoding the pancreatic β-cell KATP channel subunits Kir6.2 (KCNJ11) and SUR1 (ABCC8) confirm that the KCNJ11 E23K variant is associated with type 2 diabetes. Diabetes 2003; 52(2):568–572.

20. van Dam RM, Hoebee B, Seidell JC, Schaap MM, de Bruin TW, Feskens EJ. Common variants in the ATP-sensitive K+ channel genes KCNJ11 (Kir6.2) and ABCC8 (SUR1) in relation to glucose intolerance: population-based studies and meta-analyses. Diabet Med 2005; 22(5):590–598.

21. Florez JC, Burtt N, de Bakker PI, et al. Haplotype structure and genotype-phenotype correlations of the sulfonylurea receptor and the islet ATP-sensitive potassium channel gene region. Diabetes 2004; 53(5):1360–1368.

22. Hansen T, Echwald SM, Hansen L, et al. Decreased tolbutamide-stimulated insulin secretion in healthy subjects with sequence variants in the high-affinity sulfonylurea receptor gene. Diabetes 1998; 47(4):598–605.

23. Inoue H, Ferrer J, Welling CM, et al. Sequence variants in the sulfonylurea receptor (SUR) gene are associated with NIDDM in Caucasians. Diabetes 1996; 45:825–831.

24. Laukkanen O, Pihlajamaki J, Lindstrom J, et al. Polymorphisms of the SUR1 (ABCC8) and Kir6.2 (KCNJ11) genes predict the conversion from impaired glucose tolerance to type 2 diabetes. The Finnish diabetes prevention study. J Clin Endocrinol Metab 2004; 89(12):6286–6290.

25. Walston J, Silver K, Bogardus C, et al. Time of onset of non-insulin-dependent diabetes mellitus and genetic variation in the β-3-adrenergic-receptor gene. N Engl J Med 1995; 333(6): 343–347.

26. Widen E, Lehto M, Kanninen T, Walston J, Shuldiner AR, Groop LC. Association of a polymorphism in the β-3-adrenergic-receptor gene with features of the insulin resistance syndrome in Finns. N Engl J Med 1995; 333(6):348–351.

27. Allison DB, Heo M, Faith MS, Pietrobelli A. Meta-analysis of the association of the Trp64Arg polymorphism in the β-3 adrenergic receptor with body mass index. Int J Obes Relat Metab Disord 1998; 22(6):559–566.

28. Walston J, Silver K, Hilfiker H, et al. Insulin response to glucose is lower in individuals homozygous for the Arg 64 variant of the β-3-adrenergic receptor. J Clin Endocrinol Metab 2000; 85(11): 4019–4022.

29. Walston J, Andersen RE, Seibert M, et al. Arg64 β-(3)-adrenoceptor variant and the components of energy expenditure. Obes Res 2003; 11(4):509–511.

30. Perfetti R, Hui H, Chamie K, et al. Pancreatic β-cells expressing the Arg64 variant of the β-(3)-adrenergic receptor exhibit abnormal insulin secretory activity. J Mol Endocrinol 2001; 27(2): 133–144.

31. Horikawa Y, Oda N, Cox NJ, et al. Genetic variation in the gene encoding calpain-10 is associated with type 2 diabetes mellitus. Nat Genet 2000; 26(2):163–175.

32. Baier LJ, Permana PA, Traurig M, et al. Mutations in the genes for hepatocyte nuclear factor (HNF)-1α, -4α, -1β, and -3β; the dimerization cofactor of HNF-1; and insulin promoter factor 1 are not common causes of early-onset type 2 diabetes in Pima Indians. Diabetes Care 2000; 23(3):302–304.

33. Malecki MT, Moczulski DK, Klupa T, et al. Homozygous combination of calpain 10 gene haplotypes is associated with type 2 diabetes mellitus in a Polish population. Eur J Endocrinol 2002; 146(5): 695–699.

34. Orho-Melander M, Klannemark M, Svensson MK, Ridderstrale M, Lindgren CM, Groop L. Variants in the calpain-10 gene predispose to insulin resistance and elevated free fatty acid levels. Diabetes 2002; 51(8):2658–2664.
35. Garant MJ, Kao WH, Brancati F, et al. SNP43 of CAPN10 and the risk of type 2 diabetes in African-Americans: the Atherosclerosis Risk in Communities Study. Diabetes 2002; 51(1):231–237.
36. Horikawa Y, Oda N, Yu L, et al. Genetic variations in calpain-10 gene are not a major factor in the occurrence of type 2 diabetes in Japanese. J Clin Endocrinol Metab 2003; 88(1):244–247.
37. Cassell PG, Jackson AE, North BV, et al. Haplotype combinations of calpain 10 gene polymorphisms associate with increased risk of impaired glucose tolerance and type 2 diabetes in South Indians. Diabetes 2002; 51(5):1622–1628.
38. Tsai HJ, Sun G, Weeks DE, et al. Type 2 diabetes and three calpain-10 gene polymorphisms in Samoans: no evidence of association. Am J Hum Genet 2001; 69(6):1236–1244.
39. Bosque-Plata L, Aguilar-Salinas CA, Tusie-Luna MT, et al. Association of the calpain-10 gene with type 2 diabetes mellitus in a Mexican population. Mol Genet Metab 2004; 81(2):122–126.
40. Rasmussen SK, Urhammer SA, Berglund L, et al. Variants within the calpain-10 gene on chromosome 2q37 (NIDDM1) and relationships to type 2 diabetes, insulin resistance, and impaired acute insulin secretion among Scandinavian Caucasians. Diabetes 2002; 51(12):3561–3567.
41. Fingerlin TE, Erdos MR, Watanabe RM, et al. Variation in three single nucleotide polymorphisms in the calpain-10 gene not associated with type 2 diabetes in a large Finnish cohort. Diabetes 2002; 51(5):1644–1648.
42. Elbein SC, Chu W, Ren Q, et al. Role of calpain-10 gene variants in familial type 2 diabetes in Caucasians. J Clin Endocrinol Metab 2002; 87(2):650–654.
43. Daimon M, Oizumi T, Saitoh T, et al. Calpain 10 gene polymorphisms are related, not to type 2 diabetes, but to increased serum cholesterol in Japanese. Diabetes Res Clin Pract 2002; 56(2):147–152.
44. Xiang K, Fang Q, Zheng T, et al. The impact of calpain-10 gene combined-SNP variation on type 2 diabetes mellitus and its related metabolic traits. Zhonghua Yi Xue Yi Chuan Xue Za Zhi 2001; 18(6):426–430.
45. Evans JC, Frayling TM, Cassell PG, et al. Studies of association between the gene for calpain-10 and type 2 diabetes mellitus in the United Kingdom. Am J Hum Genet 2001; 69(3):544–552.
46. Hegele RA, Harris SB, Zinman B, Hanley AJ, Cao H. Absence of association of type 2 diabetes with CAPN10 and PC-1 polymorphisms in Oji-Cree. Diabetes Care 2001; 24(8):1498–1499.
47. Song Y, Niu T, Manson JE, Kwiatkowski DJ, Liu S. Are variants in the CAPN10 gene related to risk of type 2 diabetes? A quantitative assessment of population and family-based association studies. Am J Hum Genet 2004; 74(2):208–222.
48. Tsuchiya T, Schwarz PE, Bosque-Plata LD, et al. Association of the calpain-10 gene with type 2 diabetes in Europeans: results of pooled and meta-analyses. Mol Genet Metab 2006; 89(1–2):174–184.
49. Weedon MN, Schwarz PE, Horikawa Y, et al. Meta-analysis and a large association study confirm a role for calpain-10 variation in type 2 diabetes susceptibility. Am J Hum Genet 2003; 73(5):1208–1212.
50. Wang Y, Xiang K, Zheng T, Jia W, Shen K, Li J. The UCSNP44 variation of calpain 10 gene on NIDDM1 locus and its impact on plasma glucose levels in type 2 diabetic patients. Zhonghua Yi Xue Za Zhi 2002; 82(9):613–616.
51. Johnson JD, Han Z, Otani K, et al. RyR2 and calpain-10 delineate a novel apoptosis pathway in pancreatic islets. J Biol Chem 2004; 279(23):24794–24802.
52. Sreenan SK, Zhou YP, Otani K, et al. Calpains play a role in insulin secretion and action. Diabetes 2001; 50(9):2013–2020.
53. Zhou YP, Sreenan S, Pan CY, et al. A 48-hour exposure of pancreatic islets to calpain inhibitors impairs mitochondrial fuel metabolism and the exocytosis of insulin. Metabolism 2003; 52(5):528–534.
54. Ort T, Voronov S, Guo J, et al. Dephosphorylation of β2-syntrophin and Ca2+/mu-calpain-mediated cleavage of ICA512 upon stimulation of insulin secretion. EMBO J 2001; 20(15):4013–4023.
55. Bowden DW, Sale M, Howard TD, et al. Linkage of genetic markers on human chromosomes 20 and 12 to NIDDM in Caucasian sib pairs with a history of diabetic nephropathy. Diabetes 1997; 46(5):882–886.
56. Ji L, Malecki M, Warram JH, Yang Y, Rich SS, Krolewski AS. New susceptibility locus for NIDDM is localized to human chromosome 20q. Diabetes 1997; 46(5):876–881.
57. Zouali H, Hani EH, Philippi A, et al. A susceptibility locus for early-onset non-insulin dependent (type 2) diabetes mellitus maps to chromosome 20q, proximal to the phosphoenolpyruvate carboxy-kinase gene. Hum Mol Genet 1997; 6(9):1401–1408.
58. Ghosh S, Watanabe RM, Hauser ER, et al. Type 2 diabetes: evidence for linkage on chromosome 20 in 716 Finnish affected sib pairs. Proc Natl Acad Sci U S A 1999; 96(5):2198–2203.
59. Silander K, Mohlke KL, Scott LJ, et al. Genetic variation near the hepatocyte nuclear factor-4α gene predicts susceptibility to type 2 diabetes. Diabetes 2004; 53(4):1141–1149.

60. Hara K, Horikoshi M, Kitazato H, et al. Hepatocyte nuclear factor-4α P2 promoter haplotypes are associated with type 2 diabetes in the Japanese population. Diabetes 2006; 55(5):1260–1264.
61. Muller YL, Infante AM, Hanson RL, et al. Variants in hepatocyte nuclear factor 4α are modestly associated with type 2 diabetes in Pima Indians. Diabetes 2005; 54(10):3035–3039.
62. Bagwell AM, Bento JL, Mychaleckyj JC, Freedman BI, Langefeld CD, Bowden DW. Genetic analysis of HNF4α polymorphisms in Caucasian-American type 2 diabetes. Diabetes 2005; 54(4):1185–1190.
63. Hansen SK, Rose CS, Glumer C, et al. Variation near the hepatocyte nuclear factor (HNF)-4α gene associates with type 2 diabetes in the Danish population. Diabetologia 2005; 48(3):452–458.
64. Vaxillaire M, Dina C, Lobbens S, et al. Effect of common polymorphisms in the HNF4α promoter on susceptibility to type 2 diabetes in the French Caucasian population. Diabetologia 2005; 48(3): 440–444.
65. Wanic K, Malecki MT, Wolkow PP, et al. Polymorphisms in the gene encoding hepatocyte nuclear factor-4α and susceptibility to type 2 diabetes in a Polish population. Diabetes Metab 2006; 32(1): 86–88.
66. Auboeuf D, Rieusset J, Fajas L, et al. Tissue distribution and quantification of the expression of mRNAs of peroxisome proliferator-activated receptors and liver X receptor-α in humans: no alteration in adipose tissue of obese and NIDDM patients. Diabetes 1997; 46(8):1319–1327.
67. Mukherjee R, Jow L, Croston GE, Paterniti JR Jr. Identification, characterization, and tissue distribution of human peroxisome proliferator-activated receptor (PPAR) isoforms PPARγ2 versus PPARγ1 and activation with retinoid X receptor agonists and antagonists. J Biol Chem 1997; 272(12): 8071–8076.
68. Yen CJ, Beamer BA, Negri C, et al. Molecular scanning of the human peroxisome proliferator activated receptor γ (hPPAR γ) gene in diabetic Caucasians: identification of a Pro12Ala PPAR γ2 missense mutation. Biochem Biophys Res Commun 1997; 241(2):270–274.
69. Celi FS, Shuldiner AR. The role of peroxisome proliferator-activated receptor γ in diabetes and obesity. Curr Diab Rep 2002; 2(2):179–185.
70. Deeb SS, Fajas L, Nemoto M, et al. A Pro12Ala substitution in PPARγ2 associated with decreased receptor activity, lower body mass index and improved insulin sensitivity. Nat Genet 1998; 20(3):284–287.
71. Masugi J, Tamori Y, Mori H, Koike T, Kasuga M. Inhibitory effect of a proline-to-alanine substitution at codon 12 of peroxisome proliferator-activated receptor-γ2 on thiazolidinedione-induced adipogenesis. Biochem Biophys Res Commun 2000; 268(1):178–182.
72. Oh EY, Min KM, Chung JH. Significance of Pro12Ala variant in peroxisome proliferator-activated receptor-γ2 in Korean diabetic and obese subjects. J Clin Endocrinol Metab 2000; 85:1801–1804.
73. Beamer BA, Yen CJ, Andersen RE, et al. Association of the Pro12Ala variant in the peroxisome proliferator-activated receptor-γ2 gene with obesity in two Caucasian populations. Diabetes 1998; 47(11):1806–1808.
74. Meirhaeghe A, Fajas L, Helbecque N, et al. Impact of the peroxisome proliferator activated receptor γ2 Pro12Ala polymorphism on adiposity, lipids and non-insulin-dependent diabetes mellitus. Int J Obes Relat Metab Disord 2000; 24(2):195–199.
75. Luan J, Browne PO, Harding AH, et al. Evidence for gene-nutrient interaction at the PPARγ locus. Diabetes 2001; 50(3):686–689.
76. Ek J, Urhammer SA, Sorensen TI, Andersen T, Auwerx J, Pedersen O. Homozygosity of the Pro12Ala variant of the peroxisome proliferation-activated receptor-γ2 (PPAR-γ2): divergent modulating effects on body mass index in obese and lean Caucasian men. Diabetologia 1999; 42(7):892–895.
77. Nicklas BJ, van Rossum EF, Berman DM, Ryan AS, Dennis KE, Shuldiner AR. Genetic variation in the peroxisome proliferator-activated receptor-γ2 gene (Pro12Ala) affects metabolic responses to weight loss and subsequent weight regain. Diabetes 2001; 50(9):2172–2176.
78. Neel JV. The thrifty genotype revisited. In: Kobberling J, Tattersall R, eds. The Genetics of Diabetes Mellitus. Proceedings of the Serono Symposium. London: Academic Press, 1982:283–293.
79. Korinek V, Barker N, Moerer P, et al. Depletion of epithelial stem-cell compartments in the small intestine of mice lacking Tcf-4. Nat Genet 1998; 19(4):379–383.
80. Ringel J, Engeli S, Distler A, Sharma AM. Pro12Ala missense mutation of the peroxisome proliferator activated receptor γ and diabetes mellitus. Biochem Biophys Res Commun 1999; 254(2):450–453.
81. Mancini FP, Vaccaro O, Sabatino L, et al. Pro12Ala substitution in the peroxisome proliferator-activated receptor-γ2 is not associated with type 2 diabetes. Diabetes 1999; 48(7):1466–1468.
82. Clement K, Hercberg S, Passinge B, et al. The Pro115Gln and Pro12Ala PPARγ gene mutations in obesity and type 2 diabetes. Int J Obes Relat Metab Disord 2000; 24(3):391–393.
83. Altshuler D, Hirschhorn JN, Klannemark M, et al. The common PPARγ Pro12Ala polymorphism is associated with decreased risk of type 2 diabetes. Nat Genet 2000; 26(1):76–80.
84. Gonzalez Sanchez JL, Serrano RM, Fernandez PC, Laakso M, Martinez Larrad MT. Effect of the Pro12Ala polymorphism of the peroxisome proliferator-activated receptor γ-2 gene on adiposity, insulin sensitivity and lipid profile in the Spanish population. Eur J Endocrinol 2002; 147(4):495–501.

85. Frederiksen L, Brodbaek K, Fenger M, et al. Comment: studies of the Pro12Ala polymorphism of the PPAR-γ gene in the Danish MONICA cohort: homozygosity of the Ala allele confers a decreased risk of the insulin resistance syndrome. J Clin Endocrinol Metab 2002; 87(8):3989–3992.

86. Stumvoll M, Wahl HG, Loblein K, et al. Pro12Ala polymorphism in the peroxisome proliferator-activated receptor-γ2 gene is associated with increased antilipolytic insulin sensitivity. Diabetes 2001; 50(4):876–881.

87. Jacob, et al. Horm Metab Res 2000; 32:413.

88. Mori Y, Kim-Motoyama H, Katakura T, et al. Effect of the Pro12Ala variant of the human peroxisome proliferator-activated receptor-γ 2 gene on adiposity, fat distribution, and insulin sensitivity in Japanese men. Biochem Biophys Res Commun 1998; 251(1):195–198.

89. Grant SF, Thorleifsson G, Reynisdottir I, et al. Variant of transcription factor 7-like 2 (TCF7L2) gene confers risk of type 2 diabetes. Nat Genet 2006; 38(3):320–323.

90. Cauchi S, Meyre D, Choquet H, et al. TCF7L2 variation predicts hyperglycemia incidence in a French general population: the data from an epidemiological study on the insulin resistance syndrome (desir) study. Diabetes 2006; 55(11):3189–3192.

91. Humphries SE, Gable D, Cooper JA, et al. Common variants in the TCF7L2 gene and predisposition to type 2 diabetes in UK European whites, Indian Asians and Afro-Caribbean men and women. J Mol Med 2006; 94(12 suppl):1–10.

92. Vliet-Ostaptchouk JV, Shiri-Sverdlov R, Zhernakova A, et al. Association of variants of transcription factor 7-like 2 (TCF7L2) with susceptibility to type 2 diabetes in the Dutch Breda cohort. Diabetologia 2007; 50(1):59–62.

93. Damcott CM, Pollin TI, Reinhart LJ, et al. Polymorphisms in the transcription factor 7-like 2 (TCF7L2) gene are associated with type 2 diabetes in the Amish: replication and evidence for a role in both insulin secretion and insulin resistance. Diabetes 2006; 55(9):2654–2659.

94. Malecki MT, Jhala US, Antonellis A, et al. Mutations in NEUROD1 are associated with the development of type 2 diabetes mellitus. Nat Genet 1999; 23(3):323–328.

95. Dupont S, Vionnet N, Chevre JC, et al. No evidence of linkage or diabetes-associated mutations in the transcription factors β2/NEUROD1 and PAX4 in Type II diabetes in France. Diabetologia 1999; 42(4):480–484.

96. Utsunomiya N, Ohagi S, Sanke T, Tatsuta H, Hanabusa T, Nanjo K. Organization of the human carboxypeptidase E gene and molecular scanning for mutations in Japanese subjects with NIDDM or obesity. Diabetologia 1998; 41(6):701–705.

97. Yagui K, Shimada F, Mimura M, et al. A missense mutation in the CD38 gene, a novel factor for insulin secretion: association with Type II diabetes mellitus in Japanese subjects and evidence of abnormal function when expressed in vitro. Diabetologia 1998; 41(9):1024–1028.

98. Rau H, Braun J, Donner H, et al. The codon 17 polymorphism of the CTLA4 gene in type 2 diabetes mellitus. J Clin Endocrinol Metab 2001; 86(2):653–655.

99. Ristow M, Giannakidou E, Hebinck J, et al. An association between NIDDM and a GAA trinucleotide repeat polymorphism in the X25/frataxin (Friedreich's ataxia) gene. Diabetes 1998; 47(5):851–854.

100. Dalgaard LT, Hansen T, Urhammer SA, Clausen JO, Eiberg H, Pedersen O. Intermediate expansions of a GAA repeat in the frataxin gene are not associated with type 2 diabetes or altered glucose-induced β-cell function in Danish Caucasians. Diabetes 1999; 48(4):914–917.

101. Hart LM, Ruige JB, Dekker JM, Stehouwer CD, Maassen JA, Heine RJ. Altered β-cell characteristics in impaired glucose tolerant carriers of a GAA trinucleotide repeat polymorphism in the frataxin gene. Diabetes 1999; 48(4):924–926.

102. Kubota A, Yamada Y, Hayami T, et al. Identification of two missense mutations in the GIP receptor gene: a functional study and association analysis with NIDDM: no evidence of association with Japanese NIDDM subjects. Diabetes 1996; 45(12):1701–1705.

103. Almind K, Ambye L, Urhammer SA, et al. Discovery of amino acid variants in the human glucose-dependent insulinotropic polypeptide (GIP) receptor: the impact on the pancreatic β-cell responses and functional expression studies in Chinese hamster fibroblast cells. Diabetologia 1998; 41(10): 1194–1198.

104. Velho G, Froguel P. Genetic determinants of non-insulin-dependent diabetes mellitus: strategies and recent results. Diabetes Metab 1997; 23(1):7–17.

105. Huang CN, Lee KC, Wu HP, Tai TY, Lin BJ, Chuang LM. Screening for the Gly40Ser mutation in the glucagon receptor gene among patients with type 2 diabetes or essential hypertension in Taiwan. Pancreas 1999; 18(2):151–155.

106. Lepretre F, Vionnet N, Budhan S, et al. Genetic studies of polymorphisms in ten non-insulin-dependent diabetes mellitus candidate genes in Tamil Indians from Pondicherry. Diabetes Metab 1998; 24(3):244–250.

107. Tanizawa Y, Riggs AC, Elbein SC, Whelan A, Donis-Keller H, Permutt MA. Human glucagon-like peptide-1 receptor gene in NIDDM. Identification and use of simple sequence repeat polymorphisms in genetic analysis. Diabetes 1994; 43(6):752–757.

108. Yagi T, Nishi S, Hinata S, Murakami M, Yoshimi T. A population association study of four candidate genes (hexokinase II, glucagon-like peptide-1 receptor, fatty acid binding protein-2, and

apolipoprotein C-II) with type 2 diabetes and impaired glucose tolerance in Japanese subjects. Diabet Med 1996; 13(10):902–907.

109. Janssen RC, Bogardus C, Takeda J, Knowler WC, Thompson DB. Linkage analysis of acute insulin secretion with GLUT2 and glucokinase in Pima Indians and the identification of a missense mutation in GLUT2. Diabetes 1994; 43(4):558–563.

110. Tanizawa Y, Riggs AC, Chiu KC, et al. Variability of the pancreatic islet β-cell/liver (GLUT 2) glucose transporter gene in NIDDM patients. Diabetologia 1994; 37(4):420–427.

111. Shimada F, Makino H, Iwaoka H, et al. Identification of two novel amino acid polymorphisms in β-cell/liver (GLUT2) glucose transporter in Japanese subjects. Diabetologia 1995; 38(2):211–215.

112. Matsutani A, Koranyi L, Cox N, Permutt MA. Polymorphisms of GLUT2 and GLUT4 genes. Use in evaluation of genetic susceptibility to NIDDM in blacks. Diabetes 1990; 39(12):1534–1542.

113. Baroni MG, Oelbaum RS, Pozzilli P, et al. Polymorphisms at the GLUT1 (HepG2) and GLUT4 (muscle/adipocyte) glucose transporter genes and non-insulin-dependent diabetes mellitus (NIDDM). Hum Genet 1992; 88(5):557–561.

114. Kusari J, Verma US, Buse JB, Henry RR, Olefsky JM. Analysis of the gene sequences of the insulin receptor and the insulin-sensitive glucose transporter (GLUT-4) in patients with common-type non-insulin-dependent diabetes mellitus. J Clin Invest 1991; 88(4):1323–1330.

115. Choi WH, O'Rahilly S, Buse JB, et al. Molecular scanning of insulin-responsive glucose transporter (GLUT4) gene in NIDDM subjects. Diabetes 1991; 40(12):1712–1718.

116. Groop LC, Kankuri M, Schalin-Jantti C, et al. Association between polymorphism of the glycogen synthase gene and non-insulin-dependent diabetes mellitus. N Engl J Med 1993; 328(1):10–14.

117. Shimomura H, Sanke T, Ueda K, Hanabusa T, Sakagashira S, Nanjo K. A missense mutation of the muscle glycogen synthase gene (M416V) is associated with insulin resistance in the Japanese population. Diabetologia 1997; 40(8):947–952.

118. Rissanen J, Pihlajamaki J, Heikkinen S, et al. New variants in the glycogen synthase gene (Gln71His, Met416Val) in patients with NIDDM from eastern Finland. Diabetologia 1997; 40(11):1313–1319.

119. Echwald SM, Bjorbaek C, Hansen T, et al. Identification of four amino acid substitutions in hexokinase II and studies of relationships to NIDDM, glucose effectiveness, and insulin sensitivity. Diabetes 1995; 44(3):347–353.

120. Vidal-Puig A, Printz RL, Stratton IM, Granner DK, Moller DE. Analysis of the hexokinase II gene in subjects with insulin resistance and NIDDM and detection of a Gln142 $\rightarrow$ His substitution. Diabetes 1995; 44(3):340–346.

121. Olansky L, Janssen R, Welling C, Permutt MA. Variability of the insulin gene in American blacks with NIDDM. Analysis by single-strand conformational polymorphisms. Diabetes 1992; 41(6):742–749.

122. Pugliese A, Miceli D. The insulin gene in diabetes. Diabetes Metab Res Rev 2002; 18(1):13–25.

123. Baier LJ, Sacchettini JC, Knowler WC, et al. An amino acid substitution in the human intestinal fatty acid binding protein is associated with increased fatty acid binding, increased fat oxidation, and insulin resistance. J Clin Invest 1995; 95(3):1281–1287.

124. Hayakawa T, Nagai Y, Nohara E, et al. Variation of the fatty acid binding protein 2 gene is not associated with obesity and insulin resistance in Japanese subjects. Metabolism 1999; 48(5):655–657.

125. Galluzzi JR, Cupples LA, Meigs JB, Wilson PW, Schaefer EJ, Ordovas JM. Association of the Ala54-Thr polymorphism in the intestinal fatty acid-binding protein with 2-h postchallenge insulin levels in the Framingham Offspring Study. Diabetes Care 2001; 24(7):1161–1166.

126. Yamada K, Yuan X, Ishiyama S, et al. Association between Ala54Thr substitution of the fatty acid-binding protein 2 gene with insulin resistance and intra-abdominal fat thickness in Japanese men. Diabetologia 1997; 40(6):706–710.

127. Ito K, Nakatani K, Fujii M, et al. Codon 54 polymorphism of the fatty acid binding protein gene and insulin resistance in the Japanese population. Diabet Med 1999; 16(2):119–124.

128. Rissanen J, Pihlajamaki J, Heikkinen S, Kekalainen P, Kuusisto J, Laakso M. The Ala54Thr polymorphism of the fatty acid binding protein 2 gene does not influence insulin sensitivity in Finnish nondiabetic and NIDDM subjects. Diabetes 1997; 46(4):711–712.

129. Lei HH, Coresh J, Shuldiner AR, Boerwinkle E, Brancati FL. Variants of the insulin receptor substrate-1 and fatty acid binding protein 2 genes and the risk of type 2 diabetes, obesity, and hyperinsulinemia in African-Americans: the Atherosclerosis Risk in Communities Study. Diabetes 1999; 48(9):1868–1872.

130. Agren JJ, Valve R, Vidgren H, Laakso M, Uusitupa M. Postprandial lipemic response is modified by the polymorphism at codon 54 of the fatty acid-binding protein 2 gene. Arterioscler Thromb Vasc Biol 1998; 18(10):1606–1610.

131. Hansen L, Echwald SM, Hansen T, Urhammer SA, Clausen JO, Pedersen O. Amino acid polymorphisms in the ATP-regulatable inward rectifier Kir6.2 and their relationships to glucose- and tolbutamide-induced insulin secretion, the insulin sensitivity index, and NIDDM. Diabetes 1997; 46(3):508–512.

132. Inoue H, Ferrer J, Warren-Perry M, et al. Sequence variants in the pancreatic islet β-cell inwardly rectifying K+ channel Kir6.2 (Bir) gene: identification and lack of role in Caucasian patients with NIDDM. Diabetes 1997; 46(3):502–507.

133. Sakagashira S, Sanke T, Hanabusa T, et al. Missense mutation of amylin gene (S20G) in Japanese NIDDM patients. Diabetes 1996; 45(9):1279–1281.
134. Yamada K, Yuan X, Ishiyama S, Nonaka K. Glucose tolerance in Japanese subjects with S20G mutation of the amylin gene. Diabetologia 1998; 41(1):125.
135. Chuang LM, Lee KC, Huang CN, Wu HP, Tai TY, Lin BJ. Role of S20G mutation of amylin gene in insulin secretion, insulin sensitivity, and type II diabetes mellitus in Taiwanese patients. Diabetologia 1998; 41(10):1250–1251.
136. Birch CL, Fagan LJ, Armstrong MJ, Turnbull DM, Walker M. The S20G islet-associated polypeptide gene mutation in familial NIDDM. Diabetologia 1997; 40(9):1113.
137. Shimomura H, Sanke T, Hanabusa T, Tsunoda K, Furuta H, Nanjo K. Nonsense mutation of islet-1 gene (Q310X) found in a type 2 diabetic patient with a strong family history. Diabetes 2000; 49(9): 1597–1600.
138. Barat-Houari M, Clement K, Vatin V, et al. Positional candidate gene analysis of Lim domain homeobox gene (Isl-1) on chromosome 5q11-q13 in a French morbidly obese population suggests indication for association with type 2 diabetes. Diabetes 2002; 51(5):1640–1643.
139. Wolford JK, Hanson RL, Bogardus C, Prochazka M. Analysis of the lamin A/C gene as a candidate for type II diabetes susceptibility in Pima Indians. Diabetologia 2001; 44(6):779–782.
140. Baier LJ, Wiedrich C, Hanson RL, Bogardus C. Variant in the regulatory subunit of phosphatidyl-inositol 3-kinase (p85α): preliminary evidence indicates a potential role of this variant in the acute insulin response and type 2 diabetes in Pima women. Diabetes 1998; 47(6):973–975.
141. Hansen T, Andersen CB, Echwald SM, et al. Identification of a common amino acid polymorphism in the p85α regulatory subunit of phosphatidylinositol 3-kinase: effects on glucose disappearance constant, glucose effectiveness, and the insulin sensitivity index. Diabetes 1997; 46(3):494–501.
142. Frittitta L, Ercolino T, Bozzali M, et al. A cluster of three single nucleotide polymorphisms in the 3′-untranslated region of human glycoprotein PC-1 gene stabilizes PC-1 mRNA and is associated with increased PC-1 protein content and insulin resistance-related abnormalities. Diabetes 2001; 50(8):1952–1955.
143. Pizzuti A, Frittitta L, Argiolas A, et al. A polymorphism (K121Q) of the human glycoprotein PC-1 gene coding region is strongly associated with insulin resistance. Diabetes 1999; 48(9):1881–1884.
144. Jaikaran ET, Marcon G, Levesque L, George-Hyslop PS, Fraser PE, Clark A. Localisation of presenilin 2 in human and rodent pancreatic islet β-cells; Met239Val presenilin 2 variant is not associated with diabetes in man. J Cell Sci 1999; 112(Pt 13):2137–2144.
145. Kalidas K, Dow E, Saker PJ, et al. Prohormone convertase 1 in obesity, gestational diabetes mellitus, and NIDDM: no evidence for a major susceptibility role. Diabetes 1998; 47(2):287–289.
146. Ohagi S, Sakaguchi H, Sanke T, Tatsuta H, Hanabusa T, Nanjo K. Human prohormone convertase 3 gene: exon-intron organization and molecular scanning for mutations in Japanese subjects with NIDDM. Diabetes 1996; 45(7):897–901.
147. Yoshida H, Ohagi S, Sanke T, Furuta H, Furuta M, Nanjo K. Association of the prohormone convertase 2 gene (PCSK2) on chromosome 20 with NIDDM in Japanese subjects. Diabetes 1995; 44(4): 389–393.
148. Permana PA, Kahn BB, Huppertz C, Mott DM. Functional analyses of amino acid substitutions Arg883Ser and Asp905Tyr of protein phosphatase-1 G-subunit. Mol Genet Metab 2000; 70(2): 151–158.
149. Hansen L, Hansen T, Vestergaard H, et al. A widespread amino acid polymorphism at codon 905 of the glycogen-associated regulatory subunit of protein phosphatase-1 is associated with insulin resistance and hypersecretion of insulin. Hum Mol Genet 1995; 4(8):1313–1320.
150. Xia J, Scherer SW, Cohen PT, et al. A common variant in PPP1R3 associated with insulin resistance and type 2 diabetes. Diabetes 1998; 47(9):1519–1524.
151. Maegawa H, Shi K, Hidaka H, et al. The 3′-untranslated region polymorphism of the gene for skeletal muscle-specific glycogen-targeting subunit of protein phosphatase 1 in the type 2 diabetic Japanese population. Diabetes 1999; 48(7):1469–1472.
152. Hegele RA, Harris SB, Zinman B, et al. Variation in the AU(AT)-rich element within the 3′-untranslated region of PPP1R3 is associated with variation in plasma glucose in aboriginal Canadians. J Clin Endocrinol Metab 1998; 83(11):3980–3983.
153. Prochazka M, Mochizuki H, Baier LJ, Cohen PT, Bogardus C. Molecular and linkage analysis of type-1 protein phosphatase catalytic β-subunit gene: lack of evidence for its major role in insulin resistance in Pima Indians. Diabetologia 1995; 38(4):461–466.
154. Yuan X, Yamada K, Ishiyama-Shigemoto S, Koyama W, Nonaka K. Analysis of trinucleotide-repeat combination polymorphism at the rad gene in patients with type 2 diabetes mellitus. Metabolism 1999; 48(2):173–175.
155. Sentinelli F, Romeo S, Arca M, et al. Human resistin gene, obesity, and type 2 diabetes: mutation analysis and population study. Diabetes 2002; 51(3):860–862.
156. Wang H, Chu WS, Hemphill C, Elbein SC. Human resistin gene: molecular scanning and evaluation of association with insulin sensitivity and type 2 diabetes in Caucasians. J Clin Endocrinol Metab 2002; 87(6):2520–2524.

157. Osawa H, Onuma H, Murakami A, et al. Systematic search for single nucleotide polymorphisms in the resistin gene: the absence of evidence for the association of three identified single nucleotide polymorphisms with Japanese type 2 diabetes. Diabetes 2002; 51(3):863–866.
158. Varadi A, Lebel L, Hashim Y, Mehta Z, Ashcroft SJ, Turner R. Sequence variants of the sarco(endo)plasmic reticulum Ca(2+)-transport ATPase 3 gene (SERCA3) in Caucasian type II diabetic patients (UK prospective diabetes study 48). Diabetologia 1999; 42(10):1240–1243.
159. Goksel DL, Fischbach K, Duggirala R, et al. Variant in sulfonylurea receptor-1 gene is associated with high insulin concentrations in non-diabetic Mexican Americans: SUR-1 gene variant and hyperinsulinemia. Hum Genet 1998; 103(3):280–285.
160. Hani EH, Clement K, Velho G, et al. Genetic studies of the sulfonylurea receptor gene locus in NIDDM and in morbid obesity among French Caucasians. Diabetes 1997; 46(4):688–694.
161. Baier LJ, Dobberfuhl AM, Pratley RE, Hanson RL, Bogardus C. Variations in the vitamin D-binding protein (Gc locus) are associated with oral glucose tolerance in nondiabetic Pima Indians. J Clin Endocrinol Metab 1998; 83(8):2993–2996.
162. Baynes KC, Boucher BJ, Feskens EJ, Kromhout D. Vitamin D, glucose tolerance and insulinaemia in elderly men. Diabetologia 1997; 40(3):344–347.
163. Hitman GA, Mannan N, McDermott MF, et al. Vitamin D receptor gene polymorphisms influence insulin secretion in Bangladeshi Asians. Diabetes 1998; 47(4):688–690.
164. Chiu KC, Chuang LM, Yoon C. The vitamin D receptor polymorphism in the translation initiation codon is a risk factor for insulin resistance in glucose tolerant Caucasians. BMC Med Genet 2001; 2:2.
165. Walston J, McBurnie MA, Newman A, et al. Frailty and activation of the inflammation and coagulation systems with and without clinical morbidities: results from the cardiovascular health study. Arch Intern Med 2002; 162:2333–2341.
166. Maggio M, Guralnik JM, Longo DL, Ferrucci L. Interleukin-6 in aging and chronic disease: a magnificent pathway. J Gerontol A Biol Sci Med Sci 2006; 61(6):575–584.
167. Bastard JP, Maachi M, Lagathu C, et al. Recent advances in the relationship between obesity, inflammation, and insulin resistance. Eur Cytokine Netw 2006; 17(1):4–12.
168. Shoelson SE, Lee J, Goldfine AB. Inflammation and insulin resistance. J Clin Invest 2006; 116(7):1793–1801.
169. de Maat MP, Bladbjerg EM, Hjelmborg JB, Bathum L, Jespersen J, Christensen K. Genetic influence on inflammation variables in the elderly. Arterioscler Thromb Vasc Biol 2004; 24(11):2168–2173.
170. de Craen AJ, Posthuma D, Remarque EJ, van den Biggelaar AH, Westendorp RG, Boomsma DI. Heritability estimates of innate immunity: an extended twin study. Genes Immun 2005; 6(2):167–170.
171. Achyut BR, Srivastava A, Bhattacharya S, Mittal B. Genetic association of interleukin-1β (-511C/T) and interleukin-1 receptor antagonist (86 bp repeat) polymorphisms with Type 2 diabetes mellitus in North Indians. Clin Chim Acta 2007; 377(1-2):163–169.
172. Testa R, Olivieri F, Bon AR, et al. Interleukin-6-174 G>C polymorphism affects the association between IL-6 plasma levels and insulin resistance in type 2 diabetic patients. Diabetes Res Clin Pract 2006; 71(3):299–305.
173. Qi L, van Dam RM, Meigs JB, Manson JE, Hunter D, Hu FB. Genetic variation in IL6 gene and type 2 diabetes: tagging-SNP haplotype analysis in large-scale case-control study and meta-analysis. Hum Mol Genet 2006; 15(11):1914–1920.
174. Van Houten B, Woshner V, Santos JH. Role of mitochondrial DNA in toxic responses to oxidative stress. DNA Repair (Amst) 2006; 5(2):145–152.
175. Maassen JA, van den Ouweland JM, Hart LM, Lemkes HH. Maternally inherited diabetes and deafness: a diabetic subtype associated with a mutation in mitochondrial DNA. Horm Metab Res 1997; 29(2):50–55.
176. Donovan LE, Severin NE. Maternally inherited diabetes and deafness in a North American kindred: tips for making the diagnosis and review of unique management issues. J Clin Endocrinol Metab 2006; 91(12):4737–4742.
177. Maassen JA, Hart LM, Janssen GM, Reiling E, Romijn JA, Lemkes HH. Mitochondrial diabetes and its lessons for common Type 2 diabetes. Biochem Soc Trans 2006; 34(Pt 5):819–823.
178. Bhat A, Koul A, Sharma S, et al. The possible role of 10398A and 16189C mtDNA variants in providing susceptibility to T2DM in two North Indian populations: a replicative study. Hum Genet 2007; 120(6):821–826.
179. Liou CW, Lin TK, Huei WH, et al. A common mitochondrial DNA variant and increased body mass index as associated factors for development of type 2 diabetes: additive effects of genetic and environmental factors. J Clin Endocrinol Metab 2007; 92(1):235–239.
180. Serman A, Vlahovic M, Serman L, Bulic-Jakus F. DNA methylation as a regulatory mechanism for gene expression in mammals. Coll Antropol 2006; 30(3):665–671.
181. Schumacher A, Petronis A. Epigenetics of complex diseases: from general theory to laboratory experiments. Curr Top Microbiol Immunol 2006; 310:81–115.
182. Crews D, McLachlan JA. Epigenetics, evolution, endocrine disruption, health, and disease. Endocrinology 2006; 147(6 suppl):S4–S10.

183. Vanden Berghe W, Ndlovu MN, Hoya-Arias R, Dijsselbloem N, Gerlo S, Haegeman G. Keeping up NF-kappaB appearances: epigenetic control of immunity or inflammation-triggered epigenetics. Biochem Pharmacol 2006; 72(9):1114–1131.

184. Bjornsson HT, Fallin MD, Feinberg AP. An integrated epigenetic and genetic approach to common human disease. Trends Genet 2004; 20(8):350–358.

185. UK Prospective Diabetes Study (UKPDS) Group. Intensive blood-glucose control with sulphonyl-ureas or insulin compared with conventional treatment and risk of complications in patients with type 2 diabetes (UKPDS 33). Lancet 1998; 352(9131):837–853.

186. Rincon-Choles H, Thameem F, Lehman DM, et al. Genetic basis of diabetic nephropathy. Am J Ther 2005; 12(6):555–561.

187. Uhlmann K, Kovacs P, Boettcher Y, Hammes HP, Paschke R. Genetics of diabetic retinopathy. Exp Clin Endocrinol Diabetes 2006; 114(6):275–294.

188. Rietveld I, Ikram MK, Vingerling JR, et al. An IGF-I gene polymorphism modifies the risk of diabetic retinopathy. Diabetes 2006; 55(8):2387–2391.

189. Ng DP, Warram JH, Krolewski AS. TGF-β 1 as a genetic susceptibility locus for advanced diabetic nephropathy in type 1 diabetes mellitus: an investigation of multiple known DNA sequence variants. Am J Kidney Dis 2003; 41(1):22–28.

190. Moczulski DK, Rogus JJ, Antonellis A, Warram JH, Krolewski AS. Major susceptibility locus for nephropathy in type 1 diabetes on chromosome 3q: results of novel discordant sib-pair analysis. Diabetes 1998; 47(7):1164–1169.

191. McKnight AJ, Maxwell AP, Sawcer S, et al. A genome-wide DNA microsatellite association screen to identify chromosomal regions harboring candidate genes in diabetic nephropathy. J Am Soc Nephrol 2006; 17(3):831–836.

3 | The Pathophysiology of Diabetes in the Elderly

Graydon S. Meneilly
Department of Medicine, Vancouver Hospital and the University of British Columbia, Vancouver, British Columbia, Canada

INTRODUCTION

The pathophysiology of type 2 diabetes in younger patient populations has been extensively investigated (1). However, there have been relatively few studies in the elderly. Recently, investigators have evaluated the pathophysiology of diabetes in the elderly and have found that diabetes in this age group is unique. The factors that contribute toward the high prevalence of diabetes in the aged are shown in Figure 1.

GENETIC FACTORS

There is a strong genetic predisposition to diabetes in the elderly, although the specific genes responsible have not been elucidated (2). Diabetes is more common in certain ethnic groups, and patients with a family history of type 2 diabetes are much more likely to develop the illness as they age (3,4). The concordance in identical twins is greater than 80%, and even siblings without diabetes have abnormal glucose metabolism (5). All of these lines of evidence support the idea that genetic makeup plays a pivotal role in the development of diabetes in the elderly.

AGE-RELATED CHANGES IN GLUCOSE METABOLISM

Normal aging is characterized by a number of progressive changes in carbohydrate metabolism, which explains why the incidence of diabetes increases with age in genetically susceptible individuals. Early studies found that glucose-induced insulin release was normal in the elderly, but more recent investigations demonstrate clear alterations in insulin release, particularly in response to oral glucose (6,7). Abnormal insulin secretion may be related, in part, to age-related changes in response to incretin hormones (8). Like many hormones, insulin is secreted in a pulsatile fashion. Normal aging is also characterized by subtle alterations in pulsatile insulin release, which further contribute to age-related changes in glucose metabolism (9). However, the most important mechanism contributing to abnormal carbohydrate metabolism with age is resistance to insulin-mediated glucose disposal, although there is debate as to how much of this is due to the aging process itself and how much is related to lifestyle factors that commonly occur with aging (7).

LIFESTYLE FACTORS

Despite the fact that there is a strong genetic predisposition to diabetes in the elderly, a variety of lifestyle factors contribute to the increased risk for diabetes in the aged. The prevalence of diabetes is higher in older individuals who have a diet that is high in simple sugars and saturated fats and low in complex carbohydrates (10–13). It has been suggested that deficiencies in vitamins, minerals, or trace elements may contribute to the development or progression of diabetes in the elderly (10,14). Elderly patients with diabetes have increased free-radical production and the administration of Vitamin C and E improves insulin action in elderly patients with diabetes and insulin resistance. Glucose metabolism is improved in these patients by the administration of magnesium and zinc. Increased dietary iron may be associated with an increased risk of diabetes in aged individuals (13,15). Chromium deficiency has been found to cause abnormal glucose metabolism in younger patients, but as yet, no studies have shown a

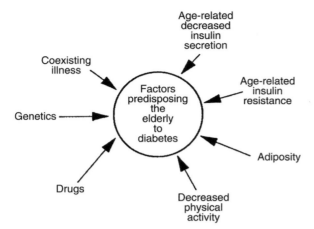

FIGURE 1 Factors contributing to the high prevalence of diabetes in the elderly.

similar effect in the elderly. Obesity, especially with a central distribution of body fat, and a reduction in physical activity occur progressively with aging, and both of these factors are associated with abnormal carbohydrate metabolism (10,12,16–19).

The above-mentioned data suggest that interventions designed to modify lifestyle may be of value in the prevention of diabetes in the aged. Indeed, the Diabetes Prevention Program found that a combined lifestyle intervention consisting of weight loss and increased physical activity was effective in reducing the incidence of diabetes in elderly patients with impaired glucose tolerance (20).

Finally, in addition to the lifestyle factors noted above, older people have multiple comorbidities including hypertension, heart failure, dyslipidemia, and various neurodegenerative diseases that can alter carbohydrate metabolism. They also take many drugs that can adversely effect carbohydrate metabolism and increase the incidence of diabetes in this age group, including thiazides, β-blockers, neuroleptics, and corticosteroids (10).

OTHER FACTORS

The presence of inflammation, as measured by C-reactive ptotein and other proinflammatory cytokines, such as tumor necrosis factor-α is associated with the development of diabetes in the elderly (21–23). Higher levels of adiponectin (an adipocytokine that increases insulin sensitivity) are associated with a reduced incidence of diabetes in the aged (22). Levels of sex steroid hormones also appear to be related to the development of diabetes in the elderly (24). In particular, lower testosterone levels in men and higher levels in women appear to be associated with an increased incidence of diabetes.

METABOLIC ALTERATIONS

Middle-aged patients with diabetes, whether lean or obese, have an increase in hepatic glucose production, a profound impairment in glucose-induced insulin release, and marked resistance to insulin-mediated glucose disposal (1). Recent studies have evaluated metabolic alterations in lean and obese older patients with diabetes and compared them to age-matched controls and middle-aged patients with diabetes (25–28). These studies have found that diabetes in the elderly is metabolically distinct. In contrast to younger subjects, older patients do not have an increase in fasting hepatic glucose production (Fig. 2). Similar to middle-aged subjects, lean older patients with diabetes have a marked impairment in glucose-induced insulin secretion (Fig. 3). However, in contrast to younger lean patients, elderly lean patients with diabetes have minimal resistance to insulin-mediated glucose disposal (Fig. 4). Middle-aged obese patients with diabetes have a marked impairment in glucose-induced insulin secretion. Overall insulin secretion is relatively preserved in obese elderly patients with diabetes (Fig. 3), although

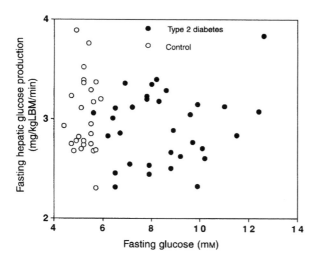

FIGURE 2 Fasting hepatic glucose production in relation to fasting glucose levels in healthy elderly controls and elderly patients with diabetes.

pulsatile insulin secretion is clearly altered (9). Finally, both middle-aged and elderly obese patients with diabetes have evidence of resistance to insulin-mediated glucose disposal (Fig. 4). In summary, diabetes in the elderly is metabolically distinct. The primary defect in obese elderly patients with diabetes is resistance to insulin-mediated glucose disposal; in lean elderly patients with diabetes, the main problem is impaired glucose-induced insulin release.

Based on the above, the therapeutic approach to diabetes in the elderly should be different than in younger patients. In middle-aged patients, many endocrinologists recommend that patients be treated with drugs that both stimulate insulin secretion and improve insulin sensitivity, on the assumption that most patients have multiple metabolic abnormalities. In obese

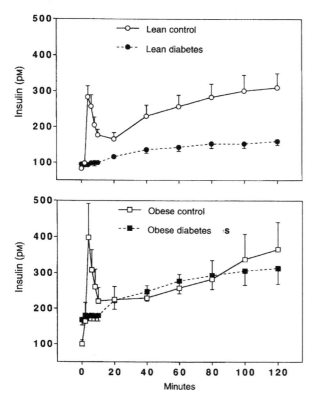

FIGURE 3 Glucose-induced insulin release in healthy lean and obese elderly controls and lean and obese elderly patients with diabetes.

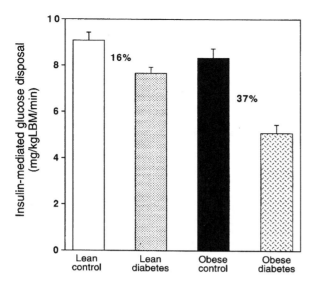

FIGURE 4 Insulin-mediated glucose disposal rates in healthy lean and obese elderly controls and lean and obese elderly patients with diabetes.

elderly subjects with diabetes, the principal defect is insulin resistance; so patients should be treated initially with drugs that enhance insulin sensitivity (such as metformin or glitazones). In contrast, in lean subjects, the principal problem is an impairment in insulin secretion. Therefore, patients should be treated with exogenous insulin or drugs that stimulate insulin secretion.

Insulin-mediated vasodilation accounts for about 30% of normal glucose disposal. Recent studies from our laboratory indicate that insulin-mediated blood flow is impaired in normal elderly subjects (26). This defect is greater in obese insulin-resistant patients with diabetes (Fig. 5), implying that drugs that enhance muscle blood flow may have a therapeutic value in the elderly (26). Indeed, angiotensin converting enzyme inhibitors have been shown to improve insulin sensitivity in elderly patients with diabetes and hypertension (29).

The destruction of β-cells is extremely important in the pathogenesis of type 1 diabetes. It has been known for several years that some middle-aged patients who were initially classified as having type 2 diabetes have high titers of antibodies to glutamic acid decarboxylase (GAD) and islet cells and have β-cell failure, which resembles type 1 diabetes (30). Older patients with diabetes who are GAD or islet cell antibody positive and who are insulin deficient have been

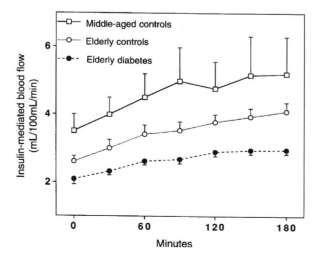

FIGURE 5 Insulin-mediated blood flow in obese middle-aged and elderly controls and obese elderly patients with diabetes.

referred to as having latent autoimmune diabetes in adults (LADA) (31–36). Some studies have found that elderly patients with diabetes who are positive for GAD have impaired β-cell function relative to controls without these markers, whereas others have not (31,37). It has been suggested that the impairment in insulin secretion in lean older patients with diabetes may be caused by autoimmune destruction of β-cells. It has been also been proposed that screening for autoimmune parameters should be performed in elderly patients with impaired glucose tolerance and newly diagnosed type 2 diabetes to predict islet cell failure. Although this is a compelling hypothesis, it would seem appropriate to begin widespread screening only when randomized studies have demonstrated that early intervention will protect β-cells and reduce the need for insulin therapy (35,36). Currently, no data are available in this regard.

GLUCOSE EFFECTIVENESS OR NON–INSULIN-MEDIATED GLUCOSE DISPOSAL

Glucose can stimulate its own uptake in cells in the absence of insulin, which is known as non–insulin-mediated glucose uptake (NIMGU) or glucose effectiveness (38). During fasting, about two-thirds of glucose uptake occurs via NIMGU, primarily in the nervous system. After a meal, about half of glucose uptake occurs via this pathway, primarily in muscle. In insulin-resistant middle-aged patients with diabetes, it is felt that over two-thirds of postprandial glucose uptake occurs via NIMGU. NIMGU is normal during fasting, but impaired during hyperglycemia in healthy elderly patients (39). We have recently shown that the defect in NIMGU is further enhanced in older patients with diabetes (Fig. 6) (40). The mechanism for this effect is unclear, but it may relate to the inability of glucose to induce glucose transporters to the cell surface. Several interventions have been shown to improve glucose effectiveness in younger patients, including reduction in free fatty acid levels, incretin peptides, exercise, and anabolic steroids (38). These interventions may ultimately be potential therapies for diabetes in the elderly.

MOLECULAR DEFECTS

Glucokinase is the glucose sensor of the β-cell. While it is possible that abnormalities in the function of the gene for glucokinase could lead to the impairment in glucose-induced insulin secretion in elderly patients, the evidence to support this hypothesis in the elderly is conflicting (41,42). After insulin binds it to its receptor, it activates tyrosine kinase and sets in motion a series of intracellular events that ultimately result in a movement of glucose transporters to the surface of the cell. In the elderly, insulin receptor number and affinity appear to be normal, but tyrosine kinase activity may be defective (43). Abnormalities in other components of the

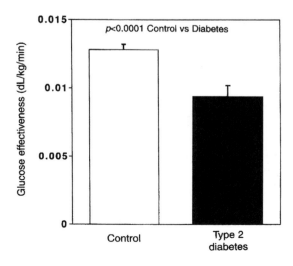

FIGURE 6 Glucose effectiveness in elderly controls and patients with diabetes.

insulin-signaling cascade have yet to be elucidated. It is clear that further investigations will be required to elucidate the molecular defects in these patients.

GLUCOSE COUNTER REGULATION

It has been known for many years that older patients with diabetes have increased frequency of severe or fatal hypoglycemia when they are treated with oral agents or insulin (10,44). There are several factors that contribute to the increased incidence of hypoglycemia. The most important hormone in the defense against acute hypoglycemia is glucagon. When glucagon secretion is deficient, epinephrine becomes important. If hypoglycemia is prolonged for several hours, growth hormone and cortisol are the most important counter-regulatory hormones. Elderly patients with diabetes have impaired glucagon and growth hormone responses to hypoglycemia (Fig. 7) (45). In addition, elderly patients with diabetes have not been taught to recognize the warning symptoms of hypoglycemia (46). Even when they have been taught about these symptoms, older people are less aware of the autonomic warning symptoms of hypoglycemia than younger patients at comparable glucose levels. Finally, elderly patients have impaired psychomotor performance during relatively modest hypoglycemia, which can prevent them from taking the necessary steps to correct low blood sugars. Therefore, the high incidence of hypoglycemia in the elderly is related to reduced knowledge and awareness of warning symptoms, altered psychomotor performance in response to hypoglycemia, and an impairment in counter-regulatory hormone secretion. To mitigate the frequency of hypoglycemia in elderly patients, these patients should be carefully educated about the warning symptoms of hypoglycemia so that they can respond appropriately to these symptoms when they occur.

CONCLUSION

Diabetes in the elderly is metabolically distinct. To properly manage this illness in the aged, the therapeutic approach should be different than in younger patient populations.

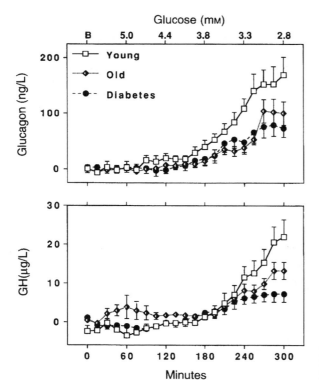

FIGURE 7 Glucagon and growth hormone responses to hypoglycemia in healthy young, healthy old, and elderly patients with diabetes.

REFERENCES

1. DeFronzo RA. Lilly Lecture 1987. The triumvirate: β-cell, muscle, liver. A collusion responsible for NIDDM. Diabetes 1988; 37:667–687.
2. Kahn CR. Banting Lecture. Insulin action, diabetogenes, and the cause of Type 2 Diabetes. Diabetes 1984; 43:1066–1084.
3. Morris RD, Rimm AA. Association of waist to hip ratio and family history with the prevalence of NIDDM among 25, 272 adult, white females. Am J Public Health 1991; 81:507–509.
4. Lipton RB, Liao Y, Cao G, et al. Determinants of incident non-insulin-dependent diabetes mellitus among blacks and white in a national sample. The NHANES 1 epidemiologic follow-up study. Am J Epidemiol 1993; 138:826–964.
5. Vaag A, Henriksen JE, Madsbad S, et al. Insulin secretion, insulin action, and hepatic glucose production in identical twins discordant for non-insulin-dependent diabetes mellitus. J Clin Invest 1995; 95:690–698.
6. Iozzo P, Beck-Nielsen J, Laakso M, et al. Independent influence of age on basal insulin secretion in non-diabetic humans. European group for the study of insulin resistance. J Clin Endocrinol Metab 1999; 84:863–868.
7. Muller DC, Elahi D, Tobin JD, et al. The effect of age on insulin resistance and secretion: a review. Semin Nephrol 1996; 16:289–298.
8. Meneilly GS, Ryan AS, Minaker KL, Elahi D. The effect of age and glycemic level on the response of the beta-cell to glucose-dependent insulinotropic polypeptide and peripheral tissue sensitivity to endogenously released insulin. J Clin Endocrinol Metab 1998; 83:2925–2932.
9. Meneilly GS, Veldhuis JD, Elahi D. Deconvolution analysis of rapid insulin pulses before and after six weeks of continuous subcutaneous administration of GLP-1 in elderly patients with type 2 diabetes. J Clin Endocrinol Metab 2005; 90:6251–6256.
10. Meneilly GS, Tessier D. Diabetes in elderly adults. J Gerontol 2001; 56A:M5–M13.
11. Feskens EJM, Virtanen SM, Rasanen L, et al. Dietary factors determining diabetes and impaired glucose tolerance. Diabetes Care 1995; 18:1104–1112.
12. van Dam RM, Rimm EB, Willett WC, et al. Dietary patterns and risk for Type 2 diabetes mellitus in U.S. men. Ann Intern Med 2002; 136:201–209.
13. Song Y, Manson JE, Buring JE, et al. A prospective study of red meat consumption and Type 2 diabetes in middle-aged and elderly women. Diabetes Care 2004; 27:2108–2115.
14. Meyer KA, Kushi LH, Jacobs DR, et al. Carbohydrates, dietary fiber, and incident type 2 diabetes in older women. Am J Clin Nutr 2000; 71:921–930.
15. Lee DH, Folsom AR, Jacobs DR. Dietary iron intake and Type 2 diabetes incidence in postmenopausal women: the Iowa Women's Health Study. Diabetologia 2004; 47:185–194.
16. The DECODE-DECODA Study Group, European Diabetes Epidemiology Group and the International Diabetes Epidemiology Group. Age, body mass index and Type 2 diabetes—associations modified by ethnicity. Diabetologia 2003; 48:1063–1070.
17. Goodpaster BH, Krishnaswami S, Resnick H, et al. Association between regional adipose tissue distribution and both Type 2 diabetes and impaired glucose tolerance in elderly men and women. Diabetes Care 2003; 26:372–379.
18. Meigs JB, Muller DC, Nathan DM, et al. The natural history of progression from normal glucose tolerance to type 2 diabetes in the Baltimore longitudinal study of aging. Diabetes 2003; 52:1475–1484.
19. Cassano PA, Rosner B, Vokonas PS, et al. Obesity and body fat distribution in relation to the incidence of non-insulin-dependent diabetes mellitus. Am J Epidemiol 1992; 136:1474–1486.
20. Diabetes Prevention Program Research Group. Reduction in the incidence of Type 2 diabetes with lifestyle intervention or metformin. N Engl J Med 2002; 346:393–403.
21. Barzilay JI, Abraham L, Heckbert S, et al. The relation of markers of inflammation to the development of glucose disorders in the elderly. Diabetes 2001; 50:2384–2389.
22. Kanaya AM, Harris T, Goodpaster BH, et al. Adipocytokines attenuate the association between visceral adiposity and diabetes in older adults. Diabetes Care 2004; 27:1375–1380.
23. Lechleitner M, Herold M, Dzien-Bischinger C, Hoppichlert F, Dzien A. Tumour necrosis factor-alpha plasma levels in elderly patients with type 2 diabetes mellitus—observations over 2 years. Diabet Med 2002; 19:949–953.
24. Oh J-Y, Barrett-Connor E, Wedick NM, et al. Endogenous sex hormones and the development of Type 2 diabetes in older men and women: the Rancho Bernardo Study. Diabetes Care 2002; 25:55–60.
25. Meneilly GS, Hards L, Tessier D, et al. NIDDM in the elderly. Diabetes Care 1996; 19:1320–1375.
26. Meneilly GS, Elliot T. Metabolic alterations in middle-aged and elderly obese patients with Type 2 diabetes. Diabetes Care 1999; 22:112–118.
27. Meneilly GS, Elahi D. Metabolic alterations in middle-aged and elderly lean patients with Type 2 diabetes. Diabetes Care 2005; 28:1498–1499.
28. Paolisso G, Gambardella A, Verza M, et al. ACE-inhibition improves insulin-sensitivity in age insulin-resistant hypertensive patients. J Hum Hypertens 1992; 6:175–179.
29. Arner P, Pollare T, Lithell H. Different Aetiologies of Type 2 (non-insulin-dependent) diabetes mellitus in obese and non-obese subjects. Diabetologia 1991; 34:483–487.

30. Zimmet PZ. Diabetes epidemiology as a tool to trigger diabetes research and care. Diabetologia 1999; 42:499–518.
31. Monge L, Brunot G, Pinach S, et al. A clinically orientated approach increases the efficiency of screening for latent autoimmune diabetes in adults (LADA) in a large clinic-based cohort of patients with diabetes onset over 50 years. Diabet Med 2004; 21:456–459.
32. Barinas-Mitchell, Pietropaolo S, Zhang Y-J, et al. Islet cell autoimmunity in a triethnic adult population of the Third National Health and Nutrition Examination Survey. Diabetes 2004; 53:1293–1302.
33. Zinman B, Kahn SE, Haffner SM, et al. Phenotypic characteristics of GAD antibody-positive recently diagnosed patients with Type 2 diabetes in North America and Europe. Diabetes 2004; 53:3193–3200.
34. Pozzilli P, Di Mario U. Autoimmune diabetes not requiring insulin at diagnosis (Latent autoimmune diabetes of the adult). Diabetes Care 2001; 24:1460–1467.
35. Gale EAM. Latent autoimmune diabetes in adults: a guide for perplexed. Diabetologia 2005; 48:2195–2199.
36. Fourlanos S, Dotta F, Greenbaum CJ, et al. Latent autoimmune diabetes in adults (LADA) should be less latent. Diabetologia 2005; 48:2206–2212.
37. Meneilly GS, Tildesley H, Elliott T, et al. Significance of GAD positivity in elderly patients with diabetes. Diabet Med 2000; 17:247–248.
38. Best JD, Kahn SE, Ader M, et al. Role of glucose effectiveness in the determination of glucose tolerance. Diabetes Care 1996; 19:1018–1030.
39. Meneilly GS, Elahi D, Minaker KL, et al. Impairment of noninsulin-mediated glucose disposal in the elderly. J Clin Endocrinol Metab 1989; 63:566–571.
40. Forbes A, Elliot T, Tildesley H, et al. Alterations in non-insulin-mediated glucose uptake in the elderly patient with diabetes. Diabetes 1998; 47:1915–1919.
41. Laakso M, Malkki M, Kekalainen P, et al. Glucokinase gene variants in subjects with late-onset NIDDM and impaired glucose tolerance. Diabetes Care 1995; 18:398–400.
42. McCarthy MI, Hitman GA, Hitchins M, et al. Glucokinase gene polymorphisms: a genetic marker for glucose intolerance in cohort of elderly Finnish men. Diabet Med 1993; 10:198–204.
43. Obermaier-Kusser B, White MF, Pongratz DE, et al. A defective intramolecular autoactivation cascade may cause the reduced kinase activity of the skeletal muscle insulin receptor from patients with non-insulin-dependent diabetes mellitus. J Biol Chem 1989; 264:9497–9504.
44. Stepka M, Rogala H, Czyzyk A. Hypoglycemia: a major problem in the management of diabetes in the elderly. Aging 1993; 5:117–121.
45. Meneilly GS, Cheung E, Tuokko H. Counter-regulatory hormone responses to hypoglycemia in the elderly patient with diabetes. Diabetes 1994; 43:403–410.
46. Thomson FJ, Masson EA, Leeming JT, et al. Lack of knowledge of symptoms of hypoglycaemia by elderly diabetic patients. Age Aging 1991; 20:404–406.

4 Diagnosis and Screening of Diabetes Mellitus in the Elderly

Seema Parikh
Division of Gerontology, Department of Medicine, Beth Israel Deaconess Medical Center, Harvard Medical School, Boston, Massachusetts, U.S.A.

Medha N. Munshi
Joslin Diabetes Center, Beth Israel Deaconess Medical Center, Boston, Massachusetts, U.S.A.

INTRODUCTION

Diabetes mellitus (DM) is a major public health problem affecting an increasing number of older individuals. The major impact of diabetes is through the increased risk of macrovascular and microvascular complications. The purpose of accurate and timely diagnosis is to identify individuals at increased risk of such complications and then to formulate therapeutic and preventative management strategies.

Among U.S. adults aged 18 to 79 years, the incidence of diagnosed diabetes increased 41% from 1997 to 2003 (1). Furthermore, estimates from the Centers for Disease Control and Prevention indicate that, in 1998, 12.7% of persons aged 70 and older had a diagnosis of DM, up from 11.6% in 1990 (2). However, national and community based studies indicate that the true prevalence of diabetes may be even higher; it is estimated that over 5.9 million individuals in the United States meet diagnostic criteria for diabetes, but remain undiagnosed (3). These undiagnosed patients with diabetes are consequently at a high risk of morbidity and mortality (4). In such patients chronic complications are often present at the time of the diagnosis. In the United States 15% to 20% of individuals with undiagnosed diabetes have been found to have diabetic retinopathy, 5% to 10% have proteinuria (5), 10% have cardiovascular disease, and 10% have neuropathy (6). Over 40% of the elderly population have some degree of impaired glucose homeostasis. The time between onset and diagnosis may be as long as 10 to 12 years during which time microvascular disease can progress in these individuals (7). In addition to traditionally known complications of diabetes such as microvascular and macrovascular diseases, diabetes in older adults is also associated with other less well-recognized comorbidities such as cognitive dysfunction (8), depression (9,10), functional disability (11), urinary incontinence (12), falls (13), polypharmacy, and chronic pain syndromes (14). Prompt diagnosis of diabetes permits lifestyle and medical interventions to control hyperglycemia and other risk factors for cardiovascular disease and thus reduce complications. Both the American Diabetes Association (ADA) and the World Health Organization (WHO) have established criteria for screening and diagnosis of diabetes. Screening and diagnosis are separate issues, as the cohorts in whom they are performed are different. While tests for diagnosis are performed in patients suspected of having diabetes, tests for screening are applied to a broader population. In this chapter we will discuss diagnosis and screening of diabetes and highlighting issues that are unique to elderly patients in this context.

DEFINITION AND NATURAL HISTORY OF DIABETES

The term "diabetes mellitus" refers to many disease processes involving carbohydrate metabolism characterized by hyperglycemia and resulting from defects in insulin secretion, insulin utilization, or both.

Hyperglycemia, which is the cardinal manifestation of diabetes, can be present for many years before symptoms appear. Polyuria, polydipsia, polyphagia, and weight loss are some of the common presenting symptoms of diabetes. The most severe form of presentation is with ketoacidosis or nonketotic hyperosmolar coma. Diabetes can also present with symptoms related to complications of diabetes. The common long-term complications of diabetes are macrovascular diseases (cardiovascular disease, cerebrovascular disease, peripheral vascular disease) and microvascular diseases (retinopathy, neuropathy, and nephropathy).

The progression of diabetes in an individual, from normal glucose regulation to diabetes, occurs over a variable time period. Patients usually develop an intermediate metabolic state, with blood glucose levels between normal and diabetic values. This state is identified as impaired fasting glucose (IFG) or impaired glucose tolerance (IGT). These individuals have a high risk of progression to diabetes and also have a higher risk of diabetes-related morbidity and mortality.

CLASSIFICATION OF DIABETES

It is important for the clinician and the patient to understand the pathogenesis of hyperglycemia as it allows effective and directed therapy. In 1997 the ADA expert committee recommended use of the terms type 1 diabetes and type 2 diabetes rather than the use of insulin dependent diabetes (IDDM) and non-insulin dependent diabetes (NIDDM) (15). This was an effort to recognize the two disease entities according to etiology, rather than time of onset or treatment of the disease. A diagnosis of DM may refer to many different entities that have hyperglycemia as a common factor. Although the most common types of diabetes are type 1 and type 2 diabetes, there are multiple other etiologies as shown in Table 1. In the elderly population, type 2 diabetes

TABLE 1 Etiologic Classification of Diabetes Mellitus

Type 1 diabetes (β-cell destruction, usually leading to absolute insulin deficiency)
    Immune-mediated
    Idiopathic
Type 2 diabetes (may range from predominantly insulin resistance with relative insulin
    deficiency to a predominantly secretory defect with insulin resistance)
Other specific types
    Genetic defects of β-cell function
        Chromosome 12, HNF-1 (MODY3)
        Chromosome 7, glucokinase (MODY2)
        Chromosome 20, HNF-4 (MODY1)
        Chromosome 13, (IPF-1; MODY4)
        Chromosome 17, HNF-1β (MODY5)
        Chromosome 2, NeuroD1 (MODY6)
        Mitochondrial DNA
        Others
    Genetic defects in insulin action
        Type A insulin resistance
        Leprechaunism
        Rabson-Mendenhall syndrome
        Lipoatrophic diabetes
        Others
    Diseases of the exocrine pancreas
        Pancreatitis
        Trauma/pancreatectomy
        Neoplasia
        Cystic fibrosis
        Hemochromatosis
        Fibrocalculous pancreatopathy
        Others
    Endocrinopathies
        Acromegaly
        Cushing's syndrome
        Glucagonoma
        Pheochromocytoma
        Hyperthyroidism
        Somatostatinoma
        Aldosteronoma
        Others

(Continued)

TABLE 1 (*Continued*)

Drug- or chemical-induced
  Vacor
  Pentamidine
  Nicotinic acid
  Glucocorticoids
  Thyroid hormone
  Diazoxide
  β-Adrenergic agonists
  Thiazides
  Dilantin
  Interferon
  Others
Infections
  Congenital rubella
  Cytomegalovirus
  Others
Uncommon forms of immune-mediated diabetes
  "Stiff-man" syndrome
  Anti–insulin receptor antibodies
  Others
Other genetic syndromes sometimes associated with diabetes
  Down's syndrome
  Klinefelter's syndrome
  Turner's syndrome
  Wolfram's syndrome
  Friedreich's ataxia
  Huntington's chorea
  Laurence–Moon–Biedl syndrome
  Myotonic dystrophy
  Porphyria
  Prader–Willi syndrome
  Others
GDM

Abbreviations: GDM, gestational diabetes mellitus; HNF, hepatocyte nuclear factor; IPF-1, insulin promoter factor-1.
Source: From Ref. 34.

is the most common variety. Some types of diabetes, pertinent to the geriatric population are discussed here.

Type 1 Diabetes

Type 1 diabetes is essentially the result of β-cell destruction, which usually leads to absolute insulin deficiency. The rate of β-cell destruction is variable. Traditionally this form of immune-mediated diabetes was thought to occur during childhood and adolescence, however it can occur at any age; rarely even in the eighth and ninth decade of life (16). Patients with type 1 diabetes ultimately become insulinopenic requiring insulin therapy for survival. The presentation of type 1 diabetes is usually acute or sub-acute with classic symptoms of polyuria, polydipsia, polyphagia, loss of weight, recurrent infections, or fatigue. Type 1 diabetes in older adults tends to present in a more sub-acute or chronic manner mimicking type 2 diabetes with fewer symptoms to none at all. This particular form of diabetes is often referred to as latent autoimmune diabetes of the adult (LADA).

Type 2 Diabetes

This type is more prevalent and comprises 90% to 95% of adults with diabetes. The cause of type 2 diabetes is a combination of resistance to insulin action and an inadequate compensatory insulin secretory response by β-cells. The degree of hyperglycemia is sufficient to cause pathological and functional changes within target tissues with or without clinical symptoms. In fact diabetes may be present for a long period of time before it is detected. During this asymptomatic period it is possible to demonstrate an abnormality in carbohydrate metabolism by measurement of plasma glucose in the fasting state or after a challenge with an oral glucose load. In most patients, at least initially, type 2 diabetes begins with insulin resistance with relative insulin deficiency and patients do not require insulin to survive. However with time, along with insulin resistance, an insulin secretory defect may predominate. Often throughout their lifetime these individuals do not need insulin treatment to survive. Most patients are obese and obesity by itself may cause some degree of insulin resistance. Patients who are not obese by traditional weight criteria may have an increased percentage of body fat distributed predominantly in the abdominal region with a high waist to hip ratio (16). Insulin resistance may improve with weight reduction and/or pharmacological treatment of hyperglycemia but usually does not revert back to normal. In this type of diabetes, ketoacidosis seldom occurs spontaneously. If it occurs, it usually arises in association with the stress of another illness such as infection. Nonetheless ketoacidosis does not exclude the diagnosis of type 2 diabetes, especially in non-Caucasian populations.

OTHER ETIOLOGIES OF DIABETES

A number of etiological factors shown in Table 1 may lead to a diabetogenic state, requiring medical intervention and lifestyle modification. Some of the more common factors in an elderly population include medications and endocrinopathies. Medications may precipitate diabetes in individuals with insulin resistance. The exact sequence or relative importance of the β-cell dysfunction and insulin resistance is unknown in these instances. Examples of such medications commonly used in the geriatric population are corticosteroids, thyroid hormones, and thiazide diuretics. Hormones such as growth hormone, cortisol, glucagon, and epinephrine antagonize insulin action and cause a hyperglycemic state. This generally occurs in individuals with pre-existing defects in insulin secretion. Resolution of hyperglycemia occurs when the hormone excess is resolved. Somatostatinoma and aldosterone induced hypokalemia can also cause diabetes, at least in part by inhibiting insulin secretion. Hyperglycemia generally resolves after successful removal of the tumor.

PRESENTATION OF DIABETES IN THE ELDERLY

Some may consider glucose intolerance almost physiological in the elderly as glucose tolerance begins to decline in the third decade, and the trend then continues throughout life. This is characterized by the moderate increase in one- or two-hour postprandial plasma glucose concentration (17).

The pathogenesis of glucose intolerance in the elderly is multifactorial involving:

1. Impaired glucose-induced insulin secretion
2. Delayed and sustained insulin-mediated suppression of hepatic glucose output
3. Delayed insulin-stimulated peripheral glucose uptake, mostly by skeletal muscle

It is important to have a high degree of suspicion, as in older adults symptoms of diabetes may be atypical (Table 2). These symptoms vary from confusion and fatigue to urinary frequency. Classical symptoms of diabetes like polyuria and thirst may be less pronounced due to the increased renal threshold for glucose excretion and the impaired thirst mechanism (18). From a practical perspective, patients may present at a later stage of disease due to under-reporting of illness, confusion as to the cause, and atypical presentations. Severe diabetes-related conditions might be the presenting illness in previously undiagnosed diabetic patients. The presenting condition may vary from painful shoulder periarthrosis to conditions as serious as acute coronary syndromes.

More importantly however, patients may be asymptomatic. Even when there are no symptoms suggestive of hyperglycemia, an assessment for risk factors for diabetes in every elderly patient is warranted because of the high prevalence of the disease in this population and the fact that the large fraction are asymptomatic. Most elderly patients have type 2 diabetes and therefore obesity is an important factor. Body mass index (BMI), in particular abdominal obesity and weight gain after the age of 18 to 20 years, predicts increased risk of diabetes and mortality.

TABLE 2 Atypical Presentations in Elderly Patients with Diabetes

Constitutional
  Fatigue
  Unexplained weight loss
Eyes
  Cataracts
  Background or proliferative retinopathy
Nervous system
  Pain
  Paresthesias
  Hypoesthesias
  Autonomic neuropathies
    Diarrhea
    Impotence
    Postural hypotension
    Overflow incontinence
  Cranial nerve palsies
  Muscle weakness
  Diabetic neuropathic cachexia and amyotrophy
  Coma (hyperosmolar nonketotic coma)
  Cognitive impairment
Cardiovascular
  Angina
  Silent ischemia
  Myocardial infarction
  Transient ischemic attack
  Stroke
  Diabetic foot ulcers
  Gangrene
Genitourinary
  Proteinuria
  Chronic renal failure
  Urinary incontinence
Metabolic
  Obesity
  Hyperlipidemia
  Osteoporosis
Skin
  Pruritus vulvae
  Intertrigo
  Bacterial infections
  Slow wound healing
Infections
  Urinary tract infections
  Reactivation of tuberculosis
  Oral thrush
  Vulvovaginitis, balanitis

Source: From Ref. 19.

All elderly persons with one or more risk factors (other than advanced age) should be screened for diabetes (Table 3).

TESTS FOR SCREENING AND DIAGNOSIS OF DIABETES

Accurate diagnosis of diabetes is essential as the medical ramifications may be far reaching. Additionally the diagnosis of a life-long illness with the possibility of multiple complications can lead to psychological trauma and a lifestyle transformation. The impact of this diagnosis in an elderly person may also affect other family members as they then have a higher risk of developing diabetes. Commonly used tests to screen and diagnose diabetes include fasting plasma glucose (FPG), oral glucose tolerance test (OGTT), casual glucose test, hemoglobin A1c, and urine dipstick test. Details of these tests are given in the following sections.

TABLE 3   Risk Factors for Type 2 Diabetes

Age ≥ 45
Overweight (BMI ≥25 kg/m^2)
Family history of diabetes
Habitual physical inactivity
Race/ethnicity
Previously identified IFG or IGT
Hypertension (≥140/90 mmHg in adults)
HDL cholesterol ≤35 mg/dL (0.90 mmol/L) and/or a triglyceride level ≥250 mg/dL
History of vascular disease
Belonging to a high-risk ethnic group (African American, Hispanic, Native American,
     Asian American, Pacific islander)

Abbreviations: BMI, body mass index; HDL, high-density lipoprotein; IFG, impaired fasting
glucose; IGT, impaired glucose tolerance.
Source: From Ref. 16.

Fasting Plasma Glucose

FPG is the most commonly used test for screening and diagnosis of diabetes because of the ease of use, acceptability to patients, and low cost. It is performed by measuring plasma glucose after fasting for at least eight hours. In 1997, the diagnostic value for the FPG was changed from 140 to 126 mg/dL. This change was made so that the prevalence of diabetes determined by the FPG more closely corresponded to that of the two-hour OGTT (>200 mg/dL) (20). The ADA expert committee has suggested that both tests reflect similar levels of hyperglycemia and risk of adverse outcomes. At this time the ADA recommends FPG as the preferred test for screening as well as diagnosis of diabetes. In a non-diabetic patient, a value of FPG ≥126 mg/dL is considered positive screening and requires further diagnostic workup.

The diagnostic categories based on the FPG are as follows (20):

- Normal fasting glucose: FPG <100 mg/dL
- IFG: FPG 100 to 125 mg/dL
- Diagnosis of diabetes: FPG ≥126 mg/dL (must be confirmed by one more reading in this range).

Oral Glucose Tolerance Test

The OGTT is performed in the morning after a fast of at least eight hours. Water is permitted. During the test the patient must remain seated and not smoke. A loading dose of 75 g glucose for non-pregnant adults is administered over five minutes. Venous plasma glucose is measured immediately before and at two hours after the load. The OGTT has a higher sensitivity, specificity, and positive predictive value for diagnosing diabetes but as can be seen from the description, requires more organization and is poorly reproducible. For these reasons the ADA does not recommend OGTT for routine use to screen or diagnose diabetes. Even though the new diagnostic criteria for FPG produce prevalence estimates closer to OGTT values, some individuals identified by FPG differ from those identified by OGTT. The latter include the elderly, the Asian population, and those who are less obese. Until 1985 the OGTT was the standard diagnostic criteria; however, now the ADA recommends FPG for routine use. The OGTT is recommended in instances when diabetes is strongly suspected but other tests are equivocal or when FPG is in the IFG range. In nondiabetic individuals screening for diabetes is considered positive using the OGTT when two-hour postload glucose ≥200 mg/dL and should be followed by diagnostic workup.

The diagnostic categories using OGTT are as follows:

- Normal glucose tolerance: Two-hour postload glucose <140 mg/dL
- IGT: Two-hour postload glucose 140 to 199 mg/dL
- Diagnosis of diabetes: Two-hour postload glucose ≥200 mg/dL

Casual Glucose

This test is defined as the measurement of blood glucose at any time of the day without regard to time since last meal. In the presence of symptoms of hyperglycemia such as polyuria, polydipsia, polyphagia, and weight loss, an unequivocally elevated casual blood glucose level (>200 mg/dL) suggests a diagnosis of diabetes. However, lack of standardization leads to low sensitivity and specificity as a screening and diagnostic test. This test is useful when it is difficult for the patient to return to the clinic or noncompliance with office visits is anticipated.

Hemoglobin A1c

Hemoglobin A1c (HbA1c) is widely used as a test to measure glycemic control in patients with diabetes. This test is not currently recommended for diagnosis or screening. HbA1c shows large inter-individual differences in nondiabetic patients and is not sufficiently sensitive as a screening or diagnostic test although it continues to be an invaluable guide to therapy and helps identify cases with relatively poor glycemic control. There are studies that suggest that other factors such as uremia may alter HbA1c, making interpretation difficult (21). Additionally, these assays are not yet standardized worldwide. Because of this, the international expert committee recommends that A1C not be used to diagnose diabetes.

Urine Dipstick Test

Measurement of glycosuria based on a urine dipstick is frequently used both in primary and in secondary care. Urine can be tested fasting, random or postprandial. However in all cases sensitivity is low (16–64%) and the predictive value of a positive test ranges from 11% to 37% (based on a prevalence of diabetes ranging 6–12%). Glycosuria should not be used as a screening instrument for diabetes, as over 65% of individuals with diabetes may be misclassified as non-diabetic. Blood glucose levels could be high enough to represent diabetes but glycosuria may not be present due to the high renal threshold in the elderly. Additionally glycosuria in the absence of hyperglycemia is not diagnostic of diabetes. Glycosuria may also be present in the absence of diabetes in disorders such as renal tubular function.

SCREENING FOR DIABETES

Type 1 diabetes presents with acute symptoms. In addition, no consensus exists on screening tests or their utility in type 1 patients. Hence, screening for this type of diabetes is not recommended at this time.

Approximately 5.9 million patients with type 2 diabetes remain undiagnosed, exposing them to increased risk of complications. At the time of diagnosis, about 20% to 30% may have microvascular complications and often the first indication of the presence of type 2 diabetes may actually be the detection of a related complication (5). In a landmark trial, the United Kingdom Prospective Diabetes Study (UKPDS), around 50% of the newly diagnosed patients with type 2 diabetes had diabetes-related tissue damage, such as retinopathy, heart disease, or microalbuminuria at the time of diagnosis (22). In this study, patients with a history of diabetes-related complications before their clinical diagnosis of diabetes carried a two-fold higher risk of developing a new complication and were at a higher risk of subsequent mortality compared to patients without such a history over a three-year period. In another study, the average latency period between onset of diabetes and diagnosis was found to be approximately four to seven years (7) and as long as 10 to 12 years. During this time between onset of the disease and diagnosis, earlier detection, initiation of lifestyle modification, and treatment may be beneficial.

During the asymptomatic period of type 2 diabetes, periodic screening is the only method of detection. Considering the significant medical and economic burden of this disease, screening becomes increasingly important. However, there are no randomized controlled trials demonstrating the effectiveness of screening an asymptomatic population, in reducing morbidity or mortality. Cost-effectiveness of routine periodic screening of such a large population is also questionable. As a result, there is no international agreement on the benefits of screening for type 2 diabetes.

In its position statement on screening for type 2 diabetes, the ADA states that there is "insufficient evidence to conclude that community screening is a cost effective approach to reduce the morbidity and mortality associated with diabetes in presumably healthy individuals." Thus general population screening was not recommended. However, the ADA does recommend screening every three years in patients over 45 years (more frequent in high-risk patients) (Table 3).

The WHO also does not advocate for screening, rather for opportunistic case finding. The WHO recommends that screening should be carried out at a time when patients are seen by healthcare professionals for a reason other than diabetes. In the United Kingdom, general population screening is not recommended; however it is advised in high-risk groups with two or more risk factors (Table 3). Diabetes UK recommends screening of 40- to 75-year olds every five years in the absence of a recognized risk factor and every three years in the presence of a risk factor.

The third United States Preventative Services Task Force concluded that there was insufficient evidence to recommend for or against screening for diabetes in non-pregnant adults without hypertension or hyperlipidemia. However, there was sufficient evidence to recommend screening in adults with hypertension or hyperlipidemia as a part of an integrated approach to reduce cardiovascular risk (23).

There are no separate guidelines for screening for diabetes in older adults. In addition to age, older adults also have coexisting medical conditions that put them into a high-risk category for developing diabetes. Many of these older adults are routinely followed by healthcare providers in clinic and thus should have periodic screening for diabetes performed at the time of the visit.

DIAGNOSIS OF DIABETES
History

Guidelines for the diagnosis of diabetes have been in existence since 1979 and were formed by the National Diabetes Data Group (NDDG) (24). Multiple organizations have played a part in stimulating discussion and generating ideas and thoughts. Two prominent contributors are the ADA and the WHO. An international expert committee working under the sponsorship of the ADA was established in May 1995. This committee reviewed all available literature since 1979 and published a report in 1997 (24). The purpose of revising the diagnostic criteria by the ADA in 1997 was to accurately predict those persons who are at risk of diabetic complications so that patients could be identified and preventative measures started earlier. The essential change was the lowering of the diagnostic FPG for diabetes to 126 mg/dL based on the equivalence to the two-hour post-OGTT level of 200 mg/dL and on the predictive power of the fasting level for microvascular complications found in cross-sectional studies. The following year, the WHO published a provisional report with similar recommendations but with some differences that will be discussed later (25).

Current Diagnostic Criteria

Unless there are unequivocal symptoms of hyperglycemia, the diagnosis of diabetes requires two diagnostic tests obtained on two separate days. The current guidelines as recommended by the ADA are shown in Table 4. There are currently no specific separate guidelines for the geriatric patients.

OGTT Vs. FPG

Significant debate exists between the utility of FPG alone and the role of the OGTT in diagnosing diabetes. The Diabetes Epidemiology: Collaborative Analysis of Diagnostic Criteria in Europe (DECODE) study was undertaken in 1997 upon the initiative of the European Diabetes Epidemiology Group (26) and has addressed a number of issues regarding utility of FPG and OGTT in the diagnosis of diabetes (20,25–27).

The DECODE study group examined epidemiological data from 20 European studies to determine if fasting glucose was sufficient to define diabetes (26). Examining over 25,000 patients

TABLE 4 ADA Criteria for Diagnosis of Diabetes

Symptoms of diabetes plus casual plasma glucose concentration ≥200 mg/dL (11.1 mol/L). Casual is defined as any time of the day without regard to time since last meal. The classic symptoms of diabetes include polyuria, polydipsia, and unexplained weight loss

or

FPG ≥ 126 mg/dL (7.00 mmol/L). Fasting is defined as no caloric intake for at least 8 hr

or

Two-hour post-load glucose ≥ 200 mg/dL (11.1 mmol/L) during the OGTT. The test should be performed as described by the WHO using a glucose load containing the equivalent of 75 g anhydrous glucose dissolved in water

Abbreviations: ADA, American Diabetes Association; FPG, fasting plasma glucose; OGTT, oral glucose tolerance test.

they concluded that when FPG was used alone, 31% of diabetic subjects with a normal fasting glucose but abnormal two-hour glucose would not be diagnosed. Furthermore the sensitivity and the specificity of the FPG in detecting abnormal two-hour plasma glucose depended on BMI such that with increasing BMI, FPG becomes a more sensitive and specific test. FPG was not helpful in identifying IGT. Because of the differences in the diagnostic criteria, the prevalence of diabetes may be altered according to the criteria utilized. A reanalysis of this very issue by the DECODE study group reported a high degree of disagreement in classification of diabetes when using FPG or OGTT; however the risk of disagreement decreased with increasing BMI and age (26). Ultimately the study concluded that prospective data are required to best identify individuals at risk of microvascular complications and cardiovascular disease (27). This same group then went on to examine data specifically for individuals in an older age group (aged 60–79) (26). One-third of older diabetic subjects who were undiagnosed at baseline had isolated postchallenge hyperglycemia in this study. In addition, OGTT screening of the subjects with IFG reduced this fraction by half. The mortality risk of patients with abnormal two-hour postchallenge glucose (normal FPG) was similar to that of other diabetic subjects (Fig. 1). These data underline the importance of identifying patients with isolated postprandial hyperglycemia.

While the OGTT is more labor intensive, its ability to detect postchallenge hyperglycemia is undeniable. Qiao et al. demonstrated that postchallenge hyperglycemia itself is associated with premature death and microvascular complications (28). In addition, the DECODE study group determined that the risk profile of impaired fasting glycemia depends on the two-hour glucose concentration. Contrasting with the ADA expert committee which gives priority to FPG, the WHO recommends OGTT for clinical purposes when random glucose levels are in the uncertain range, and the fasting level only when OGTT is impractical.

In summary, based on current knowledge, the recommendation is to use the FPG as initial diagnostic test in all nonpregnant adults including elderly persons. The OGTT may be used in the following circumstances:

1. If diabetes is strongly suspected in high-risk patients (Table 3) and other tests are equivocal.
2. When the FPG is in the IFG range (100–126 mg/dL).

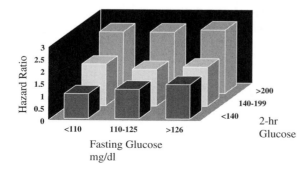

FIGURE 1 Effect of fasting and two-hour postload plasma glucose on mortality and morbidity. Hazard ratios for mortality and morbidity in patients with abnormal fasting plasma glucose and two-hour post-load glucose. *Source*: From Ref. 29.

IGT and IFG

While the definitive diagnosis of diabetes can be made using the criteria described, a grey zone remains between normal glucose homeostasis and that of diabetes. This has led to the identification of the entities of IGT and IFG. However, these diagnoses do not meet the criteria for diabetes; the level of glycemia is too high to be considered normal. They are defined as in Table 5.

IFG and IGT are not interchangeable terms as they represent different abnormalities of glucose regulation, one in the fasting state and one in the postprandial state. The DECODE study group demonstrated that IFG and IGT may not identify the same individuals. The results of large studies evaluating the use of these criteria in the elderly population have shown superiority of IGT in identifying the older adults at risk of cardiovascular disease (30). However, both the ADA and the WHO recognize both diagnostic entities as prediabetes, since they reflect an increased risk of developing overt diabetes as well as cardiovascular complications. While individuals may be asymptomatic from hyperglycemia and have normal or near normal HbA1c, it is now recognized that approximately 10% of subjects with IGT or IFT may develop microvascular complications of retinopathy, neuropathy, and nephropathy. IGT and IFT are also associated with the "metabolic syndrome,"—a term inclusive of obesity (especially abdominal or visceral obesity), dyslipidemia of the high-triglyceride and/or low high-density lipoprotein (HDL) type, and hypertension. There are means of delaying or even preventing the onset of frank diabetes in these patients with dietary modification, exercise, and certain types of yoga aimed at producing 5% to 10% loss of body weight (31,32).

Given the high prevalence of IGT or IFG in the geriatric population in comparison to their younger counterparts (Fig. 2), identifying patients with these conditions becomes important, especially in the light of possible cardiovascular complications and progression to the diabetic state.

ASSESSMENT FOR CARDIOVASCULAR RISK FACTORS AND OTHER COMORBIDITIES

When older adults are diagnosed with diabetes, it is important to screen for other risk factors for cardiovascular disease and to establish management goals. As mentioned above, elderly patients have delayed diagnosis of diabetes and may present with complications of diabetes at the time of diagnosis. Clinical and/or laboratory screening for neuropathy, retinopathy, and nephropathy and assessment of macrovascular diseases should be carried out at the time of initial diagnosis. Presence of "the geriatric syndromes" (cognitive dysfunction, depression, functional disability, falls, chronic pain, polypharmacy, and urinary incontinence) should be evaluated, as older adults with diabetes are at higher risk for these disorders. These conditions are discussed in detail in other chapters. An overall goal and strategy for management of diabetes can be formulated properly only after a diagnostic workup of all of the above conditions are performed.

SUMMARY

In summary, accurate diagnosis of diabetes is essential in a geriatric population due to high associated morbidity and mortality. Age is certainly an independent risk factor for the development of diabetes, in addition to the age-associated comorbidities that impair glucose regulation. Evaluating the patient on an individual basis, and determining the functional status and the burden of comorbidities and medications, is essential for optimal management. Diabetes

TABLE 5   Criteria for IGT and IFG

	FPG (mg/dL)	OGTT (mg/dL)
IFG	100–125	—
IGT	—	140–200 (at 2 hr)

Abbreviations: FPG, fasting plasma glucose; IFG, impaired fasting glucose; IGT, impaired glucose tolerance; OGTT, oral glucose tolerance test.

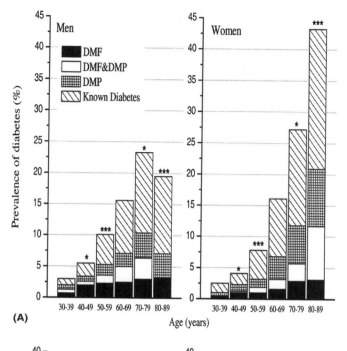

(A)

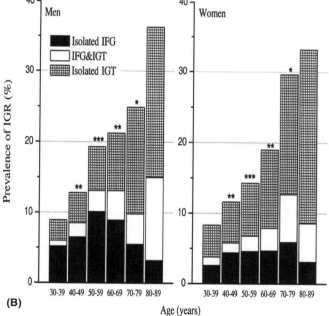

(B)

FIGURE 2 Age- and sex-specific prevalence of diabetes and IGR. *Abbreviations*: DMF, diabetes determined by fasting glucose; DMP, diabetes determined by two-hour postprandial glucose; IFG, impaired fasting glucose; IGR, impaired glucose regulation; IGT, impaired glucose tolerance. *Source*: From Ref. 33.

should be especially considered with atypical symptoms, and FPG should be performed as the diagnostic test with consideration of OGTT if uncertainty exists. Further research is needed to identify criteria for diagnosis that will detect elderly patients at risk of diabetes-related morbidity and mortality. Thus screening for diabetes should be performed periodically in elderly patients and a pro-active approach is critical to providing excellent medical care.

REFERENCES

1. Geiss LS, Pan L, Cadwell B, Gegg EW, Banjamin SM, Engelgau MM. Changes in incidence of diabetes in U.S. adults, 1997–2003. Am J Prev Med 2006; 30(5):371–377.
2. Mokdad AH, Ford ES, Bowman BA, et al. Diabetes trends in the U.S.: 1990–1998. Diabetes Care 2000; 23(9):1278–1283.
3. Cowie CC, Rust KF, Saydah S, Geiss LS, Ford ES, Gregg EN. Prevalence of diabetes and impaired fasting glucose in adults—United States, 1999-2000. MMWR Morb Mortal Wkly Rep 2003; 52(35):833–837.
4. Wild SH, et al. Criteria for previously undiagnosed diabetes and risk of mortality: 15-year follow-up of the Edinburgh Artery Study cohort. Diabet Med 2005; 22(4):490–496.
5. Ruigomez A, Garcia Rodriguez LA. Presence of diabetes related complication at the time of NIDDM diagnosis: an important prognostic factor. Eur J Epidemiol 1998; 14(5):439–445.
6. Muggeo M. Accelerated complications in Type 2 diabetes mellitus: the need for greater awareness and earlier detection. Diabet Med 1998; 15(suppl 4):S60–S62.
7. Harris MI, et al. Onset of NIDDM occurs at least 4–7 yr before clinical diagnosis. Diabetes Care 1992; 15(7):815–819.
8. Gregg EW, et al. Is diabetes associated with cognitive impairment and cognitive decline among older women? Study of Osteoporotic Fractures Research Group. Arch Intern Med 2000; 160(2):174–180.
9. Gavard JA, Lustman PJ, Clouse RE. Prevalence of depression in adults with diabetes. An epidemiological evaluation. Diabetes Care 1993; 16(8):1167–1178.
10. Peyrot M, Rubin RR. Levels and risks of depression and anxiety symptomatology among diabetic adults. Diabetes Care 1997; 20(4):585–590.
11. Songer TJ. Disability in diabetes. In: Harris M, Cowie CC, Stern MP, et al., eds. Diabetes in America. Bethesda, MD: National Institutes of Health, 1995:259–282.
12. Brown JS, et al. Urinary incontinence in older women: who is at risk? Study of Osteoporotic Fractures Research Group. Obstet Gynecol 1996; 87(5 Pt 1):715–721.
13. Kelsey JL, et al. Risk factors for fractures of the distal forearm and proximal humerus. The Study of Osteoporotic Fractures Research Group. Am J Epidemiol 1992; 135(5):477–489.
14. Greene DA, Stevens MJ, Feldman EL. Diabetic neuropathy: scope of the syndrome. Am J Med 1999; 107(2B):2S–8S.
15. Genuth S, et al. Follow-up report on the diagnosis of diabetes mellitus. Diabetes Care 2003; 26(11):3160–3167.
16. American Diabetes Association. Diagnosis and classification of diabetes mellitus. Diabetes Care 2006; 29(suppl 1):S43–S48.
17. Ho PJ, Turtle JR. Establishing the diagnosis. In: Sinclair A, Finucane P, eds. Diabetes in Old Age. 2nd ed. Chichester, New York: Wiley, 2001:viii, 274.
18. Gambert SR. Atypical presentation of diabetes mellitus in the elderly. Clin Geriatr Med 1990; 6(4):721–729.
19. Becker, et al. Principles and Practice of Endocrinology and Metabolism. 3rd ed., 2003:199–198.
20. Report of the Expert Committee on the Diagnosis and Classification of Diabetes Mellitus. Diabetes Care 1997; 20(7):1183–1197.
21. Wettre S, Lundberg M. Kinetics of glycosylated haemoglobin in uraemia determined on ion-exchange and affinity chromatography: no increase in the rate of glycosylation. Diabetes Res 1986; 3(2):107–110.
22. United Kingdom Prospective Diabetes Study (UKPDS). 13: Relative efficacy of randomly allocated diet, sulphonylurea, insulin, or metformin in patients with newly diagnosed non-insulin dependent diabetes followed for three years. Br Med J 1995; 310(6972):83–88.
23. Harris R, et al. Screening adults for type 2 diabetes: a review of the evidence for the U.S. Preventive Services Task Force. Ann Intern Med 2003; 138(3):215–229.
24. National Diabetes Data Group. Classification and diagnosis of diabetes mellitus and other categories of glucose intolerance. Diabetes 1979; 28(12):1039–1057.
25. Alberti KG, Zimmet PZ. Definition, diagnosis and classification of diabetes mellitus and its complications. Part 1: diagnosis and classification of diabetes mellitus provisional report of a WHO consultation. Diabet Med 1998; 15(7):539–553.
26. The DECODE study group. European Diabetes Epidemiology Group. Glucose tolerance and mortality: comparison of WHO and American Diabetes Association diagnostic criteria. Diabetes epidemiology: collaborative analysis of diagnostic criteria in Europe. Lancet 1999; 354(9179):617–621.
27. DECODE Study Group on behalf of the European Diabetes Epidemiology Study Group. Will new diagnostic criteria for diabetes mellitus change phenotype of patients with diabetes? Reanalysis of European epidemiological data. Br Med J 1998; 317(7155):371–375.
28. Qiao Q, Tuomilehto J, Borch-Johnsen K. Post-challenge hyperglycaemia is associated with premature death and macrovascular complications. Diabetologia 2003; 46(suppl 1):M17–M21.
29. Lancet 1999.
30. Blake DR et al. Impaired glucose tolerance, but not impaired fasting glucose, is associated with increased levels of coronary heart disease risk factors: results from the Baltimore Longitudinal Study on Aging. Diabetes 2004; 53(8):2095–2100.

31. Tuomilehto J, et al. Prevention of type 2 diabetes mellitus by changes in lifestyle among subjects with impaired glucose tolerance. N Engl J Med 2001; 344(18):1343–1350.
32. Bijlani RL, et al. A brief but comprehensive lifestyle education program based on yoga reduces risk factors for cardiovascular disease and diabetes mellitus. J Altern Complement Med 2005; 11(2):267–274.
33. DECODE Study Group. Age- and sex-specific prevalences of diabetes and impaired glucose regulation in 13 European cohorts.Diabetes Care 2003; 26(1):61–69.
34. American Diabetes Association. From Diabetes Care 2006; 29:S43–S48.

5 Insulin Resistance in the Elderly

Tina K. Thethi
Department of Medicine, Section of Endocrinology and Metabolism, Tulane University Health Sciences Center, New Orleans, Louisiana, U.S.A.

Sunil Asnani
Department of Medicine, Section of Endocrinology, UMDNJ-Robert Wood Johnson Medical School, Jersey Shore University Medical Center, Neptune, New Jersey, U.S.A.

Christina Bratcher and Vivian A. Fonseca
Department of Medicine, Section of Endocrinology and Metabolism, Tulane University Health Sciences Center, New Orleans, Louisiana, U.S.A.

INTRODUCTION

Aging is associated with metabolic alterations characterized by the development of changes in fat distribution, obesity, and insulin resistance (1). These changes are associated with a variety of age-related diseases that subsequently result in increased mortality. Sarcopenia is characterized by a decrease in the muscle mass and strength, starting as early as the fourth decade of life in humans (2), and contributes significantly to the morbidity, decrease in quality-of-life, and health-care costs in the elderly. The metabolic effects of sarcopenia include a decrease in resting metabolic rate secondary to decreased fat-free mass and decreased physical activity. These changes lead to higher prevalence of insulin resistance, type 2 diabetes mellitus (T2DM), dyslipidemia, and hypertension.

The escalating pandemic of overweight and obesity presents a major public health challenge. Whereas the prevalence of obesity among U.S. adults aged 20 through 74 years was 15% in the 1970s, it had risen to 31% in 2006 (3). Although obesity (measured by body weight) progressively decreases after the age of 60 compared to before the age of 60 years, the prevalence of obesity within the group of elderly adults has steadily increased in parallel to the overall epidemic of obesity.

Obesity is almost invariably associated with insulin resistance and its associated comorbidities, which affect all age groups. In this chapter, we highlight the problem of insulin resistance in elderly subjects. In examining the pathophysiology and correlates of this problem, we will focus on studies that have either included elderly subjects exclusively or in large numbers. (Table 1 for the factors involved in insulin resistance in elderly people, and Fig. 1 for the interaction between these factors.)

INSULIN RESISTANCE AND THE METABOLIC SYNDROME

The insulin-resistance syndrome (IRS) is a cluster of cardiovascular risk factors that are frequently, but not always, associated with obesity. The measurement of insulin resistance in epidemiological studies is difficult, especially in patients who have advanced T2DM. Several surrogates have therefore been used to define insulin resistance, all with major limitations. These include measurement of plasma insulin itself or the recognition of the various clinical components used in several definitions of the metabolic syndrome (4–6). While the IRS and the metabolic syndrome are not synonymous, and in fact we recognize that the metabolic syndrome is not sensitive or specific enough to identify insulin resistance, many studies have been carried out on patients with the metabolic syndrome—perhaps because it is clinically easier to identify. Since there is considerable overlap between the two, we will discuss the studies published in which elderly subjects with the metabolic syndrome were included and mention the definition used by the investigators. Nevertheless, it is important to recognize that while most of these patients are likely to be insulin resistant, many will not be so.

TABLE 1   Factors Associated with Insulin Resistance in the Elderly

Factors that are diminished	Factors that are increased
Vascular reactivity	FFAs
Nitrous oxide	TNF-α
Adiponectin	IL-6
ADMA	
DHEA-S	
Total testosterone	
SHBG	

Abbreviations: ADMA, asymmetric dimethylarginine; DHEA-S, dehydroepian-drosterone sulfate; FFAs, free fatty acids; IL-6, interleukin-6; SHBG, sex hormone–binding globulin; TNF-α, tumor necrosis factor-α.

Three definitions of the metabolic syndrome have been proposed, one by the WHO (6), one by the U.S. Third Report of the National Cholesterol Education Program, Adult Treatment Panel, 2001 (NCEP-ATP III) (7), and one by the International Diabetes Federation (IDF) (4).

Hyperinsulinemia is used to define insulin resistance in epidemiological studies. Fasting plasma insulin alone or formulae based on plasma insulin and glucose (such as the homeostasis model assessment commonly known as HOMA) is used. Plasma insulin measurements reflect both ambient glucose and pancreatic β-cell function (which decreases even before the onset of T2DM) (8). Hence, plasma insulin concentration is a poor marker of insulin resistance in subjects who have diabetes. Nonstandardization of the insulin assays makes it more difficult to interpret the levels. Prospective studies suggest that hyperinsulinemia may be an important risk factor for ischemic heart disease. The Quebec Heart Study studied men who were 45 to 76 years of age and who did not have ischemic heart disease (9). A first ischemic event occurred in 114 men, who were then matched for age, body mass index (BMI), smoking habits, and alcohol consumption. A control was selected from among the 1989 men who remained free of ischemic heart disease during follow-up. Case patients had fasting plasma insulin concentrations that were 18% higher than the controls at baseline. High fasting plasma insulin concentrations were an independent predictor of ischemic heart disease, plasma triglycerides, and apolipoprotein B, low-density lipoprotein (LDL) cholesterol, and high-density lipoprotein cholesterol concentrations. In the Helsinki policemen study, high fasting plasma insulin concentrations have been associated with increased all-cause and cardiovascular mortality, independent of other risk factors (10). However, the relationship between insulin resistance and plasma insulin may not be linear (11).

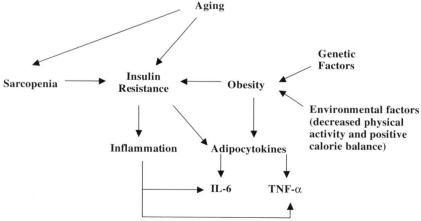

FIGURE 1   Pathophysiology of insulin resistance in the elderly: summary of the factors and their interactions in the elderly. *Abbreviations*: IL-6, interleukin-6; TNF-α, tumor necrosis factor-α.

The Uppsala Longitudinal Study of Adult Men (12) was a prospective, community-based observational study that investigated 1187 elderly (>70 years) men free from congestive heart failure (CHF) and valvular heart disease at baseline between 1990 and 1995, with follow-up until 2002. Variables such as insulin sensitivity (including euglycemic insulin clamp glucose disposal rate) and obesity, together with established risk factors for CHF, were examined as predictors of subsequent incidence of CHF. In the unadjusted Cox proportional hazards analyses, all examined variables reflecting obesity and impaired glucose regulation were found to be significant predictors of incidence of CHF. When adjusted for the presence of diabetes at baseline, the variables that remained significant were clamp glucose disposal rate, two-hour glucose level of the oral glucose tolerance test, fasting insulin levels, fasting prolinsulin levels, 23-33 split proinsulin, BMI and waist circumference. In multivariate Cox proportional hazard models adjusted for established risk factors for CHF, increased risk for CHF was associated with a one-standard deviation increase in the two-hour glucose value of a glucose tolerance test, fasting serum proinsulin level, BMI, and waist circumference. A one-standard deviation increment in the clamp glucose disposal rate decreased the risk. Thus, in this study, insulin resistance independently predicted CHF incidence.

Another study examined 3050 Mexican Americans aged 65 or older from the Hispanic Established Population for the Epidemiological Study of the Elderly conducted in five Southwestern states of the United States (13). Participants were divided into two groups: those with or without the metabolic syndrome. Metabolic syndrome was defined by the criteria established by WHO. Metabolic syndrome was significantly associated with increased incidence of heart attack (OR: 2.75, 95% CI: 1.67–4.54) and was a significant predictor for overall mortality (hazard ratio: 1.46, 95% CI: 1.16–1.84) over a seven-year period after adjusting for other demographic and clinical variables.

VASCULAR CONSEQUENCE OF INSULIN RESISTANCE

Several studies have highlighted the vascular consequences of insulin resistance either directly or through a number of "nontraditional risk factors" associated with insulin resistance, which have been extensively reviewed (8). These factors are summarized in Table 2. Insulin is a growth factor that stimulates vascular cell growth and synthesis of matrix proteins. Studies in insulin-resistant animals suggest that defects or deficiency of insulin receptor substrate results in neointimal proliferation. Neointima formation appears to be related to abnormalities induced by the altered metabolic milieu in insulin-resistant states (14). Recent studies suggest that insulin resistance is associated with endothelial dysfunction. In a study of healthy adults, soluble adhesion molecules were increased in proportion to the degree of insulin resistance (15). The insulin-signaling pathway thought to be responsible for abnormalities in glucose metabolism is also involved in nitric oxide production. A subsequent study showed that asymmetric dimethylarginine levels—an inhibitor of nitric oxide synthase—were positively correlated with impaired glucose disposal (16). Diminished nitric oxide production is a factor in endothelial dysfunction. Insulin resistance has also been found to be associated with increased reactive oxygen species in the endothelial cell, which in turn leads to the production of more inflammatory factors in the vessel wall (17).

TABLE 2 Factors Associated with Insulin Resistance and Cardiovascular Risk

PAI-1
Highly sensitive-C reactive protein
Intimal media thickness
Free fatty acids
LDL cholesterol
Triglycerides
Oxidative stress
Adipocytokines

Abbreviations: LDL, low-density lipoprotein; PAI-1, plasminogen activator inhibitor-1.

OBESITY AND INSULIN RESISTANCE IN THE ELDERLY

Obesity is frequently associated with several of the components of the IRS and may be critical for the development of the syndrome (8). Cardiovascular morbidity and mortality are increased in obese individuals independently of other risk factors. Insulin resistance is very common in obese individuals. However, some nonobese individuals demonstrate hyperinsulinemia and the other features of the IRS (18). Thus, although obesity may not be essential for the expression of the syndrome, the presence of obesity or weight gain may accentuate the pathophysiological changes associated with the syndrome. The evidence linking obesity and overweight with impaired health is abundant. Yan et al. (19) assessed hospitalization and mortality from coronary heart disease (CHD), cardiovascular disease (CVD), or diabetes beginning at age 65 in a cohort of 17,643 men and women aged 31 through 64 years, with follow-up for 32 years. The study was conducted to assess the relation of midlife BMI with morbidity and mortality outcomes in older age among individuals free of CHD, with and without other major risk factors at baseline. Individuals who were obese in middle age, those with no cardiovascular risk factors, as well as those with one or more risk factors, had a higher risk of hospitalization and mortality from CHD, CVD, and diabetes in older age than those who were normal weight.

Although obesity is usually assessed by body weight and occasionally by BMI in practice, body fat distribution rather than body mass may actually be a better predictor of insulin resistance and cardiovascular risk (20). Insulin resistance, type 2 diabetes, and hypertension are more closely associated with a central distribution of adiposity than with general increases in fat mass. Waist circumference serves as a clinical surrogate of intraabdominal fat and correlates with insulin levels and insulin resistance. Several studies have documented the value of intra-abdominal fat and increased waist circumference as a predictor of mortality (21,22) but very few have focused on the elderly. Nasir et al. (23) assessed the association of waist circumference and BMI with the presence and severity of coronary artery calcium in 451 asymptomatic men free of known CHD. The risk for increased coronary artery calcium was twofold higher among those men with a waist circumference in the highest tertile (>101 cm) compared with men with waist circumference of 92 cm or less. The relationship was independent of BMI and age. A significant association between BMI and coronary artery calcium was not observed. This study speaks of central obesity as being more strongly related to clinical and subclinical CHD end points than is BMI.

A multicenter, cross-sectional study by Lee et al. (24) looked at insulin sensitivity and abdominal adiposity in healthy, nondiabetic older (64±6 years; mean±SD) subjects. There were 23 men and 31 women. Metabolic Insulin Sensitivity Index [S(I)] was determined from a frequently sampled insulin-assisted intravenous glucose tolerance test (24). Body fat mass and abdominal fat mass were determined from dual energy X-ray absorptiometry (DXA) scans. Anthropometric measures included in the study were waist and hip circumferences, height, and body weight. In univariate analyses, S(I) was significantly inversely related with body weight, BMI, waist circumference, waist index, percentage of total body and abdominal fat, and DXA L1-L4 fat mass, but not with waist-hip-ratio. The DXA L1-L4 fat mass as a measurement of abdominal adiposity was identified as the best sex-independent predictor of S(I) in older men and women. In addition to general obesity, the distribution of body fat is independently associated with the metabolic syndrome in older men and women (25).

HYPERTENSION

The association of essential hypertension with insulin resistance is very well established. The impact of insulin resistance on blood pressure homeostasis however is a matter of debate. Hypertension is a complex disorder with multiple causes. Diminished insulin sensitivity has been documented in older hypertensive men (26). Not all patients who have hypertension have insulin resistance (8). Multiple potential mechanisms are proposed by which insulin resistance may cause hypertension (27). These include resistance to insulin-mediated vasodilatation, impaired endothelial function, sympathetic nervous system overactivity, sodium retention, increased vascular sensitivity to the vasoconstrictor effect of pressor amines, and enhanced growth factor activity leading to proliferation of smooth muscle walls. Kraus et al.

have demonstrated that aldosterone directly affects major adipose functions, including stimulation of proinflammatory adipokines. Fasting plasma insulin levels are frequently higher in hypertensive subjects, and glucose disposal during a euglycemic clamp is decreased (8). This relationship is more convincing in obese patients.

Hypertension, diabetes, obesity, and aging are associated with increased arterial stiffness. Both insulin resistance as mentioned above and hyperglycemia may contribute to the development of arterial stiffness. Sengstock et al. (28) conducted a study assessing insulin resistance, arterial stiffness, and the relationship of this association on the glucose tolerance status in 37 older (23 male, 14 female, mean age 69.4 ± 5.9 years) nondiabetic, hypertensive adults after four-week antihypertensive medication withdrawal. Aortic pulse wave velocity (PWV), pulse pressure (PP), [S(I) measured by insulin-assisted frequently sampled IV glucose test], glucose tolerance status, and abdominal fat mass were the parameters measured. PWV and PP were negatively correlated with S(I) ($r = -0.49$, $P = 0.002$, and $r = -0.38$, $P = 0.02$, respectively). In multiple regression analysis, PWV and PP remained independently correlated with S(I) ($P < 0.05$) after adjusting for age, gender, fasting glucose, glucose tolerance status, and BMI or abdominal fat mass. These results suggest that insulin resistance is associated with arterial stiffness independent of glucose tolerance status in hypertensive, nondiabetic older adults.

DYSLIPIDEMIA

Hyperlipidemia is a well-established risk factor in patients with and without diabetes. There are certain abnormalities in the lipoprotein pattern associated with insulin resistance that appear to convey risk and could be classified as nontraditional risk factors (8,29). The hallmark of the "diabetic dyslipidemia" (30) is hypertriglyceridemia and low-plasma, high-density lipoprotein cholesterol concentration. In insulin-resistant patients, there are some qualitative changes in LDL cholesterol. There is "pattern B" distribution of LDL particles—which consists of smaller LDL particles that are more susceptible to oxidation and thus potentially more atherogenic (31). An increase in the circulating free fatty acids (FFAs) has been proposed as having a causal role in the development of insulin resistance (32). Insulin resistance may result in increased activity of hormone-sensitive lipase and therefore an increased breakdown of stored triglycerides. The dyslipidemia associated with insulin resistance is likely to be an important contributor to CVD in the elderly, but the optimal treatment for this disorder (other than through lifestyle change) is unclear.

PATHOPHYSIOLOGY OF INSULIN RESISTANCE IN THE ELDERLY

Several factors contribute to insulin resistance in the elderly and are summarized in Table 1. Table 2 shows the factors involved in insulin resistance and cardiovascular risk. Figure 1 illustrates the interaction between these factors.

Adipokines and Insulin Resistance in Obesity and Aging

Adipose tissue is now recognized as a significant endocrine organ secreting a variety of hormones and cytokines. Cytokines arising from the adipose tissue may be partly responsible for the metabolic, hemodynamic, and hemostatic abnormalities associated with insulin resistance. These inflammatory factors may be the link between obesity and insulin resistance (33,34). Among the factors produced by the adipose tissue are tumor necrosis factor-X (TNF-α), interleukin (IL)-6, and leptin. Biochemical studies show that these factors interfere with insulin signaling and account for the association of insulin resistance with obesity and inflammation. Evidence is present linking TNF-α to the presentation of insulin resistance in humans, animals and in vitro systems. Hotamisligil et al. studied the relationship between TNF-α and insulin resistance using knockout mice deficient for either TNF-α or one or both of its receptors, p55 and p75. They found that deletion of TNF-α leads to increased insulin sensitivity, that is, decreased insulin resistance. The mechanism of TNF-α related insulin resistance is not completely understood, though phosphorylation of serine residues on IRS-1 has previously been shown to be important. They found an approximately two-fold increase in insulin-stimulated tyrosine phosphorylation of the insulin receptor in the muscle and adipose tissue of TNF-α knockout mice. This suggests that insulin receptor signaling is an important target for TNF-α. Other possible mediators of TNF-α induced insulin resistance include circulating free fatty acids and leptin (35–39). The increase in the FFA concentration is key to further exacerbation of inflammation and insulin resistance. Studies done in humans and rodents have demonstrated that the increase in the FFA levels in healthy subjects reduces insulin-stimulated glucose uptake (9,32) and activates the proinflammatory NF-κB. It also leads to increased formation of reactive oxygen species and oxidative stress. To test the possible acute proinflammatory effects of fatty acids, Tripathy et al. induced an increase in plasma FFA concentration after a lipid and heparin infusion for four hours in 10 healthy subjects. Reactive oxygen species generation by polymorphonuclear leucocytes (PMNs) increased significantly at two and four hours ($p < 0.005$). Plasma macrophage migration inhibitory factor increased at two ($p < 0.005$) and four hours ($p < 0.005$) respectively, and declined to baseline at six hours. There also occurs elevation of the plasma concentration of other proinflammatory mediators (34). Additionally, elevated FFA levels lead to impairment in endothelium-dependent and insulin-mediated vasodilation as a result of decreased nitric oxide production (33). This impairment in endothelium-dependent and insulin-mediated vasodilation (IMV) by FFA elevation however occurs over different time courses. Impairment of IMV occurs only if glucose metabolism is concomitantly reduced. This findings suggest that nitric oxide production in response to the different stimuli may be mediated via different signaling pathways. Reduced nitric oxide production due to elevated FFA may contribute to the higher incidence of hypertension and macrovascular disease in insulin-resistant patients.

Adiponectin is a relatively recently discovered protein that is secreted by mature adipocytes (i.e., an adipocytokine) and circulates in high concentrations in the blood (40). Evidence from animal and human studies shows that it increases insulin sensitivity (41–44) and has anti-inflammatory and antiatherogenic effects (45,46). Serum adiponectin levels are decreased in patients with obesity and T2DM (47–49) and are inversely associated with parameters of overall adiposity (42,43,47–52) as well as insulin resistance (50,51,53). Thus, one explanation for the development of insulin resistance is an imbalance between pro- and anti-inflammatory factors released by the adipose tissue.

Kanaya et al. (54) investigated the joint effects of adipocytokines and other inflammatory markers in the development of diabetes. They studied the relationships among adipocytokines, glycemia, and incident diabetes mellitus in 2356 white and black adults aged 70 to 79 years in the Health, Aging, and Body Composition Study who did not have diabetes at baseline. In their study, there were 14.1 cases of type 2 diabetes per 1000 person-years over a follow-up period of five years. Participants who developed diabetes were more likely to be black. All measurements of adiposity were significantly higher among participants who developed diabetes compared with individuals without diabetes. Median plasma leptin, IL-6, and plasminogen activator inhibitor-1 (PAI-1) levels were higher and the median adiponectin level was lower in incident cases of diabetes than in those without diabetes. However, only the associations between adiponectin, leptin, PAI-1, and incident diabetes remained significant after adjusting for age, sex, and race. The relationship between visceral adiposity and diabetes was attenuated with the addition of the adipocytokines (adiponectin, leptin, and PAI-1) to the multivariate model (from OR, 1.33; 95% CI, 1.10–1.60 to OR, 1.21; CI, 0.97–1.49 per SD). The relationship between BMI and diabetes in white individuals was also proportionately attenuated with the addition of adipocytokines (from OR, 1.65; 95% CI, 1.26–2.15 to OR, 1.42; 95% CI, 1.02–1.97 per SD). Only age and fasting glucose, fasting insulin, and PAI-1 levels remained independently associated with incident diabetes. The association between PAI-1 level and diabetes did not vary by sex or race.

Sarcopenia and Insulin Resistance

Aging causes structural and functional changes in skeletal muscles, which start in the fourth decade of life. The associated changes in body composition form the basis of many metabolic disorders such as insulin resistance (55), T2DM, hypertension, and hyperlipidemia. Insulin and amino acids have also been shown to enhance muscle mitochondrial biogenesis and mitochondrial protein synthesis. The insulin-induced increase in muscle mitochondrial ATP productive is defective in type 2 diabetic patients with insulin resistance. In the elderly, there exists dissociation between increases in muscle mitochondrial biogenesis and insulin sensitivity after exercise. It remains to be determined whether muscle mitochondrial dysfunction causes or results from insulin resistance. The structural and functional changes related to diseases that are common in the elderly are often hard to distinguish from those of the aging process.

One of the key performance measurements that declines with age is maximal oxygen uptake. Aging is associated with a decrease in muscle mass and muscle strength, along with reduced endurance, which results from reduced physical activity and produces a further decline in physical activity. The resultant reduction in muscle mass and physical activity levels decrease the overall energy expenditure in the elderly. This leads to obesity, especially abdominal fat accumulation. These alterations in body composition cause insulin resistance, which contributes to the development of type 2 diabetes in a genetically susceptible population (Fig. 1).

INFLAMMATION

Inflammation has been associated with cardiovascular events in several studies. Cytokines such as TNF-α and IL-6 facilitate a wide variety of inflammatory reactions by varying cells. They are produced chiefly by the mononuclear and endothelial cells (56). Low-grade inflammation may now be easily measured by the highly sensitive C-reactive protein (hs-CRP). Besides hs-CRP, several markers of inflammation have been used in various studies. Plasma hs-CRP has a significant predictive value in determining the risk for future coronary events (57). It is an acute-phase protein produced by the liver in response to production of cytokines such as IL-6, IL-1, and TNF-α. Production of IL-6 is also stimulated by other products such as oxidized lipids, infectious agents, and cytokines produced from adipocytes or other inflammatory cells. IL-6 then in turn serves as the "messenger" cytokine that stimulates the production of CRP by the liver (58).

Impaired fibrinolysis is recognized as an important component of the IRS and probably contributes considerably to the increased risk for cardiovascular events (59,60). Plasma PAI-1 antigen and activity are elevated in a wide variety of insulin-resistant patients, including obese patients, with or without diabetes. The greatest elevations in PAI-1 occur when there is a combination of hyperinsulinemia, hyperglycemia, and increased FFAs in obese, insulin-resistant patients (61).

PAI-1 is also one of the key genes for aging-associated thrombosis. The levels are elevated in the elderly and are induced by a variety of pathologies associated with the process of aging (62). As mentioned earlier, PAI-1 is the only adipocytokine found to be independently associated with incident diabetes in the elderly (54).

Coagulation disorders also play a role in increasing the risk for CHD in patients who have T2DM. Many of the abnormalities are nonspecific, and the association of insulin resistance with coagulation abnormalities is less robust than that with abnormal fibrinolysis (8). Increased PAI-1 levels and, to a lesser extent, increased coagulation are closely linked to CVD.

The Cardiovascular Health Study reported results from a cohort of elderly individuals in the United States, aged 65 years of age or older (63). The risk of incident DM was related to CRP levels. Those in the upper quartile of distribution at baseline were twice as likely to develop T2DM as those in the lowest quartile. Due to the fact that this cohort was elderly and the prevalence of clinical and subclinical CVD was high, analysis was adjusted for the presence of these conditions. The risk of DM associated with elevated CRP levels remained unchanged.

SEX HORMONE DECLINE AND INSULIN RESISTANCE

Sex hormone levels change during aging in both men and women, although the specific hormonal changes obviously differ between sexes. These changes, which may be associated with insulin sensitivity and the metabolic syndrome, were studied by Muller et al. (64) in cross-sectional study of 400 independently living men between the ages of 40 and 80 years. The metabolic syndrome was defined according to the NCEP definition. In this study, multiple logistic regression analyses showed an inverse relationship according to one standard deviation increase for circulating total testosterone (TT), sex hormone–binding globulin (SHBG), and dehydroepiandrosterone sulfate (DHEA-S) with the metabolic syndrome. Linear regression analyses showed that higher TT, bioavailable testosterone, and SHBG levels were related to higher insulin sensitivity, whereas no effects were found for DHEA-S and estradiol. These data suggest that these hormones may play a protective role against the development of metabolic syndrome in men. Similarly in postmenopausal women, estrogen deficiency is associated with insulin resistance, and sensitivity can be improved by hormone replacement therapy (HRT).

Li et al. (65) conducted a double-blind, randomized, prospective-controlled trial to evaluate the effect of two low doses of oral continuous-combined formulations of 17 β-estradiol [E(2)] and norethisterone acetate (NETA) on carbohydrate metabolism in 120 healthy postmenopausal women. In this study, oral low-dose E(2) 1 mg/NETA 0.5 mg did not impair carbohydrate metabolism, but seemed to improve insulin sensitivity in healthy postmenopausal women. Other studies suggest that HRT may reduce insulin sensitivity.

In a prospective, placebo-controlled study, Soranna et al. (66) evaluated the impact of a three-month continuous administration of oral E2 alone or combined with two different dosages of dydrogesterone on the glucose tolerance and insulin sensitivity in 43 postmenopausal women. The study subjects were of normal weight and normoinsulinemic. They were randomized to receive either 2 mg of oral 17β-estradiol (E2) daily (group A), or 2 mg E2 daily plus 5 mg daily oral dydrogesterone, from day 14 to 28, in a sequentially combined regimen (group B), or 2 mg of E2 and 10 mg dydrogesterone in the same sequentially combined regimen (group C) or placebo for 12 weeks. A euglycemic hyperinsulinemic clamp and an oral glucose tolerance test (OGTT) were performed before and after treatment. Total body glucose utilization for insulin sensitivity evaluation was determined in each subject. Postmenopausal women treated with unopposed 17-β E2 (group A) showed a slight but statistically significant decrease of insulin sensitivity ($p < 0.05$). A more marked deterioration of the same parameter was observed in the two groups treated with E2 plus dydrogesterone (group B and group C: $p < 0.01$). Post hoc testing for the percent change from baseline indicated that group A differed significantly from group C ($p < 0.05$) and all treated groups differed significantly from the placebo group ($p < 0.01$). Finally, after treatment in group C, there was a significant reduction of insulin and an increase of glucose responses to OGTT ($p < 0.01$) were observed.

The issue of HRT and insulin resistance is controversial. However, evidence supports the notion that the postmenopausal state is an insulin-resistant state and HRT improves insulin sensitivity. Nevertheless, due to the problems with HRT (67), it is not recommended that HRT be used as an agent to improve insulin sensitivity.

Plasma DHEA-S and testosterone levels both decline with age in healthy men. Blouin et al. (68) selected a sample of 130 nonsmoking men from the Quebec Family Study to evaluate the relationships between DHEA-S and testosterone levels with the various alterations of the metabolic profile associated with aging. They found that plasma DHEA-S and testosterone levels declined with age. The percentage of men characterized by three or more features of the metabolic syndrome increased with decreasing testosterone levels (8.9–44.2%, chi2 = 15.89, $P < 0.0005$) and DHEA-S levels (8.9–41.5%, chi2 = 13.02, $P < 0.005$). Logistic regression showed that men in the upper tertile of testosterone levels had a lower risk of being characterized by three or more features of the metabolic syndrome (OR = 0.24, $P < 0.04$) independent of age, whereas tertiles of DHEA-S levels were not related to the metabolic syndrome independent of age. Observational data suggest that the metabolic syndrome is strongly associated with hypogonadism in men (69). Multiple interventional studies have shown that exogenous testosterone has a favorable impact on body mass, insulin secretion and sensitivity, lipid profile, and blood pressure. Further research is needed in the form of randomized, clinical trials to define the role of testosterone in the metabolic syndrome.

Pitteloud et al. (70) examined the relationship between serum testosterone levels and insulin sensitivity and mitochondrial function in 60 men aged 60.5 ± 1.2 years. Insulin sensitivity was measured using a hyperinsulinemic-euglycemic clamp. Testosterone levels were positively correlated with insulin sensitivity ($r = 0.4$, $P < 0.005$). Subjects with hypogonadal testosterone levels ($n = 10$) had a BMI > 25 kg/m^2 and a threefold higher prevalence of the metabolic syndrome than their eugonadal counterparts ($n = 50$); this relationship held true even after adjusting for age and SHBG, but not BMI. Testosterone levels also correlated with VO$_2$max ($r = 0.43$, $P < 0.05$) and oxidative phosphorylation gene expression ($r = 0.57$,

$P < 0.0001$). These data indicate that low serum testosterone levels are associated with an adverse metabolic profile.

SUMMARY

The incidence and prevalence of diabetes mellitus increase with age as do the risk of complications from diabetes. While about 6.3% of the total U.S. population has T2DM, this fraction is much higher in those aged 65 to 74 (71,72). According to the Third National Health and Nutrition Examination Survey (NHANES III), over 18% of people aged 60 years and older have diabetes by the American Diabetes Association fasting plasma glucose criterion (73,74), while an equal or slightly higher proportion would have diabetes based on an OGTT. Aging is associated with changes in body composition, among which are an increase in fat mass and loss of muscle mass. Increased adiposity is associated with increased FFA levels, rate of lipolysis, and rate of lipid oxidation (75). Elevated FFA levels are key to further exacerbation of inflammation and insulin resistance. Adipocytokines interfere with insulin signaling and account for the association of insulin resistance with obesity and inflammation. Body fat distribution rather than body mass may actually be a better predictor of insulin resistance and cardiovascular risk (20). In summary, insulin resistance is a key abnormality linking T2DM and CVD.

ACKNOWLEDGMENTS

Diabetes research and education at Tulane University Health Sciences Center is supported in part by John C. Cudd Memorial Fund, the Tullis-Tulane Alumni Chair in Diabetes, and the Susan Harling Robinson Fellowship in Diabetes Research.

REFERENCES

1. Erol A. PPARalpha activators may be good candidates as antiaging agents. Med Hypotheses 2005; 65:35–38.
2. Karakelides H, Sreekumaran NK. Sarcopenia of aging and its metabolic impact. Curr Top Dev Biol 2005; 68:123–148.
3. Flegal KM, Carroll MD, Ogden CL, Johnson CL. Prevalence and trends in obesity among US adults, 1999–2000. JAMA 2002; 288:1723–1727.
4. Alberti KGMM, Zimmet P, Shaw J. The metabolic syndrome—a new worldwide definition. Lancet 2005; 366:1059–1069. International Diabetes Federation: The IDF consensus worldwide definition of the metabolic syndrome article online.
5. Third Report of the National Cholesterol Education Program (NCEP) Expert Panel on Detection, Evaluation, and Treatment of High Blood Cholesterol in Adults (Adult Treatment Panel III) final report 1. Circulation 2002; 106:3143–3421.
6. Alberti KG, Zimmet PZ. Definition, diagnosis and classification of diabetes mellitus and its complications. Part 1: diagnosis and classification of diabetes mellitus provisional report of a WHO consultation 1. Diabet Med 1998; 15:539–553.
7. Executive Summary of The Third Report of The National Cholesterol Education Program (NCEP) Expert Panel on Detection, Evaluation, And Treatment of High Blood Cholesterol In Adults (Adult Treatment Panel III). JAMA 2001; 285:2486–2497.
8. Fonseca V, Desouza C, Asnani S, Jialal I. Nontraditional risk factors for cardiovascular disease in diabetes. Endocr Rev 2004; 25:153–175.
9. Despres JP, Lamarche B, Mauriege P, et al. Hyperinsulinemia as an independent risk factor for ischemic heart disease. N Engl J Med 1996; 334:952–957.
10. Pyorala M, Miettinen H, Laakso M, Pyorala K. Plasma insulin and all-cause, cardiovascular, and non-cardiovascular mortality: the 22-year follow-up results of the Helsinki Policemen Study. Diabetes Care 2000; 23:1097–1102.
11. Perry IJ, Wannamethee SG, Whincup PH, Shaper AG, Walker MK, Alberti KG. Serum insulin and incident coronary heart disease in middle-aged British men. Am J Epidemiol 1996; 144:224–234.
12. Ingelsson E, Sundstrom J, Arnlov J, Zethelius B, Lind L. Insulin resistance and risk of congestive heart failure. JAMA 2005; 294:334–341.
13. Otiniano ME, Du XL, Maldonado MR, Ray L, Markides K. Effect of metabolic syndrome on heart attack and mortality in Mexican-American elderly persons: findings of 7-year follow-up from the Hispanic established population for the epidemiological study of the elderly. J Gerontol A Biol Sci Med Sci 2005; 60:466–470.

14. Kubota T, Kubota N, Moroi M, et al. Lack of insulin receptor substrate-2 causes progressive neointima formation in response to vessel injury. Circulation 2003; 107:3073–3080.
15. Chen NG, Holmes M, Reaven GM. Relationship between insulin resistance, soluble adhesion molecules, and mononuclear cell binding in healthy volunteers. J Clin Endocrinol Metab 1999; 84:3485–3489.
16. Stuhlinger MC, Abbasi F, Chu JW, et al. Relationship between insulin resistance and an endogenous nitric oxide synthase inhibitor. JAMA 2002; 287:1420–1426.
17. Facchini FS, Humphreys MH, DoNascimento CA, Abbasi F, Reaven GM. Relation between insulin resistance and plasma concentrations of lipid hydroperoxides, carotenoids, and tocopherols. Am J Clin Nutr 2000; 72:776–779.
18. Ruderman N, Chisholm D, Pi-Sunyer X, Schneider S. The metabolically obese, normal-weight individual revisited. Diabetes 1998; 47:699–713.
19. Yan LL, Daviglus ML, Liu K, et al. Midlife body mass index and hospitalization and mortality in older age. JAMA 2006; 295:190–198.
20. Abate N, Garg A, Peshock RM, Stray-Gundersen J, ms-Huet B, Grundy SM. Relationship of generalized and regional adiposity to insulin sensitivity in men with NIDDM. Diabetes 1996; 45:1684–1693.
21. Kuk JL, Katzmarzyk PT, Nichaman MZ, Church TS, Blair SN, Ross R. Visceral fat is an independent predictor of all-cause mortality in Men. Obes Res 2006; 14:336–341.
22. Bigaard J, Tjonneland A, Thomsen BL, Overvad K, Heitmann BL, Sorensen TI. Waist circumference, BMI, smoking, and mortality in middle-aged men and women. Obes Res 2003; 11:895–903.
23. Nasir K, Campbell CY, Santos RD, et al. The association of subclinical coronary atherosclerosis with abdominal and total obesity in asymptomatic men. Prev Cardiol 2005; 8:143–148.
24. Lee CC, Glickman SG, Dengel DR, Brown MD, Supiano MA. Abdominal adiposity assessed by dual energy X-ray absorptiometry provides a sex-independent predictor of insulin sensitivity in older adults. J Gerontol A Biol Sci Med Sci 2005; 60:872–877.
25. Goodpaster BH, Krishnaswami S, Harris TB, et al. Obesity, regional body fat distribution, and the metabolic syndrome in older men and women. Arch Intern Med 2005; 165:777–783.
26. Dengel DR, Pratley RE, Hagberg JM, Goldberg AP. Impaired insulin sensitivity and maximal responsiveness in older hypertensive men. Hypertension 1994; 23:320–324.
27. DeFronzo RA, Ferrannini E. Insulin resistance. A multifaceted syndrome responsible for NIDDM, obesity, hypertension, dyslipidemia, and atherosclerotic cardiovascular disease. Diabetes Care 1991; 14:173–194.
28. Sengstock DM, Vaitkevicius PV, Supiano MA. Arterial stiffness is related to insulin resistance in non-diabetic hypertensive older adults. J Clin Endocrinol Metab 2005; 90:2823–2827.
29. Ruige JB, Ballaux DP, Funahashi T, Mertens IL, Matsuzawa Y, Van Gaal LF. Resting metabolic rate is an important predictor of serum adiponectin concentrations: potential implications for obesity-related disorders. Am J Clin Nutr 2005; 82:21–25.
30. Sniderman AD, Scantlebury T, Cianflone K. Hypertriglyceridemic hyperapob: the unappreciated atherogenic dyslipoproteinemia in type 2 diabetes mellitus. Ann Intern Med 2001; 135:447–459.
31. Reaven GM, Chen YD, Jeppesen J, Maheux P, Krauss RM. Insulin resistance and hyperinsulinemia in individuals with small, dense low density lipoprotein particles. J Clin Invest 1993; 92:141–146.
32. Boden G, Lebed B, Schatz M, Homko C, Lemieux S. Effects of acute changes of plasma free fatty acids on intramyocellular fat content and insulin resistance in healthy subjects. Diabetes 2001; 50:1612–1617.
33. Steinberg HO, Paradisi G, Hook G, Crowder K, Cronin J, Baron AD. Free fatty acid elevation impairs insulin-mediated vasodilation and nitric oxide production. Diabetes 2000; 49:1231–1238.
34. Tripathy D, Mohanty P, Dhindsa S, et al. Elevation of free fatty acids induces inflammation and impairs vascular reactivity in healthy subjects. Diabetes 2003; 52:2882–2887.
35. Hirosumi J, Tuncman G, Chang L, et al. A central role for JNK in obesity and insulin resistance. Nature 2002; 420:333–336.
36. Hotamisligil GS, Spiegelman BM. Tumor necrosis factor alpha: a key component of the obesity-diabetes link. Diabetes 1994; 43:1271–1278.
37. Hotamisligil GS, Peraldi P, Budavari A, Ellis R, White MF, Spiegelman BM. IRS-1-mediated inhibition of insulin receptor tyrosine kinase activity in TNF-alpha- and obesity-induced insulin resistance. Science 1996; 271:665–668.
38. Hotamisligil GS. Mechanisms of TNF-alpha-induced insulin resistance. Exp Clin Endocrinol Diabetes 1999; 107:119–125.
39. Skolnik EY, Marcusohn J. Inhibition of insulin receptor signaling by TNF: potential role in obesity and non-insulin-dependent diabetes mellitus. Cytokine Growth Factor Rev 1996; 7:161–173.
40. Tsao TS, Lodish HF, Fruebis J. ACRP30, a new hormone controlling fat and glucose metabolism. Eur J Pharmacol 2002; 440:213–221.
41. Kubota N, Terauchi Y, Yamauchi T, et al. Disruption of adiponectin causes insulin resistance and neointimal formation. J Biol Chem 2002; 277:25863–25866.
42. Lindsay RS, Funahashi T, Hanson RL, et al. Adiponectin and development of type 2 diabetes in the Pima Indian population. Lancet 2002; 360:57–58.

43. Stefan N, Vozarova B, Funahashi T, et al. Plasma adiponectin concentration is associated with skeletal muscle insulin receptor tyrosine phosphorylation, and low plasma concentration precedes a decrease in whole-body insulin sensitivity in humans. Diabetes 2002; 51:1884–1888.

44. Yamauchi T, Kamon J, Waki H, et al. The fat-derived hormone adiponectin reverses insulin resistance associated with both lipoatrophy and obesity. Nat Med 2001; 7:941–946.

45. Ouchi N, Kihara S, Arita Y, et al. Novel modulator for endothelial adhesion molecules: adipocyte-derived plasma protein adiponectin. Circulation 1999; 100:2473–2476.

46. Ouchi N, Kihara S, Arita Y, et al. Adipocyte-derived plasma protein, adiponectin, suppresses lipid accumulation and class A scavenger receptor expression in human monocyte-derived macrophages. Circulation 2001; 103:1057–1063.

47. Arita Y, Kihara S, Ouchi N, et al. Paradoxical decrease of an adipose-specific protein, adiponectin, in obesity. Biochem Biophys Res Commun 1999; 257:79–83.

48. Hotta K, Funahashi T, Arita Y, et al. Plasma concentrations of a novel, adipose-specific protein, adiponectin, in type 2 diabetic patients. Arterioscler Thromb Vasc Biol 2000; 20:1595–1599.

49. Weyer C, Funahashi T, Tanaka S, et al. Hypoadiponectinemia in obesity and type 2 diabetes: close association with insulin resistance and hyperinsulinemia. J Clin Endocrinol Metab 2001; 86:1930–1935.

50. Matsubara M, Maruoka S, Katayose S. Inverse relationship between plasma adiponectin and leptin concentrations in normal-weight and obese women. Eur J Endocrinol 2002; 147:173–180.

51. Yamamoto Y, Hirose H, Saito I, et al. Correlation of the adipocyte-derived protein adiponectin with insulin resistance index and serum high-density lipoprotein-cholesterol, independent of body mass index, in the Japanese population. Clin Sci Lond 2002; 103:137–142.

52. Yang WS, Lee WJ, Funahashi T, et al. Plasma adiponectin levels in overweight and obese Asians. Obes Res 2002; 10:1104–1110.

53. Cnop M, Havel PJ, Utzschneider KM, et al. Relationship of adiponectin to body fat distribution, insulin sensitivity and plasma lipoproteins: evidence for independent roles of age and sex. Diabetologia 2003; 46:459–469.

54. Kanaya AM, Wassel FC, Vittinghoff E, et al. Adipocytokines and incident diabetes mellitus in older adults: the independent effect of plasminogen activator inhibitor 1. Arch Intern Med 2006; 166:350–356.

55. Nair KS. Aging muscle. Am J Clin Nutr 2005; 81:953–963.

56. Gabay C, Kushner I. Acute-phase proteins and other systemic responses to inflammation. N Engl J Med 1999; 340:448–454.

57. Ridker PM. Evaluating novel cardiovascular risk factors: can we better predict heart attacks? Ann Intern Med 1999; 130:933–937.

58. Jialal I, Devaraj S. Inflammation and atherosclerosis: the value of the high-sensitivity C-reactive protein assay as a risk marker. Am J Clin Pathol 2001; 116(suppl):S108–S115.

59. Haffner SM, D'Agostino R Jr, Mykkanen L, et al. Insulin sensitivity in subjects with type 2 diabetes. Relationship to cardiovascular risk factors: the Insulin Resistance Atherosclerosis Study. Diabetes Care 1999; 22:562–568.

60. Sobel BE. Insulin resistance and thrombosis: a cardiologist's view. Am J Cardiol 1999; 84:37J–41J.

61. Calles-Escandon J, Mirza SA, Sobel BE, Schneider DJ. Induction of hyperinsulinemia combined with hyperglycemia and hypertriglyceridemia increases plasminogen activator inhibitor 1 in blood in normal human subjects. Diabetes 1998; 47:290–293.

62. Yamamoto K, Takeshita K, Kojima T, Takamatsu J, Saito H. Aging and plasminogen activator inhibitor-1 (PAI-1) regulation: implication in the pathogenesis of thrombotic disorders in the elderly. Cardiovasc Res 2005; 66:276–285.

63. Barzilay JI, Abraham L, Heckbert SR, et al. The relation of markers of inflammation to the development of glucose disorders in the elderly: the Cardiovascular Health Study. Diabetes 2001; 50:2384–2389.

64. Muller M, Grobbee DE, den TI, Lamberts SW, van der Schouw YT. Endogenous sex hormones and metabolic syndrome in aging men. J Clin Endocrinol Metab 2005; 90:2618–2623.

65. Li C, Samsioe G, Borgfeldt C, Bendahl PO, Wilawan K, Aberg A. Low-dose hormone therapy and carbohydrate metabolism. Fertil Steril 2003; 79:550–555.

66. Soranna L, Cucinelli F, Perri C, et al. Individual effect of E2 and dydrogesterone on insulin sensitivity in post-menopausal women. J Endocrinol Invest 2002; 25:547–550.

67. Anderson GL, Limacher M, Assaf AR, et al. Effects of conjugated equine estrogen in postmenopausal women with hysterectomy: the Women's Health Initiative randomized controlled trial 1. JAMA 2004; 291:1701–1712.

68. Blouin K, Despres JP, Couillard C, et al. Contribution of age and declining androgen levels to features of the metabolic syndrome in men. Metabolism 2005; 54:1034–1040.

69. Makhsida N, Shah J, Yan G, Fisch H, Shabsigh R. Hypogonadism and metabolic syndrome: implications for testosterone therapy. J Urol 2005; 174:827–834.

70. Pitteloud N, Mootha VK, Dwyer AA, et al. Relationship between testosterone levels, insulin sensitivity, and mitochondrial function in men. Diabetes Care 2005; 28:1636–1642.

71. Harris MI, Flegal KM, Cowie CC, et al. Prevalence of diabetes, impaired fasting glucose, and impaired glucose tolerance in U.S. adults. The Third National Health and Nutrition Examination Survey, 1988–1994. Diabetes Care 1998; 21:518–524.

72. Centers for Disease Control and Prevention. National diabetes fact sheet: general information and national estimates on diabetes in the United States, 2003. www.cdc.gov/diabetes
73. Zinman B, Ruderman N, Campaigne BN, Devlin JT, Schneider SH. Physical activity/exercise and diabetes. Diabetes Care 2004; 27(suppl 1):S58–S62.
74. American Diabetes Association. Diabetes mellitus and exercise (Position Statement). Diabetes Care 2004; 1(27):S58–S62.
75. Bonadonna RC, Groop LC, Simonson DC, DeFronzo RA. Free fatty acid and glucose metabolism in human aging: evidence for operation of the Randle cycle. Am J Physiol 1994; 266:E501–E509.

6 | Cognitive Dysfunction and Depression in Older Adults with Diabetes

Hsu-Ko Kuo

Department of Geriatrics and Gerontology and Department of Internal Medicine, National Taiwan University Hospital, Taipei, Taiwan

INTRODUCTION

There has been a substantial increase in the total cases of diabetes mellitus (DM) in industrialized countries among elderly people. In the United States, people aged 65 and older will constitute most of the diabetic population in the next 20 years. More alarmingly, the proportion of the diabetic population 75 years or older is projected to exceed 30% in the next five decades (1,2). DM is an appalling disorder—quiet enough at onset, but with a toll on the body, causing immense and insidious damage to various organ systems. Considerable progress has been made in reducing risk for the traditionally recognized microvascular (retinopathy, nephropathy, and neuropathy) and macrovascular (coronary heart disease, stroke, and peripheral arterial disease) diabetic complications. But as DM increasingly becomes a disease of elderly people, some of the underappreciated cognitive and affective manifestations of DM must be addressed. Cognitive dysfunction and depression, imposing a direct impact on quality of life, loss of independence, and demands on caregivers, may ultimately be as great a concern to older people with diabetes as the more traditionally recognized vascular complications.

COGNITIVE DYSFUNCTION IN ELDERLY PATIENTS WITH DM

Progressive cognitive decline and dementia are common in old age. The prevalence of dementia in those aged 65 or older is estimated to range from 6% to 10% (3). Alzheimer's disease (AD) and vascular dementia (VaD) are the two most common forms of dementia, comprising approximately 70% and 20%, respectively, of all dementia cases (3,4). AD is a progressive brain disorder that gradually destroys a person's memory and ability to learn, reason, make judgments, communicate, and carry out daily activities. As AD progresses, individuals may also experience changes in personality and behavior, such as anxiety, suspiciousness or agitation, as well as delusions or hallucinations. VaD, a common form of dementia in older persons that is due to macro- and/or microcerebrovascular angiopathy, is associated with problems in the circulation of blood to the brain. The related changes in the brain are not due to AD pathology, such as β amyloid (Aβ) and neurofibrillary tangle, but due to chronic, reduced blood flow in the brain, eventually resulting in dementia. In VaD, there is usually a stepwise deterioration in cognitive function resulting from a series of small strokes. In addition to progressive decline in memory, executive dysfunction is a prominent feature in persons afflicted by VaD.

Cognitive decline has been variably related to a number of factors, including apolipoprotein E (apoE) ε4 allele, years of formal education and other lifestyle factors, depressive symptoms, as well as cardiovascular risk factors. Growing evidence suggests that the impact of DM on cognition may not entirely be due to cerebrovascular damage that often accompanies DM. Recent population-based studies have provided compelling evidence that DM should be added to the relatively short list of risk factors associated with cognitive decline and dementia among older adults.

Relation of DM to Cognitive Dysfunction
Global Cognition and Individual Cognitive Domains
A multitude of cross-sectional studies has been performed to examine the association between DM and cognitive performance among older persons. These studies, most of which were

case-control design and with small sample sizes, suggested that older diabetic adults generally performed more poorly than controls on a variety of cognitive function tests (5). In particular, DM was frequently associated with impaired declarative memory, attention, mental flexibility, information processing speed, and frontal lobe/executive functions (5,6). However, some concerns have been raised regarding the methodological limitations, generally due to inadequate statistical power and unbalanced matching between diabetes cases and controls. Recently, the evidence for the association between DM and cognitive impairment has been extended from small case-control studies to large population-based epidemiological surveys. Elias et al. by analyzing 1811 individuals aged from 55 to 89 years from the Framingham Heart Study population (7) suggested that a diagnosis of DM was associated with impairment in delayed verbal memory. The cross-sectional Nurses' Health Study (NHS), examining 2374 women aged 70 to 78 years, found that women with type 2 DM performed worse than those without type 2 DM on tests measuring general cognitive function, immediate and delayed verbal memory, and verbal fluency. Moreover, longer duration of DM and recent lack of treatment seemed to be associated with worse cognitive performance (8). Arvanitakis et al. analyzed 882 elderly participants from retirement facilities in Chicago metropolitan area and suggested that DM was associated with cognitive impairment, especially in semantic memory and perceptual speed (9).

The notion that DM is in association with cognitive impairment is further supported by a series of large prospective epidemiological studies (Table 1) (10–19). Many studies have reported a relationship between DM and decline in frontal lobe–mediated executive function, including psychomotor speed and attention, abstract thinking, mental flexibility, and multitasking. The Trail Making Tests (A&B), Digit Symbol Substitution test, and the word-list generation test (verbal fluency), requiring strategy formation, behavioral spontaneity, and to some extent retrieval ability from long-term memory, assess frontal lobe–mediated cognitive abilities and are characterized as traditional measures of executive function. Gregg et al. firstly reported a longitudinal relationship of self-reported, physician-diagnosed type 2 DM to decline of executive function among 9679 ambulatory, community-dwelling older women in the Study of Osteoporotic Fractures (10). Specifically, DM was associated with the development of major decline in the Trail Making B test [odds ratio (OR) = 1.74, 95% confidence interval (CI) 1.27–2.39] and Digit Symbol Substitution test (OR = 1.63, CI 1.20–2.23). Knopman et al. from the population-based Atherosclerosis Risk in Communities (ARIC) study prospectively followed up 10,963 individuals for six years and suggested that DM was associated with faster decline in executive cognitive function as reflected from scores on the Digit Symbol Substitution test and the first-letter word fluency (verbal fluency) test (11). By analyzing data from the Advanced Cognitive Training for Independent and Vital Elderly (ACTIVE) cognitive intervention trial, we also suggested that DM was associated with accelerated decline in executive function (19). Many other studies showed that decline in executive function was an important feature in DM-related cognitive decline (12,14,16). In addition to frontal executive function, DM has been reported to be associated with decline in other cognitive systems, including visuospatial ability (12), verbal memory (12,16), and global cognitive function (14–17).

Dementia

Diabetic complications and comorbidities such as stroke and hypertension have been implicated as risk factors for dementia and AD (20,21). Moreover, older diabetic adults typically score lower on certain cognitive tests and have a faster pace of cognitive decline than those without DM. Whether the accelerated cognitive decline implies increased risk of dementia has been rigorously examined in recent geriatric studies. Cross-sectionally, there is relatively few population-based data examining the relation of DM to dementia as an outcome. The Rotterdam population-based study, examining 6330 elderly participants aged 55 to 99 years, has demonstrated a positive association between DM and prevalent dementia (age, sex-adjusted OR = 1.3, and CI 1.0–1.9) (22). In particular, strong associations were found between dementia and DM treated with insulin (OR = 3.2, CI 1.4–7.5). The relation was strongest with VaD, but was also observed with AD.

Unlike the relatively scarce amount of data from population-based cross-sectional study, a growing body of large-scale longitudinal studies have been performed to elucidate the role of DM in the development of incident dementia, AD, or VaD (Table 2) (18,23–30). In the six studies

TABLE 1 Major Prospective Studies for the Association Between Diabetes Mellitus and Changes in Cognitive Performance

Study	Study population	Follow-up (yr)	Mean age or age range at baseline (yr)	Ascertainment of diabetes	Cognitive tests	Covariates	Results (Diabetic individuals had faster decline in …)
Gregg 2000 (10)	9679 Community-dwelling elderly white women from the Study of Osteoporotic Fractures	3–6	72 (>65)	Hx, Med	Modified MMSE, visuospatial/motor speed of processing (trails making B, DSST)	Age, education, depression, visual impairment, stroke, and baseline cognitive score	Visuospatial/motor speed of processing (trails making B and DSST)
Knopman 2001 (11)	10963 Individuals from the population-based Atherosclerosis Risk in Communities study	6	47–70	Hx, Med, FG, NFG	Speed of processing (DSST), verbal memory test (delayed word recall test), and verbal fluency	Age, sex, race, education, use of antipsychotics, antidepressants, anxiolytics, narcotics, anticonvulsants or antineoplastic agents	DSST and verbal fluency (for those age 58–70 yr or those < 58 yrs)
Fontbonne 2001 (12)	961 Community-dwelling elders from the Epidemiology of Vascular Aging study	4	65 (59–71)	Hx, Med, FG	MMSE, visuospatial/motor speed of processing (trails making B, DSST, finger trapping test), verbal memory (auditory verbal learning test), visuospatial ability (test of facial recognition), immediate visual memory, logical reasoning, and auditory attention	Age, sex, education, baseline cognitive score, systolic blood pressure	Verbal memory, speed of processing (DSST, finger trapping test), and visuospatial ability (test of facial recognition)
Wu 2003 (13)	1789 Older Mexican Americans from the population-based Sacramento Area Latino Study on Aging project	2	71	Hx, Med, FG	Modified MMSE, and verbal memory	Age, sex, education, depression, acculturation, and history of hypertension	No significant changes
Yaffe 2004 (14)	7027 Osteoporotic postmenopausal women from the Multiple Outcomes of Raloxifene Evaluation trial	4	66	Hx, Med, FG	Visuospatial/motor speed of processing and sequencing (trails making A and B), verbal memory, and word list fluency test	Age, race, education, BMI, depression, and intervention group	Trails making A and B, word list fluency, and the overall cognitive composite score

(Continued)

TABLE 1 Major Prospective Studies for the Association Between Diabetes Mellitus and Changes in Cognitive Performance (*Continued*)

Study	Study population	Follow-up (yr)	Mean age or age range at baseline (yr)	Ascertainment of diabetes	Cognitive tests	Covariates	Results (Diabetic individuals had faster decline in …)
Hassing 2004 (15)	258 Elderly individuals from the population-based Origins of Variance in the Old-Old study (OCTO-twin study)	2	83	Rec	MMSE	Age, sex, education, smoking, and vascular diseases	MMSE (0.29 points per 2-yr interval compared to those without diabetes; $p < 0.05$)
Hassing 2004 (16)	274 Elderly individuals from the population-based Origins of Variance in the Old-Old study (OCTO-Twin Study)	6	83	Rec	MMSE, speed of processing (DSST), visuospatial ability, verbal memory, and attention (Digit Span test)	Age, sex, education	MMSE, speed of processing, and verbal memory
Logroscino 2004 (17)	18999 Elderly women from the Nurses' Health Study	2	74	Hx, Med, Rec	TICS, and a global composite score combining TICS, test of verbal fluency, delayed recall, digit backwards test, and immediate/ delayed of East Boston memory test	Age, education, BMI, smoking, alcohol intake, history of high cholesterol and high blood pressure, age at menopause, use of aspirin, NSAID, antidepressant, postmenopausal hormone, vitamin E, as well as general health perception	TICS
Arvanitakis 2004 (18)	824 Catholic nuns, priests, and brothers from the Religious Orders Study	9	75	Hx, Med	Episodic memory, semantic memory, working memory, perceptual speed, visuospatial ability	Age, sex, education	Perceptual speed
Kuo 2005 (19)	2802 Elderly subjects from a cognitive intervention trial	2	74	Hx	MMSE, verbal memory, reasoning tests, motor and visual speed of processing (DSST and UFOV)	Age, sex, race, education, BMI, smoking, blood pressure, intervention group, and history of high cholesterol and vascular diseases	DSST

Abbreviations: TICS, telephone interview for cognitive status; MMSE, Minimental State Examinations; NSAID, nonsteroidal anti-inflammatory drug; BMI, body mass index; DSST, digit symbol substitution test; FG, fasting glucose test; Hx, self-report history of diabetes or a physician's diagnosis of diabetes; Med, antidiabetes medications; NFG, nonfasting glucose test; OCTO, octogenarian; Rec, diabetes mellitus ascertained from medical records; UFOV, useful field of view test.

TABLE 2 Population-Based Longitudinal Studies of Nondemented Individuals at Baseline with Diabetes Mellitus as a Risk Factor for Dementia

Study	Study population	Follow-up (yr)	Mean age or age range at baseline (yr)	Ascertainment of diabetes	Ascertainment of dementia	Covariates	Results RR (95% CI)		
							All dementia	Alzheimer's disease	Vascular dementia
Yoshitake 1995 (30)	828 Elderly residents in Hisayam town, Kyushu, Japan (Japan)	7	74	Hx	DSM-III R (dementia); NINCDS-ADRDA (AD); NINDS-AIREN (VaD)	Age	NP	2.18 (0.97–4.90)	2.77 (2.59–2.97)
Leibson 1997 (24)	1455 Persons of adult-onset diabetes residing in Rochester between 1970 and 1984 compared with the general Rochester population (1970–1984) (U.S.A.)	15	≥45	Rec	DSM-III (dementia); clinical, laboratory, and autopsy information for AD	Age, sex	1.66 (1.34–2.05)	Men: 2.27 (1.55–3.31); Women: 1.37 (0.94–2.01)	NP
Ott 1999 (27)	6370 Elderly persons from the community-based Rotterdam study (Netherlands)	2.1	68.9	Med, NFG, OGTT	DSM-III (dementia); NINCDS-ADRDA (AD); NINDS-AIREN (VaD)	Age, sex	1.9 (1.3–2.8)[a]	1.9 (1.2–3.1)[a]	2.0 (0.7–5.6)[a]
Luchsinger 2001 (25)	1262 Healthy Medicare beneficiaries residing in northern Manhattan (U.S.A.)	4.3	75.6	Hx, Med	DSM-IV (dementia); NINCDS-ADRDA (AD); clinical judgment for stroke-associated dementia (VaD)	Gender, race, education, smoking, history of hyper-tension/heart disease, LDL level	NP	1.3 (0.8–1.9)	3.4 (1.7–6.9)
Hassing 2002 (23)[b]	702 Elderly individuals from the population-based Origins of Variance in the Old-Old study (OCTO-Twin Study) (Sweden)	6	83	Rec	DSM-III R (dementia); NINCDS-ADRDA (AD); NINDS-AIREN (VaD)	Age, sex, education, smoking, vascular diseases	1.16 (0.79–1.71)	0.83 (0.46–1.48)	2.54 (1.35–4.78)
MacKnight 2002 (26)	5574 Elderly participants from the Canadian Study of Health and Aging (Canada)	5	74	Hx, Med, Rec, NFG	DSM-III R (dementia); NINCDS-ADRDA (AD); ICD-10 (VaD)	Age, sex, education, history of stroke, hypertension, and heart disease	1.26 (0.90–1.76)	1.30 (0.83–2.03)	2.03 (1.15–3.57)

(Continued)

TABLE 2 Population-Based Longitudinal Studies of Nondemented Individuals at Baseline with Diabetes Mellitus as a Risk Factor for Dementia (*Continued*)

Study	Study population	Follow-up (yr)	Mean age or age range at baseline (yr)	Ascertainment of diabetes	Ascertainment of dementia	Covariates	Results RR (95% CI)		
							All dementia	Alzheimer's disease	Vascular dementia
Peila 2002 (28)	2574 Japanese-American elderly men from the fourth exam cohort (1991–1993) of the Honolulu-Asia Aging Study (U.S.A.)	2.9	77	Hx, Med, FG, OGTT	DSM-III R (dementia); NINCDS-ADRDA (AD); CADDTC (VaD)	Age, education, apolipoprotein E ε4 status, diabetes medications, alcohol/smoking status, midlife systolic blood pressure, cholesterol, BMI, ABI, stroke, and CHD	1.5 (1.01–2.2)	1.8 (1.1–2.9)	2.3 (1.1–5.0)
Arvanitakis 2004 (18)	824 Catholic nuns, priests, and brothers from the Religious Orders Study (U.S.A.)	5.5	75	Hx, Med	NINCDS-ADRDA (AD)	Age, sex, education, stroke	NP	1.58 (1.05–2.38)	NP
Xu 2004 (29)	1301 Community elderly dwellers from the Kungsholmen project (Sweden)	4.7	81	Registered with diabetes (ICD code 250), Med, NFG	DSM III R (dementia), NINCDS-ADRDA (AD), NINDS-AIREN (VaD)	Age, sex, education, heart disease, stroke, BMI, SBP, DBP, antihypertensive medications	1.5 (1.0–2.1)	1.3 (0.9–2.1)	2.6 (1.2–6.1)

aAdditional adjustments for education, BMI, alcohol/smoking status, hypertension, ABI, heart disease, stroke did not result in substantial changes of the estimates.
bFive hundred and five individuals in the Hassing et al. were nondemented at baseline. The provided risk estimates, however, were based on total population.
Abbreviations: ABI, ankle-to-brachial index; AD, Alzheimer's disease; BMI, body mass index; CADDTC, California Alzheimer's Disease Diagnostic and Treatment Centers; CHD, coronary heart disease; CI, confidence interval; DBP, diastolic blood pressure; DSM, Diagnostic Statistical Manual; FG, fasting glucose test; HDL, high-density lipoprotein cholesterol; Hx, self-report history of diabetes or a physician's diagnosis of diabetes; ICD, International Classification of Disorders; LDL, low-density lipoprotein cholesterol; Med, antidiabetes medications; NFG, nonfasting glucose test; NINCDS-ADRDA, National Institute of Neurological and Communicative Disorders and Stroke–Alzheimer's Disease and Related Disorder Association; NINDS-AIREN, National Institute of Neurological Disorders and Stroke-Association Internationale Pour la Recherche et l'Enseignement en Neurosciences; NP, not performed; OGTT, oral glucose tolerance test; Rec, diabetes mellitus ascertained from medical records; RR, risk ratio; SBP, systolic blood pressure; SMR, standardized morbidity ratios; VaD, vascular dementia.

assessing the relationship between DM and incident all-cause dementia, four studies reported a positive association (24,27–29) while the remaining two studies did not find such relationship (23,26). Leibson et al. from the Rochester study found that diabetic individuals had higher risk of developing dementia [relative risk (RR) 1.66 and CI 1.34–2.05] compared to age- and sex-specific rates calculated from the general Rochester population (24). Following 6370 elderly individuals from the Rotterdam Study for an average of 2.1 years, Ott et al. suggested that DM almost doubled the risk of dementia (RR = 1.9 and CI 1.3–2.8). Patients treated with insulin were at the highest risk of dementia (RR = 4.3 and CI 1.7–10.5), reflecting greater risk of dementia in more severe DM (27). Hassing et al. prospectively examined 702 elderly individuals from the Swedish Twin Registry ["Origins of Variance in the Old-Old" (OCTO-Twin Study)], 505 of whom were nondemented at baseline. The authors did not imply an association between DM and dementia (RR = 1.16, CI 0.79–1.71) (23). However, interpretation of the results of Hassing et al. should be done with caution because risk estimate of "incident" dementia was not provided. Moreover, the sample size was relatively small and the ascertainment of DM totally relied on the review of medical records. Although a trend of higher risk of obtaining dementia in diabetes individuals has been demonstrated by the Canadian Study of Health and Aging 26, the association did not achieve statistical significance (RR = 1.26; 95% CI 0.90–1.76). Peila et al. (28) and Xu et al. (29) from the Honolulu-Asia Aging Study and the Kungsholmen Project, respectively, suggested that DM significantly increased the risk of incident dementia by 50% among older adults after comprehensive adjustment for basic demographics and cardiovascular risk factors. A recent systematic review of population-based studies suggested that the risk of dementia is generally increased in patients with DM (31). Cukierman et al., by using meta-analytic technique, demonstrated that people with diabetes were 1.6 times more likely to develop all-cause dementia than people without diabetes (CI: 1.4–1.8) (32). Studies addressing the potential underlying mechanisms from DM to dementia could provide insight into both the prevention and treatment of cognitive dysfunction in diabetic patients.

Given that DM is associated with increased risk of developing dementia, some prospective studies have designed to investigate the relation of DM to common subtypes of dementia, specifically AD and VaD. Yoshitake et al. followed 828 community-dwelling elders from the Hisayam study for seven years and reported that the age-adjusted RRs (95% CIs) for AD and VaD were 2.18 (0.97–4.90) and 2.77 (2.59–2.97) (30). The Rochester study reported a raised risk of developing AD associated with DM, especially in men (24). These associations, which are predictable on the basis of the strong association between DM and cerebrovascular disease, are probably mediated, at least to some extent, through the competing risks of other cardiovascular disease and risk factors. This issue was carefully addressed by subsequent studies. The prospective Rotterdam Study by Ott et al. suggested that DM doubled the risk of both AD and VaD and that adjustment for other vascular risk factors made little difference to the association (27). A prospective study with a mean follow-up of 4.3 years enrolling 1262 elderly Medicare beneficiaries in northern Manhattan, most of whom were Hispanic (45%) and Black (32%), suggested that DM was associated with incident stroke-associated dementia after controlling for demographics, smoking, hypertension, heart disease, and cholesterol levels (RR 3.4, CI 1.7–6.9) (25). However, DM was not strongly associated with AD (RR 1.3, CI 0.8–1.9). The conclusion that DM is associated with VaD, but not with AD, independent of other vascular disease, can also be confirmed from the following studies: the Origins of Variance in the Old-Old Study (OCTO-Twin Study) of Sweden (AD: RR 0.83, CI 0.46–1.48; VaD: RR 2.54, CI 1.35–4.78) (23), the Canadian Study of Health and Aging of Canada (AD: RR 1.30, CI 0.83–2.03; VaD: RR 2.03, CI 1.15–3.57) (26), as well as the Kungsholmen Project of Sweden (AD: RR 1.3, CI 0.9–2.1; VaD: RR 2.6, CI 1.2–6.1) (29). On the contrary, the Honolulu-Asia Aging Study suggested that DM was a strong risk factor for both AD (RR 1.8, CI 1.1–2.9) and VaD (RR 2.3, CI 1.1–5.0) independent of health-related behaviors and cardiovascular risk factors. A significant relation of DM to incident AD was similarly demonstrated from a group of Catholic elderly nuns, priests, and brothers (RR: 1.58, CI: 1.05–2.38).

In conclusion, diabetes, a strong risk factor for the development of VaD after comprehensive adjustment of various cardiovascular disease and risk factors, is consistently associated with a 2.0- to 2.6-fold increase in risk of incident VaD among older adults (23,26,28,29). Although studies with DM as an exposure generally suggested a 30% to 100% increased risk of AD, the evidence was less consistent and the statistical significance varied. More population-based, longitudinal studies, or a formal meta-analysis of the AD risk estimates of older adults, are needed.

Pathophysiological Mechanisms of Diabetes-Related Cognitive Dysfunction
Hyperglycemia
Chronic hyperglycemia is a key feature for elderly people afflicted by DM. Early reaction between glucose and protein amino acids proceeds from nonenzymatic glycosylation (post-translational modification) to reversible Schiff bases, and to stable, covalently bonded Amadori rearrangement products (33). Over weeks and months, these early products evolve further chemical reactions, including rearrangement, dehydration, cleavage, and addition, into irreversibly bonded advanced glycation end products (AGEs) (34). Immunohistochemically, AGE modification was identified in both senile plaques and neurofibrillary tangles (35). It was also reported that AGE-modified $A\beta$ promotes $A\beta$ aggregation, thus contributing to amyloidosis in AD (36).

In addition to forming AGEs, three major mechanisms have been implicated in glucose-mediated toxicity: increase flux of glucose through polyol pathway, activation of protein kinase C, and increased flux of glucose through hexosamine pathway (37). Each of the above-mentioned mechanisms, along with the AGE modification, reflects the hyperglycemia-induced oxidative stress: overproduction of superoxide by the electron-transport chain (38). Many studies have shown that DM and hyperglycemia increase oxidative stress, thus resulting in vascular endothelial damage and macro-/microvascular angiopathy. DM and chronic hyperglycemia, by provoking more generalized and widespread vascular changes in the brain, may lead to lacunes, white matter changes (leukoaraiosis), large ischemic stroke, or brain atrophy. DM in the elderly usually develops in the context of a cluster of cardiovascular diseases or risk factors, including atherosclerosis, hypertension, obesity, insulin resistance, or dyslipidemia. The risks of ischemic cerebrovascular disease, not entirely attributable to DM, are typically associated with a combination of various cardiovascular risk factors. The diabetes-related cerebral structural changes, specifically cortical atrophy and cerebrovascular disease, are documented risk factors for the development of cognitive impairment and dementia.

Hypoglycemia
The most common cause of hypoglycemia in diabetic patients is the use of antidiabetic medications including exogenous insulin and oral hypoglycemic agents. Under normal conditions, the brain is fueled by glucose. Depending on the magnitude and duration, hypoglycemia causes varying levels of cognitive and neurological impairment. As a result, hypoglycemia has been one of the most fearful consequences of diabetes management and many diabetic patients worry about the impact of hypoglycemia on their future cognitive function.

Extensive evidence in human studies demonstrated that *acute* hypoglycemia impaired cognitive performance in attentional flexibility (39,40), logical reasoning (41) as well as speed of information processing (39,41–43). However, reports of the cognitive impact of *recurrent* hypoglycemia are mixed and highly variable. Some researchers even postulated that prolonged and recurrent hypoglycemia results in a beneficial effect in cognition because of an adaptive increase in brain glucose supply across the blood–brain barrier, thus enhancing ability to provide glucose supply to the brain. Study of the cognitive impact of recurrent hypoglycemia in diabetic patients has been hampered by difficulty in controlling for prior hypoglycemic history, diabetes status as well as competing influences such as chronic exposure to hyperglycemia, cerebrovascular disease, depression, and other chronic comorbidities. Unfortunately, the majority of studies were conducted in animals or middle-aged type 1 diabetic patients. The generalizability toward the elderly diabetic population would be a serious concern. More studies will be needed to elucidate the role of hypoglycemia in the development of cognitive dysfunction in elderly diabetic patients.

Hyperinsulinemia and Insulin Resistance
Insulin increases glucose utilization and is a modulator of energy homeostasis, essential functions for neuronal survival and cerebral activity. Through its action on insulin receptors

widely distributed throughout the brain, rise in insulin level is followed shortly by improved cognitive function, particularly learning and memory (44). Over the past decade, neuroscientists have implied that insulin, by promoting neuronal health, is an essential element to enhance mental prowess.

However, cerebral and cognitive effects of insulin have been greatly challenged in the context of aging, chronic hyperinsulinemia, and insulin resistance. Elderly diabetes patients, most of them type 2, are known to have abnormal insulin metabolism, specifically insulin resistance and chronic, compensatory hyperinsulinemia. Abnormally high insulin levels have been associated for decades with heart disease and obesity. Recent lines of research have even cast excess insulin in a dark light. Over the past few years, the role of hyperinsulinemia in implicating the metabolism of $A\beta$ as well as the development of cognitive dysfunction and dementia has been enthusiastically explored. Senile plaque, the hallmark of AD, contains an extracellular aggregation of heterogeneous $A\beta$ peptides derived from amyloid precursor protein (APP). APP undergoes proteolytic β-secretase and γ-secretase activities to generate $A\beta40$ and $A\beta42$ peptides, the predominant $A\beta$ variants. An important hypothesis of AD, the amyloid hypothesis, states that $A\beta$ initiates a process resulting in AD (45). $A\beta$ is cleared through microglia low-density lipoprotein cholesterol (LDL)-receptor–mediated uptake or through proteolytic degradation. The proteolytic degradation of $A\beta$ involves insulin-degrading enzyme (IDE). In addition to the degrading of Alzheimer's protein ($A\beta$), IDE also degrades insulin and in fact demonstrates a strong preference for insulin over $A\beta$. Gasparini et al. by incubating neurons in vitro with insulin, suggested that insulin increased extracellular $A\beta$ both by reducing IDE-mediated $A\beta$ degradation and by stimulating $A\beta$ secretion (46). An animal study by Farris et al. demonstrated that transgenic mouse with IDE gene entirely knocked out developed typical features of AD and type 2 DM, namely hyperinsulinemia, glucose intolerance, and increased brain levels of $A\beta$ (47). The next level of evidence of insulin and amyloid metabolism has moved from cell cultures and animal models to human study. By experimentally raised plasma insulin to levels commonly encountered in many patients with type 2 DM, Watson et al. found that insulin infusion led to an increase in cerebrospinal fluid $A\beta$ levels, most notably in older subjects (48).

Findings of basic research were corroborated by recently published epidemiological studies. C-peptide, cleaved in a 1:1 ratio in the conversion of proinsulin to insulin, not excreted by the liver, and having a half-life two to five times longer than insulin, provides a stable and accurate representation of insulin secretion. Okereke et al. cross-sectionally examined the NHS cohort and found that cognitive function was worse among elderly women with high levels of C-peptide, suggesting that higher insulin secretion may be related to worse cognition (49). Independent of age, sex, education, body mass index, apoE $\varepsilon4$, diabetes, hypertension, heart disease, and stroke, Luchsinger et al. suggested that hyperinsulinemia (fasting insulin >27 µIU/mL) was a strong predictor for both AD (hazard ratio 2.1, CI 1.5–3.1) and all-cause dementia (hazard ratio 1.9, CI 1.3–2.7) after following 683 elderly people in northern Manhattan for a mean of 5.4 years (50). Hyperinsulinemia was also related to a significant decline in memory-related cognitive scores. Chronic hyperinsulinemia, through its connection to amyloid metabolism, is an important pathophysiological mechanism for diabetes-related cognitive dysfunction.

In short, diabetes in older adults, by chronic elevation of both serum glucose and insulin, may lead to excess oxidative stress and abnormal amyloid metabolism, thus resulting in generalized cerebral macro-/microvasculopathy, brain atrophy, and dementia.

Strategies for Prevention and Management

DM in older adults, seldom found in isolation, is usually encountered in the context of multiple metabolic syndromes as well as cardiovascular disease and risk factors, namely hypertension, coronary heart disease, stroke, smoking, physical inactivity, dyslipidemia, and obesity. Studies suggested that vascular risk factors modified the association between diabetes and cognitive dysfunction and that aggregation of vascular risk factors significantly increased the risk of developing dementia. A two-year prospective study of 258 community-dwelling older adults suggested an interactive effect of hypertension and DM on cognitive decline by demonstrating the greatest cognitive decline among persons with comorbid DM and hypertension (16). Whitmer et al. by conducting a retrospective cohort study demonstrated that the presence of multiple cardiovascular risk factors at midlife substantially increases risk of late-life dementia in a dose-dependent manner (51). Kivipelto et al. followed 1449 population-based individuals for an average of 21 years and suggested that midlife cardiovascular risk factors were strong predictors for the development of dementia in late-life. Moreover, clustering of vascular risk factors increases the risk in an additive manner (52). Therefore, it is plausible to aggressively manage DM, along with other vascular risk factors, in midlife in order to prevent late-life cognitive dysfunction.

Recent studies supported the notion that cardiovascular risk modification is associated with reduced risk of cognitive decline and dementia. Data from the Syst-Eur trial, a randomized, controlled trial recruiting 2412 elderly subjects without dementia at baseline, showed that active treatment of hypertension with antihypertensive medications reduced the incidence of dementia by 50% after two years of follow-up (53). Another randomized, controlled trial of 6105 people with prior stroke or transient ischemic attack showed that active treatment of high blood pressure was associated with reduced risks of dementia and cognitive decline (54). An observational study of 1037 postmenopausal women with coronary heart disease suggested that high cholesterol levels were associated with cognitive impairment and that statin users had higher modified Mini-Mental State Examination (MMSE) scores and a trend for a lower likelihood of cognitive impairment compared with nonusers (55). Hajjar et al., by analyzing patients in a community-based geriatric, clinic implied that the use of statins is associated with a lower prevalence of dementia and has a positive impact on the progression of cognitive impairment (56). A controlled clinical trial conducted by Gradman et al. found that after two months of treatment with glipizide, older DM patients were able to perform better in tests of verbal learning and memory (57). In a prospective pre-/post study of older adults with untreated DM, Meneilly et al. suggested that improved glycemic control after a stable dose of oral hypoglycemic agent for six months was associated with improved performance on a variety of cognitive tests (58). In a two-year prospective analysis of 718 old diabetic Mexican Americans, antidiabetic medications appeared to be useful in alleviating the decline in both physical and cognitive functioning, especially for those with a longer duration of the disease (59). Regular exercise, an essential approach for cardiovascular health, has also been advocated as a crucial preventive strategy for cognitive impairment. The NHS demonstrated that long-term physical activity, including walking, is associated with significantly better cognitive function and less cognitive decline in older women (60). The Honolulu Asia-Aging Study suggested that physically capable elderly men who walked more regularly were less likely to develop dementia (61).

Many prospective studies reported DM as an important predictor for decline in frontal executive function, including perceptual speed, attention, abstract thinking, and mental flexibility as assessed by such tests as the Trail Making Tests, Digit Symbol Substitution test, and verbal fluency test. Executive functions, abilities for multitasking, planning, and organizing, are essential for DM management as well as cardiovascular risk modification, which typically involves management of multiple medications, dietary and lifestyle changes, self-monitoring of blood sugar, and frequent follow-up. Although there is increasing evidence showing that DM has a negative effect on cognition, relatively few studies have addressed such effect on diabetes self-management. By analyzing 60 elderly diabetic patients, Munshi et al. demonstrated that cognitive dysfunction in this population was associated with poor diabetes control and that old diabetic adults had a high risk of depression and functional disabilities (62). Perlmuter et al. concluded that cognitive impairment might complicate adherence to medical regimens in people with diabetes (63). Sinclair et al. studied a large number of community-dwelling older adults and found that subjects with diabetes had a worse performance on MMSE and clock-drawing test than nondiabetic controls. Further, a within-group analysis of diabetic subjects revealed that those with cognitive impairment were significantly more dependent on health/ social services, scored lower on activities of daily living (ADL) measures, and were less involved with DM self-management, including self-medication, self-monitoring, and follow-up in a diabetes clinic (64).

Therefore, unable to adhere to medical advice and be sufficiently involved in self-care, diabetic patients with overlooked cognitive impairment especially executive dysfunction are

TABLE 3 Behavior Signs of Executive Dysfunction

Problems	Examples
Stopping	Disinhibited behaviors such as blurting out socially inappropriate remarks; frontal release signs such as the grasp and palmomental reflex
Starting	Lack of spontaneous retrieval of previously learned information; needing repeated reminder and monitoring for treatment plans; problems with initiation; lack of motivation; unable to maintain effortful behavior, mutism as most extreme example
Switching	Lack of mental flexibility; unable to change strategies for solving problems; difficulty in switching habitual behavior such as diet and life-style; self-management difficulty when there is a change in medical regimen such as dosage and schedule
Socialization	Poor interpretation of social cues; difficulties in socializing due to lack of motivation, personality changes, or uninhibited behaviors
Planning	Inability of volition, multitasking, and organizing; unable to manage polypharmacy and complex dosing regimen; unable to be compliant to suggestions from health care providers; "stubborn" or "uncooperative" patients not compliant with treatment advice
Judgment	Failure to anticipate consequences of behavior such as unable to self-monitor blood sugar and get hypoglycemia; unable to identify signs of medication adverse effects

often labeled as noncompliant or unmotivated. Clinician is recommended to assess the older adult with DM for cognitive impairment using a standardized instrument during the initial evaluation period and with any significant decline in clinical status, including increased difficulty with self-care. Although MMSE, a commonly used screening instrument, has been recommended by the American Geriatric Society (AGS) "Guidelines for improving the care of the older person with DM" as a tool to detect cognitive impairment (65), the fact that such test generally lacks sensitive measures of executive functions should be considered. In addition to performing a cognitive screening instrument like MMSE, clinicians should learn to recognize signs of executive dysfunction, including problems with stopping, starting, switching, socialization, planning, and judgment (Table 3). Some tests such as the Clock Drawing Test, Trail Making Tests, or word list generation are easily administered and useful in identifying subtle executive dysfunction. It is crucial to be aware of a patient's cognitive status when formulating treatment plan or prescribing antidiabetes medications. Newly developed difficulties of participating in diabetes self-care should be considered as an indicator of cognitive decline. If cognitive dysfunction is suspected from the associated behavioral signs or confirmed through cognitive tests, therapy should be simplified and prescribed in a clear step-by-step fashion in order to achieve best possible outcomes.

DM AND DEPRESSION

Depression is a highly prevalent and chronically relapsing illness among patients with DM. A recent meta-analysis of 42 studies suggested that the odds of major depression among people with DM were roughly twice that of those without (66). The chronic, relapsing nature of depression in diabetic patients has been suggested by a five-year follow-up study with 25 diabetic patients with depression. In that study, Lustman et al. found that recurrence or persistence of depression occurred in 92% of the patients with an average of 4.8 depression episodes over the follow-up period (67). The high prevalence and chronicity of depression in diabetic patients place a heavy burden on the current health-care system, as reflected in the increased health-care cost and utilization (68). This chapter will attempt to discuss the following questions: (*i*) prevalence of depression in older diabetic adults; (*ii*) temporal relationship between DM and depression; (*iii*) clinical significance of depression in diabetic adults; and (*iv*) screening and treatment of depressive disorders in persons with DM.

Prevalence of Depression in Older Adults with Diabetes

Several studies have described the prevalence of depression among older adults with DM. Bell et al. analyzed 696 elderly diabetic adults (≥65 years of age) from the Evaluating Long-term Diabetes Self-management Among Elder Rural Adults Study and reported that 15.8% of the sample had depressive symptoms, defined as 20-item modified Center for Epidemiologic Studies Depression Scale (CES-D) score of nine or above (69). Bruce et al. by using Even Briefer Assessment Scale for depression, reported that the prevalence for clinically significant depression among 223 community-dwelling diabetic elders was 14.2% (70). Chou and Chi analyzed 2003 community-dwelling elderly Chinese adults in Hong Kong by using census data and found that the prevalence for depression, defined as a 15-item Geriatric Depression Scale (GDS) score >7, among diabetic elders was 26% while that among nondiabetic elders was 19.7% ($p < 0.05$) (71). Finkelstein and coworkers analyzed 1997 Medicare claim data and found that the diagnosed annual prevalence of major depression among older claimants with diabetes was 2.85% compared with 1.88% among claimants without diabetes. The elderly claimants with diabetes were 1.58 times more likely to have major depression compared to the nondiabetic claimants (72).

Clinically significant depression is common among older diabetic patients. Unfortunately, the estimates of depression prevalence seemed not stable and varied widely across different studies. There are several reasons for the questionable estimates. First, there was a historically low reimbursement rates associated with mental illness and it is likely that major depression in the study by Finkelstein et al. was underreported (72). Second, different instruments for depression were used by different studies, leading to heterogeneous depression estimates. Moreover, the number of controlled studies was very small. Depression prevalence in older adults with diabetes would be more precise in population-based studies using standardized depression assessment tool and comparisons would be strengthened by inclusion of control subjects without diabetes.

Relationship Between Diabetes and Depression

Recently, the strength and causal direction of the association between DM and depression have been rigorously investigated. Metabolic consequences of DM may lead to changes in brain structure and function, thus leading to the development of depression. Increased burden of cardiovascular risks along with the associated metabolic derangements has been linked to neurostructural changes such as stroke, lacunar infarction, as well as cerebral white changes (leukoaraiosis). These cerebral macro- as well as microangiopathic changes have been proposed as important predictors of late-life depression (73). However, it is unknown whether such metabolic derangements or cerebral vascular pathology are specific to DM or are manifestations or interactions of multiple cardiovascular risk factors, comorbidities, and certain sociocultural factors. Prospective studies have been conducted to elucidate the independent role of DM in the development of depression or changes of depressive symptoms over time. Kessing et al., by using data from the Danish National Hospital Register from 1977 to 1993, suggested that older diabetic patients did not seem to have an increased risk of developing severe depression compared with patients with other chronic illness (74). Palinkas et al. by following 971 community-dwelling older adults aged 50 and older in Rancho Bernardo, California for an averaged eight years, did not find a predictive role of diabetes in the development of depressive symptoms (75). Bisschop et al. from the Longitudinal Aging Study Amsterdam prospectively followed 2288 community-dwelling older adults for a maximum of six years had suggested that multiple comorbidities including lung disease, arthritis, cardiac disease, and cancer were predictive of increased depressive symptoms. Diabetes was not independently associated with change of depressive symptom over time (76). The notion that diabetes per se as an independent predictor of late-life depression seemed not to be supported by evidence from recent epidemiological studies.

On the other hand, there has been speculation for a long time that mental illness specifically depression is related to the onset and the course of DM. In 1684, Thomas Willis wrote about diabetes: "Sadness, or long sorrow … and other depressions and disorders of the animal spirits, are used to generate or foment this morbid disposition" (77). A growing body of longitudinal epidemiological studies has supported this notion by demonstrating that depression constitutes a major risk factor in the development of DM. Eaton et al. followed 1715 individuals for 13 years and suggested that major depressive disorder signals increased risk for type 2 DM (78). Kawakami et al. analyzing data from an eight-year prospective cohort of Japanese male employees indicated that subjects who had moderate or severe depressive symptoms ($\geq$48 on the Zung Self-Rating Depression Scale) at baseline had a 2.3 times higher risk of developing type 2 DM than those not depressed (79). The Study of Women's Health Across the Nation (80), the NHS (81), as well as the ARIC Study (82) suggested that depressive symptoms independently predicted incident type 2 DM (80–82). Persons with psychiatric disorders generally have multiple risk factors, such as physical inactivity, medical comorbidities, and obesity, for the development of type 2 DM (83). In these studies, depression remained a significant risk factor for diabetes even after consideration of potential confounders (78–82). Recently, Talbot and Nouwen systematically reviewed the temporal relationship between depression and diabetes (84). They found that there was no solid evidence to indicate that the initial occurrence of clinically significant depression resulted either from biochemical changes directly attributable to type 2 DM or its treatment. Depression in diabetes may merely result from the increased strain of having a chronic medical condition rather than directly from the disease itself. On the contrary, a reverse pattern of temporal relation was suggested because depression or depressive symptomatology may increase the risk for onset of type 2 DM and that the onset of major depressive disorder typically preceded the diagnosis of type 2 DM by many years. However, the majority of studies were not designed to examine the relationship between depression and diabetes in older adults. Thus, the generalizability of the above studies for the elderly population remains a serious concern for geriatric practitioners. In a population-based nested case-control study using the administrative databases of Saskatchewan Health in Canada, Brown et al. took extra efforts by performing age-stratified analyses for the association between depression and the risk of diabetes. They found that depression appeared to increase the risk of developing DM by 23% in adults aged 20 to 50 years. The association did not exist in those aged greater than 51 years (85). More population-based prospective studies will be needed to elucidate the role of depression in the development of DM among older adults.

Clinical Significance of Depression in Diabetes
Glycemic Control and Diabetes Complications
Chronic hyperglycemia, a hallmark of DM closely associated with depression, is a well-established predictor of the onset and exacerbation of diabetes complication. Maintenance of good glycemic control is the focus of care for diabetes patients, and the importance of depression will be judged based on its effect on this parameter. In a recent meta-analysis, Lustman et al. suggested that depression is significantly associated with higher levels of glycated hemoglobin (86). The effect size calculated from 24 studies was modest yet consistent and clinically important. The authors also reviewed data of the clinical trials and suggested that active treatment of depression was beneficial to the mood, as well as to glycemic control.

Studies during 1980s and 1990s have actively examined the correlation of depression to a variety of diabetic complications such as neuropathy, nephropathy, and retinopathy. However, many of these studies had limited power with very small sample sizes and thus the magnitude and consistency of the correlation remained undetermined. De Groot et al. by performing a meta-analysis of 27 studies indicated a positive and consistent association between depression and various diabetes complications (diabetic retinopathy, nephropathy, neuropathy, macrovascular complications, and sexual dysfunction) (87).

Mortality
Many studies suggested that depression is associated with increased mortality in general population. A recent meta-analysis of 25 community studies found that the hazard ratio for all-cause mortality in depressed subjects was 1.81 (CI 1.58–2.07) compared with that for nondepressed subjects (88). The association became more evident when subjects have certain medical diseases such as coronary artery disease (89), myocardial infarction (90), stroke (91), and congestive heart failure (92), or have an unfavorable socioeconomic status (93).

Recently, the interrelationships between diabetes, depression, and mortality have been rigorously examined. Using data from the National Health and Nutrition Examination Survey (NHANES) Epidemiologic Follow-up Study (1982–1992), Zhang et al. found that depression played a significant role in mortality risk among people with DM (94). Among diabetic population and independent of sociodemographic, lifestyle, and health-status variables, the hazard ratio for mortality was 1.54 (CI 1.15–2.07) compared adults with CES-D scores of 16 or higher to those with scores less than 16. Using the same database, that is, NHANES I Epidemiologic Follow-up Study (1982–1992), Egede et al. performed a different analysis to investigate the interactive effect of DM and depression on mortality. The risk of death was 2.5-fold higher for people with both DM and depression compared to the reference group (individuals without both DM and depression) after multivariate adjustment (95). Moreover, coexistence of DM and depression was associated with significantly increased risk of death beyond that due to having both conditions alone. In a prospective study conducted in a large health maintenance organization (HMO), Katon et al. also suggested that patients with comorbid depression and type 2 DM had a higher mortality rate over a three-year period compared with patients with DM alone (96).

Compliance to Diabetes Care
Self-care regimens, including medication-taking, self-monitoring of blood glucose, diet control, regular exercise, and smoking cessation, are essential for high-quality diabetes care. Depression, abating the patients' ability and willingness to comply with medical advice, seems to present a major obstacle for diabetic care by affecting self-care behaviors. Ciechanowski et al. analyzed 367 type 1 and type 2 DM patients from two HMO clinics and suggested that depressive symptoms were associated with poorer diet and medication adherence (97). In another population survey of HMO enrollees with DM, Lin et al. reported that patients with major depression were more likely to lack self-care activities such as healthy diet, regular exercise, and smoking cessation compared with patients without major depression (98). When compared to diabetic patients without depression, depressed diabetic patients also demonstrated less adherence to prescribed medications. In a subsequent study at a Veterans Administration facility, depression has also been shown to adversely influence diabetes medication adherence in a group of old, diabetic patients (99).

Disability, Performance Status, and Quality of Life
Disability, highly prevalent in individuals with chronic diseases, affects the quality of life and is associated with frequent use of health and social services. DM and depression are common chronic conditions that are significantly associated with functional disability (100,101). Recently, epidemiological studies began to investigate the impact of depression on functional status among diabetic patients as well as a possible joint effect of both DM and depression on outcomes related to functional implication and quality of life. Using the Short-Form 12 Health Survey, researchers demonstrated that depressive symptoms had a significant negative effect on physical and mental functioning in a group of diabetic patients (97). Data from the 1999 National Health Interview Survey (NHIS) indicated that the odds of functional disability were significantly higher in individuals with DM and comorbid major depression than in individuals with either condition alone, suggesting a synergistic effect of diabetes and depression on disability (102). In a subsequent analysis, the author found that people with coexisting depression and diabetes had the highest disability burden, including work loss and disability bed days (103). Similarly, Goldney et al. analyzed 3010 individuals living in South Australia and demonstrated a negative, additive effect of both DM and depression on each of the eight domains of the Short Form Health-Related Quality-of-Life Questionnaire (104). Black et al., prospectively examining 2830 elderly Mexican Americans for seven years, found that the interaction of DM and depression was synergistic, predicting a greater incidence of disability in ADL after controlling for potential confounders (105).

In conclusion, once depression is established, it may affect glycemic control as well as patients' compliance to diabetic care, leading to the development of diabetes-related complications and disability regardless of whether or not the depression is developed preceding or following the course of diabetes. Both conditions need to be managed in proper manner to enhance quality of care.

Screening for Depression in Elderly Diabetics

It is well known that a major proportion of chronically ill patients with depression are most often not treated optimally or not treated at all. Experts currently estimate that less than 25% of depression in diabetic patients is effectively identified and treated in clinical practice (106). The problem is partly due to the fact that a significant number of patients who suffer from depression do not consult a doctor. Also, a correct diagnosis of depression in diabetic patients is frequently encumbered with the similarity between manifestations of uncontrolled DM and depressive symptoms (e.g., fatigue; changes in weight, appetite, and libido). Moreover, primary-care physicians are generally less equipped to perform a psychodiagnostic interview and often lack sufficient clinical time (107). Depression in diabetic patients, associated with poor glucose regulation, medical noncompliance, and diabetic complications, will eventually affect performance status as well as quality of life. Thus, timely identification and effective treatment of comorbid depression, an essential component of high-quality care of diabetic patients, seem to be a great challenge in routine diabetes care.

AGS guidelines for the treatment of DM in geriatric populations suggested that depression should be screened by using a standardized screening tool during the initial evaluation and if there is any unexplained decline in clinical status (65). A number of instruments have been reported in the literatures to screen for depression in diabetic patients. Lustman et al. performed a study, recruiting 172 diabetic outpatients, to determine the utility of the Beck Depression Inventory (BDI) as a screening tool for major depression in diabetic patients (108). The BDI contains 21 self-administered questionnaires and each of the 21 items measures the presence and severity of a symptom of depression by rating from zero to three. The authors suggested that the BDI is an effective screening test for major depression in diabetic patients and they recommended using a BDI cutoff equal to or greater than 16 for referral to a mental health specialist or treatment. Another study conducted in Australia also suggested that it is feasible to utilize the BDI to screen for depression in primary-care type 2 DM patients (109). The World Health Organization (WHO) 5-item Well-Being Index (WB5), a short screening instrument for the detection of depression in the general population, is recommended in the WHO DiabCare Basic Information Sheet. Rakovac et al. suggested that WB5 scores below 13 can be used as a cutoff value to define depression and the estimates of depression prevalence were comparable to the prevalence reported by Anderson et al. The WB5 questionnaire can be completed in less than five minutes and "should be more widely used for depression screening among persons with diabetes (110)." Although GDS is widely used as a basic screening measure for depression in older adults, the validity of GDS as a screening measure for depression among diabetic older adults has not been examined. Some other instruments such as the Hospital Anxiety and Depression Scale and the concise assessment for depression have been shown to be effective as screening tools in measuring depression in medically ill patients. Likewise, more studies are needed to determine the usefulness of depression screening among older diabetic patients.

An old diabetic adult should be screened for depression during the initial evaluation period and if there is any unexplained decline in clinical status. If an old diabetic adult presents with new-onset or recurrent depression, medications should be evaluated to determine whether any of them are associated with depression. If therapy is initiated, targeted symptoms should be identified and documented in the record.

Treatment

Affective outcomes in diabetic patients with depression respond to antidepressants or depression-specific psychotherapies. Selective serotonin reuptake inhibitor (SSRI) is the first choice of antidepressant to treat depressed older patients because of its better side effect profile (e.g., few anticholinergic, orthostatic, and cardiovascular side effects). Furthermore, SSRI has been demonstrated to be effective in the treatment of depression in diabetic patients. A 10-week, open label study of 28 depressed type 2 DM patients treated with sertraline at the dose of 50 mg/day showed significant improvements in both the Hamilton Rating Scale for Depression (HAMD) and the BDI (111). In a eight-week, randomized controlled trial of 34 diabetic patients with major depression, Lustman et al. found that reduction in depression symptoms was significantly greater in patients treated with fluoxetine (up to 40 mg/day) compared with those receiving placebo (BDI, -14.0 vs. -8.8, $p = 0.03$; HAMD, -10.7 vs. -5.2, $p = 0.01$) (112). They also found trends toward greater improvement in glycemic control as well as a better rate of depression remission in patients treated with fluoxetine. In addition, SSRI such as fluoxetine has been demonstrated in animals as well as in humans to increase insulin action, induce weight loss, as well as exhibit a hypoglycemic effect (113–116).

Tricyclic antidepressants (TCAs) should be used cautiously in older people because of their anticholinergic/antihistaminic property as well as potential adverse effects on cardiovascular systems (e.g., orthostatic hypotensive effect and ventricular conduction delay). An eight-week, randomized controlled trial of 68 diabetic patients with major depression found that patients receiving nortriptyline demonstrated greater reductions in depressive symptoms compared with those receiving placebo (BDI, –10.2 vs. –5.8, $p = 0.03$). However, they did not observe any superior glycemic effect of nortriptyline in the depressed subjects. In fact, TCAs may potentially induce hyperglycemia, carbohydrate craving, as well as weight gain (117,118) and should be used very judiciously in diabetic patients. At the time of this writing, treatment studies using other newer antidepressants such as mirtazapine or venlafaxine in diabetic patients are not available.

In addition to antidepressants, numerous randomized trials have demonstrated the efficacy of psychotherapies such as cognitive behavioral therapy (CBT) for patients with depression (119). The cognitive therapist, using techniques to increase pleasurable and productive activities, works with the depressed patient to abate self-perpetuating cycles of negative thoughts, low mood, and inactivity. In a randomized controlled trial of 10-week CBT for depression in patients with type 2 DM, the researchers found that 85% of patients in the intervention group (subjects receiving CBT and diabetic education) achieved remission while only 27.3% of controls (subjects receiving diabetic education only) achieved remission ($p < 0.001$) (120). Furthermore, the effect of CBT carried through a follow-up period of six months with 70% of patients in the CBT group compared with 27.3% of controls remained remitted ($p < 0.03$). Mean glycosylated hemoglobin levels were lower in the CBT group (9.5% vs. 10.9%; $p = 0.03$) after six months of follow-up. Further analysis indicated that responders of CBT, defined as patients whose depression remitted (BDI score ≤ 9) at both post-treatment and six months follow-up evaluations, had lower glycosylated hemoglobin levels compared with nonresponders (those manifest depression with BDI scores ≥ 14 at both evaluations). CBT combined with diabetic education seems an effective nonpharmacologic treatment for depression in patients with DM.

Most patients with DM and depression are managed by their primary-care physicians. Despite the potential efficacy of depression treatment, diabetic patients with depression still experienced considerable gaps in their care. In addition to the underdetection of depression, depression-specific strategies were often not initiated even after depression is identified. Additionally, patients may be unwilling to be compliant with depression treatment because of antidepressants side effect or concerns about labeling. Health services research in primary-care systems has improved the quality of care with telephone or in-person case management intervention (121). Recently, efficacy of managed care in diabetic patients with depression has attracted significant research interest. The Improving Mood-Promoting Access to Collaborative Treatment (IMPACT) study is a randomized controlled trial of care management of depression with a total of 1801 depressed patients aged 60 years or older (122). In the IMPACT intervention, a care manager offered education, problem-solving treatment, or support for antidepressant management by the patient's primary-care physician. In the diabetes-specific subanalyses confined to 417 subjects with coexisting DM, care management of depression has been found to be effective in improving the quality of depression care as well as affective and functional status outcomes. However, glycemic control was unaffected by intervention, probably due to a much better mean glycosylated hemoglobin levels at baseline than did patients in other studies (112,120) that showed benefits on glycemic control. Another randomized, controlled trial of depression care management, the Pathways Study, recruited a total of 329 patients with DM and comorbid depression (123). Similarly, the Pathways intervention provided care management including enhanced education and support of antidepressant medication treatment prescribed by the primary-care physician or problem-solving therapy delivered in primary care. Subjects who received Pathways intervention showed greater improvement in adequacy of antidepressant dosage, less depression severity, higher self-rating global improvement, and higher satisfaction with care compared with controls. Likewise, no differences in glycosylated hemoglobin levels were observed.

Given that diabetic patients with depression have more severe disease and higher numbers of behavioral risk factors than diabetic patients without depression, a coherent view of patients' clinical problems that encompasses both disorders is required. Thus, treatment extending beyond traditional scope of antidepressant, behavioral therapy, or diabetic therapy, such as an integration between medical and mental services or an incorporated biopsychosocial intervention program, may be required to improve clinical outcomes in both of these chronic illnesses.

SUMMARY

DM is associated with cognitive dysfunction in older adults. Many studies suggested a relationship between DM and decline in frontal executive function, including psychomotor speed, attention, abstract thinking, mental flexibility, and multitasking. In addition to frontal executive function, DM has been reported to be associated with decline in other cognitive systems, including visuospatial ability, verbal memory, and global cognitive function. The accelerated cognitive decline associated with DM implies increased risk of dementia. Studies showed elderly diabetic people generally had a 50% to 90% increase in risk of developing incident dementia. Moreover, DM was consistently associated with a 2.0- to 2.6-fold increase in risk of incident VaD among older adults after comprehensive adjustment of various cardiovascular disease and risk factors. The evidence for the association between DM and AD is less consistent and more population-based prospective studies are needed. The clinician should assess elderly diabetic adults for cognitive impairment using a standardized screening instrument during the initial evaluation period and with any significant decline in clinical status because unrecognized cognitive impairment may interfere with the patient's ability to implement lifestyle modifications and take medications recommended by the clinician. In addition to performing a cognitive screening instrument like MMSE, clinicians should learn to recognize signs of executive dysfunction. If cognitive dysfunction is suggested, therapy should be simplified and prescribed in a clear step-by-step fashion in order to achieve best possible outcomes. Involvement of a caregiver in diabetic education and management can be critical to the successful management of the cognitively impaired older diabetic person.

In addition to cognitive impairment, depression is also a highly prevalent and chronically relapsing condition among diabetic patients. The odds of major depression among diabetic people were roughly twice that of those without. Although metabolic consequences of DM may lead to changes in brain structure and function, which leads to the development of depression, prospective studies did not suggest an independent role of DM in the development of depressive disorder in older adults. Metabolic derangements or cerebral vascular pathology, not necessarily specific to DM, are probably due to interactions between various cardiovascular disease and risk factors. The increased risk of depression in diabetes may merely result from the interactions between multiple vascular risk factors, increased strain of having chronic comorbidities, and certain sociocultural factors. On the other hand, a growing body of epidemiological studies of middle-aged adults demonstrated that the onset of major depressive disorder typically preceded the diagnosis of DM by many years and that depression seemed to be a major risk factor for the development of DM. Whether the association exists in older adults needs to be explored.

On initial presentation of an older diabetic adult, the clinician should assess the patient for symptoms of depression using a single screening question or consider using a standardized screening tool because a major proportion of depression are not correctly identified or optimally treated. Moreover, among older diabetic adults, depression is associated with poor glycemic control, increased diabetic complications, impaired compliance to diabetes care, as well as disability and impaired performance status. If depression is identified, treatment or referral should be initiated as soon as possible. There is strong evidence that pharmacological and psychobehavioral treatment of older diabetic adults is effective in reducing depressive symptoms. If therapy is started, targeted symptoms should be identified, documented, and regularly reevaluated. In addition to traditional depression management, care management, involving education, problem-solving treatment, or support for antidepressant management, of depression in older diabetic patients has also been found to be effective in improving the quality of depression care and affective and functional status outcomes. A biopsychosocial integration care model may be required for better care.

REFERENCES

1. Boyle JP, Honeycutt AA, Narayan KM, et al. Projection of diabetes burden through 2050: impact of changing demography and disease prevalence in the U.S. Diabetes Care 2001; 24(11):1936–1940.
2. King H, Aubert RE, Herman WH. Global burden of diabetes, 1995–2025: prevalence, numerical estimates, and projections. Diabetes Care 1998; 21(9):1414–1431.
3. Leifer BP. Early diagnosis of Alzheimer's disease: clinical and economic benefits. J Am Geriatr Soc 2003; 51(5 suppl Dementia):S281–S288.
4. Roman GC. Vascular dementia: distinguishing characteristics, treatment, and prevention. J Am Geriatr Soc 2003; 51(5 suppl Dementia):S296–S304.
5. Stewart R, Liolitsa D. Type 2 diabetes mellitus, cognitive impairment and dementia. Diabet Med 1999; 16(2):93–112.
6. Vanhanen M, Soininen H. Glucose intolerance, cognitive impairment and Alzheimer's disease. Curr Opin Neurol 1998; 11(6):673–677.
7. Elias PK, Elias MF, D'Agostino RB, et al. NIDDM and blood pressure as risk factors for poor cognitive performance. The Framingham study. Diabetes Care 1997; 20(9):1388–1395.
8. Grodstein F, Chen J, Wilson RS, Manson JE. Type 2 diabetes and cognitive function in community-dwelling elderly women. Diabetes Care 2001; 24(6):1060–1065.
9. Arvanitakis Z, Wilson RS, Li Y, Aggarwal NT, Bennett DA. Diabetes and function in different cognitive systems in older individuals without dementia. Diabetes Care 2006; 29(3):560–565.
10. Gregg EW, Yaffe K, Cauley JA, et al. Is diabetes associated with cognitive impairment and cognitive decline among older women? Study of osteoporotic fractures research group. Arch Intern Med 2000; 160(2):174–180.
11. Knopman D, Boland LL, Mosley T, et al. Cardiovascular risk factors and cognitive decline in middle-aged adults. Neurology 2001; 56(1):42–48.
12. Fontbonne A, Berr C, Ducimetiere P, Alperovitch A. Changes in cognitive abilities over a 4-year period are unfavorably affected in elderly diabetic subjects: results of the epidemiology of vascular aging study. Diabetes Care 2001; 24(2):366–370.
13. Wu JH, Haan MN, Liang J, Ghosh D, Gonzalez HM, Herman WH. Impact of diabetes on cognitive function among older Latinos: a population-based cohort study. J Clin Epidemiol 2003; 56(7):686–693.
14. Yaffe K, Blackwell T, Kanaya AM, Davidowitz N, Barrett-Connor E, Krueger K. Diabetes, impaired fasting glucose, and development of cognitive impairment in older women. Neurology 2004; 63(4):658–663.
15. Hassing LB, Grant MD, Hofer SM, et al. Type 2 diabetes mellitus contributes to cognitive decline in old age: a longitudinal population-based study. J Int Neuropsychol Soc 2004; 10(4):599–607.
16. Hassing LB, Hofer SM, Nilsson SE, et al. Comorbid type 2 diabetes mellitus and hypertension exacerbates cognitive decline: evidence from a longitudinal study. Age Ageing 2004; 33(4):355–361.
17. Logroscino G, Kang JH, Grodstein F. Prospective study of type 2 diabetes and cognitive decline in women aged 70–81 years. BMJ 2004; 328(7439):548.
18. Arvanitakis Z, Wilson RS, Bienias JL, Evans DA, Bennett DA. Diabetes mellitus and risk of Alzheimer disease and decline in cognitive function. Arch Neurol 2004; 61(5):661–666.
19. Kuo HK, Jones RN, Milberg WP, et al. Effect of blood pressure and diabetes mellitus on cognitive and physical functions in older adults: a longitudinal analysis of the advanced cognitive training for independent and vital elderly cohort. J Am Geriatr Soc 2005; 53(7):1154–1161.
20. Kokmen E, Whisnant JP, O'Fallon WM, Chu CP, Beard CM. Dementia after ischemic stroke: a population-based study in Rochester, Minnesota (1960–1984). Neurology 1996; 46(1):154–159.
21. Skoog I, Lernfelt B, Landahl S, et al. 15-year longitudinal study of blood pressure and dementia. Lancet 1996; 347(9009):1141–1145.
22. Ott A, Stolk RP, Hofman A, van Harskamp F, Grobbee DE, Breteler MM. Association of diabetes mellitus and dementia: the Rotterdam Study. Diabetologia 1996; 39(11):1392–1397.
23. Hassing LB, Johansson B, Nilsson SE, et al. Diabetes mellitus is a risk factor for vascular dementia, but not for Alzheimer's disease: a population-based study of the oldest old. Int Psychogeriatr 2002; 14(3):239–248.
24. Leibson CL, Rocca WA, Hanson VA, et al. Risk of dementia among persons with diabetes mellitus: a population-based cohort study. Am J Epidemiol 1997; 145(4):301–308.
25. Luchsinger JA, Tang MX, Stern Y, Shea S, Mayeux R. Diabetes mellitus and risk of Alzheimer's disease and dementia with stroke in a multiethnic cohort. Am J Epidemiol 2001; 154(7):635–641.

26. MacKnight C, Rockwood K, Awalt E, McDowell I. Diabetes mellitus and the risk of dementia, Alzheimer's disease and vascular cognitive impairment in the Canadian study of health and aging. Dement Geriatr Cogn Disord 2002; 14(2):77–83.
27. Ott A, Stolk RP, van Harskamp F, Pols HA, Hofman A, Breteler MM. Diabetes mellitus and the risk of dementia: the Rotterdam study. Neurology 1999; 53(9):1937–1942.
28. Peila R, Rodriguez BL, Launer LJ. Type 2 diabetes, APOE gene, and the risk for dementia and related pathologies: the Honolulu-Asia aging study. Diabetes 2002; 51(4):1256–1262.
29. Xu WL, Qiu CX, Wahlin A, Winblad B, Fratiglioni L. Diabetes mellitus and risk of dementia in the Kungsholmen project: a 6-year follow-up study. Neurology 2004; 63(7):1181–1186.
30. Yoshitake T, Kiyohara Y, Kato I, et al. Incidence and risk factors of vascular dementia and Alzheimer's disease in a defined elderly Japanese population: the Hisayama study. Neurology 1995; 45(6):1161–1168.
31. Biessels GJ, Staekenborg S, Brunner E, Brayne C, Scheltens P. Risk of dementia in diabetes mellitus: a systematic review. Lancet Neurol 2006; 5(1):64–74.
32. Cukierman T, Gerstein HC, Williamson JD. Cognitive decline and dementia in diabetes—systematic overview of prospective observational studies. Diabetologia 2005; 48(12):2460–2469.
33. Brownlee M, Vlassara H, Cerami A. Nonenzymatic glycosylation and the pathogenesis of diabetic complications. Ann Intern Med 1984; 101(4):527–537.
34. Monnier VM, Cerami A. Nonenzymatic browning in vivo: possible process for aging of long-lived proteins. Science 1981; 211(4481):491–493.
35. Smith MA, Taneda S, Richey PL, et al. Advanced Maillard reaction end products are associated with Alzheimer disease pathology. Proc Natl Acad Sci U S A 1994; 91(12):5710–5714.
36. Vitek MP, Bhattacharya K, Glendening JM, et al. Advanced glycation end products contribute to amyloidosis in Alzheimer disease. Proc Natl Acad Sci U S A 1994; 91(11):4766–4770.
37. Brownlee M. Biochemistry and molecular cell biology of diabetic complications. Nature 2001; 414(6865):813–820.
38. Du XL, Edelstein D, Rossetti L, et al. Hyperglycemia-induced mitochondrial superoxide overproduction activates the hexosamine pathway and induces plasminogen activator inhibitor-1 expression by increasing Sp1 glycosylation. Proc Natl Acad Sci U S A 2000; 97(22):12222–12226.
39. McAulay V, Deary IJ, Ferguson SC, Frier BM. Acute hypoglycemia in humans causes attentional dysfunction while nonverbal intelligence is preserved. Diabetes Care 2001; 24(10):1745–1750.
40. McAulay V, Deary IJ, Sommerfield AJ, Frier BM. Attentional functioning is impaired during acute hypoglycaemia in people with Type 1 diabetes. Diabet Med 2006; 23(1):26–31.
41. Warren RE, Allen KV, Sommerfield AJ, Deary IJ, Frier BM. Acute hypoglycemia impairs nonverbal intelligence: importance of avoiding ceiling effects in cognitive function testing. Diabetes Care 2004; 27(6):1447–1448.
42. Ewing FM, Deary IJ, McCrimmon RJ, Strachan MW, Frier BM. Effect of acute hypoglycemia on visual information processing in adults with type 1 diabetes mellitus. Physiol Behav 1998; 64(5):653–660.
43. Strachan MW, Ewing FM, Frier BM, McCrimmon RJ, Deary IJ. Effects of acute hypoglycaemia on auditory information processing in adults with Type I diabetes. Diabetologia 2003; 46(1):97–105.
44. Zhao WQ, Alkon DL. Role of insulin and insulin receptor in learning and memory. Mol Cell Endocrinol 2001; 177(1–2):125–134.
45. Hardy J, Selkoe DJ. The amyloid hypothesis of Alzheimer's disease: progress and problems on the road to therapeutics. Science 2002; 297(5580):353–356.
46. Gasparini L, Gouras GK, Wang R, et al. Stimulation of β-amyloid precursor protein trafficking by insulin reduces intraneuronal β-amyloid and requires mitogen-activated protein kinase signaling. J Neurosci 2001; 21(8):2561–2570.
47. Farris W, Mansourian S, Chang Y, et al. Insulin-degrading enzyme regulates the levels of insulin, amyloid β-protein, and the β-amyloid precursor protein intracellular domain in vivo. Proc Natl Acad Sci U S A 2003; 100(7):4162–4167.
48. Watson GS, Peskind ER, Asthana S, et al. Insulin increases CSF Aβ42 levels in normal older adults. Neurology 2003; 60(12):1899–1903.
49. Okereke O, Hankinson SE, Hu FB, Grodstein F. Plasma C peptide level and cognitive function among older women without diabetes mellitus. Arch Intern Med 2005; 165(14):1651–1656.
50. Luchsinger JA, Tang MX, Shea S, Mayeux R. Hyperinsulinemia and risk of Alzheimer disease. Neurology 2004; 63(7):1187–1192.
51. Whitmer RA, Sidney S, Selby J, Johnston SC, Yaffe K. Midlife cardiovascular risk factors and risk of dementia in late life. Neurology 2005; 64(2):277–281.
52. Kivipelto M, Ngandu T, Fratiglioni L, et al. Obesity and vascular risk factors at midlife and the risk of dementia and Alzheimer disease. Arch Neurol 2005; 62(10):1556–1560.
53. Forette F, Seux ML, Staessen JA, et al. Prevention of dementia in randomised double-blind placebo-controlled systolic hypertension in Europe (Syst-Eur) trial. Lancet 1998; 352(9137):1347–1351.
54. Tzourio C, Anderson C, Chapman N, et al. Effects of blood pressure lowering with perindopril and indapamide therapy on dementia and cognitive decline in patients with cerebrovascular disease. Arch Intern Med 2003; 163(9):1069–1075.

55. Yaffe K, Barrett-Connor E, Lin F, Grady D. Serum lipoprotein levels, statin use, and cognitive function in older women. Arch Neurol 2002; 59(3):378–384.

56. Hajjar I, Schumpert J, Hirth V, Wieland D, Eleazer GP. The impact of the use of statins on the prevalence of dementia and the progression of cognitive impairment. J Gerontol A Biol Sci Med Sci 2002; 57(7):M414–M418.

57. Gradman TJ, Laws A, Thompson LW, Reaven GM. Verbal learning and/or memory improves with glycemic control in older subjects with non-insulin-dependent diabetes mellitus. J Am Geriatr Soc 1993; 41(12):1305–1312.

58. Meneilly GS, Cheung E, Tessier D, Yakura C, Tuokko H. The effect of improved glycemic control on cognitive functions in the elderly patient with diabetes. J Gerontol 1993; 48(4):M117–M121.

59. Wu JH, Haan MN, Liang J, Ghosh D, Gonzalez HM, Herman WH. Impact of antidiabetic medications on physical and cognitive functioning of older Mexican Americans with diabetes mellitus: a population-based cohort study. Ann Epidemiol 2003; 13(5):369–376.

60. Weuve J, Kang JH, Manson JE, Breteler MM, Ware JH, Grodstein F. Physical activity, including walking, and cognitive function in older women. JAMA 2004; 292(12):1454–1461.

61. Abbott RD, White LR, Ross GW, Masaki KH, Curb JD, Petrovitch H. Walking and dementia in physically capable elderly men. JAMA 2004; 292(12):1447–1453.

62. Munshi M, Grande L, Hayes M, et al. Cognitive dysfunction is associated with poor diabetes control in older adults. Diabetes Care 2006; 29(8):1794–1799.

63. Perlmuter LC, Hakami MK, Hodgson-Harrington C, et al. Decreased cognitive function in aging non-insulin-dependent diabetic patients. Am J Med 1984; 77(6):1043–1048.

64. Sinclair AJ, Girling AJ, Bayer AJ. Cognitive dysfunction in older subjects with diabetes mellitus: impact on diabetes self-management and use of care services. All Wales Research into Elderly (AWARE) Study. Diabetes Res Clin Pract 2000; 50(3):203–212.

65. Brown AF, Mangione CM, Saliba D, Sarkisian CA. Guidelines for improving the care of the older person with diabetes mellitus. J Am Geriatr Soc 2003; 51(5 suppl Guidelines):S265–S280.

66. Anderson RJ, Freedland KE, Clouse RE, Lustman PJ. The prevalence of comorbid depression in adults with diabetes: a meta-analysis. Diabetes Care 2001; 24(6):1069–1078.

67. Lustman PJ, Griffith LS, Freedland KE, Clouse RE. The course of major depression in diabetes. Gen Hosp Psychiatry 1997; 19(2):138–143.

68. Egede LE, Zheng D, Simpson K. Comorbid depression is associated with increased health care use and expenditures in individuals with diabetes. Diabetes Care 2002; 25(3):464–470.

69. Bell RA, Smith SL, Arcury TA, Snively BM, Stafford JM, Quandt SA. Prevalence and correlates of depressive symptoms among rural older African Americans, Native Americans, and whites with diabetes. Diabetes Care 2005; 28(4):823–829.

70. Bruce DG, Casey GP, Grange V, et al. Cognitive impairment, physical disability and depressive symptoms in older diabetic patients: the Fremantle cognition in diabetes study. Diabetes Res Clin Pract 2003; 61(1):59–67.

71. Chou KL, Chi I. Prevalence of depression among elderly Chinese with diabetes. Int J Geriatr Psychiatry 2005; 20(6):570–575.

72. Finkelstein EA, Bray JW, Chen H, et al. Prevalence and costs of major depression among elderly claimants with diabetes. Diabetes Care 2003; 26(2):415–420.

73. Alexopoulos GS, Meyers BS, Young RC, Campbell S, Silbersweig D, Charlson M. "Vascular depression" hypothesis. Arch Gen Psychiatry 1997; 54(10):915–922.

74. Kessing LV, Nilsson FM, Siersma V, Andersen PK. No increased risk of developing depression in diabetes compared to other chronic illness. Diabetes Res Clin Pract 2003; 62(2):113–121.

75. Palinkas LA, Lee PP, Barrett-Connor E. A prospective study of Type 2 diabetes and depressive symptoms in the elderly: the Rancho Bernardo study. Diabet Med 2004; 21(11):1185–1191.

76. Bisschop MI, Kriegsman DM, Deeg DJ, Beekman AT, van Tilburg W. The longitudinal relation between chronic diseases and depression in older persons in the community: the longitudinal aging study Amsterdam. J Clin Epidemiol 2004; 57(2):187–194.

77. Geringer E. Affective disorders and dibetes mellitus. In: Neuropsychological and Behavioral Aspect of Diabetes. New York: Springer-Verlag, 1990.

78. Eaton WW, Armenian H, Gallo J, Pratt L, Ford DE. Depression and risk for onset of type II diabetes. A prospective population-based study. Diabetes Care 1996; 19(10):1097–1102.

79. Kawakami N, Takatsuka N, Shimizu H, Ishibashi H. Depressive symptoms and occurrence of type 2 diabetes among Japanese men. Diabetes Care 1999; 22(7):1071–1076.

80. Everson-Rose SA, Meyer PM, Powell LH, et al. Depressive symptoms, insulin resistance, and risk of diabetes in women at midlife. Diabetes Care 2004; 27(12):2856–2862.

81. Arroyo C, Hu FB, Ryan LM, et al. Depressive symptoms and risk of type 2 diabetes in women. Diabetes Care 2004; 27(1):129–133.

82. Golden SH, Williams JE, Ford DE, et al. Depressive symptoms and the risk of type 2 diabetes: the atherosclerosis risk in communities study. Diabetes Care 2004; 27(2):429–435.

83. Hayward C. Psychiatric illness and cardiovascular disease risk. Epidemiol Rev 1995; 17(1):129–138.

84. Talbot F, Nouwen A. A review of the relationship between depression and diabetes in adults: is there a link? Diabetes Care 2000; 23(10):1556–1562.

85. Brown LC, Majumdar SR, Newman SC, Johnson JA. History of depression increases risk of type 2 diabetes in younger adults. Diabetes Care 2005; 28(5):1063–1067.

86. Lustman PJ, Anderson RJ, Freedland KE, de Groot M, Carney RM, Clouse RE. Depression and poor glycemic control: a meta-analytic review of the literature. Diabetes Care 2000; 23(7):934–942.

87. de Groot M, Anderson R, Freedland KE, Clouse RE, Lustman PJ. Association of depression and diabetes complications: a meta-analysis. Psychosom Med 2001; 63(4):619–630.

88. Cuijpers P, Smit F. Excess mortality in depression: a meta-analysis of community studies. J Affect Disord 2002; 72(3):227–236.

89. Sheps DS, McMahon RP, Becker L, et al. Mental stress-induced ischemia and all-cause mortality in patients with coronary artery disease: results from the psychophysiological investigations of myocardial ischemia study. Circulation 2002; 105(15):1780–1784.

90. Lesperance F, Frasure-Smith N, Talajic M, Bourassa MG. Five-year risk of cardiac mortality in relation to initial severity and one-year changes in depression symptoms after myocardial infarction. Circulation 2002; 105(9):1049–1053.

91. Lewis SC, Dennis MS, O'Rourke SJ, Sharpe M. Negative attitudes among short-term stroke survivors predict worse long-term survival. Stroke 2001; 32(7):1640–1645.

92. Jiang W, Alexander J, Christopher E, et al. Relationship of depression to increased risk of mortality and rehospitalization in patients with congestive heart failure. Arch Intern Med 2001; 161(15):1849–1856.

93. Berkman LF, Melchior M, Chastang JF, Niedhammer I, Leclerc A, Goldberg M. Social integration and mortality: a prospective study of French employees of electricity of France-Gas of France: the GAZEL cohort. Am J Epidemiol 2004; 159(2):167–174.

94. Zhang X, Norris SL, Gregg EW, Cheng YJ, Beckles G, Kahn HS. Depressive symptoms and mortality among persons with and without diabetes. Am J Epidemiol 2005; 161(7):652–660.

95. Egede LE, Nietert PJ, Zheng D. Depression and all-cause and coronary heart disease mortality among adults with and without diabetes. Diabetes Care 2005; 28(6):1339–1345.

96. Katon WJ, Rutter C, Simon G, et al. The association of comorbid depression with mortality in patients with type 2 diabetes. Diabetes Care 2005; 28(11):2668–2672.

97. Ciechanowski PS, Katon WJ, Russo JE. Depression and diabetes: impact of depressive symptoms on adherence, function, and costs. Arch Intern Med 2000; 160(21):3278–3285.

98. Lin EH, Katon W, Von Korff M, et al. Relationship of depression and diabetes self-care, medication adherence, and preventive care. Diabetes Care 2004; 27(9):2154–2160.

99. Kilbourne AM, Reynolds CF III, Good CB, Sereika SM, Justice AC, Fine MJ. How does depression influence diabetes medication adherence in older patients? Am J Geriatr Psychiatry 2005; 13(3):202–210.

100. Wray LA, Ofstedal MB, Langa KM, Blaum CS. The effect of diabetes on disability in middle-aged and older adults. J Gerontol A Biol Sci Med Sci 2005; 60(9):1206–1211.

101. Lyness JM, King DA, Cox C, Yoediono Z, Caine ED. The importance of subsyndromal depression in older primary care patients: prevalence and associated functional disability. J Am Geriatr Soc 1999; 47(6):647–652.

102. Egede LE. Diabetes, major depression, and functional disability among U.S. adults. Diabetes Care 2004; 27(2):421–428.

103. Egede LE. Effects of depression on work loss and disability bed days in individuals with diabetes. Diabetes Care 2004; 27(7):1751–1753.

104. Goldney RD, Phillips PJ, Fisher LJ, Wilson DH. Diabetes, depression, and quality of life: a population study. Diabetes Care 2004; 27(5):1066–1070.

105. Black SA, Markides KS, Ray LA. Depression predicts increased incidence of adverse health outcomes in older Mexican Americans with type 2 diabetes. Diabetes Care 2003; 26(10):2822–2828.

106. Rubin RR, Ciechanowski P, Egede LE, Lin EH, Lustman PJ. Recognizing and treating depression in patients with diabetes. Curr Diab Rep 2004; 4(2):119–125.

107. Lustman PJ, Harper GW. Nonpsychiatric physicians' identification and treatment of depression in patients with diabetes. Compr Psychiatry 1987; 28(1):22–27.

108. Lustman PJ, Clouse RE, Griffith LS, Carney RM, Freedland KE. Screening for depression in diabetes using the Beck depression inventory. Psychosom Med 1997; 59(1):24–31.

109. Wright MJ, White A, Glover M, Lewin TJ, Harmon KD. Patients with diabetes and impaired glucose tolerance—is it feasible to screen for depression? Aust Fam Physician 2005; 34(7):607–608.

110. Rakovac I, Gfrerer RJ, Habacher W, et al. Screening of depression in patients with diabetes mellitus. Diabetologia 2004; 47(8):1469–1470.

111. Goodnick PJ, Kumar A, Henry JH, Buki VM, Goldberg RB. Sertraline in coexisting major depression and diabetes mellitus. Psychopharmacol Bull 1997; 33(2):261–264.

112. Lustman PJ, Freedland KE, Griffith LS, Clouse RE. Fluoxetine for depression in diabetes: a randomized double-blind placebo-controlled trial. Diabetes Care 2000; 23(5):618–623.

113. Furman BL. The hypoglycaemic effect of 5-hydroxytryptophan. Br J Pharmacol 1974; 50(4): 575–580.
114. Wilson GA, Furman BL. Effects of inhibitors of 5-hydroxytryptamine uptake on plasma glucose and their interaction with 5-hydroxytryptophan in producing hypoglycaemia in mice. Eur J Pharmacol 1982; 78(3):263–270.
115. Potter van Loon BJ, Radder JK, Frolich M, Krans HM, Zwinderman AH, Meinders AE. Fluoxetine increases insulin action in obese nondiabetic and in obese non-insulin-dependent diabetic individuals. Int J Obes Relat Metab Disord 1992; 16(2):79–85.
116. Ferguson JM, Feighner JP. Fluoxetine-induced weight loss in overweight non-depressed humans. Int J Obes 1987; 11(suppl 3):163–170.
117. Harris B, Young J, Hughes B. Changes occurring in appetite and weight during short-term antidepressant treatment. Br J Psychiatry 1984; 145:645–648.
118. Paykel ES, Mueller PS, De la Vergne PM. Amitriptyline, weight gain and carbohydrate craving: a side effect. Br J Psychiatry 1973; 123(576):501–507.
119. Practice Guideline for Major Depressive Disorder in Adults. Washington, DC: American Psychiatric Association, 1993.
120. Lustman PJ, Griffith LS, Freedland KE, Kissel SS, Clouse RE. Cognitive behavior therapy for depression in type 2 diabetes mellitus. A randomized, controlled trial. Ann Intern Med 1998; 129(8): 613–621.
121. Walsh EG, Osber DS, Nason CA, Porell MA, Asciutto AJ. Quality improvement in a primary care case management program. Health Care Financ Rev 2002; 23(4):71–84.
122. Williams JW Jr, Katon W, Lin EH, et al. The effectiveness of depression care management on diabetes-related outcomes in older patients. Ann Intern Med 2004; 140(12):1015–1024.
123. Katon WJ, Von Korff M, Lin EH, et al. The pathways study: a randomized trial of collaborative care in patients with diabetes and depression. Arch Gen Psychiatry 2004; 61(10):1042–1049.

7 | Falls Risk and Prevention in the Diabetic Patient

Lewis A. Lipsitz[a] and Attila Priplata
Hebrew SeniorLife Institute for Aging Research, Beth Israel Deaconess Medical Center, Harvard Medical School, Boston, Massachusetts, U.S.A.

EPIDEMIOLOGY

Falls are a common occurrence among elderly people that often result in serious injury and loss of independent function. Approximately 30% of community-dwelling elders and 50% of those living in nursing homes fall each year. Two-thirds of accidental deaths in the United States are due to falls, nearly three quarters of which occur among people over 65 years of age. Approximately 10% to 15% of falls lead to fractures and many more are associated with lacerations, bruises, hemorrhage, fear of falling, and a decline in functional status. Falls often result in hospitalization, restricted activity, and nursing home admission, costing the United States over $32 billion annually.

Older people with diabetes are particularly vulnerable to falls and related complications. In the large prospective Study of Osteoporotic Fractures, community-dwelling women with diabetes aged 67 years and older had an increased risk of recurrent falls during an average follow-up of 7.2 years (1). Those with non–insulin-treated diabetes had an age-adjusted odds ratio of 1.68 [95% confidence interval (CI) = 1.37–2.07] for more than one fall per year, while those with insulin-treated diabetes had an age-adjusted odds ratio of 2.78 (CI = 1.82–4.24). The risk of falls was attributable to an increased rate of known falls risk factors in the non–insulin-treated group, but not in women treated with insulin. Therefore, insulin-treated diabetes appears to be an independent risk for falls in elderly women.

Diabetes is also a powerful independent predictor of falls in disabled populations. In the Women's Health and Aging Study I (2), women with diabetes had a higher risk of any fall during the three-year follow-up period (odds ratio adjusted for traditional risk factors = 1.38, 95% CI = 1.04–1.81) as well as of two or more falls (adjusted odds ratio = 1.69, CI = 1.18–2.43), compared with women without diabetes. Also, those on insulin therapy were at higher risk compared with those on oral hypoglycemic agents. There were interactions between diabetes and lower extremity pain, and diabetes and body mass index, such that diabetics with more pain or higher body mass index had the greatest risk of falls. Insulin-treated diabetics with multiple sites of pain were at the highest risk, with an odds ratio of 6.5 (95% CI = 2.98–14.2).

In another prospective cohort study of 139 nursing home residents followed for an average of 299 days, diabetes treated with either oral agents or insulin was again independently associated with an increased risk of falls (adjusted hazard ratio 4.03, 95% CI = 1.96–8.28) (3). In all of the above studies, the subjects were predominantly women. Therefore, the results may not be generalizable to older men.

Diabetes increases not only the risk of falls, but also the risk of fractures. In the Health, Aging, and Body Composition Study, diabetes (but not impaired fasting glucose) was associated with an increased incidence of nontraumatic fractures over a 4.5-year (± 1.1 SD) follow-up period, independent of hip bone mineral density and fracture risk factors [relative risk (RR) = 1.64; 95% CI = 1.07–2.51] (4). Diabetic subjects with fractures had lower hip bone mineral density and lean body mass and were more likely to have impaired peripheral sensation, transient ischemic attacks or strokes, lower physical performance scores, and falls, compared with those without fractures in this study. The higher incidence of fractures in diabetic white women than

---

[a]Dr. Lipsitz holds the Irving and Edyth S. Usen and Family Chair in Geriatric Medicine at Hebrew SeniorLife.

in those with normal glucose may be due to a more rapid bone loss at the femoral neck (5). The more rapid bone loss has not been observed in diabetic men or black women.

PATHOPHYSIOLOGY OF FALLS

The increased risk of falling in older age is associated with (*i*) age-related changes in postural control, blood pressure (BP) regulation, and cerebral perfusion, and (*ii*) disease-related conditions, including medications that accumulate with aging and impair an older person's adaptive capacity. Type II diabetes is a common disease of elderly people that interacts with normal aging to further compromise adaptive capacity. Thus, when exposed to common everyday physical stresses, such as environmental hazards or other perturbations, elderly people with diabetes may not be able to mount the normal compensatory mechanisms that ordinarily would prevent them from falling. Age- and diabetes-related causes of falls are reviewed in the following section.

Age-Related Changes in Postural Control

There are many physiologic changes believed to be associated with human aging that impair postural control and predispose older people to falling (6). These include loss of muscle mass and strength (7); more cocontraction of antagonist muscles in the lower extremities (8); reduced nerve conduction velocity and reflex response time; loss of neurons, dendritic connections, and neurotransmitters (e.g., dopamine) in the frontal cortex and basal ganglia (9); reductions in visual acuity, depth perception, contrast sensitivity, and dark adaptation in the visual system (10); proprioceptive sensory loss in the lower extremities (11); and loss of hair cells, ganglion neurons, and otoconia in the vestibular system (12).

As a result of these changes older people demonstrate an increase in postural sway when their center of pressure is recorded on a balance platform. Using traditional center of pressure analysis and a dynamic technique called "stabilogram diffusion analysis" (SDA), which treats the moment-to-moment changes in center of pressure as a random walk, the postural strategies used to maintain upright balance can be identified and explained (13). The traditional sway parameters, computed relative to the geometric center of pressure, include the mean stabilogram radius (in mm), the area swept by the stabilogram over time (in mm^2), the maximum radius of sway (in mm), and the range of the anteroposterior (AP) and mediolateral (ML) excursions (in mm). Any increase in these traditional measures would indicate an increase in postural sway.

The SDA technique demonstrates that the postural control system uses two types of control mechanisms while standing. The first is an open-loop control mechanism, manifest as a random drift away from the base of support over a very short time period (less than a second) or for a very small distance. This short-term stochastic behavior does not use sensory feedback to keep the body upright and relies on the mechanical interactions of muscles and joints. But over longer time periods and greater distances, a closed-loop, feedback-driven system is operative that corrects postural deviations and returns the center of pressure toward the base of support. This mechanism relies on visual, vestibular, and somatosensory feedbacks (13).

Earlier studies that compared healthy elderly with healthy young subjects showed that elderly people travel farther in distance and longer in time before switching from open-loop to closed-loop feedback postural control mechanisms [indicated by an increase in the critical mean square displacement, $\langle\Delta r^2\rangle_c$ (mm^2)] (14). Moreover, elderly subjects show a stronger tendency to return toward their base of support when they sway beyond the switching threshold (indicated by a decrease in the long-term scaling exponent, H_l, usually less than 0.5). However, before reaching the switching threshold, elderly subjects are more likely to sway further away from their base of support (indicated by an increase in the short-term scaling exponent, H_{rs}, usually greater than 0.5). These changes are exaggerated in elderly subjects at risk of falls and in subjects with diabetes. Within the modeling framework of traditional and SDA measures, these findings suggest that elderly subjects, particularly those with falls or diabetes, have greater postural sway, a higher feedback threshold, and a stiffer, less finely tuned control system when compared with healthy young individuals (Table 1) (15,16).

A recent study found that muscle activity in elderly fallers is highly correlated with increases in postural sway over short-term time intervals (8). Moreover, there is more

TABLE 1 Dimensionless Values of the Traditional and SDA Sway
Parameters at Baseline for 42 Subjects

Parameters	Young	Elderly	Diabetics
Traditional			
Mean radius	5.1 ± 0.4	5.5 ± 0.5	6.1 ± 0.4
Swept area	335.5 ± 24.5	477.6 ± 64.0	472.0 ± 58.0
Max radius	12.3 ± 0.6	13.9 ± 1.3	15.2 ± 1.0^{a}
Range anteroposterior	19.9 ± 1.0	22.5 ± 1.9	25.3 ± 1.5^{a}
Range mediolateral	13.5 ± 0.7	15.7 ± 1.8	16.5 ± 1.9
SDA			
$<\Delta r^2>_c$	42.3 ± 3.9	68.3 ± 10.9	78.0 ± 11.9^{a}
H_{rs}	0.74 ± 0.01	0.78 ± 0.02	0.83 ± 0.02^{c}
H_{rl}	0.24 ± 0.02	0.14 ± 0.03^{b}	0.15 ± 0.03^{a}

Note: 15 Healthy young, aged 19–27, mean 23 years; 12 healthy elderly, aged 68–78, mean
73 years; and 15 diabetics, aged 38–81, mean 60 years. The group mean and standard error
for each parameter are shown.
[a]Significant difference between young subjects and subjects with diabetes ($P < 0.05$).
[b]Significant difference between young subjects and elderly subjects ($P < 0.05$).
[c]Significant difference among young subjects, elderly subjects, and subjects with diabetes
($P < 0.05$).
Abbreviation: SDA, stabilogram diffusion analysis.
Source: From Refs. 15, 16.

cocontraction of lower extremity antagonistic muscles in the elderly (8), which may lead to
stiffness, delays in appropriate muscle activation, and failure to rapidly develop lower extremity joint torque in response to a postural disturbance (17,18). Thus, increases in lower extremity
muscle activity and short-term postural sway may compromise an individual's ability to maintain upright stance.

Another difference in postural control that has been observed between healthy young and
old subjects is the pattern of muscle activation in response to a perturbation of the surface of
support. While young subjects compensate by activating distal muscles, such as the tibialis
anterior and soleus, before proximal hip muscles, elderly subjects tend to show the opposite
pattern (19). This is an inefficient strategy that may also lead to falls.

Age-Related Changes in BP Regulation and Cerebral Blood Flow
Baroreflex Impairment
The ability to stand and walk upright is dependent on maintaining an adequate BP to perfuse
the brain and other vital organs. Ordinarily, the baroreflex maintains a normal BP by increasing
heart rate and vascular resistance in response to transient reductions in stretch of arterial baroreceptors in the carotid arteries and aorta, and by decreasing these parameters in response to an
increase in stretch of baroreceptors. Normal human aging is associated with a reduction in
baroreflex sensitivity. This is evident in the blunted cardioacceleratory response to stimuli such
as upright posture, nitroprusside infusion, and lower-body negative pressure which all lower
arterial pressure, as well as a reduced bradycardic response to drugs such as phenylephrine
that elevate pressure. Furthermore, baroreflex impairment is manifest by an increase in BP variability during common daily activities (20), often with potentially dangerous BP reductions
during hypotensive stresses such as upright posture or meal digestion. With the superimposi-
tion of conditions such as diabetic autonomic neuropathy, or medications with hypotensive
effects, orthostatic and postprandial hypotension may result, causing falls and syncope in
elderly people.

Dehydration
Dehydration is another physiologic change that predisposes older people to falls and syncope.
Older people are particularly vulnerable to dehydration due to impairment in renal salt and
water conservation. When exposed to a salt-restricted diet, elderly individuals excrete
larger quantities of salt and water than their younger counterparts, leading to volume contraction (21). This is probably due to the reductions in renin and aldosterone concentrations, as well

as the elevations in natriuretic peptide associated with aging (22). Consequently, elderly people may rapidly become dehydrated when exposed to fluid restriction, diuretics, or hot weather. The development of diabetes and glucosuria further increases this risk by causing an osmotic diuresis.

Diastolic Dysfunction

One more important age-related change that affects cardiac output and BP is diastolic dysfunction. With aging, the heart stiffens due to increased cross-linking of myocardial collagen and prolongation of ventricular relaxation time. As a result, early diastolic ventricular filling is impaired, and the heart becomes dependent on adequate preload to fill the ventricle and on atrial contraction during late diastole to maintain stroke volume. Consequently, orthostatic hypotension and syncope occur commonly in older persons as a result of volume contraction or venous pooling, which reduce cardiac preload, or at the onset of atrial fibrillation when the atrial contribution to cardiac output is suddenly lost.

Cerebral Blood Flow

Resting cerebral blood flow declines with aging (23), placing elderly people closer to the threshold for cerebral ischemia if perfusion pressure suddenly falls. Although cerebral autoregulation remains intact in most healthy elderly people (24), a rapid fall in BP may not leave adequate time for cerebral autoregulatory mechanisms to respond. Furthermore, many elderly individuals have a resting cerebral perfusion that is further compromised by diabetes and/or vascular disease, making them even more vulnerable to cerebral ischemic symptoms such as falls.

Diabetes-Related Causes of Falls

A myriad of comorbid conditions and complications associated with diabetes are largely responsible for the high prevalence of falls among this population. The conditions associated with diabetes that may result in falls are listed in Table 2.

Peripheral sensory neuropathy is one of the most salient effects of diabetes that can result in falls (25). People with diabetic peripheral neuropathy have impaired peripheral sensation, reaction time, and balance; reduced walking speed, cadence, and step length; and less rhythmic acceleration patterns at the head and pelvis while walking (26). These abnormalities are exaggerated while walking on an irregular surface. During quiet standing, patients with diabetic sensory neuropathy also demonstrate greater center of pressure displacement (sway) in the AP and ML directions than healthy age-matched controls, both with eyes open and closed (27). Even in mild diabetic patients with early peripheral neuropathy there is an increase in whole body reaction time to lateral platform movement, which may lead to falls (28).

Autonomic neuropathy is another important cause of falls that is particularly relevant to the diabetic population (29). It can appear subclinically and may affect all parts of the autonomic nervous system. Although it produces falls most commonly via orthostatic hypotension, autonomic neuropathy may also cause exercise intolerance, silent cardiac ischemia, diarrhea, urinary incontinence, hypoglycemia unawareness, and dehydration, which may all result in falls. Autonomic neuropathy is reviewed in Chapter 17 of this book.

TABLE 2   Causes of Falls in Patients with Diabetes

Metabolic: hyper- and hypoglycemia, dehydration, ketoacidosis (rare in the elderly)
Vascular
Cardiovascular: ischemic heart disease, congestive heart failure, arrhythmias
Peripheral vascular disease: claudication, ischemic ulcers, foot lesions
Cerebrovascular: stroke, TIAs, microvascular disease
Peripheral nervous system:
Peripheral neuropathy
Autonomic neuropathy, orthostatic, and postprandial hypotension
Lumbar polyradiculopathy (diabetic amyotrophy)
Visual: diabetic retinopathy
Musculoskeletal: deconditioning and atrophy
Environmental hazards

Abbreviation: TIA, transient ischemic attack.

Each of the conditions in Table 2 makes it difficult for the elderly diabetic patient to adapt to environmental hazards such as poor lighting, slippery floors or walkways, throw rugs, loose objects, thresholds, steps, and glare. In most cases, it is not acceptable to blame falls on an environmental hazard alone without seeking the underlying disease or physical condition that impaired the patient's adaptive response.

PREDICTORS OF FALLS IN ELDERLY DIABETICS

A few studies have examined risk factors for falls in a variety of populations with diabetes (Table 3). Among them, peripheral neuropathy and poor lower extremity function are consistent predictors. Other risk factors including poor mobility, multiple medications (especially psychotropic medications), and musculoskeletal pain are common to all fallers, regardless of the presence of diabetes.

EVALUATION OF THE FALLER

Since hypoglycemia is a common condition that can present as a fall in the elderly diabetic, it should be ruled out by evaluation of a fingerstick blood glucose whenever possible at the time of the fall. Once acute hypoglycemia is excluded or no longer assessable, the evaluation should proceed with a thorough history and a physical examination, which, in most cases, are sufficient to identify the cause.

History

The patient and any witnesses should be asked to describe the events preceding the fall, including activities, medication administration, symptoms, and circumstances occurring during the hour preceding the fall. In particular, a physician should note whether the episode occurred after a change in posture from lying down or sitting to standing or after a long period of standing; either event suggests orthostatic hypotension as a cause. If a fall occurred within an hour or two of eating a meal, it might represent postprandial hypotension or hypoglycemia. A history of cognitive dysfunction may suggest the possibility of a skipped meal that can result in hypoglycemia and falling. If a fall occurred during exercise, tachyarrhythmias such as ventricular tachycardia and reduced cardiac output due to aortic stenosis should be considered possible causes. A seizure disorder is suggested when a fall is preceded by an olfactory or a gustatory

TABLE 3 Independent Predictors of Falls in Elderly Diabetics

Study	Elder	SOF	WHAS	Puget sound
Population:	Multiethnic rural	Community cohort	Disabled women	History of foot ulcers
Male sex	X	—	—	—
Peripheral neuropathy	X	X	—	X
Previous stroke or cardiovascular disease	X	X	—	—
Longer duration of diabetes mellitus	X	—	—	—
Impaired physical function	X	—	—	—
Poor mobility	X	—	—	—
Greater number of medications	X	—	—	—
Widespread musculoskeletal pain or arthritis	—	X	X	—
Insulin therapy	—	—	X	—
Overweight	—	—	X	X
Poor lower extremity performance	—	—	X	—
Poor balance	—	X	—	—

Source: From Refs. 1, 2, 30, and 31.

aura or is accompanied by tongue biting, tonic-clonic movements, or incontinence, followed by postictal confusion.

The patient or caregiver should be asked about all medications the patient may be taking, including those prescribed by consultants, eye medications, and over-the-counter (OTC) drugs. Many OTC drugs, especially antihistamines and medications for sleep or gastrointestinal symptoms, have anticholinergic properties, which can cause confusion, postural instability, tachycardia, or orthostatic hypotension.

The nature of recovery from a fall can also provide important clues to its etiology and outcome. Often patients are unable to get up after a fall, which portends a poor prognosis (32). This may not only lead to dehydration, renal failure, and hypothermia if the patient is not found promptly, but also signal a seizure disorder, stroke, or cardiac event.

A full review of symptoms is also important. Specifically, the patient should be asked about symptoms of peripheral and autonomic neuropathies, including burning, tingling, or decreased sensation of the feet and hands for the former and poor night vision, early satiety, diarrhea, constipation, urinary frequency or retention, sexual dysfunction, abnormal sweating, or postural dizziness for the latter.

Physical Examination

To diagnose orthostatic hypotension, BP and heart rate should be measured with the patient supine after resting for five minutes; then with the patient upright after standing (or sitting, if the patient is unable to stand) for one minute and three minutes. Orthostatic hypotension is diagnosed if systolic BP decreases by at least 20 mmHg or diastolic BP decreases by 10 mmHg. A small (<10 beats/min) or no increase in heart rate with standing or sitting may indicate autonomic impairment or a drug effect; tachycardia (heart rate>100 beats/min), which is rare in response to postural change in elderly people, may indicate volume depletion.

The carotid arteries are palpated and auscultated for bruits to look for evidence of flow abnormalities and to determine whether the patient may be a candidate for carotid sinus massage. The heart is auscultated for murmurs of aortic stenosis, mitral regurgitation, mitral stenosis, or hypertrophic cardiomyopathy, which are the most common structural cardiac causes of syncopal falls. A neurologic examination is essential for detecting the rigidity, bradykinesia, and abnormal gait of Parkinsonism or multiple systems atrophy; focal abnormalities that may indicate cerebrovascular disease or space-occupying lesions; and signs of peripheral neuropathy.

One of the most revealing examination techniques is to watch the patient perform the activity that was associated with the fall. One can often observe physical impairments or risky behaviors while reaching for objects, turning in a circle, stepping over obstacles, opening a door, or transferring from a bed or chair. If the patient fell or fainted after a meal, medication, and/or change in posture, BP should be measured under similar circumstances. This can be done in the outpatient setting by obtaining a baseline BP, then asking the patient to take their medications in the office or eat a meal in the waiting room or cafeteria and returning for repeated measurements 30 and 60 minutes later. If the patient fell after standing up, taking medications, and eating, measurements should be taken after this sequence of hypotensive events.

Finally, a "Get up and go test" should be performed to assess muscle strength, balance, and gait. This involves asking the patient to stand up from an armchair without using his or her own arms to push off. They should cross their arms in front of them and try to stand. Inability to do so suggests they have weak extensor muscles of the thighs (gluteus maximu) and knees (quadriceps), which may be remediable with strengthening exercises. Next, the patient is asked to stand still for a Romberg test with eyes open and then closed. An increase in sway with eyes closed indicates reliance on visual input to maintain balance. This can be remedied with treatment of cataracts or improved environmental lighting. A wide-based, unsteady stance with eyes open may indicate cerebellar deficits. Next, the patient is asked to walk 20 ft, turn in a circle, and return while the examiner observes their gait and balance. In Table 4, the different abnormalities in gait that can be detected and the specific treatments for each are listed. The "Get up and go test" can be timed to quantify the extent of a patient's mobility impairment and assess the response to treatment (33).

TABLE 4 Abnormalities of Gait and Their Treatment

Gait abnormality	Common cause	Treatment
Shuffle and festination	Parkinson's disease	Dopamine agonists
Start hesitation and petit-pas	Frontal subcortical microvascular disease and stroke	CV risk reduction
Hemiparetic	Stroke	CV risk reduction, physical therapy
Ataxic	Cerebellar degeneration, alcohol, stroke	Avoid alcohol, CV risk reduction, physical therapy
Antalgic	Osteoarthritis of hip and knee	Nonsteroidal anti-inflammatory agents, PT
Spastic	Cervical spondylosis	Cervical collar, PT
Foot drop	Peroneal palsy	Foot brace
Sensory	Peripheral neuropathy	Control of diabetes mellitus, cane, foot care

Abbreviations: CV, cardiovascular; PT, physical therapy.

Laboratory Testing

Laboratory testing is often necessary in elderly diabetic fallers because falls may be the atypical presentation of conditions not ordinarily expected to produce them. A resting electrocardiogram (ECG) should be done to detect arrhythmias, conduction abnormalities, ischemia, or infarction. Pulse oximetry should be done if patients are evaluated immediately after a fall. Other routine tests should include a white blood cell count to detect occult infection and hematocrit to detect anemia. Electrolytes, blood urea nitrogen, and creatinine should be measured to help assess hydration status and rule out electrolyte disorders. Review of self-monitored blood glucose records or measurements of plasma glucose may help exclude hypoglycemia or hyperglycemia. A fall may be the first sign of hyperosmolar dehydration with hyperglycemia.

Other, more specialized laboratory tests are done only if indicated by the history and physical examination. If the patient was exercising or experiencing chest pain or dyspnea just before the fall or if ECG abnormalities are present, cardiac enzymes should be measured to rule out myocardial infarction. If the patient is taking an antiarrhythmic medication, an anticonvulsant, or digoxin, measuring drug concentration levels may help determine whether the drug level is subtherapeutic, therapeutic, or toxic. If the drug level is subtherapeutic, the fall may have resulted from inadequate treatment of a known predisposing disorder, such as a seizure disorder. If the drug level is toxic (sometimes even within the usual therapeutic range), a syncopal fall may have resulted from a drug-induced proarrhythmia.

Ambulatory ECG monitoring (with a Holter, loop, or implantable recorder) should be done only when the history strongly suggests arrhythmia as the cause (e.g., when the fall is associated with otherwise unexplained syncope), and the patient is a candidate for treatment. Even in such circumstances, results can be difficult to interpret because monitoring usually detects no arrhythmias or so many asymptomatic arrhythmias that their relationship to a fall is uncertain. Loop event recorders can be worn continuously for one month or implanted for longer periods and activated when symptoms occur. A memory function records several minutes of cardiac rhythm before the recorder is activated; thus, patients can document an arrhythmia by activating the recorder after recovering from a fall or syncope. Similarly, electrophysiologic studies should be reserved for elderly patients who have recurrent unexplained syncope and who have ECG or other clinical evidence of coronary artery disease or a structural cardiac disorder.

Ambulatory BP monitoring should be done to detect hypotension if falls occur soon after activities that potentially predispose to hypotension (e.g., eating meals, taking drugs, postural changes). Because BP monitors are often heavy and cumbersome, patients may prefer to use a portable automated device and diary to record BP at certain times of day, including early morning after arising from bed, one hour after taking drugs or eating, and at the time the fall occurred.

Recent studies suggest that carotid hypersensitivity is an often-overlooked cause of falls, particularly among patients with risk factors for cardiovascular disease, including diabetes (34).

Therefore, carotid sinus massage should be done to detect carotid sinus hypersensitivity when no other cause of a fall or syncope is apparent, but only in patients who have no evidence of cerebrovascular disease (e.g., carotid bruit, previous stroke, transient ischemic attacks) or cardiac conduction abnormalities. The technique involves a circular five-second massage of one carotid sinus at a time while an ECG is recording the patient's cardiac rhythm. BP is measured before and immediately after each massage. Carotid sinus massage is usually safe when done for five seconds in carefully screened patients. Serious complications (e.g., stroke) can occur in patients with underlying cerebrovascular disease or during vigorous, prolonged massage.

Doppler echocardiography should be done in patients with exercise-induced syncope or with previously undetected murmurs to check for hemodynamically significant valvular heart disease and hypertrophic cardiomyopathy.

Tilt-table testing should be reserved for patients whose fall history suggests reflex-mediated syncope or orthostatic hypotension when the physical examination is not diagnostic. A head-up tilt at 60° to 80° for up to 45 minutes can precipitate neurally mediated (vasova-gal) syncope with associated bradycardia and hypotension. Using isoproterenol can increase the test's sensitivity. However, isoproterenol is often contraindicated in elderly patients with known or suspected coronary artery disease. The development of vasovagal syncope during the tilt table test only suggests that vasovagal syncope may have caused the unexplained episode. Usually, vasovagal syncope can be readily diagnosed without the tilt test from a history of typical vagal prodromes (e.g., nausea; light-headedness; pale, cold, clammy skin). The tilt test may also help identify delayed orthostatic hypotension as the cause of a fall or syncope.

An electro encephalogram (EEG) should be performed only when a seizure is suspected. Clinical experience suggests that this test has little value unless the history yields evidence of a seizure or underlying focal neurologic abnormality. Similarly, brain imaging with computed tomography or magnetic resonance (MR) imaging is useful for the evaluation of focal neuro-logic abnormalities when a stroke, intracranial hemorrhage, brain tumor, or hydrocephalus is suspected. MR imaging of the spine is helpful in the hyperreflexic, spastic patient to rule out cervical spondylosis or spinal cord compression.

Finally, patients with vertigo, hearing loss, or unexplained dizziness may benefit from referral to an otolaryngologist for vestibular testing, an audiogram, and appropriate treatment.

PREVENTION OF FALLS

The prevention of falls requires the identification of all potential risk factors and efforts to eradi-cate or lessen the impact of those that are modifiable. Several previous studies have shown that multifactorial interventions that target modifiable risks can reduce the annual incidence of falls by 25% to 39% (35). Consensus guidelines for the prevention of falls in older persons have been published previously (36). Interventions shown to be effective in preventing falls are listed in Table 5.

Preventive efforts can generally be targeted to four categories of risk: (*i*) lower extremity leg extension weakness, (*ii*) poor balance, (*iii*) medication toxicity (including alcohol), and (*iv*) hypotension. In addition, the environment should be made safe by eliminating hazards and installing adaptive equipment. There are several promising new approaches to the treatment of

TABLE 5   Interventions Shown to Prevent Falls in Elderly People

Intervention	Risk or odds ratio
Muscle strengthening and balance training	0.80
Tai Chi Chuan	0.51
Home hazard assessment and modification	0.64
Withdrawal of psychotropic medications	0.34
Multidisciplinary multifactorial intervention	0.75
Vitamin D	0.78

Source: From Refs. 35, 37.

peripheral neuropathy that may be particularly relevant to elderly fallers with diabetes. Each of these interventions is summarized in the following section.

Leg Extension Weakness

Leg extension strength is essential for rising from a chair, climbing stairs, and walking—three activities that may precipitate falls if strength is inadequate to perform them. Leg extension weakness is diagnosed if a patient cannot rise from a chair without pushing off. Several studies have shown that resistance exercises can increase quadriceps strength and size in patients well into their 90s (38) and that muscle strengthening and balance exercises can reduce the incidence of falls (39). Therefore, lower extremity strengthening exercises are recommended for the prevention of falls.

Poor Balance

Poor balance is evident in a patient with a positive Romberg test or unstable gait. It can be successfully treated with balance training by a physical therapist or Tai Chi Chuan exercises. Other helpful interventions include the use of hard wide-soled shoes with ankle support, a cane or walker, and correction of visual deficits.

Medication Toxicity

Both the overall number of medications and specific agents that impair alertness or reduce BP are associated with falls. A meta-analysis published in 1999 showed that use of any psychotropic medications was associated with a 73% increase, diuretics with an 8% increase, class 1a antiarrhythmics with a 59% increase, and digoxin with a 22% increase in risk of falling (40). Therefore, efforts should be made to reduce the number of medications a patient is taking, or if this is not possible, substitute dangerous drugs with safer alternatives and use the lowest effective dose.

Hypotension

Orthostatic and postprandial hypotension are particularly common in elderly diabetics. At the time of a fall, orthostatic hypotension may be due to acute dehydration, medications, or adrenocortical insufficiency. Therefore, it is important to assess and replete intravascular volume, stop hypotensive medications, and, if these interventions are not successful, measure plasma cortisol levels.

If the patient has chronic orthostatic or postprandial hypotension, the initial treatment is nonpharmacologic. This includes reducing hypotensive medications, separating meals, and medications, maintaining lower extremity muscle tone, pumping the legs, and standing up slowly, avoiding prolonged standing, increasing salt and water intake, wearing thigh or waist-high pressurized stockings, and elevating the head of the bed at night while sleeping.

If nonpharmacologic measures fail, fludrocortisone is usually the first line of pharmacologic therapy. Fludrocortisone is a synthetic mineralocorticoid, whose principal mode of action is to reduce renal salt loss and expand blood volume. The initial dose is 0.1 mg per day with increments of 0.1 mg every week until either there is development of trace pedal edema or the maximal dose of 1 mg per day is reached. Common side effects include hypokalemia, supine hypertension, congestive heart failure, and headache. Elderly patients should be monitored for fluid overload and hypokalemia. In patients taking higher doses, potassium supplements are usually required.

If the patient remains symptomatic, Midodrine, an α-agonist with selective vasopressor properties, is often effective. The starting dose is 2.5 mg three times per day. This is titrated upwards at 2.5 mg increments per week until a maximum of 10 mg three times per day is achieved. For best results, the morning dose should be given early and the evening dose no later then 6:00 P.M. Combination therapy of fludrocortisone and midodrine at lower doses of both agents (due to synergistic effects) is also beneficial. Adverse effects include supine hypertension, piloerection, pruritus, and paresthesia. This drug is contraindicated in patients with coronary heart diseases, heart failure, urinary retention, thyrotoxicosis, and acute renal failure.

Midodrine should be used cautiously in elderly patients who are taking medications that decrease heart rate, such as β-blockers, calcium channel blockers, and cardiac glycosides.

Other second-line treatments for autonomic failure include prostaglandin inhibitors, caffeine, and erythropoietin. These are reviewed elsewhere.

Environmental Hazards

For elderly diabetic patients with multiple pathologic conditions that make them vulnerable to falls, it is particularly important to eliminate environmental hazards, prescribe assistive devices, and install adaptive equipment in the home. Often visiting nurses can be sent to the patient's home to do an environmental assessment and make appropriate recommendations. These recommendations include improvements in lighting; removal of loose throw rugs, electrical cords, and clutter; repair of broken steps or banisters; installation of handrails on stairs and in bathrooms; and use of nonslip bathmats and tub seats. Beds and toilet seats should be lowered or raised to assure an optimal height for safe transfers. Patients should also be referred to physical therapists for the proper assessment and fitting of canes and walkers.

Experimental Treatments for Diabetic Peripheral Neuropathy
Monochromatic Near-Infrared Phototherapy
Recently, monochromatic near-infrared phototherapy of the lower limbs has shown promise for improving pain, sensation, and balance in patients with diabetic peripheral neuropathy (41). This noninvasive treatment involves six 40-minute applications of gallium aluminum arsinide diodes to the feet and calves over a two-week period. Each diode emits 890 nm near-infrared photo energy, which is thought to dilate arteries and veins under the exposed area. When compared with a sham device that generates the same heat without the photo energy, this treatment improved sensitivity to Semmes Weinstein monofilaments and subjective reports of pain and balance (41). Experience is limited with this device and it has not yet been shown to prevent falls or improve measures of gait and balance.

Noise-Enhanced Sensory Detection
Within the last decade, a novel mechanism known as stochastic resonance (42–44) has been used to enhance sensory detection in individuals with age- or disease-related sensory loss. This mechanism involves the application of imperceptible vibrations to the fingertip or soles of the feet. The applied vibrations are not of a finely tuned frequency, but rather white noise—a signal comprising all frequencies within a certain band, typically less than 1 kHz. The concept of enhancing sensory perception with noise is counterintuitive because noise is usually thought to interfere with signal transmission and detection. However, in many neurophysiological and perceptual systems, including rat cutaneous afferents (45) and human muscles spindles (46), there is an optimal level of noise at which signal transmission is maximized.

Recently, a psychophysical study involving healthy elderly people, patients with stroke, and patients with diabetic neuropathy demonstrated that the ability of an individual to detect a subthreshold (imperceptible) mechanical cutaneous stimulus was significantly enhanced by introducing a particular level of mechanical noise (90% of the sensory threshold to noise vibration) (47). As part of the protocol, each healthy elderly subject was tested on the middle digit of their right hand for their ability to detect a weak vibrotactile stimulus. Each stroke patient was tested on the middle digit of their affected hand and each diabetic patient was tested on the middle digit of their right hand and the first metatarsal head of their left foot. The findings showed that the noise-mediated decreases in vibrotactile detection threshold at the fingertip were on average 29%, 16%, and 32% for the group means in the elderly subjects, patients with stroke, and patients with diabetes, respectively. A significant decrease in the group mean for the detection threshold at the foot (31%) was also found in the patients with diabetes.

Motivated by the above findings, subsequent work examined the effects of noise input to the somatosensory system on posture control in humans (15). In a series of quiet standing experiments, healthy young and elderly subjects stood on a pair of vibrating insoles to introduce subsensory mechanical noise (90% of the sensory threshold) to the sole of each foot (Fig. 1).

A Vicon motion analysis system recorded the displacement of a marker placed on the shoulder. Using a plot of the shoulder displacement, called a stabilogram, to quantify postural

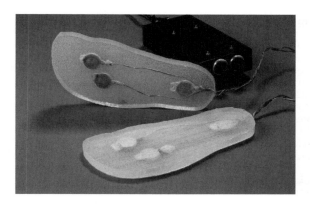

FIGURE 1 Two gel insoles contain three vibrating actuators called tactors embedded into a viscoelastic silicone gel. The tactors were controlled by the noise signal generated from the black box. The box was battery operated. Potentiometers on the outside of the box allowed the user to adjust the intensity of the vibration independently for each insole.

sway, the study showed a significant improvement in balance control in both young and elderly subjects with the application of noise. Various measures of postural sway showed reductions of 4.9% to 8.5% in young subjects and 4.9% to 14.6% in elderly subjects. The improvements were more pronounced for the older adults in whom the application of vibratory noise produced sway values similar to those of young subjects during baseline conditions. Furthermore, SDA measures demonstrated that when the insoles were vibrating, subjects swayed a shorter distance before feedback mechanisms (e.g., somatosensation) helped correct their posture.

In a follow-up study, the vibrating insoles were tested on patients with diabetic neuropathy and diminished sensation in the soles of their feet, and also patients with stroke, whose sensory loss in the feet was caused by brain damage (16). On average, all subjects showed a 2.9% to 53.8% reduction in both traditional and SDA measures of sway. In fact, those subjects with the greatest postural sway at baseline had the greatest benefit.

These laboratory-based data suggest that imperceptible mechanical noise applied to the soles of the feet can improve balance control in elderly people and patients with sensory deficits due to diabetic peripheral neuropathy or stroke. Future studies are needed to determine whether noise-based devices, such as randomly vibrating shoe insoles, are effective in enhancing functional performance and reducing the incidence of falls.

ACKNOWLEDGMENT

Supported by grants P01-AG004390, P60-AG08812, and T32-AG023480 from the National Institute on Aging, Bethesda, Maryland.

REFERENCES

1. Schwartz AV, Hillier TA, Sellmeyer DE, et al. Older women with diabetes have a higher risk of falls: a prospective study. Diabetes Care 2002; 25(10):1749–1754.
2. Volpato S, Leveille SG, Blaum C, Fried LP, Guralnik JM. Risk factors for falls in older disabled women with diabetes: the women's health and aging study. *J Gerontol A Biol Sci Med Sci* 2005; 60(12): 1539–1545.
3. Maurer MS, Burcham J, Cheng H. Diabetes mellitus is associated with an increased risk of falls in elderly residents of a long-term care facility. J Gerontol A Biol Sci Med Sci 2005; 60(9):1157–1162.
4. Strotmeyer ES, Cauley JA, Schwartz AV, et al. Nontraumatic fracture risk with diabetes mellitus and impaired fasting glucose in older white and black adults: the health, aging, and body composition study. Arch Intern Med 2005; 165(14):1612–1617.
5. Schwartz AV, Sellmeyer DE, Strotmeyer ES, et al. Diabetes and bone loss at the hip in older black and white adults. J Bone Miner Res 2005; 20(4):596–603.
6. Lipsitz LA. An 85-year-old woman with a history of falls. JAMA 1996; 276(1):59–66.
7. Lipsitz LA, Nakajima I, Gagnon M, Hirayama T, Connelly CM, Izumo H. Muscle strength and fall rates among residents of Japanese and American nursing homes: an International Cross-Cultural Study. J Am Geriatr Soc 1994; 42(9):953–959.
8. Laughton CA, Slavin M, Katdare K, et al. Aging, muscle activity, and balance control: physiologic changes associated with balance impairment. Gait Posture 2003; 18(2):101–108.

9. Scheibel AB. Falls, motor dysfunction, and correlative neurohistologic changes in the elderly. Clin Geriatr Med 1985; 1(3):671–677.
10. Lord SR, Dayhew J. Visual risk factors for falls in older people. J Am Geriatr Soc 2001; 49(5):508–515.
11. Lipsitz LA, Jonsson PV, Kelley MM, Koestner JS. Causes and correlates of recurrent falls in ambulatory frail elderly. J Gerontol 1991; 46(4):M114–M122.
12. Rauch SD, Velazquez-Villasenor L, Dimitri PS, Merchant SN. Decreasing hair cell counts in aging humans. Ann N Y Acad Sci 2001; 942:220–227.
13. Collins JJ, De Luca CJ. Open-loop and closed-loop control of posture: a random-walk analysis of center-of-pressure trajectories. Exp Brain Res 1993; 95(2):308–318.
14. Collins JJ, De Luca CJ, Burrows A, Lipsitz LA. Age-related changes in open-loop and closed-loop postural control mechanisms. Exp Brain Res 1995; 104(3):480–492.
15. Priplata AA, Niemi JB, Harry JD, Lipsitz LA, Collins JJ. Vibrating insoles and balance control in elderly people. Lancet 2003; 362(9390):1123–1124.
16. Priplata AA, Patritti BL, Niemi JB, et al. Noise-enhanced balance control in patients with diabetes and patients with stroke. Ann Neurol 2006; 59(1):4–12.
17. Maki BE, McIlroy WE. Postural control in the older adult. Clin Geriatr Med 1996; 12(4):635–658.
18. Thelen DG, Ashton-Miller JA, Schultz AB, Alexander NB. Do neural factors underlie age differences in rapid ankle torque development? J Am Geriatr Soc 1996; 44(7):804–808.
19. Woollacott MH, Shumway-Cook A, Nashner LM. Aging and posture control: changes in sensory organization and muscular coordination. Int J Aging Hum Dev 1986; 23(2):97–114.
20. Jonsson PV, Lipsitz LA, Kelley M, Koestner J. Hypotensive responses to common daily activities in institutionalized elderly. A potential risk for recurrent falls. Arch Intern Med 1990; 150(7):1518–1524.
21. Epstein M, Hollenberg NK. Age as a determinant of renal sodium conservation in normal man. J Lab Clin Med 1976; 87(3):411–417.
22. Miller M. Nocturnal polyuria in older people: pathophysiology and clinical implications. J Am Geriatr Soc 2000; 48(10):1321–1329.
23. Lipsitz LA, Mukai S, Hamner J, Gagnon M, Babikian V. Dynamic regulation of middle cerebral artery blood flow velocity in aging and hypertension. Stroke 2000; 31(8):1897–1903.
24. Serrador JM, Sorond FA, Vyas M, Gagnon M, Iloputaife ID, Lipsitz LA. Cerebral pressure-flow relations in hypertensive elderly humans: transfer gain in different frequency domains. J Appl Physiol 2005; 98(1):151–159.
25. Simoneau GG, Ulbrecht JS, Derr JA, Becker MB, Cavanagh PR. Postural instability in patients with diabetic sensory neuropathy. Diabetes Care 1994; 17(12):1411–1421.
26. Menz HB, Lord SR, St George R, Fitzpatrick RC. Walking stability and sensorimotor function in older people with diabetic peripheral neuropathy. Arch Phys Med Rehabil 2004; 85(2):245–252.
27. Lafond D, Corriveau H, Prince F. Postural control mechanisms during quiet standing in patients with diabetic sensory neuropathy. Diabetes Care 2004; 27(1):173–178.
28. Richerson SJ, Robinson CJ, Shum J. A comparative study of reaction times between type II diabetics and non-diabetics. Biomed Eng Online 2005; 4(1):12.
29. Vinik AI, Maser RE, Mitchell BD, Freeman R. Diabetic autonomic neuropathy. Diabetes Care 2003; 26(5):1553–1579.
30. Quandt SA, Stafford JM, Bell RA, Smith SL, Snively BM, Arcury TA. Predictors of falls in a multiethnic population of older rural adults with diabetes. J Gerontol A Biol Sci Med Sci 2006; 61(4):394–398.
31. Wallace C, Reiber GE, LeMaster J, et al. Incidence of falls, risk factors for falls, and fall-related fractures in individuals with diabetes and a prior foot ulcer. Diabetes Care 2002; 25(11):1983–1986.
32. Wild D, Nayak US, Isaacs B. How dangerous are falls in old people at home? Br Med J (Clin Res Ed) 1981; 282(6260):266–268.
33. Podsiadlo D, Richardson S. The timed "Up & Go": a test of basic functional mobility for frail elderly persons. J Am Geriatr Soc 1991; 39(2):142–148.
34. Kenny RA, Richardson DA, Steen N, Bexton RS, Shaw FE, Bond J. Carotid sinus syndrome: a modifiable risk factor for nonaccidental falls in older adults (SAFE PACE). J Am Coll Cardiol 2001; 38(5):1491–1496.
35. Gillespie LD, Gillespie WJ, Robertson MC, Lamb SE, Cumming RG, Rowe BH. Interventions for preventing falls in elderly people. Cochrane Database Syst Rev 2003(4):CD000340.
36. American Geriatrics Society, British Geriatrics Society, and American Academy of Orthopaedic Surgeons Panel on Falls Prevention. Guideline for the prevention of falls in older persons. J Am Geriatr Soc 2001; 49(5):664–672.
37. Bischoff-Ferrari HA, Dawson-Hughes B, Willett WC, et al. Effect of Vitamin D on falls: a meta-analysis. JAMA 2004; 291(16):1999–2006.
38. Fiatarone MA, O'Neill EF, Ryan ND, et al. Exercise training and nutritional supplementation for physical frailty in very elderly people. N Engl J Med 1994; 330(25):1769–1775.
39. Province MA, Hadley EC, Hornbrook MC, et al. The effects of exercise on falls in elderly patients. A preplanned meta-analysis of the FICSIT trials. Frailty and Injuries: Cooperative Studies of Intervention Techniques. JAMA 1995; 273(17):1341–1347.

40. Leipzig RM, Cumming RG, Tinetti ME. Drugs and falls in older people: a systematic review and meta-analysis: II. Cardiac and analgesic drugs. J Am Geriatr Soc 1999; 47(1):40–50.
41. Leonard DR, Farooqi MH, Myers S. Restoration of sensation, reduced pain, and improved balance in subjects with diabetic peripheral neuropathy: a double-blind, randomized, placebo-controlled study with monochromatic near-infrared treatment. Diabetes Care 2004; 27(1):168–172.
42. Hanggi P. Stochastic resonance in biology. How noise can enhance detection of weak signals and help improve biological information processing. Chemphyschem 12 2002; 3(3):285–290.
43. Moss F, Ward LM, Sannita WG. Stochastic resonance and sensory information processing: a tutorial and review of application. Clin Neurophysiol 2004; 115(2):267–281.
44. Wiesenfeld K, Moss F. Stochastic resonance and the benefits of noise: from ice ages to crayfish and SQUIDs. Nature 1995; 373(6509):33–36.
45. Collins JJ, Imhoff TT, Grigg P. Noise-enhanced information transmission in rat SA1 cutaneous mechanoreceptors via aperiodic stochastic resonance. J Neurophysiol 1996; 76(1):642–645.
46. Cordo P, Inglis JT, Verschueren S, et al. Noise in human muscle spindles. Nature 1996; 383(6603): 769–770.
47. Liu W, Lipsitz LA, Montero-Odasso M, Bean J, Kerrigan DC, Collins JJ. Noise-enhanced vibrotactile sensitivity in older adults, patients with stroke, and patients with diabetic neuropathy. Arch Phys Med Rehabil 2002; 83(2):171–176.

8 | Polypharmacy

Sudeep S. Gill
Departments of Medicine and Community Health and Epidemiology, Queen's University, Kingston, and Institute for Clinical Evaluative Sciences, Toronto, Ontario, Canada

Lorraine L. Lipscombe
Department of Medicine, University of Toronto, and Institute for Clinical Evaluative Sciences, Toronto, Ontario, Canada

Paula A. Rochon
Departments of Medicine and Health Policy, Management and Evaluation, University of Toronto, and Institute for Clinical Evaluative Sciences, Toronto, Ontario, Canada

INTRODUCTION

The management of older adults with diabetes involves a number of challenges. An important challenge in this patient population is the appropriate prescribing of medications. Medications are used to treat a host of problems: hyperglycemia, common comorbid conditions (such as hypertension and hyperlipidemia), and microvascular and macrovascular complications of diabetes. Each of these conditions may require several medications; new drug development (such as the introduction of incretin mimetics) will likely further add to this medication burden (1,2). In addition, elderly patients with diabetes are often at risk of developing certain geriatric syndromes (including cognitive impairment, injurious falls, urinary incontinence, and depression) that warrant additional drug treatment (3). As a result, older individuals with diabetes are often prescribed many medications. But how many medications are "too many"?

The concept of polypharmacy as it applies to the management of older adults with diabetes is of great clinical importance, but this concept is complex and continues to evolve (4). For example, the term polypharmacy has traditionally suggested suboptimal prescribing and has been linked to a heightened risk of drug interactions, adverse drug events, and reduced overall medication adherence (5,6). More recent research, however, has emphasized the underuse of beneficial medications by high-risk patient groups such as those with diabetes, and this research suggests that polypharmacy may be necessary in some individuals to permit the optimal management of their diabetes, its complications, and associated comorbidities (7,8).

Despite the fact that polypharmacy is commonly encountered by physicians who care for elderly patients with diabetes, the medical literature provides limited guidance on the appropriate clinical approach to this issue. Clinicians may struggle to harmonize the individual needs of their patients with the recommendations of clinical practice guidelines (9–11). Several recent articles have attempted to provide practical strategies to prioritize and individualize the medication portfolios for older patients with diabetes (3,12).

This chapter briefly reviews age-related changes in the body's handling of medications (i.e., pharmacokinetics) and the body's response to medications (i.e., pharmacodynamics). With this background, the chapter then goes on to discuss the definition, epidemiology, and consequences of polypharmacy; the related concepts of appropriate prescribing, errors of commission, and errors of omission; important drug–drug and drug–disease interactions in diabetes; and the epidemiology and predictors of drug adherence in diabetes. The chapter ends by reviewing strategies to optimize the appropriate prescribing of medications for elderly individuals with diabetes.

PHARMACOKINETICS

Pharmacokinetics is the study of the processes involved in the body's handling of drugs. Traditionally, pharmacokinetics is subdivided into four major components: absorption, distribution, metabolism, and elimination. Aging and associated factors (such as the effects of common age-related diseases and concomitant drug use) can influence the pharmacokinetics of drugs in generally predictable ways. Understanding age-associated changes in pharmaco-kinetics can help guide rational prescribing of drugs for older patients with diabetes.

Drug absorption is largely unaffected by normal aging, despite well-documented changes in gastric motility and blood flow to the gut. In particular, the overall extent of drug absorption is generally unaffected by age, although the rate of absorption and time-to-peak serum concentrations may be delayed with advancing age. Factors other than aging have a greater influence on the absorption of a drug. Such factors include the concomitant use of certain drugs and the patient's comorbid illness profile. For example, the absorption of antibiotics such as fluoroquinolones and tetracycline is decreased when they are taken together with calcium or iron supplements. As another example, the use of acid-lowering medications such as histamine-2 receptor blockers and proton pump inhibitors has been linked to an increased risk of developing vitamin B_{12} deficiency (13). Drug absorption (and elimination) may be affected in some cases by drug interactions mediated by P-glycoprotein, a multidrug efflux pump located on the luminal surface of the epithelial cells of the small intestine as well as several other locations (including the liver, kidneys, and blood–brain barrier) (14). Delayed gastric emptying (gastroparesis) due to autonomic neuropathy is common in diabetics and may be an important cause of alterations in drug absorption and blood glucose control (15).

Drug distribution involves the body tissues that drugs penetrate into, and the binding of drugs to carrier proteins such as albumin. Age-associated changes in body composition can affect a drug's volume of distribution, which is the theoretical fluid compartment in a patient that is occupied by the drug. A drug with a large volume of distribution has good tissue pene-tration, while a drug with a smaller volume of distribution has poorer tissue penetration. With increasing age, drugs that are water-soluble (hydrophilic) have relatively lower volumes of distribution, as older people have less body water and lean body mass. Hydrophilic drugs such as ethanol and lithium are affected by these changes. Furthermore, fat-soluble (lipophilic) drugs such as diazepam have an increased volume of distribution because older persons typically have greater fat stores than do younger persons.

These age-related changes in body composition and drug distribution can have important implications for both the steady-state concentration and the half-life (i.e., the rate of clearance) of many medications. For example, the increase in the volume of distribution for a lipophilic drug such as diazepam means that it takes longer for it to reach a steady-state concentration and longer for it to be eliminated from the body once it has been discontinued. The impact of these alterations in drug distribution can be further pronounced by age-related changes in drug metabolism and elimination that are discussed below. A drug's volume of distribution can also be influenced by the extent to which it is bound to plasma proteins. Albumin is the primary plasma protein to which many drugs bind. (Some lipophilic and cationic drugs bind instead to α-1 acid glycoprotein, another plasma protein, but age-related changes in α-1 acid glycoprotein levels and drug binding are not thought to be clinically significant.) Albumin's concentration is typically decreased in older persons, especially when they suffer from malnutrition or severe chronic disease. For a drug that is usually highly bound to albumin, the age-associated decline in albumin concentration results in a higher proportion of unbound (free)—and thus pharma-cologically active—amount of drug. Thus, for extensively protein-bound drugs whose binding is reduced as a result of hypoalbuminemia (such as phenytoin), clinicians should anticipate both therapeutic and toxic drug effects at lower total serum concentrations in older adults with chronic illnesses. In elderly patients with malnutrition or chronic illness, it can therefore be difficult to interpret serum drug levels (such as those commonly reported for phenytoin) that reflect total drug concentrations rather than free drug concentrations.

Although drug metabolism is carried out in many places throughout the body (including the intestinal wall, lungs, kidneys, and skin), the primary site for the metabolic conversion of drugs is the liver. Normal aging is associated with a reduction in liver mass and hepatic blood flow. As a result, metabolic clearance of certain drugs is reduced with aging. This reduced clear-ance is particularly evident for drugs that are metabolized through phase I reactions, such as hydroxylation, dealkylation, oxidation, and reduction. In contrast, drugs subject to phase II metabolic reactions (such as glucuronidation, conjugation, and acetylation) are generally less affected by aging. Factors other than age may have a profound influence on drug metabolism. For example, the rapidly expanding knowledge base related to specific drug metabolic pathways, such as those involving the cytochrome P450 (CYP450) system, is improving our understanding of genetic differences in drug metabolism and important pharmacokinetic drug–drug interactions (which are discussed in greater detail below) (14,16,17).

Elimination involves a drug's exit from the body. Renal clearance is the most common pathway for the elimination of drugs, although hepatobiliary clearance is also an important pathway for some medications. Elimination can involve removal of the parent compound or metabolites of the parent compound. On average, aging is associated with a linear decline in renal function, such that the average reduction in glomerular filtration rate from young adulthood to old age is roughly one-third. However, it is important to realize that there can be significant heterogeneity in the decline of renal function with age—some subjects have minimal changes in renal function with aging, and a few subjects even appear to have improvements in renal function over time. Thus, the effects of age on renal function can be quite variable in individual patients. This is especially true of diabetic patients, who are at risk for subtle and overt nephropathy. Serum creatinine measurements provide a limited perspective on the level of renal function. Cystatin C, a non-glycosylated basic protein that is freely filtered by the glomerulus, is under investigation as a possible alternative to serum creatinine for estimating the glomerular filtration rate (18). At present, however, cystatin C measurements are not commonly available for clinical use. Several formulae have been suggested to better estimate renal function. For example, the Cockcroft–Gault formula (19) is one useful approach for estimating renal function and requires only a few easily obtained measurements:

$$\text{Estimated creatinine clearance (in mL/min)} = \frac{(140 - \text{Age in yr}) \times (\text{Ideal body weight in kg})}{\text{Serum creatinine (in mg/dL)} \times 72}$$

(For women, multiply $\times 0.85$. When using serum creatinine measurements in micromoles per liter, replace 72 in the denominator with 0.84.)

Clinicians should interpret the results of this estimating equation or other similar equations with caution, as they may overestimate the measured glomerular filtration rate. Nevertheless, estimating creatinine clearance from the Cockcroft-Gault formula can facilitate dose adjustment of drugs that are primarily cleared by the kidneys (such as digoxin) and nephrotoxic medications (such as aminoglycosides). Estimation of creatinine clearance can also promote appropriate prescribing decisions for the older diabetic patient. For example, it is generally recommended that metformin should be avoided in patients with significant renal dysfunction (e.g., creatinine clearance less than 30–60 mL/min) to avoid the risk of lactic acidosis. The evidence to support this recommendation, however, has been questioned (20,21). Also, it is important to remember that there is an increased risk of hypoglycemia due to drug-drug interactions in patients with renal insufficiency, as oral hypoglycemic medications and their active metabolites can accumulate when there is less effective renal clearance of these substances.

PHARMACODYNAMICS

The pharmacodynamic action of a given medication relates to its end-organ effects. In contrast to pharmacokinetics, it is more difficult to make general predictions about the effects of aging on the pharmacodynamics of medications. While aging is associated with a diminished action for some drugs (e.g., a reduced heart rate response to β-blockers), the activity of other drugs is typically enhanced with increasing age (e.g., significantly lower doses of benzodiazepines are needed to achieve sedation in elderly individuals as compared to younger individuals). It is probably fair to say that for many drug classes, the interplay of age-related changes in pharmacokinetics and pharmacodynamics results in an increased sensitivity to medications by older adults. Thus, it is often advisable to initiate medications at the lowest possible dose and titrate the dose upward slowly to target levels in order to minimize the opportunity for medication intolerance or adverse effects.

POLYPHARMACY
Definition of Polypharmacy

The term "polypharmacy" is commonly used, but there is no consensus on the definition of this concept. A simple definition is based on the total number of medications concomitantly taken by a patient. For patients who take more than some arbitrarily determined total number, polypharmacy can be said to exist. The number of medications constituting polypharmacy using this approach has been variably defined in the literature as between 5 and 10 (4). This definition has been proposed because the number of potential drug–drug interactions rises dramatically with more than five or six drugs (22). Nonetheless, this sort of definition is fraught with problems: for example, which drugs should take priority and which should be excluded if the "appropriate target" number is set at five drugs but the patient is potentially eligible to receive eight drugs? Should the number of medications include over-the-counter products or herbal therapies? What about other drug preparations that can have systemic effects, such as eye drops for glaucoma or inhaled insulin? (23). Thus, although defining polypharmacy in terms of an arbitrary numerical threshold is appealing in its simplicity, it does not address the appropriate or inappropriate use of medications and could promote the exclusion of potentially useful drug treatments for some patients ("errors of omission," discussed below). A more practical definition of polypharmacy is, "the prescription, administration, or use of more medications than are clinically indicated" (4). This definition emphasizes the fact that the problems of polypharmacy involve unnecessary medications, inappropriate drug combinations, and inappropriate drugs for specific patients. As a result, patients taking only two medications could have polypharmacy according to this definition depending on the specific profile of the medications and the patient.

Epidemiology of Polypharmacy

Regardless of the definition used for polypharmacy, it is highly prevalent in older adults, particularly in those with chronic diseases such as diabetes. A national survey in Finland found that patients with diabetes used significantly more medications, with significantly higher costs, than nondiabetic patients who were matched for age, sex, and area of residence (24).

Reasons for Polypharmacy

Many factors conspire together to promote polypharmacy in older diabetic patients (4). First, multidrug regimens are often emphasized to achieve tight glycemic control in order to prevent diabetic complications. The latest guidelines promote combination hypoglycemic treatment rather than monotherapy even at diabetes diagnosis (25). Second, successful treatment of comorbidities that are common in diabetes (such as hypertension and hyperlipidemia) and complications of diabetes (such as painful neuropathies, coronary artery disease, and congestive heart failure) often requires the use of additional sets of medications. In fact, antihypertensive and lipid-lowering therapies are now indicated for the majority of patients with diabetes to reduce cardiovascular events and mortality (25).

Consequences of Polypharmacy

Although the intentions of prescribing multidrug regimens to manage diabetes and its complications are usually good, unintended negative consequences become progressively more common as the number of medications prescribed to frail elderly diabetic patients increases. Such consequences include increasing costs, adverse drug reactions to a single drug, drug–drug interactions, drug–disease interactions, reduced overall medication adherence, and the development of geriatric syndromes. Geriatric syndromes associated with the inappropriate use of medications include cognitive impairment, falls and consequent injuries, and urinary incontinence (3). Older patients who have had diabetes for many years are at particular risk for these adverse events, because of underlying neuropathy, dysautonomia, renal dysfunction, and vascular disease and because of the greater number of drugs required with advanced disease (4).

APPROPRIATE PRESCRIBING—ERRORS OF COMMISSION AND OMISSION

In order to highlight the importance of adverse drug events in older patients, several expert-based consensus panels have developed guidelines for appropriate prescribing in the elderly (26,27). The lists of inappropriate medications generated by these panels have been widely employed in studies that assess the prevalence of inappropriate prescribing in a variety of settings, and these studies have documented persistently high rates of inappropriate medication prescribing for older adults (28). However, these figures only reflect one part of the problem. While the guidelines have generally included only "errors of commission" in drug prescribing, other investigators have highlighted the fact that elderly patients with multiple chronic diseases are often undertreated with potentially useful medications (i.e., "errors of omission") (7,8). An example of a common error of omission is the underprescribing of osteoporosis treatments to patients who have suffered a hip fracture. Potential undertreatment is particularly relevant to older adults with diabetes, for whom multiple drug therapies are indicated for the primary and secondary prevention of complications. For example, other comorbidities such as hypertension and dyslipidemia may be less diligently treated than dysglycemia, despite good evidence of benefit for drug therapy (29). Thus, concerns over polypharmacy must be balanced against the need to adequately treat diabetes and associated comorbid conditions in order to reduce the risk of diabetic complications.

Other potentially useful approaches to assessing the quality of drug prescribing have been identified, including the medication appropriateness index (MAI), which uses 10 criteria to assess the appropriateness of each prescription drug (30). The MAI has been used primarily in research settings, but may also be valuable in clinical settings when trying to assess patients who are taking complex multidrug regimens (12).

DRUG–DRUG INTERACTIONS

A clinically relevant drug–drug interaction takes place when the efficacy or toxicity of one drug is altered by the coadministration of a second drug (14). This interaction can result in enhanced benefit to the patient and is one reason why certain drugs are used in combination. Interactions can become problematic, however, when the combination causes either reduced therapeutic effect or increased toxicity. There are two basic mechanisms of drug–drug interactions: pharmacokinetic interactions arise when the concentration of a drug is altered at its site of action by another drug (typically, through changes in absorption, distribution, metabolism, or elimination), while pharmacodynamic interactions develop when a change in drug effect occurs without altering drug concentration at the site of action (14,16,31). Table 1 highlights clinically important drug-drug interactions involving oral hypoglycemic medications.

Pharmacokinetic Drug–Drug Interactions

Pharmacokinetic interactions are more common than pharmacodynamic ones. Although pharmacokinetic drug–drug interactions can result from changes in drug absorption or distribution, the more frequent cause is an alteration in drug metabolism and/or elimination. Induction of elimination of one drug by another can result in dramatically reduced drug effects and reduced therapeutic benefits. On the other hand, inhibition of drug elimination can produce excessive drug effects and dose-related toxicity. Drug elimination is often determined by drug-metabolizing enzymes (such as the CYP450 enzymes) and/or drug-transporting proteins (such as P-glycoprotein) (14). CYP450 is a superfamily of enzymes coded by different genes. Over 50 different isoforms of CYP450 have been identified in humans, but only a few account for the majority of the oxidative reactions involved in drug metabolism. Some of the most important isoforms are CYP1A2, CYP2C9, CYP2C19, CYP2D6, CYP2E1, and CYP3A4. A clinically important example of a pharmacokinetic drug–drug interaction involves the sulfonylurea drugs and sulfonamide antibiotics. Sulfonylureas, such as glyburide and glipizide, are extensively metabolized by CYP2C9. Sulfonamide antibiotics inhibit the metabolism of sulfonylureas by CYP2C9 and can therefore promote potentially life-threatening hypoglycemia. One large case-control study examined the importance of this drug–drug interaction. Elderly patients taking glyburide who had been admitted to hospital with a diagnosis

TABLE 1   Oral Hypoglycemic Medications and Potentially Important Drug-Drug Interactions

Drug class (examples)	Primary mechanism of action	Common or severe adverse effects	Potential drug–drug interactions
Sulfonylureas (glyburide, glipizide, glimepiride)	Increase insulin secretion	Hypoglycemia, weight gain	Documented increase in risk of hypoglycemia from sulfonylureas when taken together with CYP2C9 inhibitors (e.g., sulfonamide antibiotics such as cotrimoxazole, antifungals such as fluconazole) Reduced glucose-lowering effect from sulfonylureas when taken together with rifampin (a CYP2C9 inducer)
Glitinides (repaglinide, nateglinide)	Increase insulin secretion	Hypoglycemia, weight gain	Documented substantial increase in risk of hypoglycemia from repaglinide when taken together with gemfibrozil (a CYP2C8 inhibitor); risk does not appear to exist with other fibrates (e.g., bezafibrate, fenofibrate) Potential increased risk of hypoglycemia from repaglinide when taken together with CYP3A4 inhibitors (e.g., ketoconazole, clarithromycin), and potential reduced glucose-lowering effect from repaglinide when taken together with CYP3A4 inducer (e.g., rifampin) Potential increased risk of hypoglycemia from nateglinide when taken together with fluconazole (a CYP2C9 inhibitor)
Biguanides (metformin)	Decrease hepatic glucose output	Gastrointestinal upset Lactic acidosis	Metformin has few clinically relevant drug-drug interactions, as it undergoes little metabolism once it is absorbed Although acarbose can reduce metformin absorption from the small intestine, the combination of these two oral hypoglycemic agents is still thought to be safe and effective
Alpha-glucosidase inhibitors (acarbose, miglitol)	Delay gastrointestinal absorption of carbohydrates	Flatulence, gastrointestinal upset, weight gain	Potential interactions with digoxin (reduced absorption of digoxin), warfarin (increased absorption of warfarin), metformin (reduced absorption of metformin); the clinical relevance of these interactions is unclear
Thiazolidinediones (rosiglitazone, pioglitazone)	Increase insulin sensitivity	Edema, weight gain Fluid retention may precipitate new-onset heart failure or exacerbate pre-existing heart failure	Increased risk of hypoglycemia from rosiglitazone when taken together with gemfibrozil (a CYP2C8 inhibitor). A similar risk may exist with other CYP2C8 inhibitors (e.g., cotrimoxazole) Reduced glucose-lowering effect from rosiglitazone when taken together with rifampin (a CYP2C8 inducer) No documented clinically relevant drug-drug interactions between either pioglitazone or rosiglitazone and other oral hypoglycemic medications (e.g., sulfonylureas, glitinides, metformin, alpha-glucosidase inhibitors)

Note: Cotrimoxazole is the combination of sulfamethoxazole with trimethoprim. Rifampin is also known as rifampicin.
Abbreviation: CYP, cytochrome P450.
Source: From Refs. 31, 34, 35.

of hypoglycemia were more than six times as likely as control subjects to have been treated with co-trimoxazole in the week preceding hospitalization (adjusted odds ratio, 6.6; 95% confidence interval 5.8–12.4) (32).

Pharmacodynamic Drug–Drug Interactions

Pharmacodynamic interactions between drugs can occur when they operate by different mechanisms to produce a shared effect on the same target organ. An obvious example is the increased risk of hypoglycemia produced by the co-administration of two oral hypoglycemic drugs with different mechanisms of action and no pharmacokinetic drug-drug interactions (e.g., glyburide and metformin). A second example of a pharmacodynamic drug-drug interaction that is relevant to elderly patients with diabetes involves the adverse renal effects of coadministering nonsteroidal anti-inflammatory drugs (NSAIDs) and angiotensin-converting enzyme (ACE) inhibitors. Adequate glomerular blood flow depends in part on prostaglandin-mediated afferent arteriolar vasodilatation and angiotensin II–mediated efferent arteriolar vasoconstriction. NSAID therapy inhibits cyclooxygenase, thereby decreasing prostaglandin production; as a result, afferent arteriolar flow is reduced and glomerular filtration falls. On the other hand, ACE inhibitors depress angiotensin II and thus inhibit angiotensin II–mediated efferent arteriolar vasoconstriction. This also lowers glomerular filtration pressure and decreases the glomerular filtration rate. The concomitant use of NSAIDs and ACE inhibitors has been frequently cited as a cause for acute renal failure (33). Avoidance of this interaction is complicated by the fact that many NSAIDs are available over-the-counter. In this example, NSAIDs and ACE inhibitors have shared effects on the kidney but they are achieved by different mechanisms, and neither the concentration of the NSAID nor that of the ACE inhibitor is affected. This example therefore represents a pharmacodynamic drug–drug interaction.

DRUG–DISEASE INTERACTIONS
Drugs Associated with Hyperglycemia and Hypoglycemia

A wide variety of commonly prescribed medications can influence glucose metabolism, and Pandit et al. have provided an excellent review on this topic (34). In the years since this review was published, the list of medications that can cause dysglycemia has continued to grow, with evidence implicating protease inhibitors, second generation ("atypical") antipsychotics, and gatifloxacin (35,36). Multiple mechanisms of action on glucose metabolism exist through pancreatic, hepatic, and peripheral effects. Based on circumstances at the time of use, a drug may cause both hyper- and hypoglycemia in a patient (34–37). The patient's previous pancreatic reserve, nutritional state, use of other medication, or exposure to alcohol may influence the direction of the plasma glucose alterations. Table 2 details the medications that have been associated with hypoglycemia, hyperglycemia, or both.

Although some physicians avoid β-blockers in patients with diabetes because of concerns that these drugs might mask the symptoms of hypoglycemia, there is little evidence to support this notion (16). Hypoglycemia-induced sweating is not affected by β-blocker use as it is not under sympathetic control. In the United Kingdom Prospective Diabetes Study, there was no significant increase in the incidence of hypoglycemia among patients treated with β-blockers. β-blockers (and in particular cardioselective agents) can be used safely and with good effect in patients with diabetes who require control of hypertension, angina, and/or congestive heart failure.

Diabetes Drugs and Their Drug–Disease Interactions

Drugs used to treat diabetes may be contraindicated when certain comorbid conditions exist. However, a major challenge to appropriate drug prescribing in this context is the fact that some drugs are on the market for many years before the full range of their adverse effects and interactions are known (38). Many examples relevant to the management of diabetes exemplify this situation, and three are highlighted here: first, the use of thiazolidinediones in patients with heart failure; second, the use of metformin in patients with renal insufficiency; and third, the safety of sulfonylureas. Evidence has linked use of thiazolidinediones to the

TABLE 2   Nondiabetes Medications Associated with Hypoglycemia, Hyperglycemia, or Both

Medications associated with hypoglycemia
  Analgesics
    Acetaminophen
    Salicylates
    Propoxyphene
  Antidepressants
    Tricyclic antidepressants
    Monoamine oxidase inhibitors
    Selective serotonin reuptake inhibitors (sertraline, fluoxetine)
  Antihypertensives
    Angiotensin converting enzyme (ACE) inhibitors
  Miscellaneous
    Antiarrhythmic drugs (cibenzoline, disopyramide)
    Clotrimoxazole—may exert its hypoglycemic effects via drug–drug interactions with some oral hypoglycemic drugs
      (see Table 1)
    Fibric acid derivatives (fibrates)—especially gemfibrozil, via drug–drug interactions with some oral hypoglycemic drugs
      (see Table 1)
    Ganciclovir
    Mebendazole
    Quinine and quinidine
    Stanozolol
    Streptozotocin
    Tetracycline
    Tromethamine

Medications associated with hyperglycemia
  Antibiotics
    Dapsone
    Isoniazid
    Rifampin—may exert its hyperglycemic effects via drug–drug interactions with certain oral hypoglycemic drugs
      (see Table 1)
  Antihypertensives
    Thiazide diuretics
    Loop diuretics
    Calcium channel blockers
    Central alpha blockers
    Potassium channel agonists (minoxidil, diazoxide)
  Hormones
    Corticosteroids and adrenocorticotrophic hormone (ACTH)
    Oral contraceptives
    Thyroid hormones
  Psychotropic medications
    Amoxapine
    Antipsychotics—including both first-generation (e.g., droperidol, loxapine) and second-generation (e.g., clozapine,
      olanzapine) agents
    Chlordiazepoxide
    Phenytoin
  Miscellaneous
    Asparaginase
    Doxapram
    Encainide
    Indomethacin
    Morphine
    Nicotinic acid and niacin
    Protease inhibitors

Medications associated with both hypoglycemia and hyperglycemia
  Antibiotics
    Fluoroquinolones (gatifloxacin, temafloxacillin both withdrawn from the market due to adverse glycemic effects), nalidixic acid
    Pentamidine
  Miscellaneous
    Beta agonists
    Beta-blockers
    Ethanol
    Lithium
    Octreotide

Source: From Refs. 31, 34, 35.

development and worsening of heart failure. A consensus statement from the American Heart Association and the American Diabetes Association has detailed the appropriate use of thiazolidinediones in the context of left ventricular dysfunction (39). In general, the guidelines recommend that these drugs should be avoided when a patient has advanced heart failure and used only with caution when milder heart failure exists. A second example involves the role of metformin in patients with significant renal dysfunction. As discussed above, it is generally recommended that metformin should be avoided in patients with advanced renal insufficiency due to a potential increase in the risk of lactic acidosis. However, some investigators have questioned the evidence for this recommendation (19,20). Finally, the safety of sulfonylureas is a subject with a long history. Results from the University Group Diabetes Project published in 1970 showed that subjects treated with tolbutamide had a significantly higher risk of cardiovascular mortality than subjects given placebo. This effect may be due to the influence of certain sulfonylureas on a phenomenon known as ischemic preconditioning (40). The UKPDS did not find an association between sulfonylurea treatment (chlorpropamide or glibenclamide) and cardiovascular events or mortality. However, a recent cohort study found that exposure to higher daily doses of either a first-generation sulfonylurea (chlorpropamide or tolbutamide) or the second-generation sulfonylurea glyburide was associated with a higher risk of all-cause mortality or death from an acute ischemic event, while metformin monotherapy was not associated with an increased risk of mortality (41). No consensus has yet emerged on this important issue and further research is needed to clarify the safety profile of sulfonylureas.

ADHERENCE
Definitions of Persistence, Compliance, Adherence

Unfortunately, consensus has not yet been reached on these terms. In general, however, persistence refers to the accumulation of time during which a medication is taken, from the time it is initiated until the time it is discontinued. Compliance is the proportion of medication taken at a given time according to instructions while a patient is persistent. The term compliance has been viewed as having paternalistic overtones, and therefore more recently many authors have preferred to use the term adherence, which is thought to better reflect a therapeutic alliance between the prescribing physician and the patient (42).

Inadequate adherence to medications is a substantial problem among older adults with diabetes (43). The level of adherence necessary to achieve benefit from a medication varies by drug class, but many studies use a cutoff of 80% to separate high from low adherence rates (44). Inadequate adherence is associated with failure to reach therapeutic goals (such as target blood glucose levels, lipid levels, or blood pressure measurements), and worse clinical outcomes including mortality (42,45–48). Although diabetes control tends to worsen over time even with good adherence, physicians should consider suboptimal adherence as an explanation for patients who do not achieve treatment goals.

Epidemiology of Adherence

Studies have shown that adherence to oral hypoglycemic drugs and insulin therapy ranges widely (in one review, adherence ranged from 36% to 93% in patients remaining on treatment for 6–24 months) (43). Furthermore, adherence to other beneficial treatments such as lipid-lowering drugs is suboptimal: Only 52% of men and 37% of women with diabetes achieved target lipid levels, and much of this could be explained by suboptimal adherence to statin therapy (49).

Reasons for Nonadherence

Factors associated with inadequate drug adherence in patients with diabetes include the patient's comprehension of the treatment regimen and its benefits, adverse effects, medication costs, and regimen complexity, as well as their comorbid conditions (especially untreated depression, cognitive impairment, and the overall burden of comorbid disease) (6,42,50,51). To improve long-term drug adherence, particularly for elderly patients with diabetes who have complex drug regimens, effective communication between the prescribing physician and the patient is critical. It is important to set time aside to collaborate with the patient in order to reach goals of treatment tailored to the individual and to adequately educate them about the benefits of medications, particularly those medications that are used for preventative reasons rather than immediate symptom control (3,10,12,52). Ongoing communication should also explore reasons such as adverse drug effects, low mood, cognitive impairment, and socioeconomic factors that might impact drug adherence. Simple strategies to improve adherence such as the use of pharmacy-issued blister packs or dosette boxes can also provide some support for patients with complex medication regimens. Successful interventions for long-term treatment are labor-intensive but can provide significant benefits in terms of clinical outcomes and cost-effectiveness (52).

STRATEGIES TO OPTIMIZE APPROPRIATE MEDICATION PRESCRIBING

- Emphasize the additive benefits of nonpharmacological treatments (e.g., diet, exercise, sleep hygiene, and smoking cessation).
- Obtain a complete medication history on each patient visit—include all prescription drugs, over-the-counter drugs, herbal and complementary therapies, and supplements (e.g., calcium and vitamin D)—ask the patient to "brown bag" all of their medications to bring to each clinic visit, along with any aids they might use (e.g., blister packs and dosette boxes) to see if they are being filled properly.
- Recognize that patients with diabetes often have cognitive impairment (either subtle executive dysfunction or more overt impairment such as dementia). As executive dysfunction may impair the ability to plan, organize, sequence, and perform complex tasks (and thereby upset proper diabetes monitoring and management), patients with diabetes should undergo regular cognitive assessment with an instrument that includes measures of executive function, to ensure that they are capable of complying with their diabetes management plans.
- Encourage patients to maintain an up-to-date list of medications (generic name, trade name, dose, frequency, and timing for each drug)—many pharmacies may be able to help generate these lists for patients.
- Consider the possibility that any new symptoms may be related to an adverse drug effect before starting new medication (in order to avoid creating a "prescribing cascade").
- Regularly review all medications—does each medication have an appropriate indication? Any contraindications? Has the drug achieved its therapeutic goals?
- Discontinue medications that have no clear indication or that have not achieved a therapeutic goal.
- Regularly review patients' renal function to ensure that drug doses are being adjusted when necessary (e.g., metformin, digoxin, and antibiotics).
- When prescribing a new medication, take time to educate the patient about the indications for use, likely duration of use, potential adverse effects, and what to do if adverse effects develop (e.g., stopping the medication and seeking medical attention).
- Consider drug costs and substitute low-cost alternatives (e.g., generics) whenever possible.
- When prescribing a new long-term drug treatment, consider the patient's remaining life expectancy; time until benefit from the drug treatment; the goals of care as expressed by the patient; and whether treatment targets are preventative or palliative (12).
- When possible, use once daily or once weekly dosing to reduce the overall pill burden.
- Consider investing in software programs to help prevent drug–drug interactions.
- Avoid potentially inappropriate medications such as those associated with a high risk of adverse outcomes in the elderly (26).
- Coordinate care with all health-care providers including specialists to eliminate conflicting advice and duplicate prescriptions.
- Involve the patient in therapeutic decision-making to ensure that the patient's goals are being met and to optimize adherence.

REFERENCES

1. Kuehn BM. New diabetes drugs target gut hormones. JAMA 2006; 296(4):380–381.
2. Riddle MC, Drucker DJ. Emerging therapies mimicking the effects of amylin and glucagon-like peptide 1. Diabetes Care 2006; 29(2):435–449.

3. Brown AF, Mangione CM, Saliba D, Sarkisian CA. Guidelines for improving the care of the older person with diabetes mellitus. J Am Geriatr Soc 2003; 51(suppl 5 Guidelines):S265–S280.
4. Good CB. Polypharmacy in elderly patients with diabetes. Diabetes Spectr 2002; 15(4):240–248.
5. Mateo JF, Gil-Guillen VF, Mateo E, Orozco D, Carbayo JA, Merino J. Multifactorial approach and adherence to prescribed oral medications in patients with type 2 diabetes. Int J Clin Pract 2006; 60(4): 422–428.
6. Rubin RR. Adherence to pharmacologic therapy in patients with type 2 diabetes mellitus. Am J Med 2005; 118(suppl 5A):27S–34S.
7. Higashi T, Shekelle PG, Solomon DH, et al. The quality of pharmacologic care for vulnerable older patients. Ann Intern Med 2004; 140(9):714–720.
8. Winkelmayer WC, Fischer MA, Schneeweiss S, Wang PS, Levin R, Avorn J. Underuse of ACE inhibitors and angiotensin II receptor blockers in elderly patients with diabetes. Am J Kidney Dis 2005; 46(6):1080–1087.
9. Boyd CM, Darer J, Boult C, Fried LP, Boult L, Wu AW. Clinical practice guidelines and quality of care for older patients with multiple comorbid diseases: implications for pay for performance. JAMA 2005; 294(6):716–724.
10. Durso SC. Using clinical guidelines designed for older adults with diabetes mellitus and complex health status. JAMA 2006; 295(16):1935–1940.
11. Tinetti ME, Bogardus ST Jr, Agostini JV. Potential pitfalls of disease-specific guidelines for patients with multiple conditions. N Engl J Med 2004; 351(27):2870–2874.
12. Holmes HM, Hayley DC, Alexander GC, Sachs GA. Reconsidering medication appropriateness for patients late in life. Arch Intern Med 2006; 166(6):605–609.
13. Mitchell SL, Rockwood K. The association between antiulcer medication and initiation of cobalamin replacement in older persons. J Clin Epidemiol 2001; 54(5):531–534.
14. Dresser GK, Bailey DG. A basic conceptual and practical overview of interactions with highly prescribed drugs. Can J Clin Pharmacol 2002; 9(4):191–198.
15. Horowitz M, Su YC, Rayner CK, Jones KL. Gastroparesis: prevalence, clinical significance and treatment. Can J Gastroenterol 2001; 15(12):805–813.
16. Kroner BA. Common drug pathways and interactions. Diabetes Spectr 2002; 15(4):249–255.
17. Wilkinson GR. Drug metabolism and variability among patients in drug response. N Engl J Med 2005; 352(21):2211–2221.
18. Stevens LA, Coresh J, Greene T, Levey AS. Assessing kidney function—measured and estimated glomerular filtration rate. N Engl J Med 2006; 354(23):2473–2483.
19. Cockcroft DW, Gault MH. Prediction of creatinine clearance from serum creatinine. Nephron 1976; 16(1):31–41.
20. Holstein A, Stumvoll M. Contraindications can damage your health—is metformin a case in point? Diabetologia 2005; 48(12):2454–2459.
21. Salpeter S, Greyber E, Pasternak G, Salpeter E. Risk of fatal and nonfatal lactic acidosis with metformin use in type 2 diabetes mellitus. Cochrane Database Syst Rev 2003; (2):CD002967.
22. Ferner RE, Aronson JK. Communicating information about drug safety. Br Med J 2006; 333(7559): 143–145.
23. Weiss SR, Cheng SL, Kourides IA, Gelfand RA, Landschulz WH. Inhaled insulin provides improved glycemic control in patients with type 2 diabetes mellitus inadequately controlled with oral agents: a randomized controlled trial. Arch Intern Med 2003; 163(19):2277–2282.
24. Reunanen A, Kangas T, Martikainen J, Klaukka T. Nationwide survey of comorbidity, use, and costs of all medications in Finnish diabetic individuals. Diabetes Care 2000; 23(9):1265–1271.
25. American Diabetes Association. Standards of Medical Care in Diabetes—2006. Diabetes Care 2006; 29(suppl 1):S4–S42.
26. Fick DM, Cooper JW, Wade WE, Waller JL, Maclean JR, Beers MH. Updating the Beers criteria for potentially inappropriate medication use in older adults: results of a US consensus panel of experts. Arch Intern Med 2003; 163(22):2716–2724.
27. McLeod PJ, Huang AR, Tamblyn RM, Gayton DC. Defining inappropriate practices in prescribing for elderly people: a national consensus panel. CMAJ 1997; 156(3):385–391.
28. Curtis LH, Ostbye T, Sendersky V, et al. Inappropriate prescribing for elderly Americans in a large outpatient population. Arch Intern Med 2004; 164(15):1621–1625.
29. Shah BR, Mamdani M, Jaakkimainen L, Hux JE. Risk modification for diabetic patients. Are other risk factors treated as diligently as glycemia? Can J Clin Pharmacol 2004; 11(2):e239–e244.
30. Shelton PS, Fritsch MA, Scott MA. Assessing medication appropriateness in the elderly: a review of available measures. Drugs Aging 2000; 16(6):437–450.
31. Scheen AJ. Drug interactions of clinical importance with antihyperglycaemic agents: an update. Drug Saf 2005; 28(7):601–631.
32. Juurlink DN, Mamdani M, Kopp A, Laupacis A, Redelmeier DA. Drug-drug interactions among elderly patients hospitalized for drug toxicity. JAMA 2003; 289(13):1652–1658.
33. Adhiyaman V, Asghar M, Oke A, White AD, Shah IU. Nephrotoxicity in the elderly due to co-prescription of angiotensin converting enzyme inhibitors and nonsteroidal anti-inflammatory drugs. J R Soc Med 2001; 94(10):512–514.

34. Pandit MK, Burke J, Gustafson AB, Minocha A, Peiris AN. Drug-induced disorders of glucose tolerance. Ann Intern Med 1993; 118(7):529–539.

35. Luna B, Feinglos MN. Drug-induced hyperglycemia. JAMA 2001; 286(16):1945–1948.

36. Park-Wyllie LY, Juurlink DN, Kopp A, et al. Outpatient gatifloxacin therapy and dysglycemia in older adults. N Engl J Med 2006; 354(13):1352–1361.

37. Seltzer HS. Drug-induced hypoglycemia. A review of 1418 cases. Endocrinol Metab Clin North Am 1989; 18(1):163–183.

38. Lasser KE, Allen PD, Woolhandler SJ, Himmelstein DU, Wolfe SM, Bor DH. Timing of New Black Box Warnings and Withdrawals for Prescription Medications. JAMA 2002; 287(17):2215–2220.

39. Nesto RW, Bell D, Bonow RO, et al. Thiazolidinedione use, fluid retention, and congestive heart failure: a consensus statement from the American Heart Association and American Diabetes Association. Diabetes Care 2004; 27(1):256–263.

40. Bell DSH. Do sulfonylurea drugs increase the risk of cardiac events? Can Med Assoc J 2006; 174(2):185–186.

41. Simpson SH, Majumdar SR, Tsuyuki RT, Eurich DT, Johnson JA. Dose-response relation between sulfonylurea drugs and mortality in type 2 diabetes mellitus: a population-based cohort study. Can Med Assoc J 2006; 174(2):169–174.

42. Badamgarav E, Fitzpatrick LA. A new look at osteoporosis outcomes: the influence of treatment, compliance, persistence, and adherence. Mayo Clin Proc 2006; 81(8):1009–1012.

43. Cramer JA. A systematic review of adherence with medications for diabetes. Diabetes Care 2004; 27(5):1218–1224.

44. Granger BB, Swedberg K, Ekman I, et al. Adherence to candesartan and placebo and outcomes in chronic heart failure in the CHARM programme: double-blind, randomised, controlled clinical trial. Lancet 2005; 366(9502):2005–2011.

45. Kogut SJ, Andrade SE, Willey C, Larrat EP. Nonadherence as a predictor of antidiabetic drug therapy intensification (augmentation). Pharmacoepidemiol Drug Saf 2004; 13(9):591–598.

46. Pladevall M, Williams LK, Potts LA, Divine G, Xi H, Lafata JE. Clinical outcomes and adherence to medications measured by claims data in patients with diabetes. Diabetes Care 2004; 27(12):2800–2805.

47. Simpson SH, Eurich DT, Majumdar SR, et al. A meta-analysis of the association between adherence to drug therapy and mortality. Br Med J 2006.

48. Sokol MC, McGuigan KA, Verbrugge RR, Epstein RS. Impact of medication adherence on hospitalization risk and healthcare cost. Med Care 2005; 43(6):521–530.

49. Parris ES, Lawrence DB, Mohn LA, Long LB. Adherence to statin therapy and LDL cholesterol goal attainment by patients with diabetes and dyslipidemia. Diabetes Care 2005; 28(3):595–599.

50. Katon W, Cantrell CR, Sokol MC, Chiao E, Gdovin JM. Impact of antidepressant drug adherence on comorbid medication use and resource utilization. Arch Intern Med 2005; 165(21):2497–2503.

51. Kilbourne AM, Reynolds CF III, Good CB, Sereika SM, Justice AC, Fine MJ. How does depression influence diabetes medication adherence in older patients? Am J Geriatr Psychiatry 2005; 13(3):202–210.

52. Haynes RB, McDonald HP, Garg AX. Helping patients follow prescribed treatment: clinical applications. JAMA 2002; 288(22):2880–2883.

9 | Urinary Incontinence in Older Adults with Diabetes

Catherine E. DuBeau
Section of Geriatrics, The University of Chicago, Chicago, Illinois, U.S.A.

INTRODUCTION

Any discussion of the impact of diabetes mellitus (DM) on voiding function and symptoms in older persons faces enormous challenges. First, the literature is fraught with definitional disarray and imprecision that not only predates but also continues after the establishment of standardized terminology for lower urinary tract (LUT) function (1). Second, the prevalence of age-related LUT changes, comorbid conditions, and functional and cognitive impairment that affect the LUT and the functional ability to toilet in older persons makes it difficult to sort out the independent effect of DM. Finally, changes in DM-related disease factors (type, duration, treatment, glycemic control, and complications) in the population over the past decades have likely affected the epidemiology and indeed the pathophysiology of DM-related voiding dysfunction. The assertion over 25 years ago that "the clinical picture and therapy (of bladder involvement in DM) have been clearly delineated" (2) could not be further from the truth today.

In general, the understanding of the effect of DM on voiding has moved from that of a highly symptomatic late-stage "diabetic cystopathy" with "progression of the bladder paralysis" leading to poor prognosis with urinary retention and frequent urinary tract infections (UTIs) (2) to one of earlier and asymptomatic cystometric abnormalities (3), reflecting pathophysiologic changes in the detrusor smooth muscle, urothelium, central and autonomic nervous systems, and blood supply. For older persons, the effect of DM on voiding is more complex. Even in the presence of a normal LUT, urinary incontinence (UI) may occur because of functional, cognitive, or affective impairment, medical conditions, and medications. Thus, effects of DM, DM-related complications, and DM treatment have important roles in the etiology of UI in older persons with DM.

This chapter will review the epidemiology of voiding symptoms in older persons with DM; the pathophysiologic impact of DM on voiding; DM-related factors that affect toileting and micturition; asymptomatic bacteriuria (ASB) and UTIs; assessment and treatment of UI in older persons with DM; and the effects of DM treatment on UI.

EPIDEMIOLOGY OF VOIDING SYMPTOMS IN PERSONS WITH DM

An early review reported that LUT symptoms (LUTS) as determined by "careful questioning... (regarding) bladder dysfunction" were present in 37% to 50% of DM patients (primarily insulin treated) (4). More recent estimates of the prevalence of LUTS in older persons with DM are difficult to codify because of wide variation in LUTS definitions, survey methods, source populations, and DM-related factors. For example, a case control study of 176 older women found that nocturia and voiding difficulty were more common with DM [for nocturia, 37% vs. 22% ($P < 0.001$); for voiding difficulty, odds ratio (OR) 4.8 (95% confidence interval CI, 2.3–10.4)] (5); however, UI was not reported, and the source population (Taiwanese, mean age 63, mean duration DM 11 years, 84% on oral agents) is difficult to generalize (5). At the same time, this study was unusual in its examination of a range of LUTS because many studies examine only UI. Prevalence of UI with DM in broader population-based studies may be affected by selection bias; for example, among 28,000 Scandinavian women aged 20 and above, the crude prevalence of UI was 38% with DM versus 24% without; yet the study included only 731 diabetics (6). Data regarding men are scant and often confounded by coexistent prostate disease.

Table 1 summarizes the estimated odds of UI with DM from cross-sectional and longitudinal cohort studies and secondary analyses of intervention trials.

TABLE 1 Epidemiology of UI in Older Persons with DM

Study (Ref.)	Method	Population	Definition of UI	Risk of UI with DM	DM-related covariates
Nurses Health Study (7)	Cross-sectional and longitudinal (4 yr followup) survey	Community-dwelling married female nurses, $n = 81,845$, mean age ~63, 5% with self-reported type 2 DM; followup available in 58%	Self-reported leakage at least weekly in past 12 mo; incident UI = UI in previously dry women at 4 yr followup	Prevalent UI: any, adjusted RR 1.28 (95% CI, 1.18–1.39); very severe UI, adjusted RR 1.78 (95% CI, 1.49–2.12). Incident UI: any, RR 1.21 (95% CI, 1.02–1.43); very severe, RR 1.97 (95% CI, 1.24–3.12)	DM duration >10 yr and microvascular complications increased UI risk
Study of Women's Health Across the Nation (8)	Cross-sectional population-based survey	Community-based perimenopausal women aged 42–54, $n = 3302$, 7.6% with DM	Self-reported urine leakage of any amount in past 12 mo	Any UI: adjusted OR 1.53 (95% CI, 1.12–2.1), moderate–severe UI: adjusted OR 1.55 (95% CI, 1.07–2.25)	NA
Health, Aging, and Body Composition Study (9)	Cross-sectional survey from two clinical sites with large minority populations (49% black)	Community-dwelling healthy women aged 70–79, $n = 1584$, 20% with DM	Self-reported urine leakage of any amount in past 12 mo	Insulin-treated DM: urge UI OR 3.50 (95% CI, 1.55–7.91); no association with DM treated by diet or oral medication; no association with stress UI	No interaction between race and DM despite the higher prevalence of DM in blacks
Study of Osteoporotic Fractures (10)	Cross-sectional analysis of prospective cohort study	Community-dwelling, healthy, nonblack women aged ≥65, $n = 7949$, mean age 77, 6.5% with DM	Self-reported urine leakage of any amount in past 12 mo	Daily UI: OR 1.7 (95% CI, 1.2–2.4); risk of daily UI attributable to DM 4%	NA
EPESE (11)	Cross-sectional survey	Community-dwelling residents of East Boston, Massachusetts aged ≥65, $n = 3809$, 16% with DM	Self-report of frequency of difficulty holding urine until one can reach toilet	Among men aged 65–74, for mild difficulty holding, OR 1.8 ($P < 0.001$); no association for severe difficulty. Among men 75+ no association for mild or severe difficulty	NA

Study	Design	Population	Measure of UI	Results	
Iowa 65+ Rural Health Study of EPESE (12)	Cross-sectional analysis of longitudinal cohort study	Community-based women aged ≥65 in two rural counties, n = 2025, 11% with DM	Self-report of frequency of difficulty holding urine until one can reach toilet (urge UI); leakage of urine with cough, sneeze or laugh (stress UI)	Among women aged 65–74, for mild difficulty, OR 1.9 ($P < 0.001$); for severe difficulty, OR 3.7 ($P < 0.001$) Among women aged 75+, no association for mild or severe difficulty	NA
Washtenaw County, Michigan (13)	Cross-sectional survey	Probability sample of community-based persons aged ≥60, n = 1956	Self-reported involuntary loss of urine, at least days in the preceding 12 mo or with urgency and stress leakage symptoms	All prevalent UI, OR (controlled for age and parity) 1.38 ($P = 0.02$); no assessment of incident UI. UI in 20.3% of men ($P = 0.07$) and 13.6% of women ($P = 0.55$) who reported DM	NA
Heart and Estrogen/ Progestin Replacement Study (14,15)	Cross-sectional baseline (14) and longitudinal (4.2 yr) (15) data from randomized controlled trial of estrogen + progestin	Postmenopausal women with age <80 with coronary heart disease and intact uterus, n = 2763, mean age 67, 23% with DM; follow-up data available for 44%	Self-report of frequency of unintentional leakage during previous week: with coughing, etc (stress UI); before reaching toilet (urge UI)	Urge UI, adjusted OR 1.49 (95% CI, 1.11–2.00); mixed UI, 1.32 (95% CI, 1.04–1.67); no association with stress UI; DM did not modify the increased risk of incident UI with hormone therapy	NA
Health and Retirement Study (16)	Cross-sectional analysis of longitudinal cohort study	Community-dwelling women aged 50–90 yr from probability sample of U.S. national households oversampled for minority populations, n = 10,497, 8% with DM	Self-reported urine leakage of any amount beyond one's control at least once in the preceding month	For insulin-requiring DM, adjusted OR 1.63 (95% CI, 1.28–2.09); non-insulin-requiring DM, OR 1.20 (95% CI, 1.00–1.45)	NA

Abbreviations: CI, confidence interval; DM, diabetes mellitus; EPESE, Established Populations for Epidemiologic Study of the Elderly; NA, not available; OR, odds ratio; RR, relative risk; UI, urinary incontinence.

Despite the heterogeneity of the studies, several trends are evident. Clearly, DM increases the risk of UI, although the attributable risk (that is, the proportion of all UI in a population primarily due to DM) varies widely, from 4% (10) to 17% (7) among women. The risk of severe UI (more frequent and/or large volume) is at least as great or greater than the risk of less-severe UI (7,8,11). The risk of UI appears to increase with DM duration (7) and with insulin-treated DM (9,16). In the trial that reported types of UI, DM was associated with urge but not with stress UI (14,15). The impact of age on the risk of UI from DM was usually obscured by controlling for age in the analyses. One study did find that the odds of UI were increased among women and men with DM aged 65 to 75 but not those aged ≥75 (11), possibly due to the confounding of the association by higher comorbidity and cognitive and functional impairments.

Further data are anticipated from ongoing large studies, including the Action for Health in Diabetes (Look AHEAD), a randomized trial of weight loss in obese women with type 2 DM aged 45 to 75; the Diabetes Prevention Program Outcome Program; and the Epidemiology of Diabetes Interventions & Complications, a prospective cohort study of persons with type 1 DM (17).

PATHOPHYSIOLOGIC IMPACT OF DIABETES ON VOIDING
Diabetes and Continence

Continence in the older persons depends not only on intact LUT and neurological function but also on cognitive and functional status, manual dexterity, motivation, and absence of medical conditions and medications that can affect the LUT, either directly or through any of the domains determining continence. UI is a classic geriatric syndrome and has, with other such syndromes, shared risk factors, including lower and upper extremity impairment, decreased vision and hearing, and affective impairment (18). Because the risk of UI increases with the number of predisposing factors present (18) and because DM may result in many of these predisposing factors, the association between DM and UI in older persons is driven as much by DM-associated comorbidity as by direct effects on detrusor smooth muscle and nerves.

Thus, DM-associated comorbidity can impair UI in multiple and additive ways (Table 2).

Constipation, which affects nearly 60% of diabetics (20), can impair bladder emptying. Congestive heart failure from DM-related coronary artery disease can cause pedal edema and nocturnal polyuria, leading to the nocturia and nighttime UI. Stroke can impair cerebral areas affecting bladder sensation and ability to inhibit voiding; associated cognitive impairment can impair the functional ability to toilet independently (and when severely advanced, even impair toileting with

TABLE 2   Diabetic Comorbidity Associated with Incontinence

System/condition	Effect on continence
Cardiovascular	
Coronary heart disease with congestive heart failure	Nocturnal diuresis from CHF
Arteriosclerosis	Detrusor underactivity or areflexia from ischemic myopathy or neuropathy
Neurologic	
Cerebrovascular disease; stroke	DO from damage to upper motor neurons; impaired sensation to void from interruption of subcortical pathways; impaired function and cognition
Delirium	Impaired function and cognition
Dementia	DO from damage to upper motor neurons; impaired function and cognition
Peripheral neuropathy	Impaired ambulation
Infectious disease	
Urinary tract infections	Urgency, frequency, and UI
Psychiatric	
Affective disorders	Decreased motivation to toilet
Gastrointestinal	
Constipation	Retention and overflow UI
Musculoskeletal	Mobility impairment
Ophthalmologic	Retinopathy causing impaired vision and ability to safely set to a toilet

Abbreviations: CHF, congestive heart failure; DO, detrusor overactivity; UI, urinary incontinence.
Source: From Ref. 19.

assistance). Diabetic neuropathy, associated Charcot joints, peripheral vascular disease, and amputation can impair mobility, which is a key determinant of UI in older persons.

In addition, some medications for the treatment of DM and its complications can impair continence or complicate its treatment. The thiazolidinediones, as well as gabapentin and pregabalin (used to treat DM neuropathy), may cause pedal edema and congestive heart failure, thereby leading to nocturia and nighttime UI. The cough associated with angiotensin converting enzyme inhibitors can exacerbate stress UI. Calcium channel blockers (CCBs) used for hypertension can impair detrusor contraction through direct effects on calcium-mediated smooth muscle contraction and indirectly through exacerbation of constipation. In addition, pyridine CCBs can cause pedal edema. Other agents used for DM neuropathy with potential LUT effect include duloxetine, which has been shown to decrease stress UI (21), and tricyclic antidepressants, the anticholinergic effects of which can impair detrusor contractility and cause constipation. Pioglitazone, diltiazem, sildenafil and tadalafil (for DM-associated erectile dysfunction), losartan, and statins (atorvastatin, lovastatin, and simvastatin) may interfere with the hepatic metabolism of the bladder-relaxant drugs oxybutynin, tolterodine, darifenacin, and solifenacin, all of which are metabolized via CYP450-2D6 and 3A4. Metformin may compete for renal clearance with the bladder-relaxant trospium.

Overview of Normal Micturition
Physiology
Normal micturition requires low-pressure urine storage with urethral closure and effective emptying through bladder contraction and urethral relaxation at the desired time and place. Micturition is coordinated through the central, peripheral, and autonomic nervous systems. The parietal lobes and thalamus receive and coordinate detrusor afferent stimuli while the frontal lobes and basal ganglia provide modulation with inhibitory signals. Central coordination occurs in the pontine micturition center, and peripheral coordination in the sacral-cord micturition center (S2–S4). The detrusor receives efferent stimulation via the parasympathetic pelvic nerve, which acts on muscarinic receptors in detrusor smooth muscle and possibly also in the urothelium. The urethral smooth-muscle sphincter receives efferent stimulation via the sympathetic hypogastric nerve arising from spinal levels T11–L2, and act on α-adrenergic receptors. Sphincter closure is augmented by striated sphincter muscle contraction with somatic nicotinic cholinergic stimulation via the pudendal nerve. Maintenance of urethral closure also depends on a fascial and muscular "hammock" which supports the urethra by compressing it when there is increased abdominal pressure or when the pelvic muscles are contracted (22).

When detrusor afferent stimuli indicate the need to void, the pontine center coordinates efferent parasympathetic signaling, resulting in preganglionic inhibition of sympathetic tone, leading to urethral relaxation and the stimulation of detrusor contraction.

Afferent and efferent signaling in the bladder depends, however, on more than muscarinic receptors. Purinergic, β-adrenergic, and vanilloid-receptor systems, plus transmitters and second messengers (such as nitric oxide, prostaglandins, substance P, and ATP/cAMP) in both the smooth muscle and, possibly more importantly, the urothelium also play a role in mediating normal and uninhibited bladder contractions (23). Recent work highlights a growing emphasis on the role of the urothelium in both normal micturition and generation of uninhibited contractions and impaired contractility (23).

As noted above, a key difference between younger and older persons is that in the latter, an intact LUT is insufficient to assure normal voiding. In older persons, "continence" additionally depends on the "ability to toilet oneself"—requiring physical function, cognition, motivation, and toilet availability—and the absence of medical conditions, medications, or other factors that affect LUT function, volume status, urine excretion, and/or physical and cognitive function. A full discussion of all of these factors is outside of the scope of this chapter; the reader is referred to reviews of this topic (24,25).

Pathophysiology and LUT Symptoms
UI is grouped into five main types:

1. In older persons, UI may be due to "potentially reversible conditions" that can contribute to UI. This has also been called "transient" or "functional" UI (24,26). The associated conditions

can be categorized into four main types: (*i*) inflammation or irritation in or around the LUT; (*ii*) increased urine production; (*iii*) medication side effects; and (*iv*) conditions that impair the functional and/or cognitive ability or willingness to toilet (26).

2. "Urge UI" is characterized by leakage associated with urgency, an abrupt compelling need to void (1). Urgency, with or without UI, is often accompanied by frequency and nocturia, a symptom complex termed overactive bladder. Uninhibited detrusor contractions (termed detrusor overactivity) are often found on cystometry. However, because detrusor overactivity (DO) is found in healthy continent older persons (27), failure of LUT and functional compensatory mechanisms may play an important etiologic role in urge UI in older persons. DO may coexist with impaired detrusor contractility, a condition called detrusor hyperactivity with impaired contractility (DHIC) (28). Persons with DHIC have urge UI with an elevated postvoid residual (PVR) in the absence of outlet obstruction.

3. "Stress UI" is characterized by leakage associated with increased abdominal pressure (e.g., from coughing, sneezing, or physical activity). It results from failure of the sphincter mechanism(s) to preserve outlet closure during bladder filling.

4. "Mixed UI" is the combination of urge and stress UI symptoms and is common in women.

5. "UI due to impaired bladder emptying" (also known as "overflow" UI) results from impaired detrusor contractility, bladder outlet obstruction, or both. Leakage is typically small in volume but continual. The PVR is elevated, and associated LUTS may include dribbling, weak urinary stream, intermittency, hesitancy, frequency, or nocturia.

Age-Related Changes

The prevalence of DO increases with age, and it can be found in 21% of healthy, continent, community-dwelling older persons (27). The ability to postpone voiding decreases and the total bladder capacity may diminish, leading to increased frequency of normal voiding and urge UI. An age-related decrease in detrusor contractility (29) leads to lower urinary flow rates in both older men and women with a modest increase in PVR (up to 50 mL). Most older men have benign prostatic hyperplasia, with about one-half developing hypertrophy with the potential for bladder outlet obstruction and voiding symptoms. Obstruction also is associated with the development of uninhibited detrusor contractions. The diurnal pattern of fluid excretion can shift toward later in the day and into the night (30).

Urodynamic Observations

Urodynamic evaluation, including cystometry, urethral pressure measurement, and pressure-flow studies, provide quantitative data on bladder sensation, contractility, compliance, uninhibited contractions, and sphincter function. Table 3 lists commonly used standardized (1) urodynamic terminology and definitions.

Urodynamic studies dating to the 1940s describe impaired bladder sensation and large cystometric capacity in patients with DM (3). The term "diabetic cystopathy" is attributed to Frimodt-Moller (31) and is generally described as the combination of impaired bladder sensation, large bladder capacity, and impaired contractility (including areflexia). Early reviews cited urodynamic (largely cystometric) abnormalities in 26% to 87% of diabetics, with an association between cystopathy and DM duration but not age or gender (4). Later reports stress that urodynamic abnormalities may be more subtle, asymptomatic, and occur earlier in the course of DM (3,32,33).

There have been numerous case series describing urodynamic findings among selected and unselected persons with DM. They are difficult to summarize because of the heterogeneity of the populations, subject selection criteria [even some purportedly "nonselected" general care DM patients were referred for evaluation (32)], symptoms, DM duration and complications, comorbidity [e.g., prostate disease and stroke (32)], and urodynamic definitions. Many of these case series are relatively small. The lack of control groups makes these studies especially difficult to interpret in regard to older patients because normal urodynamic findings are the exception even among healthy asymptomatic elders (27). Moreover, the correlation between laboratory cystometric findings, usual voiding function, symptoms is

TABLE 3 Standardized Terminology of Urodynamically Defined Lower Urinary Tract Function

Bladder sensation during filling cystometry	Normal bladder sensation	Judged by three defined points (first sensation of filling, first desire to void, and strong desire to void) and evaluated in relation to the bladder volume at that moment and in relation to the patient's symptomatic complaints
	First sensation of bladder filling	The feeling the patient has when he/she first becomes aware of the bladder filling
	First desire to void	The feeling that would lead the patient to pass urine at the next convenient moment, but voiding can be delayed if necessary
	Strong desire to void	A persistent desire to void without the fear of leakage
	Increased bladder sensation	An early first sensation of bladder filling (or an early desire to void) and/or an early strong desire to void, which occurs at low bladder volume and which persists
	Reduced bladder sensation	Diminished sensation throughout bladder filling
	Absent bladder sensation	The individual has no bladder sensation
	Urgency	A sudden compelling desire to void
Bladder function during filling cystometry	Normal detrusor function	Allows bladder filling with little or no change in pressure. No involuntary phasic contractions occur despite provocation
	Detrusor overactivity[a]	Involuntary detrusor contractions during the filling phase that may be spontaneous or provoked
	Detrusor overactivity incontinence	Incontinence due to an involuntary detrusor contraction
	Neurogenic detrusor overactivity[b]	Detrusor overactivity in the setting of a relevant neurological condition
	Idiopathic detrusor overactivity	Detrusor overactivity with no defined cause
	Detrusor underactivity	A contraction of reduced strength and/or duration, resulting in prolonged bladder emptying and/or a failure to achieve complete bladder emptying within a normal time span
	Acontractile detrusor	Cannot be demonstrated to contract during urodynamic studies
Bladder capacity	Cystometric capacity	The bladder volume at the end of the filling cystometrogram, when "permission to void" is usually given. The endpoint should be specified, for example, if filling is stopped when the patient has a normal desire to void. The cystometric capacity is the volume voided together with any residual urine
	Maximum cystometric capacity	In patients with normal sensation, the volume at which the patient feels he/she can no longer delay micturition (has a strong desire to void); in patients with impaired sensation, the volume at which the clinician decides to terminate filling[c]

[a]Replaced the term "detrusor instability"; the new definition specifically does not specify the amplitude of the involuntary contraction.
[b]Replaced the term "detrusor hyperreflexia."
[c]The reason(s) for terminating filling should be defined, for example, high detrusor filling pressure, large infused volume or pain, and uncontrollable voiding. In the presence of sphincter incompetence, the cystometric capacity may be significantly increased by occlusion of the urethra, for example, by Foley catheter.
Source: From Ref. 1.

imprecise. For example, in one series of 109 patients who had abnormally high maximum bladder volumes (>800 mL) during cystometry (which might suggest impaired detrusor compliance and contractility) one-third had otherwise normal urodynamic findings, including compliance and contractility (34).

In a widely cited study, Kaplan et al. reviewed the urodynamic results in a case series of 182 DM patients referred for urological evaluation (age 48–93 years, mean DM duration 58 ± 16 months, 37% diet controlled, and 28% on insulin). DO was present in 52%, 23% had impaired contractility, 10% had areflexia, 24% had poor bladder compliance, and 57% of the men had outlet obstruction (35). DO may have been underestimated because the definition used required a phasic increase in detrusor pressure of ≥ 15 cmH$_2$O, whereas current criteria allow for any phasic increase (1). Although mean volumes at first sensation of filling and bladder capacity were high (298 and 485 mL, respectively), it is not clear what proportion of patients had abnormal sensation and increased capacity. Similar findings of impaired sensory threshold, increased bladder capacity, and impaired contractility have been confirmed by others (32). Classic cystopathic findings of reduced or absent contractility appear more common in patients with abnormal sacral sensation or reflexes (35), autonomic neuropathy (abnormal sympathetic skin response) (32), peripheral neuropathy (4), and longer DM duration (4). Sphincter function in DM has not been well evaluated; an older, small, case series using voiding cystourethrograms found impaired internal sphincter relaxation in 23%, which correlated with symptomatic neuropathy (33).

There has been one small study in frail older persons with DM ($n = 23$), but the results are difficult to interpret because of selection (all referred for urodynamics, including four with retention), comorbidity (e.g., 13 had stroke), and use of CO_2 rather than fluid cystometry (36).

Pathophysiological Effects of DM on the LUT

Yoshimura et al. have postulated a multifactoral, three-component model of DM-related detrusor dysfunction involving the detrusor smooth muscle, urothelium, and peripheral nerves (37). However, another element, especially for patients with poorly controlled or long-standing DM, may be ischemia affecting the bladder and its innervation. Therefore, an expanded model may be more appropriate (Fig. 1), in which DM and/or its associated hyperglycemia affect detrusor muscle cells through four main pathways: alterations to nerves innervating the LUT; ischemic damage to the detrusor and its innervation; alterations in the urothelium and its function; and/or direct effects on smooth muscle.

These pathways lead to the observed DM-related changes in detrusor smooth muscle: altered ionic mechanisms (leading to changes in excitability and/or intercellular communication); molecular changes in gene expression and contractile proteins; pharmacological changes in receptors and signal transduction; and structural changes, particularly hypertrophy and fibrosis.

Many of the insights regarding the effects of DM on the LUT come from animal models, especially the streptozotosin-induced diabetic (STZ-DM) rat and the alloxan-induced diabetic

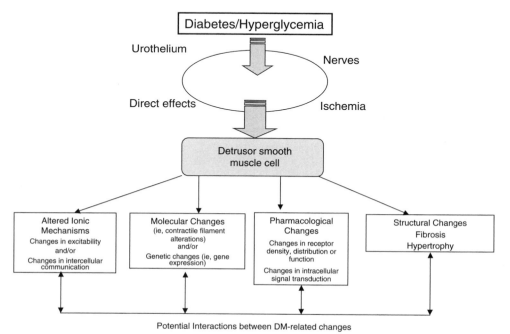

FIGURE 1 Pathways and mechanisms of the effects of DM on detrusor smooth muscle. *Abbreviation*: DM, diabetes mellitus. *Source*: From Ref. 37.

rabbit. A number of studies have used sucrose-fed animals as a control, to distinguish the impact of DM from that of osmotic diuresis, which puts a mechanical stretch load on the bladder that independently may affect motor and sensory function (38).

Detrusor
Smooth Muscle
The major changes found in animal models are hypertrophy (39,40) (which may be driven at least as much by osmotic diuresis as by DM itself) (40,41), increased responsiveness to electric field stimulation (contraction independent of specific receptor mechanisms) (37), and variable and contradictory responses to agonist stimulation (37,42,43). These changes, especially the increased stimulatory response, are thought to possibly underlie the development of DM-related DO. The variable findings in agonist-induced contractility may be due to: whether results were normalized to account for increases in tissue mass; treatment with insulin (44); duration of STZ-DM; or more receptor-specific alterations. Smooth-muscle changes thought to account for DM-related DO are complex and multiple. They include altered signaling mechanisms (membrane ion handling, decrease in Na^+-K^+-ATPase pump activity) (45), alterations in prostaglandins and second messengers such as cAMP (46), or alterations in transmitter density (e.g., substance P and vasointestinal peptide) (47); changes in myosin phosphorylation, leading to decreased force generation (48,49); changes in Aδ and C-fiber afferents (from the bladder to the dorsal root ganglia) due to a time-dependent decrease in nerve growth factor (50); and oxidative stress (51). Cytosolic calcium levels do not appear to change (52).

Urothelium
As noted above, the sensory and pharmacological properties of the urothelium are increasingly recognized as key factors in normal and pathological micturition. In STZ-DM models, the urothelium undergoes progressive hypertrophy (37), which together with injury and inflammation appears to increase release of ATP and bradykinins, resulting in urothelium-dependent smooth-muscle excitability and contraction (37) that could contribute to the development of DM-related DO. Many of the same factors mentioned above causing impaired contractility also may occur in the urothelium and alter urothelial smooth muscle–interstitial cell interactions.

Afferent and Efferent Nerves
The prominence of neuropathic complications in DM suggests a likely role for DM neuropathies in DM-related voiding dysfunction. Peripheral motor and sensory neuropathy in peroneal and sural nerves has been correlated with impaired bladder sensation and contractility in humans (53). However, STZ-DM animal studies have overall found no changes in detrusor efferent nerve function (38). Increased cross-sectional area of efferent neurons in STZ-DM has been attributed to osmotic diuresis alone (38). Sensory afferent function, however, is clearly affected by DM (37,38) and the cross-sectional area of afferent nerves to the dorsal root ganglia decreases (47). Impaired production of nerve-growth factor in the bladder, and/or its axonal transport to the dorsal root ganglia, appear to be an important underlying mechanism causing impaired sensory function (37). Many of the detrusor muscle and urothelium changes noted above are closely tied to and may affect afferent nerve function.

Ischemia
Severe atherosclerosis affects ganglia and small nerve bundles, raising the possibility that with DM degeneration in the intrinsic detrusor ganglia may be due to ischemic injury (54). However, no studies of ischemia in DM animal or human models exist; inferences are from non-DM animal models in which the experimental ischemia may not reflect what occurs in human DM.

Ischemia effects may be mediated by changes in the detrusor smooth muscle, intracellular tissue, and urothelium (38,55,56). Although in vivo, animal models demonstrate ischemia-related impaired contractility (55), in vitro studies show no decrease in contractility with nonspecific and cholinergic (bethanecol) stimulation (57). Other models suggest that ischemia/reperfusion alterations affect contractility (primarily through nerve and not smooth-muscle damage) (58) and that hypertrophied bladders may be relatively protected (59). Variability in the observed effects of ischemia on contractility may be related to the extent of ischemic injury (55) and the degree of ischemia-induced detrusor fibrosis (60).

Urethra

The detrusor may not be the only LUT site affected by DM. Anderson and Bradley first identified slowed sphincter nerve conduction velocity using electromyography in 27 DM patients (61). Twenty years later, it was shown that cerebral evoked potentials could not be elicited by stimulation of the vesicourethral junction in 31 of 46 men with DM (mean age 46), and that this abnormality was not related to peripheral neuropathy (62). Studies in STZ-DM rats demonstrate impaired urethral relaxation (which is partially reversed by the α-blocker terazosin) (63), possibly mediated by changes in nitric oxide synthetase (NOS) (63,64); others have found no change in contractile and relaxation responses to acetylcholine and capsaicin, respectively (65). Studies in alloxan-DM rabbits also found changes in sphincter NOS (46).

ASYMPTOMATIC BACTERIURIA AND URINARY TRACT INFECTION

Both UTI and asymptomatic bacteriuria ASB are well-recognized complications of DM in women. Very little is known, however, about UTI in older DM men (66,67). The following discussion therefore applies only to women.

Asymptomatic Bacteriuria

ASB is defined as two consecutive voided urine specimens with isolation of the same bacterial strain in quantitative counts of $\geq 10^5$ data colony-forming units/mL from a patient without fever or other UTI symptoms (e.g., dysuria, frequency) (68). Although it is frequently quoted that ASB is three times more common in DM than in non-DM women, this figure was derived by comparing the rate of ASB in a case series of DM women (7.9%) (69) with population-based data. More recent population-based studies, however, have found higher ASB rates of 5% in healthy young women (70). Also, the relevance of the case series to older women with DM is unclear, because the prevalence of ASB in women aged 65 and older is estimated at 20%. One case-control study found ASB in 26% of DM women (aged 18–75) versus 6% of control subjects, but it defined ASB by only one positive asymptomatic culture (71). Another found the incidence of ASB (definition not specified) was 6.7/100 person-years in DM women versus 3.0 in nondiabetics [adjusted hazard ratio (HR) 2.1 (95% CI, 1.2–3.5)] (72). ASB was related to poor glycemic control [HgbA1c at baseline and one year >7.9% (HR 2.6; 95% CI, 1.1–6.0)], insulin treatment (HR 2.7; 95% CI, 1.0–6.6), and DM duration (≥ 10 years, HR 2.8; 95% CI, 1.4–5.7) (72). Others also have found ASB related to DM duration and racial/ethnic group (69). Pathogenesis of bacteriuria in women with DM has been attributed to lower urinary IL-6 concentration, altered production and structure of Tamm-Horsfall glycoproteins (which prevents bacterial attachment to epithelium), glycosuria, and the relationship of poor DM control with enhanced adherence of Escherichia coli type I fimbriae (66).

Not all diabetic women with ASB may be at increased risk of developing UTI, as some have suggested (67). In a prospective study of 589 DM women (mean age 52, all aged ≤ 75 years), 25% had baseline ASB (based on a single and not consecutive cultures), which was associated with development of symptomatic UTI in those with type II but not type I DM (73). Women with type I DM and ASB had a faster decline in renal function (based on serum creatinine) over 18 months (73). A randomized trial of antimicrobial treatment of ASB in DM women ($n = 105$, mean age ~56) did not reduce the frequency of or the time to UTI, and treatment was associated with higher rates of reinfection and adverse effects (74). Based on these results, the Infectious Disease Society of America guideline on ASB recommends against both routine screening for and treatment/prophylaxis of ASB in women with DM (68).

Urinary Tract Infection

Patients with DM carry a higher risk of UTIs, especially complicated ones. In a prospective case-control study, UTI incidence was 12.2/100 person-years in DM women versus 6.7 in nondiabetics; however, the association was no longer significant after controlling for age, sexual activity, and previous UTIs (72). Nonetheless, a risk remained for women with poor glycemic control (HgbA1c at baseline and one year >7.9%, adjusted HR 2.2; CI, 1.1–4.3), insulin treatment (HR 3.7; 95% CI, 1.8–7.3), and DM duration ≥10 years, (HR 2.6; CI, 1.3–5.1). While some authors assert that infection is a "chief complication" of diabetic bladder dysfunction (2), others have not found a consistent association between cystopathy and UTIs (4).

Diabetics with a UTI are more likely to develop bacteremia, pyelonephritis (including emphysematous), papillary necrosis, renal abscess, acute renal failure, and metastatic complications such as septic arthritis, osteomyelitis, and endopthalmytitis (67). Complicated pyelonephritis occurs in at least 10% (67). Reasons for these complications are unclear. Suggested etiologies include higher rates of upper track involvement (based on presence of antibody-coated bacteria) in diabetic women with ASB (69,72), elevated PVR (67), and the factors facilitating bacterial adherence and bacteriuria discussed above. Others have not found PVR to be a factor (72). To date, type of urinary pathogens, renal function, and immunity have not been found to contribute to the higher rate of complicated UTIs in DM (67).

Given the high complication rate, the evaluation of DM patients with UTI symptoms should include clinician examination, collection of a urine specimen for urinalysis and culture, and assessment of renal function and glycemic status (67). Patients with symptoms of pyelonephritis (e.g., flank pain, rigors, fever) should have blood cultures, and, if systemically ill, should have an ultrasound or computed tomography scan to evaluate the upper tracks for renal emphysema, obstruction, edema, abscess, or calculi (67,75). Treatment of uncomplicated UTI in diabetic women is the same as that for nondiabetics, that is a three-day course of trimethoprim-sulfa or seven days of nitrofurantoin; fluroquinolones also are effective in a three-day course but there are increasing concerns about resistance with widespread use (76,77). Antibiotics should be adjusted based on culture results. Follow-up urinalysis and culture should not be done, given the high prevalence of ASB in this population and lack of evidence that ASB treatment prevents recurrent UTIs.

ASSESSMENT AND TREATMENT OF UI IN DIABETES

Given the high prevalence of voiding dysfunction with DM and the fact that many persons with UI never mention it to a health-care provider, all older persons with DM should be screened for UI and other LUTS (78). Questions about "leakage" and "bladder control" may elicit more positive responses than those about "incontinence." Patients also should be asked specifically about frequency, urgency, and nocturia. History and exam is similar to that for other older persons with UI (79), but with special attention to constipation, diabetic control, medications, cognitive and functional status (including vision), and neurological changes. At the same time, providers should consider that not all UI in persons with DM is due to DM or its complications. Postvoiding residual volume, by ultrasound or catheter, should be performed (26,79). Urinalysis should be done, looking especially for glycosuria, but urine culture should not be done in the absence of UTI symptoms because of the high prevalence of ASB. A bladder diary can be very useful for evaluating whether polyuria, especially nocturnal, contributes to symptoms. Urodynamics are not necessary in the initial evaluation (26) but should be considered if the patient has a very large PVR (e.g., >300 mL), has failed empiric therapy, or desires surgical treatment for stress incontinence.

There have been essentially no robust studies regarding the impact of DM on the efficacy of UI treatment. Therefore, DM patients should be treated the same as others, starting with remediation of contributing factors and/or medications, followed by behavioral interventions, and then addition of a bladder relaxant if there is persistent urgency or urge UI (80) or referral for surgical treatment of stress UI, if desired. The association between poor glucose control, glycosuria, and worsening of LUTS should be explicitly described to patients because UI may be a motivating factor for better glycemic control. Weight loss should be encouraged for obese women (81). Table 4 lists the behavioral and pharmacological treatments for urge incontinence.

TABLE 4 Evidence-Based Efficacy of Treatments for Urge Incontinence[a]

Treatment	Target population	Efficacy	Level of evidence
Behavioral			
Bladder retraining	Cognitively intact	>35% decrease in UI episodes	A
Prompted voiding	Dependent, cognitively impaired	Average reduction 0.8–1.8 UI episodes daily; cure rare, caregiver dependent	A
Habit training	Voiding record available	≥25% decrease in UI episodes in one-third of patients; caregiver dependent	B
Scheduled toileting (timed voiding)	Unable to toilet independently	30–80% decrease in UI episodes	C
Pelvic muscle exercises	Women	Up to 80% decrease in episodes; motivated patients; more effective for stress UI	B
Medications			
All antimuscarinics	Unresponsive to behavioral treatment alone	Weighted mean difference in daily UI episodes 0.6 (95% CI, 0.4–0.8); dry mouth RR 2.56 (95% CI, 2.24–2.92)	A
Oxybutynin	—	Immediate release 2.5–5 mg b.i.d–q.i.d: extended release 5–20 mg daily: 71% mean reduction in weekly UI episodes, cure rate 23%, dry mouth 30%; topical patch 3.7 mg every 3 days	A
Tolterodine	—	Extended release 2–4 mg daily: 69% mean reduction in weekly UI episodes, cure rate 17%, dry mouth 22%	A
Trospium	—	20 mg b.i.d (20 mg qHS in persons with renal impairment): 59% mean reduction in daily UI episodes, cure rate 21%, dry mouth 22%, constipation 10%. Must be taken on empty stomach	A
Darifenacin	—	7.5–15 mg daily; 68% and 73%, respectively, median reduction in weekly UI episodes; dry mouth 19% and 31%, respectively; constipation 14% (both doses)	A
Solifenacin	—	5–10 mg daily; 61% and 52%, respectively, mean reduction in daily UI episodes; dry mouth 8% and 23%, respectively; constipation 4% and 9%, respectively	A
Estrogen	Vaginal atrophy	Oral ineffective, especially when combined with progestin; topical possibly of some benefit	A (oral), B (topical)
Botulinum toxin	Refractory to multiple trials of antimuscarinics	Under investigation	D

[a]Evidence strength: A—randomized controlled studies; B—case-control studies; C—case descriptions/expert opinion; D—no recommendation possible.
Abbreviations: CI, confidence interval; RR, relative risk; UI, urinary incontinence.
Source: From Ref. 80.

It is not known whether persons with DM are at a higher risk of developing high PVR with bladder relaxants; if the patient does not have a normal PVR (<50 mL) before treatment, the PVR should be monitored. Choice of bladder relaxant should consider potential drug–drug interactions with the patient's other medications (see above).

Unfortunately, treatment for impaired detrusor contractility is largely supportive. Earlier recommendations to use bethanecol (82) have been superceded by a lack of evidence for efficacy (83). Clean intermittent catheterization may be considered if the patient is willing. Indwelling or intermittent catheterization should be a last resort, particularly because of the very high risk of UTI from both catheters and DM.

IMPACT OF DIABETES TREATMENT ON UI

One would hope that comprehensive DM treatment, including good glycemic control, lifestyle interventions, and prevention of microvascular and neuropathic complications, would prevent or delay LUT pathology and symptoms. However, there is yet little evidence. In a secondary analysis of the Diabetes Prevention Program, prediabetic obese women (mean age 50) randomized to the intensive life style intervention had a lower UI prevalence at the end of the trial (38%) than women treated with metformin (48%) or placebo (46%) ($P = 0.001$) (84). Of note, UI rates were not determined at the start of the trial. Furthermore, the lower prevalence of UI was attributable entirely to a decrease in stress UI, which in turn was almost entirely attributable to weight loss. Hopefully, analyses of UI in the ongoing Look AHEAD trial and the Diabetes Prevention Program Outcome Program will provide more answers (17).

SUMMARY

UI is a common complication of DM in older persons, reflecting DM-specific effects on the LUT as well as the impact of DM complications and treatment on the functional ability to toilet. Older persons with DM also are at higher risk for UTIs, especially complicated UTIs. The effects of DM on the LUT are multifactoral, including interactions between the urothelium, autonomic and peripheral nervous systems, LUT blood flow, and detrusor smooth muscle, resulting in uninhibited bladder contractions, impaired bladder sensation, and decreased bladder contractility. Insights from animal models regarding the role of osmotic diuresis in mediating some of the detrusor changes underscores the importance of good glycemic control in ameliorating and potentially even preventing LUT dysfunction. At the same time, addressing the impact on continence of DM complications such as congestive heart failure and impaired functional status should be the cornerstone of treatment of DM-related UI and LUTS.

REFERENCES

1. Abrams P, Cardozo L, Fall M, et al. The standardisation of terminology in lower urinary tract function. Neurourol Urodynam 2002; 21:167–178.
2. Ellenberg M. Development of urinary bladder dysfunction in diabetes mellitus. Ann Intern Med 1980; 92(2 Pt 2):321–323.
3. Buck A, McRae C, Chisholm G. The diabetic bladder. Proc R Soc Med 1974; 67:81–83.
4. Frimodt-Moller C. Diabetic cystopathy: epidemiology and related disorders. Ann Intern Med 1980; 92(2 Pt 2):318–321.
5. Yu HJ, Lee WC, Liu SP, Tai TY, Wu HP, Chen J. Unrecognized voiding difficulty in female type 2 diabetic patients in the diabetes clinic: a prospective case-control study. Diabetes Care 2004; 27:988–989.
6. Ebbesen M, Hannestad Y, Midthjell K, Hunskaar S. Does diabetes increase the prevalence of urinary incontinence in women? Annual Meeting International Continence Society. Available at: http://www.continet.org/publications/2004/pdf/0182.pdf. Accessed April 10, 2006.
7. Lifford KL, Curhan GC, Hu FB, Barbieri RL, Grodstein F. Type 2 diabetes mellitus and risk of developing urinary incontinence. J Am Geriatr Soc 2005; 53:1851–1857.
8. Sampselle CM, Harlow SD, Skurnick J, Brubaker L, Bondarenko I. Urinary incontinence predictors and life impact in ethnically diverse perimenopausal women. Obstet Gynecol 2002; 100:1230–1238.
9. Jackson RA, Vittinghoff E, Kanaya AM, et al. Urinary incontinence in elderly women: findings from the Health, Aging, and Body Composition Study. Obstet Gynecol 2004; 104:301–307.
10. Brown J, Seeley D, Fong J, Black D, Ensrud K, Grady D. Urinary incontinence in older women: who is at risk? Obstet Gynecol 1996; 87(5 Pt 1):715–721.
11. Wetle T, Scherr P, Branch L, et al. Difficulty with holding urine among older persons in a geographically defined community: prevalence and correlates. J Amer Geriatr Soc 1995; 43:349–355.
12. Nygaard I, Lemke J. Urinary incontinence in rural older women: prevalence, incidence, and correlates. J Amer Geriatr Soc 1996; 44:1049–1054.
13. Diokno A, Brock B, Herzog A, Bromberg J. Medical correlates of urinary incontinence in the elderly. Urology 1990; 36:129–138.
14. Brown J, Grady D, Ouslander J, Herzog A, Varner R, Posner S. Prevalence of urinary incontinence and associated risk factors in postmenopausal women. Obstet Gynecol 1999; 94:66–70.
15. Steinauer J, Waetjen L, Vittinghoff E, et al. Postmenopausal hormone therapy: does it cause incontinence? Obstet Gynecol 2005; 106(5 Pt 1):940–945.

16. Lewis C, Schrader R, Many A, Mackay M, Rogers R. Diabetes and urinary incontinence in 50- to 90-year-old women: a cross-sectional population-based study. Amer J Obstet Gynecol 2005; 193:2154–2158.

17. Brown J, Nyberg L, Kusek J, et al. Proceedings of the National Institute of Diabetes and Digestive and Kidney Diseases International Symposium on epidemiologic issues in urinary incontinence in women. Am J Obstet Gynecol 2003; 188:S77–S88.

18. Tinetti M, Inouye S, Gill T, Doucette J. Shared risk factors for falls, incontinence, and functional dependence: unifying the approach to geriatric syndromes. JAMA 1995; 273:1348–1353.

19. DuBeau CE. Interpreting the effect of common medical conditions on voiding dysfunction in the elderly. Urol Clin North Amer 1996; 23:11–18.

20. Vinik AI, Freeman R, Erbas T. Diabetic autonomic neuropathy. Semin Neurol 2003; 23:365–372.

21. Millard R, Moore K, Rencken R, et al. Duloxetine vs placebo in the treatment of stress urinary incontinence: a four-continent randomized clinical trial. BJU Int 2004; 93:311.

22. DeLancey J. Structural aspects of the extrinsic continence mechanism. Obstet Gynecol 1988; 72:296.

23. Andersson K-E, Amer A. Urinary bladder contraction and relaxation: physiology and pathophysiology. Physiol Rev 2004; 84:935–986.

24. Ouslander J. Management of overactive bladder. N Engl J Med 2004; 350:786.

25. DuBeau C. Epidemiology, risk factors, and pathogenesis of urinary incontinence. Up To Date. Available at: www.uptodate.com. Accessed April 12, 2006.

26. Fonda D, DuBeau C, Harari D, et al. Incontinence in the frail elderly. In: Abrams PCL, Khoury S. Wein A, eds. Incontinence: 3rd International Consultation on Incontinence. Vol. 2. Plymouth, U.K.: Health Publication Ltd, 2005:1163–1240.

27. Resnick N, Elbadawi A, Yalla S. Age and the lower urinary tract: what is normal? Neurourol Urodyn 1995; 14:577–578.

28. Resnick N, Yalla S. Detrusor hyperactivity with impaired contractile function. An unrecognized but common cause of incontinence in elderly patients. JAMA 1987; 257:3076–3081.

29. Elbadawi A, Yalla S, Resnick N. Structural basis of geriatric voiding dysfunction. II. Normal versus impaired contractility. J Urol 1993; 150:1657.

30. Kirkland J, Lye M, Levy D, Banerjee A. Patterns of urine flow and excretion in healthy elderly people. Br Med J 1983; 287:1665.

31. Frimodt-Moller C. Diabetic cystopathy: I. A clinical study of the frequency of bladder dysfunction in diabetics. Dan Med Bull 1976; 23:267–268.

32. Ueda T, Yoshimura N, Yoshida O. Diabetic cystopathy: relationship to autonomic neuropathy detected by sympathetic skin response. J Urol 1997; 157:580–584.

33. Bartley O, Brolin I, Fagerberg SE, Wilhelmsen L. Neurogenic disorders of the bladder in diabetes mellitus. A clinical-roentgenological investigation. Acta Med Scand 1966; 180:187–198.

34. Weir J, Jaques P. Large-capacity bladder. A urodynamic survey. Urology 1974; 4:544–548.

35. Kaplan SA, Te AE, Blaivas JG. Urodynamic findings in patients with diabetic cystopathy. J Urol 1995; 153:342–344.

36. Starer P, Libow L. Cystometric evaluation of bladder dysfunction in elderly diabetic patients. Arch Intern Med 1990; 150:810–813.

37. Yoshimura N, Chancellor MB, Andersson KE, Christ GJ. Recent advances in understanding the biology of diabetes-associated bladder complications and novel therapy. BJU Int 2005; 95:733–738.

38. Turner WH, Brading AF. Smooth muscle of the bladder in the normal and the diseased state: pathophysiology, diagnosis and treatment. Pharmacol Ther 1997; 75:77–110.

39. Pitre DA, Ma T, Wallace LJ, Bauer JA. Time-dependent urinary bladder remodeling in the streptozotocin-induced diabetic rat model. Acta Diabetol 2002; 39:23–27.

40. Eika B, Levin RM, Longhurst PA. Comparison of urinary bladder function in rats with hereditary diabetes insipidus, streptozotocin-induced diabetes mellitus, and nondiabetic osmotic diuresis. J Urol 1994; 151(2):496–502.

41. Tammela TL, Leggett RE, Levin RM, Longhurst PA. Temporal changes in micturition and bladder contractility after sucrose diuresis and streptozotocin-induced diabetes mellitus in rats. J Urol 1995; 153:2014–2021.

42. Kodama M, Takimoto Y. Influence of 5-hydroxytryptamine and the effect of a new serotonin receptor antagonist (sarpogrelate) on detrusor smooth muscle of streptozotocin-induced diabetes mellitus in the rat. Int J Urol 2000; 7:231–235.

43. Dahlstrand C, Dahlstrom A, Ahlman H, et al. Effect of substance P on detrusor muscle in rats with diabetic cystopathy. Br J Urol 1992; 70:390–394.

44. Longhurst PA. Urinary bladder function 6 months after the onset of diabetes in the spontaneously diabetic BB rat. J Urol 1991; 145:417–422.

45. Gupta S, Yang S, Cohen RA, Krane RJ, Saenz De Tejada I. Altered contractility of urinary bladder in diabetic rabbits: relationship to reduced Na+ pump activity. Am J Physiol 1996; 271(6 Pt 1): C2045–C2052.

46. Mumtaz F, Sullivan M, Thompson C, Dashwood M, et al. Alterations in the nitric oxide synthase binding sites and non-adrenergic, non-cholinergic mediated smooth muscle relaxation in the diabetic

rabbit bladder outlet: possible relevance to the pathogenesis of diabetic cystopathy. J Urol 1999; 162:558–566.

47. Steers WD, Mackway-Gerardi AM, Ciambotti J, de Groat WC. Alterations in neural pathways to the urinary bladder of the rat in response to streptozotocin-induced diabetes. J Auton Nerv Syst 1994; 47(1–2):83–94.

48. Su X, Changolkar A, Chacko S, Moreland RS. Diabetes decreases rabbit bladder smooth muscle contraction while increasing levels of myosin light chain phosphorylation. Am J Physiol Renal Physiol 2004; 287:F690–F699.

49. Mannikarottu AS, Changolkar AK, Disanto ME, Wein AJ, Chacko S. Over expression of smooth muscle thin filament associated proteins in the bladder wall of diabetics. J Urol 2005; 174:360–364.

50. Sasaki K, Chancellor MB, Phelan MW, et al. Diabetic cystopathy correlates with a long-term decrease in nerve growth factor levels in the bladder and lumbosacral dorsal root Ganglia. J Urol 2002; 168:1259–1264.

51. Changolkar AK, Hypolite JA, Disanto M, Oates PJ, Wein AJ, Chacko S. Diabetes-induced decrease in detrusor smooth muscle force is associated with oxidative stress and overactivity of aldose reductase. J Urol 2005; 173:309–313.

52. Waring JV, Wendt IR. Effects of streptozotocin-induced diabetes mellitus on intracellular calcium and contraction of longitudinal smooth muscle from rat urinary bladder. J Urol 2000; 163:323–330.

53. Mitsui T, Kakizaki H, Kobayashi S, Morita H, Matsumura K, Koyanagi T. Vesicourethral function in diabetic patients: association of abnormal nerve conduction velocity with vesicourethral dysfunction. Neurourol Urodyn 1999; 18:639–645.

54. Mastri AR. Neuropathology of diabetic neurogenic bladder. Ann Intern Med 1980; 92(2 Pt 2): 316–318.

55. Azadzoi K, Tarcan T, Kozlowski R, Krane R, Siroky M. Overactivity and structural changes in the chronically ischemic bladder 1999; 62:1768–1778.

56. Saito M, Yokoi K, Ohmura M, Kondo A. Effects of ligation of the internal iliac artery on blood flow to the bladder and detrusor function in rat. Internatl Urol Nephrol 1998; 30:283–292.

57. Shenfeld O, Meir K, Yutkin V, Gofrit O, Landau E, Pode D. Do atherosclerosis and chronic bladder ischemia really play a role in detrusor dysfunction of old age? Urology 2005; 65:181–184.

58. Lorenzi B, McMurray G, Jarvis G, Brading A. Preconditioning protects the guinea-pig urinary bladder against ischaemic conditions in vitro. Neurourol Urodyn 2003; 22:687–692.

59. Levin R, English M, Barretto M, et al. Normal detrusor is more sensitive than hypertrophied detrusor to in vitro ischemia followed by re-oxygenation. Neurourol Urodyn 2000; 19:701–712.

60. Azadzoi K, Tarcan T, Siroky M, Krane R. Atherosclerosis-induced chronic ischemia causes bladder fibrosis and non-compliance in the rabbit. J Urol 1999; 161:1626–1635.

61. Andersen JT, Bradley WE. Early detection of diabetic visceral neuropathy. An electrophysiologic study of bladder and urethral innervation. Diabetes 1976; 25:1100–1105.

62. Sarica Y, Karastas M, Bozdemir H, Karacan I. Cerebral responses elicited by stimulation of the vesicourethral junction in diabetes. Electroencephalography Clin Neurophysiol 1996; 55–61.

63. Torimoto K, Hirao Y, Matsuyoshi H, de Groat W, Chancellor M, Yoshimura N. Alpha1-adrenergic mechanism in diabetic urethral dysfunction in rats. J Urol 2005; 173:1027–1032.

64. Podlasek C, Zelner D, Bervig T, Gonzalez C, McKenna K, McVary K. Characterization and localization of nitric oxide synthase isoforms in the BB/WOR diabetic rat. J Urol 2001; 166:746–755.

65. Maggi C, Santicioli P, Manzini S, et al. Functional studies on the cholinergic and sympathetic innervation of the rat proximal urethra: effect of pelvic ganglionectomy or experimental diabetes. J Autonomic Pharm 1989; 9:231–241.

66. Geerlings S, Meiland R, Hoepelman A. Pathogenesis of bacteriuria in women with diabetes mellitus. Internatl J Antimicrobial Agents 2002; 19:539–545.

67. Ronald A, Ludwig E. Urinary tract infections in adults with diabetes. Internatl J Antimicrobial Agents 2001; 17:287–292.

68. Nicolle L, Bradley S, Colgan R, et al. Infectious Diseases Society of America guidelines for the diagnosis and treatment of asymptomatic bacteriuria in adults. Clin Infect Dis 2005; 40:643–654.

69. Zhanel G, Nicolle L, Harding G. Prevalence of asymptomatic bacteriuria and associated host factors in women with diabetes mellitus. Clin Infect Dis 1995; 21:316–322.

70. Hooton T, Scholes D, Stapleton A, et al. A prospective study of asymptomatic bacteriuria in sexually active young women. N Engl J Med 2000; 343:992.

71. Geerlings S, Stolk R, Camps M, et al. Asymptomatic bacteriuria may be considered a complication in women with diabetes. Diabetes Mellitus Women Asymptomatic Bacteriuria Utrecht Study Group. Diabetes Care 2000; 23:744–749.

72. Boyko EJ, Fihn SD, Scholes D, Abraham L, Monsey B. Risk of urinary tract infection and asymptomatic bacteriuria among diabetic and nondiabetic postmenopausal women. Am J Epidemiol 2005; 161:557–564.

73. Geerlings SE, Stolk RP, Camps MJ, et al. Consequences of asymptomatic bacteriuria in women with diabetes mellitus. Arch Intern Med 2001; 161:1421–1427.

74. Harding G, Zhanel G, Nicolle L, Cheang M. Antimicrobial treatment in diabetic women with asymptomatic bacteriuria. N Engl J Med 2002; 347:1576–1583.

75. Segal A, Choyke P, Bluth E, et al. Expert panel on urologic imaging. Recurrent lower urinary tract infections in women. American College of Radiology. Available at: http://www.acr.org/s_acr/bin.asp?CID=1202&DID=11824&DOC=FILE.PDF. Accessed April 5, 2006.

76. Katchman E, Milo G, Paul M, Christiaens T, Baerheim A, Leibovici L. Three-day vs longer duration of antibiotic treatment for cystitis in women: systematic review and meta-analysis. Am J Med 2005; 118:1196–1207.

77. Warren J, Hebel J, Johnson J, Schaeffer A, Stamm W. Guidelines for antimicrobial treatment of uncomplicated acute bacterial cystitis and acute pyelonephritis in women. Infectious Disease Society of America. Available at: http://www.journals.uchicago.edu/IDSA/guidelines/p745.pdf. Accessed April 5, 2006.

78. Guidelines for improving the care of the older person with diabetes mellitus. California Healthcare Foundation/American Geriatrics Society Panel of Improving Care for Elders with Diabetes. J Amer Geriatr Soc 2003; 51:S265–S280.

79. DuBeau C. Evaluation of urinary incontinence. Up To Date. Available at: www.uptodate.com. Accessed April 12, 2006.

80. DuBeau C. Treatment of urinary incontinence. Up To Date. Available at: www.uptodate.com. Accessed April 12, 2006.

81. Subak L, Whitcomb E, Shen H, Saxton J, Vittinghoff E, Brown J. Weight loss: a novel and effective treatment for urinary incontinence. J Urol 2005; 174:190–195.

82. Frimodt-Moller C, Mortensen S. Treatment of diabetic cystopathy. Ann Int Med 1980; 92(2 Pt 2): 327–328.

83. Andersson K-E, Appell R, Cardozo L, et al. Pharmacological treatment of urinary incontinence. In: Abrams PCL, Khoury S. Wein A, eds. Incontinence: 3rd International Consultation on Incontinence. Vol. 2. Plymouth, U.K.: Health Publication Ltd, 2005:809–854.

84. Brown JS, Wing R, Barrett-Connor E, et al. Lifestyle intervention is associated with lower prevalence of urinary incontinence: the Diabetes Prevention Program. Diabetes Care 2006; 29:385–390.

10 | Chronic Pain and Disability in Diabetes

Suzanne G. Leveille
Department of Medicine, Beth Israel Deaconess Medical Center, Harvard Medical School, Boston, Massachusetts, U.S.A.

Stefano Volpato
Department of Clinical and Experimental Medicine, Section of Internal Medicine, Gerontology, and Geriatrics, University of Ferrara, Ferrara, Italy

CAUSES OF PAIN

Chronic pain is a common condition in the general population, and its prevalence increases with advancing age (1,2). The prevalence of chronic pain in older patients with diabetes has not been extensively evaluated thus far. However chronic pain is considered an important problem in older persons with diabetes; one recent survey reported that almost 55% of diabetic patients aged 60 and older reported chronic pain (3). There are several potential sources of acute and chronic pain in older diabetic patients (Table 1) and often two or more painful conditions coexist in the same patients.

Peripheral Neuropathy

Diabetic neuropathies encompass a wide range of nerve abnormalities and are common, with prevalence estimated between 5% and 100% of diabetics, depending on sampling methods and diagnostic criteria. Although chronic pain is not associated with all clinical presentations of diabetic neuropathy, in older diabetic patients, painful peripheral neuropathies (PNs) are especially disabling due to their detrimental effects on balance, sensorimotor function, gait, and functional autonomy (4). In the U.S. population aged 40 and older that has PN, persons with diabetes have twice the prevalence of symptoms (foot pain or numbness) compared with nondiabetics (42% and 21%, respectively) (5).

Chronic sensorimotor distal polyneuropathy, also called distal symmetrical polyneuropathy, is the most common and widely recognized form of diabetic neuropathy and, although not limited to patients with diabetes, probably accounts for 75% of all diabetic neuropathies (6). It may be sensory or motor and may involve small or large fibers. Pain is usually rare in large-fiber neuropathy, which is mainly characterized by reduced vibration and position sense, weakness, muscle wasting, and depressed tendon reflexes. When present, pain may be described as deep or "gnawing." Small-fiber neuropathies manifest first in the lower limbs with pain and hyperalgesia followed by reduction or loss of thermal sensitivity and diminished light-touch and pinprick sensation. Patients with damage of small unmyelinated C-fibers might complain of burning sensation, dysesthetic pain, hyperalgesia, and allodynia. Patients with late-stage small-fiber neuropathy might not have pain or might experience pain relief due to depletion of substance P.

Other less common forms of painful neuropathies can affect patients with diabetes mellitus. Focal neuropathies include mononeuropathies and entrapment syndromes. Mononeuropathies are frequent in older adults and are typically associated with pain. Their onset is usually acute but clinical remission is spontaneous and short-term (usually six to eight weeks). Common entrapment sites in patients with diabetes involve the upper extremities (median and ulnar nerves) and the lower extremities (lateral cutaneous nerve of the thigh and the tibial nerve in the tarsal canal). The onset of clinical signs is usually gradual and limited to a single nerve. Proximal motor neuropathy, also referred to as diabetic amyotrophy or diabetic neuropathic cachexia, is a clinical entity that primarily affects the elderly. This is a painful and highly disabling condition, characterized by pain in the hips, buttocks, or thighs,

TABLE 1   Common Types and Characteristics of Pain Due to Diabetic Complications

Diabetic complication	Pain characteristics
Peripheral neuropathy	
Generalized symmetrical polyneuropathies	
Chronic sensorimotor distal polyneuropathy	
Large fiber	Pain is rare
Small fiber	Prominent pain: burning, associated with allodynia and hyperalgesia
Diffuse neuropathies	
Proximal motor	Pain in low back, hip, thigh (typically unilateral), followed by significant muscle weakness
Focal neuropathies	
Mononeuritis	Acute onset, short-lasting
Entrapment syndromes	Gradual onset, progressive
Diabetic foot	
Charcot neuroarthropathy	Pain is unusual due to loss of pain perception
Foot ulcer	Moderate to severe pain. Onset can be acute, but chronic pain is common
Peripheral arterial disease	
Intermittent claudication	Calf pain or weakness with walking, which is relieved with rest
Critical lower extremity ischemia	Rest pain in the toes or foot with progression to ulceration or gangrene

with sudden or gradual presentation, followed by weakness of the proximal muscles of the lower extremities that impairs the ability to rise from a sitting position.

Peripheral Arterial Disease

Diabetes increases the incidence and severity of limb ischemia approximately two- to fourfold. Data from epidemiological studies show increased rates of absent pedal pulses, femoral bruits, and diminished ankle-brachial indices among persons with diabetes compared to others without diabetes (7). For example, in the Women's Health and Aging Study, a sample of the one-third most disabled women aged 65 and older living in the community, the age-adjusted prevalence of peripheral arterial disease (PAD) was 48.7% among diabetic women and 27.5% in the nondiabetic women (8). Diabetic PAD often affects distal limb vessels, such as the tibial and peroneal arteries, limiting the potential for collateral vessel development and reducing options for revascularization. As such, patients with diabetes are more likely than others to develop symptomatic forms of PAD, such as intermittent claudication and critical limb ischemia, and are more likely to undergo amputations. In the Framingham cohort, the presence of diabetes increased the frequency of intermittent claudication by more than threefold in men and more than eightfold in women (9). In addition, the clinical picture of PAD is different in older patients with and without diabetes. Older patients with diabetes have worse PAD below the knee and are at higher risk of lower extremity amputation. However, clinical and epidemiological studies demonstrated that despite a more severe PAD, diabetic patients are less likely to have classical exertional calf pain (intermittent claudication), and, conversely, they more often complain of atypical leg pain with exertion and rest. This atypical clinical presentation can be explained by the concomitant presence of diabetes-related neuropathy and altered foot architecture (10,11).

Foot Ulcers

Foot ulcers are another prevalent and painful complication of diabetes. In fact, epidemiologic studies suggest that 2.5% of diabetic patients develop diabetic foot ulcers each year and that 15% of all diabetic patients develop foot ulcers at some point during their lifetime (12). Patients are particularly susceptible to acute pain during wound care or when foot ulcer dressings are changed, or as a result of Charcot arthropathy. Chronic ulcer-related pain can result from arterial insufficiency, chronic infectious processes, or osteomyelitis (13). Clinical experience suggests that the pain associated with diabetic foot ulcers can be moderate to severe in intensity. Recent research showed that three out of four patients with diabetic foot ulcers experienced pain and more than 50% reported pain while walking or standing and also while in bed at night (14).

Comorbid Conditions

Older adults who have diabetes often have comorbid conditions that are generally unrelated to diabetes, which may contribute to chronic pain and physical disability. There are common pathways through which diabetes and other chronic conditions may contribute to chronic pain. These include obesity, age, and possibly also through inflammatory processes. Although, PAD and PN are related to diabetes in young and middle-aged adults, both conditions increase in prevalence with age in both diabetic and nondiabetic persons (Fig. 1) (5). In addition, we know that PN and PAD are associated with lower extremity mobility difficulty and more commonly so among persons with diabetes than those without diabetes (52% and 40%, respectively) (15).

In general, obese older persons suffer a greater burden of the major chronic diseases than their nonobese counterparts (16). The prevalence of musculoskeletal pain such as knee, hip, and back pain is higher in persons with a higher body mass index (BMI), and it generally increases with age into the ninth decade of life (17). Older persons with diabetes have a higher prevalence of range of motion impairments, for example, limited hip and knee flexion, though the association is generally related to the higher prevalence of obesity among diabetic versus nondiabetic elders (18).

Osteoarthritis is one of the most prevalent disabling conditions affecting older adults and the major cause of musculoskeletal pain in the older population (19,20). Arthritis and diabetes share the common major risk factor of obesity, though the pathway from obesity to either of these chronic conditions remains unclear. Osteoarthritis of the knees, hips, and, to some extent, the hands has been linked to obesity (21). Thus, persons with diabetes who are obese are more likely than other persons to have osteoarthritis. And the reverse is true as well, that persons with arthritis who also have diabetes face higher risks for functional decline even after controlling for obesity (22). Methodologic issues in arthritis research continue to complicate our understanding of pain and arthritis. For example, when arthritis is assessed by self-report, researchers have shown that it is primarily a marker for musculoskeletal pain rather than radiographic evidence of disease (23). Musculoskeletal pain is very common in older persons and it is often difficult to diagnose the underlying pathology. In the absence of a definitive diagnosis, symptom management to prevent functional decline becomes paramount in the care of older patients.

Other Neuropathic Pain

Other causes of neuropathic pain in older persons regardless of diabetes status include postherpetic neuralgia, tumors, nerve trauma, and multiple sclerosis. Persons with diabetes have increased risk for cerebrovascular disease and stroke, which can lead to chronic pain.

Clinically, neuropathic pain is distinguished from non-neuropathic pain by pain characteristics. Typical descriptors used by patients to describe pain of neuropathic origin include burning, painful cold, electric shocks, tingling, numbness, and "pins and needles"

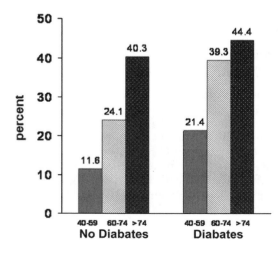

FIGURE 1 Prevalence of lower extremity disease (peripheral arterial disease and peripheral neuropathy) according to age and diagnosed diabetes in adults aged more than 40 years from the National Health and Nutrition Examination Survey, 1999–2002. *Source*: From Ref. 5.

(24). Treatments for neuropathic pain include a broad range of pharmacologic, rehabilitative, and nonpharmacologic therapies, described later in this chapter.

DISABILITY

Several epidemiologic studies in older populations have shown that diabetes is among the major chronic conditions that predict disability in a number of domains of function. In the Third National Health and Nutrition Examination Survey (NHANES III), women and men aged 60 years or more with diagnosed diabetes were approximately two to three times more likely to be unable to walk one-fourth of a mile, climb stairs, and do housework than similarly aged adults without diabetes (25). Women with diabetes also had significantly slower walking speed, worse balance, and almost a 60% greater likelihood of falling than did nondiabetic women (25). Among the nearly 7000 participants in the Established Populations for Epidemiologic Studies in the Elderly (EPESE), self-reported diabetes and cardiovascular diseases present at baseline predicted loss of lower extremity mobility over the four-year follow-up (26). Also, number of chronic conditions was associated with functional loss.

In a two-year study of incident disability from the Longitudinal Study of Aging (LSOA), among over 4000 nondisabled older persons at baseline, 10% developed inability to perform one or more activities of daily living (ADL) in the follow-up (27). Major chronic conditions were assessed by self-report and the results showed that the total number of chronic conditions at baseline was strongly predictive of incident disability. Diabetes, arthritis, and cerebrovascular disease were the chronic diseases with the greatest impact on functional decline. Incontinence and vision impairment were also strong risk factors for disablement. In the LSOA study, the relationship between black race and disability was largely accounted for by number of chronic conditions (27).

Reports from the Hispanic EPESE, a more recent EPESE study of Mexican Americans living in the Southwestern United States, have examined the role of diabetes in disability in older persons. Diabetes and arthritis were the most common chronic diseases reported at baseline (22% and 41%, respectively) and were each associated with a twofold increased risk for disability in walking and stair climbing (28). Evidence from this study showed higher rates of disability related to chronic diseases than has been reported in studies of Non-Hispanic populations. The authors concluded this was in part related to lower institutionalization rates among Hispanics and thus more ill persons remain in the community cared for by family members. A longitudinal study from the Hispanic EPESE showed that persons with diabetes and stroke had increased risk for ADL and instrumental activities of daily living disability and this risk was increased in the presence of other chronic diseases including arthritis (29).

In the Women's Health and Aging Study, a prospective study of older women with mild to moderate physical disability, women with diabetes were at greater risk for decline in measures of lower extremity performance and for transition to severe mobility and ADL disability than nondiabetic women over a three-year period (30). These results suggest that the disabling effect of diabetes on physical function is still present and measurable even in the subgroup of frail, physically impaired older women.

The biological mechanisms explaining the association between diabetes and physical disability in older adults are not completely elucidated and are probably multifactorial. The relative roles of several comorbidities associated with diabetes have been evaluated in different studies and results vary according to the population studied and research protocols used. In NHANES III, coronary heart disease (CHD) and high BMI were the strongest explanatory factors among women, accounting for more than 50% of their excess risk for disability (25). Among men, conversely, CHD and stroke were the most important explanatory factors, explaining 25% and 21% of the excess disability risk, respectively. In the Study of Osteoporotic Fractures, age, CHD, arthritis, physical inactivity, BMI, and visual impairment were key predictors of disability among the women with diabetes (31). Alternatively, in the Women's Health and Aging Study, where standardized objective information on lower-extremity disease was collected, peripheral nerve dysfunction, PAD, and depression were the main predictors of physical disability (8). Noteworthily, however, in each of these studies, a significant excess risk of disability associated with diabetes remained, even after controlling for diabetes-related complications. Globally taken, these results suggest either that diabetes has a direct intrinsic effect on disability or that other unmeasured or undiscovered diabetes-related complications influence the risk for disability. For example, none of the above-mentioned studies evaluated the role of chronic pain as potential mediator of the association between diabetes and physical disability.

Pain-Related Disability

In the Nagi model describing the pathway from pathology to disability, physical impairments such as muscle weakness, balance problems, and gait limitations are considered as steps in the process leading to disability (32,33). The very few population-based studies examining the impact of pain on physical impairments in older persons generally have been limited to pain associated with knee osteoarthritis or peripheral vascular disease. Declines in strength and balance have been observed in older persons with knee pain, independent of other factors (34,35). Reports from clinical studies showed that gait problems were associated with intermittent claudication, an important cause of leg pain in older persons (36,37). However, controversy exists about the role of physical impairments in pain-related disability with evidence suggesting that pain has a direct impact on disability regardless of other impairments (38). Further work in this area is continuing.

The theoretical model shown in Figure 2 portrays the role of chronic pain as a mediator or effect modifier in the biological pathway leading from diabetes to functional limitation and disability. Regardless of the underlying conditions that cause pain (i.e., diabetes-related or diabetes-associated conditions), the presence of persistent pain, and particularly back and lower-extremity pain, will have a detrimental effect on multiple steps of the disablement process. Moreover this direct disabling effect of pain might interact with other diabetes-related mechanisms, greatly enhancing the risk for functional limitation or disability. From this point of view, accurate assessment and appropriate management of pain would help older diabetic patients to maintain their independence.

Rarely has chronic pain been studied as a unique chronic comorbidity contributing to disability in older patients with diabetes. In the Health Aging and Body Composition (ABC) Study of nondisabled adults aged 70 and older, diabetes and obesity were more common among those with the most severe back pain compared to those without back pain (39). In that study, persons with most severe back pain had lowest scores on mobility performance tests and self-reported functioning, suggesting that coexisting pain might, at least in part, explain the association between diabetes and functional decline.

Further indirect evidence for a possible link between diabetes, pain, and physical function comes from studies on falls in older persons. Using data from the Women's Health and Aging Study, the authors investigated the relationship between diabetes and risk of falls related to lower-extremity pain (40). The study showed that older women with diabetes had an increased independent risk of falling and that the excess risk of falls associated with diabetes was greater among women with chronic musculoskeletal pain compared to those without this comorbidity. Figure 3 (41) shows the graded relationship between pain level and risk of recurrent falls according to diabetes status, with highest risk observed among women receiving insulin therapy who also had multisite pain (OR 6.5; 95% CI, 2.98–14.2) (40). Notably, among women without pain, there was no relationship between diabetes status and risk of recurrent falls. Regardless of the underlying causes of lower-extremity pain, a synergistic effect between diabetes and lower-extremity pain was observed.

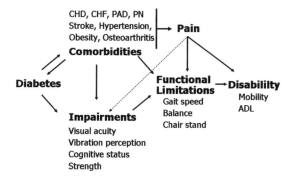

FIGURE 2 Theoretical model of the pathway from diabetes to disability. *Abbreviations*: ADL, activities of daily living; CHD, coronary heart disease; CHF, congestive heart failure; PAD, peripheral arterial disease; PN, peripheral neuropathy.

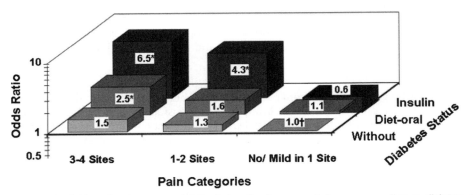

FIGURE 3 Odds ratios for recurrent falls during the three-year follow-up according to diabetes status and pain categories, The Women's Health and Aging Study, 1992–1998. Odds ratios are adjusted for age, race, presence of hand pain and chest pain, and lower-extremity physical performance score. *Note*: *, $p < 0.05$; †, reference group. *Source*: From Ref. 40.

Since older patients with diabetes are characterized by a number of comorbidities and functional impairments predisposing to gait abnormalities and lower-extremity weakness, it is conceivable that diabetic patients might be less able to buffer and compensate for the pathophysiological and psychological factors associated with chronic pain, including reflex inhibition, joint instability, fear of falling, and reduced attention. This pathway might be further exacerbated in elderly individuals who are, independent of disease status, experiencing a multisystemic reduction of functional reserve. Researchers have recently reported that two painful conditions such as arthritis and PN are significant contributors to mobility decline over time among older persons with diabetes, indirectly supporting this hypothesis (42).

These findings show that the functional consequence of pain place older adults with diabetes at high risk for loss of independence. Effective assessment and management of pain in this group of patients require careful attention to physical functioning. Appropriate rehabilitative therapies to improve muscle strength and balance, resulting in lower risk for falls and mobility limitations, are an important component of chronic care of older adults with diabetes and comorbid conditions. Further research is needed to define the optimal rehabilitative approaches to enhance physical functioning in diabetic patients.

ASSESSMENT OF PAIN
General Pain Assessment Measures

Pain management depends on a comprehensive assessment; inadequate assessment results in inadequate pain treatment. This is especially true for patients with persistent pain and patients with multiple causes of pain. Multiple comorbid conditions may alter what may be considered a typical pain presentation and influence treatment decisions. Painful neuropathy may be compounded by claudication related to PAD or pain from common musculoskeletal conditions affecting the feet and knees such as osteoarthritis. As a result of the pain assessment, the clinician should understand the nature of the pain in terms of its etiology, pathophysiology, syndrome, and its impact on many domains of functioning. It is important to perform a careful history and physical examination, use appropriate pain assessment instruments (discussed below), and consider the potential role of comorbidity, mental health, and cognitive status. With older diabetic patients, clinicians should inquire about the presence of associated symptoms and physical signs that might orient them toward a specific diabetes-related pain etiology. Physical examination should emphasize an evaluation of the neurological and cardiovascular systems.

Several approaches to the assessment of pain have been recommended for the care of older primary-care patients. The method advocated by the American Geriatrics Society (AGS), consistent with The Joint Commission standards, is to assess all patients for pain through use of a single question such as, "on a scale of 0 to 10, with zero meaning no pain and 10 meaning worst pain, as bad as you can imagine, how much pain are you having right now?"(43). Showing patients a card depicting the 11-point numeric rating scale is helpful. The AGS guidelines caution that many elders may have difficulty using the numeric rating scale and that it is important to have a variety of instruments available including pain "thermometers" and questions with descriptive or non-numeric response options. An initial question to determine the presence of pain is useful primarily for screening purposes. Instruments such as the faces scale (with pictures of faces ranging from happy to severely distressed) and the pain thermometer have been shown to be useful in older persons who may have difficulty with the standard numeric rating scale (43). Pain assessment for patients who have cognitive impairments is discussed below.

If the pain screen is positive, a more detailed follow-up assessment should include pain history information and a detailed description of the pain including frequency, duration, location, characteristics, associations with movement or position, and impact on functioning, social activities, and mood. In addition, the assessment should include a history of pain management strategies: use of analgesics and nonpharmacologic measures that may or may not have relieved the pain. A few multidimensional pain assessments that address many of these factors are available. The Brief Pain Inventory (BPI) and the McGill Pain Questionnaire (MPQ) are well-tested and reliable instruments that have been validated in several languages (44–46). A European Expert Panel recommended the BPI and the MPQ over a number of other pain measurement tools for use in clinical and research environments (47). A newer instrument, the Pain Outcomes Questionnaire-VA, is available in a long and short version and has been useful in clinical and research settings for monitoring pain outcomes of treatment (48).

Patients who have mild to moderate cognitive impairment may be able to use the faces scale, the pain thermometer, or numeric rating scales to describe their level of pain (43). Pain assessment is challenging in patients who have cognitive impairment, particularly those with moderate or severe dementia. Although a number of instruments have been developed for assessing pain-related behaviors in persons with severe dementia, further evaluation and research is needed before the currently available instruments could be recommended for clinical use (49). The AGS Guidelines recommend observation of facial expressions and behaviors in patients who have moderate or severe cognitive impairment (43). Agitation or behavior changes in persons with dementia may be related to pain symptoms. It is important to involve the family and caregivers in ascertaining history of pain and behavior patterns. A trial of analgesic therapy may be needed to evaluate whether pain is contributing to agitation or depressive symptoms (49).

Most elders who have chronic pain have pain in multiple sites (50,51). In studies that specifically examined pain in relation to functioning in older persons, pain severity and location were each found to be independently associated with disability (50,52). Thus, in caring for older patients who report chronic pain, it is essential to assess location and intensity of pain as part of the overall pain history and assessment. Instruments that include a homunculus, such as the McGill Pain Map (Fig. 4), allow the patient to identify all sites of current or recent pain (46,53). The patient is asked to identify sites of pain on a blank version of the homunculus shown in Figure 4; the clinician can record sites of pain referring to the numbered areas shown in the figure (53).

Patterns of pain location, with the worst pain being widespread pain, have been shown to predict disability and falls in older persons (54,55). The American College of Rheumatology defines widespread pain as pain present in each of the following areas: pain above the waist, below the waist, on the left and right sides of the body, and axial pain (56). Our understanding of underlying causes of pain syndromes especially in older adults is limited. Despite the serious consequences of persistent pain and the availability of a broad range of treatment options, pain is often undertreated in older persons (57,58). Nonetheless, management of chronic pain is critical to the well-being and independence of elders who struggle with the burden of daily pain.

Pain Assessment: Neuropathies and PAD

The diagnosis of diabetes-related painful neuropathies rests heavily on a careful clinical history; a number of questionnaires have been developed and validated for clinical and research use

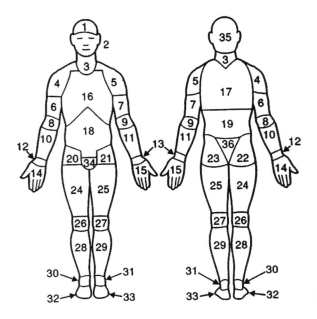

FIGURE 4 McGill Pain Map, scoring template for use in assessing patient's locations of pain. *Source*: From Ref. 53.

(24,59–61). The initial step should be directed toward the definition of the specific part of the nervous system affected. The bedside neurologic examination is relatively quick and easy but contains substantial interindividual and intraindividual variability. The American Academy of Neurology and the American Diabetes Association recommends that at least one variable from each of the following categories is measured to classify diabetic neuropathy: symptom profiles, neurologic examination, quantitative sensory test, nerve conduction study, and autonomic function testing. The quantitative sensory test and the quantitative autonomic function test are objective indices of neurologic functional status that together cover vibratory, proprioceptive, tactile, pain, and thermal and autonomic function (62,63). Two summary scales, the recently validated Leeds Assessment of Neuropathic Symptoms and Signs pain scale and the French, DN4 scale, each combine self-report symptoms assessments with a brief set of sensory tests to measure neuropathic pain in clinical or research settings (24,59,60).

Persons with PAD of the lower extremities have diminished or absent arterial pulses. Among these patients, initial assessment should aim to identity PAD risk factors, symptoms of claudication, resting pain, and functional limitation. Alternative or coexisting causes of leg pain during exercise, including spinal stenosis, should be excluded with computed tomography or magnetic resonance imaging (64). Noninvasive tests used to assess lower extremity arterial blood flow include measurement of ankle and brachial artery systolic blood pressures, characterization of velocity wave form, and duplex ultrasonography.

Measurement of ankle and brachial artery systolic blood pressures using a Doppler stethoscope and blood pressure cuffs allows calculation of the ankle/brachial index (ABI), which is normally 0.9 to 1.2. An ABI of less than 0.90 is 95% sensitive and 99% specific for the diagnosis of PAD. The lower the ABI, the more severe the restriction of arterial blood flow, and the more serious the ischemia. With ABIs between 0.25 and 0.4, resting pain and tissue loss are often found. Patients with calcified arteries from diabetes mellitus or renal failure occasionally have relatively noncompressible arteries leading to falsely elevated ABI values in the normal range. In addition to measuring arterial pressure in nonpalpable arteries, Doppler ultrasound methods allow characterization of the flow velocity waveform. Finding biphasic flow at the groin or monophasic flow more distally is evidence of arterial obstruction even when ABI measurements are falsely increased to normal levels because of calcification. Duplex ultrasonography combines Doppler frequency measurements with two-dimensional images of blood vessels. The severity of flow restriction induced by an arterial stenosis can be accurately assessed by this most comprehensive noninvasive method.

MANAGEMENT OF PAIN
Pharmacologic Treatment

Pharmacotherapy is the most common treatment to control pain in older patients. There is wide variability in the extent to which older patients may experience relief or, conversely, side effects in response to the same pain-relieving drugs. Compared with younger patients, elderly patients show measurable pharmacokinetic differences that result in higher and more prolonged plasma drug concentrations, which may increase risk for adverse effects, toxicity, and drug–drug interactions. In older patients, the risk of adverse drug reactions is strongly associated with age and number of medications (65). Persons who have cognitive impairments are particularly vulnerable to psychoactive effects of medications used to treat pain. However, it is particularly important to effectively manage pain in patients with cognitive impairments who may have difficulty in describing their discomfort or may express their pain through behaviors including agitation or depressive symptoms.

In addition, older patients, and particularly older diabetic patients, are more likely to have "concealed" renal impairment (i.e., reduction of the glomerular filtration rate despite normal serum creatinine levels, due to reduced muscle mass). In a study of hospitalized older patients, as many as 16% of older diabetic patients with normal creatinine level had a decreased glomerular filtration rate, a condition associated with increased risk for adverse drug reactions to renally excreted drugs (66). Therefore, individually tailored therapeutic trials starting with low doses of medication and titrating upward in dose are the hallmark of effective pharmacotherapy for persistent pain. This careful clinical approach is particularly well suited for older diabetic patients (43).

An important step in pain management is the correct classification of the pain syndrome according to pathophysiologic mechanisms. Treatment strategies that specifically target underlying pain mechanisms are more likely to be effective. It is important to establish whether the pain is neuropathic (e.g., diabetic neuropathy) or nociceptive (e.g., arthritis pain or other somatic or visceral pain), although other common conditions may have a mixed pathogenesis.

Treatment of Painful Neuropathic Symptoms

Glucose control is of paramount importance to prevent PN and should be considered the first therapeutic target in neuropathic pain management. Although sudden reduction of glucose levels may trigger acute painful neuritis, good glycemic control often improves symptoms and improves motor conduction velocity (67).

Antidepressants

Antidepressants have been the traditional first-line therapy for pain related to PN. A systematic review of eight randomized, double-blinded clinical trials that used tricyclic antidepressants found that 69% of patients treated with tricyclic antidepressants achieved at least 50% pain reduction compared with 39% of those randomized to placebo (68). However, side effects, most notably anticholinergic effects such as confusion, dry mouth, fatigue, constipation, headache, and orthostatic hypotension, limit their usefulness in older diabetic patients. Selective serotonin reuptake inhibitors have fewer side effects than tricyclic antidepressants but their efficacy is lower than that of tricyclic agents (69). Duloxetine, an inhibitor of both serotonin and norepinephrine reuptake, has been approved for the treatment of diabetic neuropathy. Approved dosages for treatment of diabetic PN pain are 60 or 120 mg once daily. Short-term clinical trials demonstrated that nondepressed diabetic patients experienced significant and graded reduction in 24-hour average pain when given 60 and 120 mg per day of duloxetine as compared to those receiving placebo; however, the 120 mg dose resulted in more side effects (70,71). Common side effects of duloxetine include nausea, tiredness, dizziness, constipation, dry mouth, increased sweating, and muscle weakness (asthenia). These side effects may be of greater concern in older diabetic patients with functional impairments (72).

In addition, postmarketing surveillance recently reported increased rates of hepatotoxicity (abdominal pain, hepatomegaly, cholestatic jaundice, and marked elevation of transaminase levels) with Cymbalta® (duloxetine hydrochloride). Patients with substantial alcohol use or with preexisting liver disease are at higher risk of additional liver damage. According to Food and

Drug Administration and pharmaceutical manufacturer Eli Lilly, duloxetine should not be prescribed to patients with heavy alcohol use or evidence of chronic liver disease. Uncontrolled studies of other antidepressants for diabetic PN demonstrate the need for further research in this area using better study designs.

Anticonvulsants

Anticonvulsants are frequently prescribed to treat painful diabetic PN. Although the pain-relieving mechanism is not fully understood, several clinical trials demonstrated that anti-convulsants are effective and superior to placebo and comparable to the effect of the antidepressant, amitriptyline (68,73). Of the many anticonvulsant available, gabapentin, lamotrigine, and pregabalin have the more convincing scientific evidence and are the most commonly prescribed. With regards to side effects, gabapentin and pregabalin are generally well-tolerated but some patients may experience minor side effects including dizziness, somnolence, and confusion. In the United States, however, only the newer drug, pregabalin, is approved for the treatment of diabetic PN.

Other Agents

Capsaicin is a natural colloid extracted from red chilli peppers, which depletes substance P from afferent nerves. Randomized clinical trials suggest that topical application of capsaicin cream is more effective than placebo and as effective as amitriptyline in the treatment of painful diabetic neuropathy (74). Capsaicin cream may be a useful adjunct to neuropathy treatment with amitriptyline.

Lidocaine, a local anesthetic and antiarrhythmic, blocks sodium channels, reducing both peripheral nociceptor stimulation and central nervous system hyperexcitability. Early studies suggested that intravenous lidocaine administration might be beneficial in relieving neuropathic pain, but the potential side effects and the need for intravenous administration precluded extensive clinical application. More recently, a small open-label, pre-post-clinical trial in patients with painful diabetic neuropathy, suggested that the local use of a 5% lidocaine patch (up to four lidocaine patches 18 hours per day for three weeks) was effective in relieving neuropathic symptoms without serious adverse effects in diabetic polyneuropathy (75).

Treatment of Nociceptive Pain

Nociceptive (non-neuropathic) pain often responds to nonopioid analgesia, such as nonsteroi-dal anti-inflammatory drugs (NSAIDs). NSAIDs work primarily by inhibiting cyclo-oxygenase, thereby inhibiting prostaglandin production. Adverse effects include dyspepsia, gastrointestinal ulceration, interference with platelet aggregation, renal failure, and central nervous system tox-icity. In older diabetic patients, the potential for renal impairment and gastrointestinal hemor-rhage must be carefully considered (76). The risk of renal failure and gastrointestinal bleeding is amplified by the common and concomitant use of antiplatelet agents, particularly aspirin. Acetaminophen does not adversely affect gastric mucosa or platelet aggregation. Therefore, according to the American Geriatric Society guideline, acetaminophen is the treatment of choice for mild to moderate musculoskeletal pain in older patients (43). However, it can cause serious hepatic toxicity at dosages that exceed 4000 mg per day.

Opioid analgesics are often the first line of treatment for pain associated with malignancy but are also used effectively for other types of pain, especially when other agents have not worked. Opioid agonists, such as morphine, codeine, oxycodone, and hydrocodone, commonly cause sedation, nausea, and constipation; these side effects may be particularly problematic for older patients. Respiratory depression is a serious, dose-limiting side effect. For all opioids, physical dependence with repeated usage is expected. However, opioid abuse is relatively uncommon when these drugs are appropriately prescribed and managed (43).

Tramadol is a centrally acting analgesic that both binds to opioid receptors and inhibits the uptake of catecholamines. Despite its mechanism of action, it is not scheduled as an opioid medication. Respiratory depression is not a side effect, and the drug has little potential for abuse. The major side effects, nausea, dizziness, and agitation, occur early in therapy and are often diminished by slow titration. Administration of tramadol may enhance the risk of seizure when administered to patients taking other medications that lower seizure threshold, such as neuroleptics, monoamine oxidase inhibitors, and other psychotropic agents. Tramadol is effective for several pain conditions, including osteoarthritis as well as painful diabetic PN (77). However in older adults, long-term prescription requires careful follow-up for adverse events.

Over-the-Counter Pharmacologic Approaches

An important concern is the degree to which medications used to treat pain are prescribed by a medical provider versus taken ad lib from the vast array of over-the-counter choices. Research in this area is limited because of time-consuming data collection efforts needed to determine both prescription and nonprescription medication use. A study of older persons in rural Pennsylvania found that two-thirds of participants were taking over-the-counter analgesics (78). In an Iowa study, nearly half of participants aged 65 and older reported using one or more analgesic medications, though it was unclear what proportion of these were over-the-counter (79). Use of nonprescription over-the-counter analgesic medications in older persons may help to explain the apparent undertreatment of pain in this population. The reverse also may be true; undertreatment of pain may lead to increased use of over-the-counter analgesics. Adherence is another factor in the undertreatment of pain; older people are less likely to take medications as prescribed for symptom management particularly if they are ordered to be taken three or more times in a day (80,81). Management of medications for pain relief including routine review of all medications used at home is a critical component of safe and effective management of persistent pain in older diabetic patients.

Nonpharmacologic Approaches

Surveys show that more than half of older persons with arthritis use complementary and alternative medicine (CAM) therapies (82,83). Chiropracty, acupuncture, and dietary supplements are among the more common CAM modalities used by older adults (84,85) and pain management is one of the most frequently reported reasons for using CAM therapies (86,87). However, very little is known about the impact of CAM use on pain and pain-related disability. In the general population, CAM therapies are often taken by persons who also use conventional medical approaches (88) and most do not report CAM use to their medical doctors (89). Thus, assessment of CAM use is essential in planning a pain management strategy for older patients who have persistent pain.

The AGS guidelines for pain management emphasize use of an interdisciplinary approach that is central to quality care of older patients (43). Referrals to pain specialists, pain clinics, and rehabilitation specialists are important and often underutilized components of chronic pain management for older patients. However, physicians report that lack of such resources for consultation and referral influences their care of patients with chronic nonmalignant pain (90).

Promoting Self-Management

Goal setting and monitoring of progress, with appropriate adjustments to treatment, are essential elements of chronic care. Strategies that reinforce effective coping and build confidence in pain management skills are important complements to medical therapies. The development of self-management approaches for chronic conditions have brought innovation and optimism to the management of chronic pain conditions in older adults. The Arthritis Self-Management Program (ASMP), developed by Lorig et al. at Stanford University, was among the first effective community-based self-management programs led by trained lay-leaders (91,92). The ASMP, a six-week series of classes that meets weekly and is based on a workbook (93), is now widely disseminated by the Arthritis Foundation (http://www.arthritis.org) (94). In an expansion of the ASMP, Lorig et al. developed and successfully tested the Chronic Disease Self-Management Program to address the many chronic conditions experienced particularly by older persons (95). This program is disseminated through the Stanford Patient Education Research Center.

In recent years, several other approaches for chronic care management have been developed and tested, some based in medical practices and others available in the community or through home-based programs (96,97). More research is needed in this area to address the problems of older persons with diabetes and comorbid conditions that contribute to pain and disability. However, many organized efforts within primary-care practices to promote better patient self-management of their chronic conditions may be beneficial for older adults who are striving to maintain their independence.

SUMMARY

There are several potential sources of acute and chronic pain in older diabetic patients, many of whom have two or more painful conditions. Major contributors to chronic lower extremity pain in older diabetic patients include PN and PAD. Although chronic pain is not always present in neuropathies, painful PNs are especially disabling in older patients because of detrimental effects on balance, sensorimotor function, gait, and functional autonomy. Older diabetic patients have worse PAD below the knee than their nondiabetic peers and higher risk of amputation. Research has demonstrated that diabetics have more severe PAD but complain more of atypical leg pain with exertion and rest, rather than the classic intermittent claudication.

Musculoskeletal pain is very common in older persons and it is often difficult to diagnose the underlying pathology. In the absence of a definitive diagnosis, symptom management to prevent functional decline becomes paramount in the care of older patients. Among patients who score positive on a simple pain screen, a more detailed follow-up assessment should include pain history and a detailed description of pain frequency, duration, location, and impact on mood and functioning.

Correct classification of the pain syndrome according to pathophysiologic mechanisms will establish whether pain is neuropathic (e.g., diabetic neuropathy) or nociceptive (e.g., arthritis pain or other somatic or visceral pain), or of mixed pathogenesis. Regardless of the underlying conditions that cause pain, the presence of persistent pain, particularly back pain, and lower-extremity pain, has a marked disabling effect, adding to the risk for functional limitation or worsening disability and further reducing the quality of life of older patients with diabetes. From this point of view, accurate assessment and appropriate management of pain will help older diabetic patients to maintain their activities and independence.

Individually tailored therapeutic trials are the hallmark of effective pharmacotherapy for persistent pain in older diabetic patients. Providers face particular challenges in assessment and treatment of persons who have cognitive impairments. These patients are particularly vulnerable to medication side effects and also to undertreatment. The AGS guidelines for pain management emphasize use of an interdisciplinary approach. Referrals to pain specialists, pain clinics, and rehabilitation specialists are important and often underutilized components of chronic pain management for older patients. Efforts within primary-care practices to promote better patient self-management of chronic conditions may be beneficial for older adults with diabetes.

REFERENCES

1. Centers for Disease Control. Prevalence of self-reported arthritis or chronic joint symptoms among adults—United States, 2001. MMWR Morb Mortal Wkly Rep 2002; 51:948–950.
2. Elliott AM, Smith BH, Penny KI, et al. The epidemiology of chronic pain in the community. Lancet 1999; 354(9186):1248–1252.
3. Krein SL, Heisler M, Piette JD, et al. The effect of chronic pain on diabetes patients' self-management. Diabetes Care 2005; 28(1):65–70.
4. Witzke KA, Vinik AI. Diabetic neuropathy in older adults. Rev Endocr Metab Disord 2005; 6(2):117–127.
5. Centers for Disease Control. Lower extremity disease among persons aged > or =40 years with and without diabetes—United States, 1999–2002. MMWR Morb Mortal Wkly Rep 2005; 54(45):1158–1160.
6. Bansal V, Kalita J, Misra UK. Diabetic neuropathy. Postgrad Med J 2006; 82(964):95–100.
7. Luscher TF, Creager MA, Beckman JA, et al. Diabetes and vascular disease: pathophysiology, clinical consequences, and medical therapy: part II. Circulation 2003; 108(13):1655–1661.
8. Volpato S, Blaum C, Resnick H, et al. Comorbidities and impairments explaining the association between diabetes and lower extremity disability: the Women's Health and Aging Study. Diabetes Care 2002; 25(4):678–683.
9. Kannel WB, McGee DL. Update on some epidemiologic features of intermittent claudication: the Framingham Study. J Am Geriatr Soc 1985; 33(1):13–18.
10. Jude EB, Oyibo SO, Chalmers N, et al. Peripheral arterial disease in diabetic and nondiabetic patients: a comparison of severity and outcome. Diabetes Care 2001; 24(8):1433–1437.

11. Dolan NC, Liu K, Criqui MH, et al. Peripheral artery disease, diabetes, and reduced lower extremity functioning. Diabetes Care 2002; 25(1):113–120.
12. Reiber GE, Lipsky BA, Gibbons GW. The burden of diabetic foot ulcers. Am J Surg 1998; 176(suppl 2A):S5–S10.
13. Sibbald RG, Armstrong DG, Orsted HL. Pain in diabetic foot ulcers. Ostomy Wound Manage 2003; 49(4 suppl):24–29.
14. Ribu L, Rustoen T, Birkeland K, et al. The prevalence and occurrence of diabetic foot ulcer pain and its impact on health-related quality of life. J Pain 2006; 7(4):290–299.
15. Centers for Disease Control. Mobility limitation among persons aged > or =40 years with and without diagnosed diabetes and lower extremity disease—United States, 1999–2002. MMWR 2005; 54(46): 1183–1186.
16. Himes CL. Obesity, disease, and functional limitation in later life. Demography 2000; 37(1):73–82.
17. Andersen RE, Crespo CJ, Bartlett SJ, et al. Relationship between body weight gain and significant knee, hip, and back pain in older Americans. Obes Res 2003; 11(10):1159–1162.
18. Escalante A, Lichtenstein MJ, Dhanda R, et al. Determinants of hip and knee flexion range: results from the San Antonio longitudinal study of aging. Arthritis Care Res 1999; 12(1):8–18.
19. Ettinger WH Jr, Fried LP, Harris T, et al. Self-reported causes of physical disability in older people: the Cardiovascular Health Study. CHS collaborative research group. J Am Geriatr Soc 1994; 42(10): 1035–1044.
20. Guccione AA, Felson DT, Anderson JJ, et al. The effects of specific medical conditions on the functional limitations of elders in the Framingham study. Am J Public Health 1994; 84(3):351–358.
21. Felson DT, Lawrence RC, Dieppe PA, et al. Osteoarthritis: new insights. Part 1: the disease and its risk factors. Ann Intern Med 2000; 133(8):635–646.
22. Dunlop DD, Semanik P, Song J, et al. Risk factors for functional decline in older adults with arthritis. Arthritis Rheum 2005; 52(4):1274–1282.
23. Hochberg MC, Lawrence RC, Everett DF, et al. Epidemiologic associations of pain in osteoarthritis of the knee: data from the national health and nutrition examination survey and the national health and nutrition examination-i epidemiologic follow-up survey. Semin Arthritis Rheum 1989; 18(4 suppl 2):4–9.
24. Bouhassira D, Attal N, Alchaar H, et al. Comparison of pain syndromes associated with nervous or somatic lesions and development of a new neuropathic pain diagnostic questionnaire (DN4). Pain 2005; 114(1–2):29–36.
25. Gregg EW, Beckles GL, Williamson DF, et al. Diabetes and physical disability among older U.S. adults. Diabetes Care 2000; 23(9):1272–1277.
26. Guralnik JM, LaCroix AZ, Abbott RD, et al. Maintaining mobility in late life. I. Demographic characteristics and chronic conditions. Am J Epidemiol 1993; 137(8):845–857.
27. Dunlop DD, Manheim LM, Song J, et al. Gender and ethnic/racial disparities in health care utilization among older adults. J Gerontol Soc Sci 2002; 57(4):S221–S233.
28. Markides KS, Stroup-Benham CA, Goodwin JS, et al. The effect of medical conditions on the functional limitations of Mexican-American elderly. Ann Epidemiol 1996; 6(5):386–391.
29. Otiniano ME, Du XL, Ottenbacher K, et al. The effect of diabetes combined with stroke on disability, self-rated health, and mortality in older Mexican Americans: results from the Hispanic EPESE. Arch Phys Med Rehabil 2003; 84(5):725–730.
30. Volpato S, Ferrucci L, Blaum C, et al. Progression of lower-extremity disability in older women with diabetes: the Women's Health and Aging Study. Diabetes Care 2003; 26(1):70–75.
31. Gregg EW, Mangione CM, Cauley JA, et al. Diabetes and incidence of functional disability in older women. Diabetes Care 2002; 25(1):61–67.
32. Nagi SZ. An epidemiology of disability among adults in the United States. Milbank Mem Fund Q Health Soc 1976; 54(4):439–467.
33. Verbrugge LM, Jette AM. The disablement process. Soc Sci Med 1994; 38(1):1–14.
34. Messier SP, Glasser JL, Ettinger WH Jr, et al. Declines in strength and balance in older adults with chronic knee pain: a 30-month Longitudinal, Observational, Study. Arthritis Rheum 2002; 47(2): 141–148.
35. O'Reilly SC, Jones A, Muir KR, et al. Quadriceps weakness in knee osteoarthritis: the effect on pain and disability. Ann Rheum Dis 1998; 57(10):588–594.
36. McCully K, Leiper C, Sanders T, et al. The effects of peripheral vascular disease on gait. J Gerontol A Biol Sci Med Sci 1999; 54(7):B291–B294.
37. Scherer SA, Bainbridge JS, Hiatt WR, et al. Gait characteristics of patients with claudication. Arch Phys Med Rehabil 1998; 79(5):529–531.
38. Leveille SG, Guralnik JM, Hochberg M, et al. Low back pain and disability in older women: independent association with difficulty but not inability to perform daily activities. J Gerontol Med Sci 1999; 54(10):M487–M493.
39. Weiner DK, Haggerty CL, Kritchevsky SB, et al. How does low back pain impact physical function in independent, well-functioning older adults? Evidence from the Health ABC cohort and implications for the future. Pain Med 2003; 4(4):311–320.

40. Volpato S, Leveille SG, Blaum C, et al. Risk factors for falls in older disabled women with diabetes: the Women's Health and Aging Study. J Gerontol A Biol Sci Med Sci 2005; 60(12):1539–1545.
41. http://www.geron.org/journals/repro.html.
42. Bruce DG, Davis WA, Davis TM. Longitudinal predictors of reduced mobility and physical disability in patients with type 2 diabetes: the Fremantle Diabetes Study. Diabetes Care 2005; 28(10):2441–2447.
43. American Geriatrics Society Panel. The management of persistent pain in older persons. J Am Geriatr Soc 2002; 50(suppl 6):S205–S224.
44. Cleeland C. Measurement of pain by subjective report. In: Chapman C, Loeser J, eds. Advances in Pain Research and Therapy. New York, NY: Raven Press, 1989:391–403.
45. Keller S, Bann CM, Dodd SL, et al. Validity of the brief pain inventory for use in documenting the outcomes of patients with noncancer pain. Clin J Pain 2004; 20(5):309–318.
46. Melzack R. The McGill pain questionnaire: major properties and scoring methods. Pain 1975; 1(3):277–299.
47. Caraceni A, Cherny N, Fainsinger R, et al. Pain measurement tools and methods in clinical research in palliative care: recommendations of an expert working group of the European association of palliative care. J Pain Symptom Manage 2002; 23(3):239–255.
48. Clark ME, Gironda RJ, Young RW. Development and validation of the pain outcomes questionnaire-VA. J Rehabil Res Dev 2003; 40(5):381–395.
49. Herr K, Bjoro K, Decker S. Tools for assessment of pain in nonverbal older adults with dementia: a state-of-the-science review. J Pain Symptom Manage 2006; 31:170–192.
50. Scudds R, Robertson J. Pain factors associated with physical disability in a sample of community-dwelling senior citizens. J Gerontology A biol Sci Med 2000; 55:M93–M99.
51. Leveille SG, Guralnik JM, Ferrucci L, et al. Foot pain and disability in older women. Am J Epidemiol 1998; 148(7):657–665.
52. Lichtenstein M, Dhanda R, Cornell J, et al. Disaggregating pain and its effects on physical functional limitations. J Gerontol Med Sci 1998; 53A:M361–M371.
53. Escalante A, Lichtenstein M, Lawrence V, et al. Where does it hurt? Stability of recordings of pain location using the McGill Pain Map. J Rheumatol 1996; 23:1788–1793.
54. Leveille SG, Ling S, Hochberg MC, et al. Widespread musculoskeletal pain and the progression of disability in older disabled women. Ann Intern Med 2001; 135(12):1038–1046.
55. Leveille SG, Bean J, Bandeen-Roche K, et al. Musculoskeletal pain and risk for falls in older disabled women living in the community. J Am Geriatr Soc 2002; 50(4):671–678.
56. Wolfe F, Smythe H, Yunus M, et al. The American college of rheumatology 1990 criteria for the classification of fibromyalgia. Report of the multicenter criteria committee. Arthritis Rheum 1990; 33:160–172.
57. Pahor M, Guralnik JM, Wan JY, et al. Lower body osteoarticular pain and dose of analgesic medications in older disabled women: the women's health and aging study. Am J Public Health 1999; 89(6):930–934.
58. Won A, Lapane K, Gambassi G, et al. Correlates and management of nonmalignant pain in the nursing home. SAGE study group. Systematic assessment of geriatric drug use via epidemiology. J Am Geriatr Soc 1999; 47(8):936–942.
59. Bennett M. The LANSS pain scale: the Leeds assessment of neuropathic symptoms and signs. Pain 2001; 92(1–2):147–157.
60. Bennett MI, Smith BH, Torrance N, et al. The S-LANSS score for identifying pain of predominantly neuropathic origin: validation for use in clinical and postal research. J Pain 2005; 6(3):149–158.
61. Vinik AI, Park TS, Stansberry KB, et al. Diabetic neuropathies. Diabetologia 2000; 43(8):957–973.
62. Siao P, Cros DP. Quantitative sensory testing. Phys Med Rehabil Clin N Am 2003; 14(2):261–286.
63. Hilz MJ, Dutsch M. Quantitative studies of autonomic function. Muscle Nerve 2006; 33(1):6–20.
64. American Diabetes Association. Peripheral arterial disease in people with diabetes. Diabetes Care 2003; 26(12):3333–3341.
65. Field TS, Gurwitz JH, Harrold LR, et al. Risk factors for adverse drug events among older adults in the ambulatory setting. J Am Geriatr Soc 2004; 52(8):1349–1354.
66. Corsonello A, Pedone C, Corica F, et al. Concealed renal insufficiency and adverse drug reactions in elderly hospitalized patients. Arch Intern Med 2005; 165(7):790–795.
67. Boulton AJ, Drury J, Clarke B, et al. Continuous subcutaneous insulin infusion in the management of painful diabetic neuropathy. Diabetes Care 1982; 5(4):386–390.
68. Collins SL, Moore RA, McQuay HJ, et al. Antidepressants and anticonvulsants for diabetic neuropathy and postherpetic neuralgia: a quantitative systematic review. J Pain Symptom Manage 2000; 20(6):449–458.
69. Mendell JR, Sahenk Z. Clinical practice. Painful sensory neuropathy. N Engl J Med 2003; 348(13):1243–1255.
70. Goldstein DJ, Lu Y, Detke MJ, Lee TC, Iyengar S. Duloxetine vs. placebo in patients with painful diabetic neuropathy. Pain 2005; 116(1–2):109–118.
71. Raskin J, Pritchett YL, Wang F, et al. A double-blind, randomized multicenter trial comparing duloxetine with placebo in the management of diabetic peripheral neuropathic pain. Pain Med 2005; 6(5):346–356.

72. Park SW, Goodpaster BH, Strotmeyer ES, et al. Decreased muscle strength and quality in older adults with type 2 diabetes: the Health, Aging, and Body Composition Study. Diabetes 2006; 55(6): 1813–1818.
73. Morello CM, Leckband SG, Stoner CP, et al. Randomized double-blind study comparing the efficacy of gabapentin with amitriptyline on diabetic peripheral neuropathy pain. Arch Intern Med 1999; 159(16):1931–1937.
74. Biesbroeck R, Bril V, Hollander P, et al. A double-blind comparison of topical capsaicin and oral amitriptyline in painful diabetic neuropathy. Adv Ther 1995; 12(2):111–120.
75. Barbano RL, Herrmann DN, Hart-Gouleau S, Pennella-Vaughan J, Lodewick PA, Dworkin RH. Effectiveness, tolerability, and impact on quality of life of the 5% lidocaine patch in diabetic polyneuropathy. Arch Neurol 2004; 61:914–918.
76. Gallerani M, Simonato M, Manfredini R, et al. Risk of hospitalization for upper gastrointestinal tract bleeding. J Clin Epidemiol 2004; 57(1):103–110.
77. Harati Y, Gooch C, Swenson M, et al. Double-blind randomized trial of tramadol for the treatment of the pain of diabetic neuropathy. Neurology 1998; 50(6):1842–1846.
78. Stoehr GP, Ganguli M, Seaberg EC, et al. Over-the-counter medication use in an older rural community: the MoVIES Project. J Am Geriatr Soc 1997; 45(2):158–165.
79. Chrischilles EA, Foley DJ, Wallace RB, et al. Use of medications by persons 65 and over: data from the established populations for epidemiologic studies of the elderly. J Gerontol A Med Sci 1992; 47: M137–M144.
80. Punchak S, Goodyer LI, Miskelly F. Use of an electronic monitoring aid to investigate the medication pattern of analgesics and non-steroidal anti-inflammatory drugs prescribed for osteoarthritis. Rheumatology (Oxford) 2000; 39(4):448–449.
81. Knight JR, Campbell AJ, Williams SM, et al. Knowledgeable non-compliance with prescribed drugs in elderly subjects—a study with particular reference to non-steroidal anti-inflammatory and antidepressant drugs. J Clin Pharm Ther 1991; 16(2):131–137.
82. Kaboli PJ, Doebbeling BN, Saag KG, et al. Use of complementary and alternative medicine by older patients with arthritis: a population-based study. Arthritis Rheum 2001; 45(4):398–403.
83. Jordan JM, Bernard SL, Callahan LF, et al. Self-reported arthritis-related disruptions in sleep and daily life and the use of medical, complementary, and self-care strategies for arthritis: the national survey of self-care and aging. Arch Fam Med 2000; 9(2):143–149.
84. Foster DF, Phillips RS, Hamel MB, et al. Alternative medicine use in older Americans. J Am Geriatr Soc 2000; 48(12):1560–1565.
85. Najm W, Reinsch S, Hoehler F, et al. Use of complementary and alternative medicine among the ethnic elderly. Altern Ther Health Med 2003; 9(3):50–57.
86. Astin JA, Pelletier KR, Marie A, et al. Complementary and alternative medicine use among elderly persons: one-year analysis of a Blue Shield Medicare supplement. J Gerontol A Med Sci 2000; 55(1): M4–M9.
87. Rao JK, Mihaliak K, Kroenke K, et al. Use of complementary therapies for arthritis among patients of rheumatologists. Ann Intern Med 1999; 131(6):409–416.
88. Druss BG, Rosenheck RA. Association between use of unconventional therapies and conventional medical services. JAMA 1999; 282(7):651–656.
89. Eisenberg DM, Kessler RC, Van Rompay MI, et al. Perceptions about complementary therapies relative to conventional therapies among adults who use both: results from a national survey. Ann Intern Med 2001; 135(5):344–351.
90. Potter M, Schafer S, Gonzalez-Mendez E, et al. Opioids for chronic nonmalignant pain. Attitudes and practices of primary care physicians in the UCSF/Stanford collaborative research network. University of California, San Francisco. J Fam Pract 2001; 50(2):145–151.
91. Lorig K, Lubeck D, Kraines RG, et al. Outcomes of self-help education for patients with arthritis. Arthritis Rheum 1985; 28(6):680–685.
92. Lorig KR, Mazonson PD, Holman HR. Evidence suggesting that health education for self-management in patients with chronic arthritis has sustained health benefits while reducing health care costs. Arthritis Rheum 1993; 36(4):439–446.
93. Lorig K, Fries JF. The Arthritis Helpbook: A Tested Self-Management Program for Coping with Arthritis and Fibromyalgia. 5th ed. New York: Perseus Books, 2000.
94. http://www.arthritis.org.
95. Lorig KR, Sobel DS, Stewart AL, et al. Evidence suggesting that a chronic disease self-management program can improve health status while reducing hospitalization: a randomized trial. Med Care 1999; 37(1):5–14.
96. Glasgow RE, Davis CL, Funnell MM, et al. Implementing practical interventions to support chronic illness self-management. Jt Comm J Qual Saf 2003; 29(11):563–574.
97. Glasgow RE, Funnell MM, Bonomi AE, et al. Self-management aspects of the improving chronic illness care breakthrough series: implementation with diabetes and heart failure teams. Ann Behav Med 2002; 24(2):80–87.

11 | Erectile Dysfunction in Older Adults with Diabetes

Kenneth J. Snow
Section of Adult Diabetes, Joslin Diabetes Center, and Department of Clinical Medicine, Harvard Medical School, Boston, Massachusetts, U.S.A.

EPIDEMIOLOGY

Erectile dysfunction (ED) is recognized as the inability to attain or maintain a penile erection sufficient for sexual performance. ED is a common sexual problem in men, especially those with diabetes. Various medical problems have been shown to be risk factors for ED. These include diabetes, hypertension, hyperlipidemia, and coronary artery disease. Studies have also clearly demonstrated that aging is a significant risk factor for developing ED (1).

For much of the early part of the twentieth century, ED was felt to be predominantly a psychological problem. Several factors contributed to this belief. First, cultural and religious issues prevented erectile pathophysiology from being openly discussed and investigated. Second, normal penile physiology was poorly understood. Finally, much of the research into ED that did occur involved patients at psychiatric institutions, which led to the bias that much of the etiology behind ED was found to be psychological in nature.

In 1948, Alfred Kinsey published *Sexual Behavior in the Human Male*. This ground-breaking text suggested that erectile problems may not be psychological, but rather physiologic in nature (2). These studies revealed that the rate of ED for men under 40 years of age was <2%, but by age 70, it climbed to 27%. In 1994, Feldman reported data from the Massachusetts Male Aging Study, which revealed some degree of ED in 52% of the 1300 men studied, and the most significant risk factor for developing ED was age. Men aged 70 had a sixfold increase in the incidence of ED when compared to 40-year-old men. In addition, factors such as diabetes mellitus, hypertension, hyperlipidemia, and smoking were also found to be independent risk factors (1).

In a review of ED, Braunstein found an incidence of ED in men with diabetes that was between 27.5% and 75% in the studies he identified. As the ages of the men in the studies increased, so did the incidence of ED, with up to 95% of the men over the age of 70 with diabetes having some degree of ED (3). In addition, glycemic control has been shown to be associated with the degree of ED (4). Adequate blood flow in penile sinusoids is necessary for adequate erections. With aging, there is a decrease in penile blood flow (5). This process increases the likelihood of ED in older men. These data clearly show that the likelihood of developing ED is related to the presence of other conditions that are related to endothelial dysfunction.

NORMAL PHYSIOLOGY

The penis is composed of two elongated shafts, the corpora cavernosa, running its length. Each of these shafts is composed of multiple venous pools, the penile sinusoids, surrounded by smooth muscle. The sinusoids are enclosed by a tough membrane, the tunica albuginea. The veins draining the sinusoids lie on the inside of the tunica albuginea. During the resting state of the penis, the smooth muscle surrounding the sinusoids is constricted. This vasoconstriction is mediated through numerous pathways including α-adrenergic stimulation. The vasoconstriction of the smooth muscle results in decreased blood within the corpus cavernosum, and the result is the flaccid resting state of the penis.

In the presence of sexual stimulation, cholinergic fibers in the central nervous system release acetylcholine, which partially blocks the adrenergic fibers. Nonadrenergic noncholinergic (NANC) nerve fibers are stimulated, resulting in the formation of nitric oxide (NO) through the action of nitric oxide synthase. In addition, NO is also directly produced from the endothelial cells of the corpus cavernosa.

NO leads to the stimulation of guanylyl cyclase, which converts guanosine 5′-triphosphate into cyclic guanosine 5′-monophosphate (cGMP). cGMP stimulates protein kinase C, causing a decrease in intracellular calcium. This decrease in calcium leads to relaxation of the smooth muscle on the corpus cavernosa. As the smooth muscle relaxes, the sinusoids of the corpora cavernosa fill with blood and expand. The sinusoids continue to expand until they press up against the tunica albuginea. This expansion then compresses the veins that drain the sinusoids, decreasing drainage of blood from the corporal sinusoids and thus maintaining intrasinusoidal pressure, leading to penile rigidity.

After ejaculation, epinephrine leads to intrapenile arterial constriction. Phosphodiesterase (PDE) type 5, present in penile smooth muscle, metabolizes cGMP to 5′GMP. This decrease in cGMP leads to an increase in intracellular calcium, leading to contraction of the smooth muscle of the corpora. Detumescence then occurs (Fig. 1). Any process that adversely affects the production and release of NO, endothelial function, smooth muscle responsiveness, or intrapenile blood flow will adversely affect erections (6).

Some changes that occur as men age are part of the normal aging process and independent of disease states. One change is a decreased ability to experience spontaneous erections either from visual stimuli or from fantasy. More direct genital stimulation is required as men

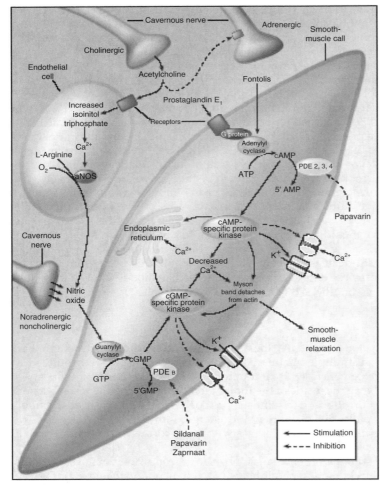

FIGURE 1   Molecular mechanism of penile smooth-muscle relaxation (6). *Abbreviations*: ATP, adenosine triphosphate; 5′AMP, adenosine 5′-monophosphate; cAMP, cyclic adenosine monophosphate; cGMP, cyclic guanosine 5′-monophosphate; 5′GMP, guanosine 5′-monophosphate; GTP, guanosine triphosphate; PDE-5, phosphodiesterase type 5.

TABLE 1   Sexual Changes Independent of Disease State

Decreased ability to experience spontaneous erections from visual stimuli
More direct genital stimulation required
Loss of focus more likely to have a negative impact
Fatigue plays a greater role
Increased refractory time
Less-forceful ejaculation

age. This fact is important for both the patient and their partner to be aware of. Some men may view inadequate stimulation as ED. In addition, a loss of focus is more likely to have a negative impact on erections. Therefore, sexual activity should be attempted at a time when there are fewer distractions. Also, fatigue plays a greater role in older men in leading to erectile problems, so that sexual activity should be attempted when well rested. Refractory time, the time from ejaculation to the next erection, is known to increase as men age. Masters and Johnson reported that the refractory period can be two days at age 70. In addition, ejaculation can be less forceful in older men (Table 1) (7).

PATHOPHYSIOLOGY

NO is the major chemical mediator of erections. The vasodilatory response to NO has been shown to be impaired in men with diabetes (8). Studies have shown that acetylcholine synthesis is reduced in men with diabetes, leading to greater difficulty for smooth muscle relaxation (9). Autonomic relaxation of smooth muscle has also been shown to be impaired in men with diabetes (10).

Aside from the ability for smooth muscle relaxation, there also needs to be an adequate penile blood supply to facilitate the development of erections. Although vascular disease of large blood vessels can lead to decreased penile blood flow, the most likely cause is problems with the intrapenile blood flow. A decrease in the flow of blood into the lacuna spaces of the penis will lead to ED (11).

TESTOSTERONE

Testosterone levels are known to decrease with age. This decrease is caused by a decrease in total testosterone production as well as by an increase in clearance of testosterone. In addition, the amount of sex hormone–binding globulin increases with age, resulting in a greater fraction of bound testosterone and a decrease in free testosterone levels. Interestingly, despite the fact that testosterone production is decreased and clearance is increased, the resulting low testosterone levels are not accompanied by increases in luteinizing hormone (LH) levels. This finding suggests that the defect may lie at the level of the hypothalamus rather than being primary testicular failure. Loss of the diurnal rhythm for LH and testosterone also occurs, along with a decrease in LH pulse amplitude and frequency. Thus, the majority of older men with testosterone deficiency have secondary, not primary, gonadal deficiency (12).

Low testosterone levels can be associated with a loss of libido, decreased muscle mass with associated weakness, impaired gait and balance, decreased bone density, loss of energy, and a lowered sense of well-being. Although a decrease in testosterone may be associated with decreased erectile function, erectile function may be unaffected by significant reductions in testosterone levels. Symptoms such as muscle weakness, loss of energy, and a decreased sense of well-being can be very vague, and failure to recognize low testosterone as a possible etiology will cause it to be overlooked. Some professionals use a testosterone level <300 ng/dL or a free testosterone level <5 ng/dL as diagnostic of male hypogonadism. Alternatively, one can consider using a level lower than the lower limit of normal for the reference lab being used (13). As discussed, LH levels are low or normal. A normal prolactin level excludes a prolactinoma as the cause of the hypogonadism.

Treatment of hypogonadism is accomplished with the use of testosterone. Various forms of testosterone therapy are available (Table 2). Although all forms are effective at increasing testosterone levels, topical gels tend to be the treatment of choice because of

TABLE 2   Available Testosterone Preparations

Route	Generic	Trade name	Dosing	Side effects
Injectable	Testosterone cypionate	Depo-testosterone	50–200 mg/wk	Pain, bleeding, sciatica
	Testosterone enanthate	Delatestryl	50–200 mg/wk	
Buccal	—	Striant	30 mg/12 hr	Gum irritation
Transdermal patch	—	Androderm	2.5–5 mg/day	Rash
		Testosderm TTS	5 mg/day	
Transdermal gel	—	Androgel	5–10 g/day	Transfer to partner
		Testim	—	

Abbreviation: TTS, testosterone transdermal system.

ease of use and minimal side effects. Oral therapy, because of the risk of hepatotoxicity, is contraindicated.

Side effects are uncommon in testosterone therapy. Since testosterone stimulates erythropoietin secretion, there is a risk for the development of polycythemia. Hence, one must monitor the hematocrit of patients on therapy. The risk of prostate cancer with testosterone use has been a subject of controversy. Evidence does not support the hypothesis that testosterone therapy induces prostate cancer (14). However, it is known that testosterone can stimulate growth of prostate cancer. Hence, all patients should undergo screening tests including a digital rectal exam and a prostate specific antigen (PSA) prior to initiation of therapy. If there is no contraindication for treatment, then patients should be followed at three months and then at least annually (13). Gynecomastia and fluid retention are rare side effects.

For those patients who are started on testosterone therapy, appropriate levels of testosterone can usually be achieved without much difficulty. It is important to assess the patient clinically and see if their initial complaints improve. If not, ongoing therapy may not be called for, and the risks and benefits of ongoing therapy need to be assessed for each patient.

DIAGNOSIS OF ED

As with other medical conditions, the hallmark of an appropriate diagnostic approach is an appropriate history, physical exam, and prudent use of laboratory evaluation (Table 3).

TABLE 3   Diagnosis of Erectile Dysfunction

Sexual health history
   Identify the sexual health problem
   Onset (sudden or gradual)
   Duration
   Progression
   Relationship to other events
   Situation
General health history
   Diabetes: duration, control, and other complications
   Hypertension
   Cardiovascular disease
   Medications: prescription and nonprescription
Physical exam
   Blood pressure
   Cardiovascular system
   Neurologic system
   Breast examination
   Genital examination
Laboratory testing
   Glucose and Hgb A_1C
   Creatinine
   CBC
   Liver function tests
   Testosterone (possibly)

Abbreviation: CBC, complete blood count.

History

When evaluating the older patient with ED, one must take a detailed history, with emphasis on the sexual history as well as comorbid conditions that are risk factors for ED. The first issue is to ascertain the sexual health condition of the patient. Patients may be less than clear on their sexual problem, feeling uncomfortable in discussing this topic. One must clarify whether the patient has a problem with ED or a problem related to ejaculation or libido. The onset (sudden or gradual), duration, and progression, and any relation to other events in the patient's life are helpful in identifying the cause of the patient's complaint. ED of organic etiology is usually of gradual onset, slowly progressive, and consistent despite various other events in the patient's life. It is usually not situational and is consistent on repeated attempts. Psychogenic etiologies are usually sudden in onset and are often situational, depending on the partner and other stressors. Although younger men may have spontaneous nocturnal erections, arguing against an organic etiology, nocturnal erections are rare in older men and as such, their absence does not argue in favor of or against an organic etiology.

Other medical problems that are risk factors for ED are much more common in the geriatric population. Diabetes mellitus, hypertension, and cardiovascular disease are common in the geriatric population. Older medications used in the treatment of hypertension were commonly associated with ED. Newer agents, such as calcium channel blockers, angiotensin-converting enzyme (ACE) inhibitors, and selective β-blockers, are not likely to contribute to ED.

Many over-the-counter medications are associated with ED. Agents such as pseudo-ephedrine, diphenhydramine, and chlorpheniramine are known to have a negative impact on erections. Many centrally acting agents such as selective serotonin reuptake inhibitors used for depression can adversely affect erections. Common agents associated with ED are listed in Table 4.

The use of survey tools is now commonly employed. These tools can complement the history, facilitate communication, and be used to monitor therapy. Two of the most widely used tools are the International Index of Erectile Function (IIEF) (16) and the Sexual Encounter Profile (SEP) (17). The IIEF is a validated tool that can be used to assess sexual function. The erectile function domain questions, numbers 1 to 5 and 15, address the ability to attain and maintain an erection. Scoring for the IIEF is from 1 to 30, with lower scores reflecting a greater degree of ED (Table 5).

The SEP is composed of seven diary questions. Patients are able to record results after each sexual encounter. Questions 2 and 3 are of utmost importance in assessing ED (Table 6). This tool can be used to quickly assess a patient's baseline function and response to therapy.

TABLE 4 Common Drugs Associated with Erectile Dysfunction

Central nervous system—acting drugs
   Antidepressants (including tricyclics and SSRIs)
   Antipsychotics
   Tranquilizers
   Anorexiants
Cardiovascular
   Digoxin
   β-blockers (especially propranolol and metoprolol)
   Certain α-blockers (prazosin)
   Central sympatholytics (clonidine, α-methyl-dopa)
   α and β-blockers (labetalol)
   Thiazide diuretics
   Spironolactone
   Calcium channel blockers (fairly low risk)
Allergy related
   Corticosteroids
   Bronchodilators
   Antihistamines (chlorpheniramine, diphenhydramine, chlortrimeton)
   Decongestants
Miscellaneous
   Metoclopramide, gemfibrozil

Abbreviation: SSRI, selective serotonin reuptake inhibitor.
Source: From Ref. 15.

TABLE 5   International Index of Erectile Function Questions and Scoring

Question	Scoring					
	0	1	2	3	4	5
How often were you able to get an erection during sexual activity?	No sexual activity	Almost never/never	A few times (much less than half the time)	Sometimes (about half the time)	Most times (much more than half the time)	Almost always/always
When you had erections with sexual stimulation, how often were your erections hard enough for penetration?	No sexual activity	Almost never/never	A few times (much less than half the time)	Sometimes (about half the time)	Most times (much more than half the time)	Almost always/always
When you attempted sexual intercourse, how often were you able to penetrate (enter) your partner?	Did not attempt intercourse	Almost never/never	A few times (much less than half the time)	Sometimes (about half the time)	Most times (much more than half the time)	Almost always/always
During intercourse, how often were you able to maintain your erection after you had penetrated (entered) your partner?	Did not attempt intercourse	Almost never/never	A few times (much less than half the time)	Sometimes (about half the time)	Most times (much more than half the time)	Almost always/always
During sexual intercourse, how difficult was it to maintain your erection to completion of intercourse?	Did not attempt intercourse	Extremely difficult	Very difficult	Difficult	Slightly difficult	Not difficult
How would you rate your confidence that you could get and keep an erection?	—	Very low	Low	Moderate	High	Very high

Score Severity of ED: 26–30, Normal; 22–25, Mild; 17–21, Mild to moderate; 11–16, Moderate; 1–10, Severe.

Physical Exam

Physical exam includes the measurement of blood pressure and an assessment of the neurologic and cardiovascular systems. A breast and genital exam must be performed. One should assess for normal virilization and any anatomic abnormalities.

Laboratory Testing

Glucose, hemoglobin A1c, liver function tests, creatinine, and a complete blood count should be checked to assess the health status of the patient. An initial testosterone level can be of value if the patient is also complaining of a decreased libido. More sophisticated testing, such as a penile vascular study, is usually not needed.

TREATMENT OF ED

If the history has uncovered any potentially reversible causes of ED, then those should be addressed first. If the patient is on a medication that may be contributing and it is safe to either stop it or switch to another, less-problematic agent, then that should be done. It may be of benefit to assess for hypogonadism, especially if other symptoms are present as well. Finally, psychological problems may need to be addressed, including potential conflicts in the relationship regarding sexual relations.

TABLE 6 Sexual Encounter Profile Questions and Scoring

SEP 2: Were you able to insert your penis into your partner's vagina?	
Yes	No
SEP 3: Did your erection last long enough for you to have successful intercourse?	
Yes	No

Abbreviation: SEP, sexual encounter profile.

Oral Therapies for ED

Sildenafil (Viagra) was approved for use in 1998 and quickly revolutionized the treatment of ED. Currently, there are three PDE-5 inhibitors available—sildenafil, vardenafil (Levitra), and tadalafil (Cialis). PDE-5 is an important enzyme involved in the erectile process. During sexual stimulation, NO is released from NANC nerves as well as from endothelial cells in the corpus cavernosum. NO activates guanylyl cyclase, which causes an increase in the level of cGMP. This increase leads to a decrease in intracellular calcium, leading to a relaxation of smooth muscle with a resulting vasodilation of the corpus cavernosum as previously discussed. PDE-5 degrades cGMP to 5'GMP, leading to vasoconstriction of the smooth muscle and detumescence. By inhibiting PDE-5, cGMP activity is increased, leading to an improved vasodilatory response (Fig. 1). Differences exist between these three agents regarding the time to peak serum concentrations and the duration of action (Table 7).

Sildenafil is available in 25, 50, and 100 mg tablets. The typical starting dose is 50 mg, with the option to increase to 100 mg if the patient does not achieve an adequate response with the 50 mg dose. Patients can decrease to 25 mg if side effects occur with the 50 mg dose. Men with more significant disease are less likely to respond to the 50 mg dose. Hence, older men and men with diabetes are much more likely to require 100 mg (19).

The time to maximal serum concentration after taking sildenafil is about one hour. Therefore, men should be advised to take the agent about one hour prior to initiating sexual activity, although some men may note a much more rapid onset of action (20). The drug has a half-life of about four hours. Thus, the period of maximal effect is between one and four hours after taking the drug. After four hours, men will notice decreasing efficacy.

Sildenafil is highly selective for the PDE-5 isoform. The only other isoform with which sildenafil has any significant cross-reactivity is PDE-6. Sildenafil has a binding affinity that is 11 times greater for PDE-5 compared to PDE-6 (21). PDE-6 is found in the retina and this cross-reactivity can account for changes that can occur in blue–green color discrimination or the presence of a bluish halo seen around objects.

Side effects are uncommon. The most common side effects include headache (16%), flushing (10%), dyspepsia (7%), and nasal congestion (4%). These side effects can be explained by the distribution of PDE-5 in other tissues. In addition, changes in vision, as discussed earlier, can occur in 3%.

Sildenafil has not been shown to increase the risk of heart attack. Rather, this agent will allow a patient to engage in a form of exercise, sexual activity, which they have not participated in for a while. As such, those with undiagnosed heart disease may uncover significant disease by initiating this form of exercise. If concern exists about the patient's cardiovascular fitness to begin sexual activity, the patient should undergo cardiac evaluation similar to any patient who planned on embarking on a new exercise routine.

Vardenafil (Levitra) is available in 2.5, 5, 10, and 20 mg tablets. The typical starting dose is 10 mg, which can be increased to 20 mg if patients do not achieve an adequate response. Lower doses are appropriate for those who have side effects with 10 mg and for those patients on

TABLE 7 Time to Peak Concentration and Half-Life

	Sildenafil	Tadalafil	Vardenafil
Time to peak concentration (hr)	1.0 (0.5–2.0)	2.0 (0.5–12.0)	0.7 (0.25–3.0)
Half-life (hr)	3.7	17.5	4.8

Source: From Ref. 18.

antifungal or antiretroviral therapy. Vardenafil reaches a maximum concentration in about 45 minutes and has a half-life of about four to five hours. Patients should be advised to take the agent about 60 minutes before intercourse. Side effects are similar to those seen with sildenafil. Headache (15%), flushing (11%), rhinitis (9%), and dyspepsia (4%) are the most common. Since the agent is much more selective for PDE-5 than for PDE-6, the effect on blue–green color discrimination observed with sildenafil is not observed with vardenafil (22).

Tadalafil (Cialis) is available in 5, 10, and 20 mg tablets. The starting dose for tadalafil is 10 mg, and it can be increased to 20 mg in patients not achieving an adequate response. The time to peak serum concentration is much longer than with either of the other two PDE-5 inhibitors, with a peak concentration reached at two hours (0.5–12 hours). The half-life of tadalafil is about 18 hours. Rather than taking this drug on demand and waiting an appropriate amount of time to reach peak concentration, this agent should be taken well in advance of sexual activity, but that the effects of the agent will last 24 hours and up to 36 hours should be taken into account (23).

Side effects are similar to those of the other two agents: headache (15%), dyspepsia (10%), nasal congestion (3%), and flushing (3%). As with vardenafil, tadalafil does not bind to PDE-6, so no visual disturbances are noted if this agent is used. Tadalafil does have a low selectivity against PDE-11, which is present in skeletal muscle, and lower back pain has been reported in 6% of men taking the drug, although a causal relationship has not been shown. PDE-11 is also present in other tissues such as the testes, prostate, and kidneys; however, no clinical effect of this distribution has been reported (24).

All three agents are contraindicated with nitrate-containing agents, because of the demonstration of the development of significant hypotension in healthy patients taking a PDE-5 inhibitor and nitrate-based vasodilators at the same time (19,22,23). Mild hypotension has been reported in patients using sildenafil and terazosin together. Hence, one should be careful in the use of α-blockers and PDE-5 inhibitors. One should start with the lowest dose of a PDE-5 inhibitor in a patient on a stable dose of an α-blocker. Newer α-blockers such as tamsulosin (Flomax) do not have as much of an effect on blood pressure and as such pose less of an issue with PDE-5 inhibitors.

All three PDE-5 inhibitors are effective in patients regardless of the severity of their ED, although patients with less-severe ED are more likely to achieve a greater response. Response to therapy can be assessed through the use of either the IIEF or the SEP 2 and SEP 3 questions. Improvements in IIEF scores of 8 to 10 points have been reported with all three agents. Positive response rates of 80% for SEP 2 and 65% for SEP 3 are achieved with PDE-5 inhibitors. To date, no good head-to-head study showing any significant difference in response rates between the three agents has been performed (19,22,23).

In July 2005, the Food and Drug Administration (FDA) approved new labeling for the three PDE-5 inhibitors based on the postmarketing reporting of several cases of nonarteritic anterior ischemic optic neuropathy (NAION) in men using all three agents. Although the majority of cases have been associated with Viagra, this greater frequency probably reflects the greater number of men using this agent. Most of these patients had underlying anatomic or vascular risk factors for the development of NAION, including a low cup-to-disc ratio, age over 50, diabetes, hypertension, coronary artery disease, hyperlipidemia, and smoking. One should quickly recognize that many of these risk factors are also risk factors for ED and that it should not be surprising that cases of NAION would occur in PDE-5 users. It must therefore be recognized that this event occurs in a similar population that does not use PDE-5 inhibitors. Given the small number of total events reported and the large number of users of PDE-5 inhibitors and the similarity of risk factors in the two groups, it is not possible to determine whether these events are related directly to the use of PDE-5 inhibitors, to the patient's underlying vascular risk factors or anatomical defects, to a combination of these factors, or to other unrelated factors. Patients should be informed that there is no firm evidence for a causal link between NAION and PDE-5 inhibitor use. Clearly, men should contact their physician immediately if they experience sudden loss of vision whether associated with PDE-5 use or not.

Yohimbine is an α2-adrenergic blocker derived from the bark of the Yohimbe tree in Africa. The agent is quite old and is now available in the United States without a prescription.

The starting dose is 5.4 mg three times each day. The agent has not shown significant benefit in men with organic ED but has shown benefit in men with psychological disease. Side effects include hypertension, nervousness, tachycardia, and urinary retention (25).

Injectable Therapies for ED

Intracavernosal injection therapy (ICI) was the primary form of therapy prior to the development of PDE-5 inhibitors. It was first demonstrated to be effective in 1983. In this method, one obtains an erection by injecting a vasodilator into the corpus cavernosum (26). Papaverine was first used, although this therapy was complicated by penile fibrosis. The addition of phentolamine improved this complication.

Although injection therapy was widely used for years, alprostadil (Caverject, Edex) became the first approved therapy when it received FDA approval in 1995. Alprostadil is a synthetic compound identical to prostaglandin E1 (PGE1). It works by increasing intracellular cyclic adenosine monophosphate, leading to vasodilation. The dosage ranges from 2.5 to 20 mcg. Studies have shown that over 80% of men achieve erections adequate for sexual activity with alprostadil therapy (27). The combination of papaverine and phentolamine, known as bimix, was used extensively prior to the approval of alprostadil. For those who do not have success, PGE1 can be added. This mix, referred to as trimix, has reported response rates of up to 80% (28). The most common side effects with this form of therapy are pain when injecting and the development of painless, fibrotic nodules. Various studies report a highly variable rate of this complication, ranging from 1.5% to 60%, depending on the frequency and duration of therapy and how nodules are identified (29). Priapism is the most worrying side effect. Although rare, it has been reported and is more likely to occur early in the course of therapy on exceeding the optimal dose for therapy either accidentally or purposely in the hope of a better response. Priapism is quite painful and requires immediate treatment to prevent damage to the corpus cavernosa. Despite high rates of success with ICI, follow-up studies have shown that half of patients who had a good response to therapy discontinued treatment by one year (30,31).

Intraurethral Therapy for ED

Alprostadil, in addition to its use in ICI, is available as an intraurethral suppository (MUSE). Alprostadil is absorbed across the urethral mucosa. Doses must be higher and the suppository is available in 125 mcg, 250 mcg, 500 mcg, and 1000 mcg doses. Success rates up to 65% have been reported (32). The most common side effects include penile and peroneal burning (30%).

Mechanical Therapies for ED

Vacuum devices for erections have been utilized in the treatment of ED for over a century. These devices consist of a plastic tube with an opening in one end so the device can fit over the penis. At the other end of the tube is a pump device that generates negative pressure. By activating the pumping mechanism, air is evacuated from the tube, creating negative pressure, which draws venous blood into the penis, resulting in an erection. A rubber constriction ring fits over the penis to maintain the erection when the vacuum pump is removed.

The devices have a high success rate, with reports of as high as 90% of men achieving an adequate erection. Erections are quite firm. Side effects are rare but can include decreased ability for ejaculation and mild bruising. A unique side effect can come about because of the lack of tumescence of the part of the penis that is proximal to the constriction band. Care must be taken to avoid a hinging injury. The major advantages of this form of therapy include a lack of pharmacologic side effects and interactions as well as the lack of a cost per use. The major disadvantage is the mechanical aspect of this treatment, which may be psychologically unacceptable to some patients. The therapy is more acceptable for those who are in long-term stable relationships (33).

Patients who are still able to attain an erection but have early detumescence can often be treated with a constriction ring. Various products are currently available. All work by compressing the penile vein without compressing either the penile artery or the urethra. In this way, the patient is able to attain an erection and maintain the erection. The patient is still able to ejaculate and can then remove the ring. The rings are inexpensive and have no side effects or drug interactions.

TABLE 8   Cost of Therapy

Agent	Retail cost per use ($)[a]
PDE-5 inhibitors	—
Sildenafil	10.00
Tadalafil	11.00
Vardenafil	9.50–9.90
Alprostadil injection therapy[b]	—
Caverject	9.15–35.50
Edex	21.85–47.78
MUSE	21.77–23.94
Vacuum pumps	0[c]

[a]Based on pricing from www.drugstore.com (35).
[b]The cost of bimix and trimix are not included since the final cost will be greatly influenced by pharmacy charges for custom mixing of the agents.
[c]There is no cost per use for a vacuum pump but there is the initial cost of acquisition.
Abbreviations: MUSE, Medicated Urethral System for Erection; PDE-5, phosphodiesterase type 5.

Penile implants are a highly successful form of therapy. As newer forms of therapy have been introduced, the number of men opting for a penile implant has decreased. Nonetheless, this option of therapy is still a good one for those who have failed other forms of therapy. There are two types of implants: The first is the semirigid rod, which creates a semierect status for the penis at all times. The second type is the inflatable rod. This type of implant has two inflatable tubes that are placed within the corpora cavernosa. The tubes are filled with a saline solution that resides in a reservoir placed in the abdomen. A small pump device is placed within the scrotum to inflate or deflate the tubes, thus achieving an erection. Current devices have a low rate of failure and a low rate of surgical complications even in patients with diabetes. Satisfaction rates can be quite high with these devices (34).

Nitric Oxide Therapy

Patients may choose not to treat their ED. They may not respond to a PDE-5 inhibitor and choose not to pursue other forms of therapy. Regardless of their reason, patients should understand that choosing to not treat their ED is an acceptable choice. Likewise, the physician evaluating and treating the patient needs to understand that all medically appropriate options for therapy should be presented to the patient and it is for the patient to accept or reject them. Physicians should not fail to mention to a patient who fails oral therapy that there are other options available to them.

COST OF THERAPIES FOR ED

The cost of each of the various therapies for ED is quite variable and can have a significant impact on the choice of an optimal therapy for a patient. Insurance coverage for therapy is quite variable. In addition, the cost of therapy can also be influenced by the frequency with which the therapy is used. Some insurance plans limit the number of therapies per month and others may provide no coverage. An overview of the cost of therapy is provided in Table 8.

REFERENCES

1. Feldman HA, Goldstein I, Hatzichristou DG, et al. Impotence and its medical and psychosocial correlates: results of the Massachusetts male aging study. J Urol 1994; 151:54–61.
2. Kinsey AC, Pomeroy WB, Martin CE. Sexual Behavior in the Human Male. WB Saunders, Co, 1948:236–238.
3. Braunstein GD. Impotence in diabetic men. Mt Sinai J Med 1987; 54:236–240.
4. Romeo JH, Seftel AD, Madhun ZT, et al. Sexual function in men with diabetes type 2: association with glycemic control. J Urol 2000; 163:788–791.

5. Corona G, Mannucci E, Mansani R, et al. Aging and pathogenesis of erectile dysfunction. Int J Impot Res 2004; 16(5):395–402.
6. Lue TF. Erectile dysfunction. NEJM 2000; 342:1802–1813.
7. Masters WH, Johnson VE. Sex after sixty-five. Reflections 1977; 12:31–43.
8. Williams SB, Cusco JA, Roddy MA, et al. Impaired nitric oxide-mediated vasodilation in patients with non-insulin-dependent diabetes mellitus. Am Coll Cardiol 1996; 27(3):567–574.
9. Blanco R, Saenz de Tejada I, Goldstein I, et al. Dysfunctional penile cholinergic nerves in diabetic impotent men. J Urol 1990; 144:278–280.
10. Saenz de Tejada I, Goldstein I, Azadzoi K, et al. Impaired neurogenic and endothelium-mediated relaxation of penile smooth muscle from diabetic men with impotence. N Engl J Med 1989; 320:1025–1030.
11. Breza J, Aboseif SR, Orvis BR, et al. Detailed anatomy of penile neurovascular structures: surgical significance. J Urol 1989; 141:437–443.
12. Liu PY, Swerdloff RS, Wang C. Relative testosterone deficiency in older men: clinical definition and presentation. Endocrinol Metab Clin North Am 2005; 34(4):957–972.
13. Bhasin S, Cunningham GR, Hayes FJ, et al. Testosterone therapy in adult men with androgen deficiency syndromes: an endocrine society clinical practice guideline. J Clin Endocrinol Metab 2006; 91(5).
14. Rhoden EL, Morgentaler A. Testosterone replacement therapy in hypogonadal men at high risk for prostate cancer: results of 1 year of treatment in men with prostatic intraepithelial neoplasia. J Urol 2003; 170:2348–2351.
15. Drugs that cause sexual dysfunction: an update. Med Lett 1992; 34:73–78.
16. Rosen RC, Riley A, Wagner G, et al. The international index of erectile function (IIEF): a multidimensional scale for assessment of erectile dysfunction. Urology 1997; 49:822–830.
17. Rosen R, Bennett A, Ferguson D, et al. Standards for clinical trials in erectile dysfunction: research designs and outcomes assessment. In: Jardin A, Wagner G, Khoury S, et al, eds. Erectile Dysfunction. Plymouth, UK: Plymbridge Distributors Heath Publications, 2000:647–768.
18. Kim S, Narayanan S, Song J. An oral selective phosphodiesterase 5 inhibitor for treatment of erectile dysfunction. Formulary 2002; 37:289–296.
19. Sildenafil-package insert. Pfizer Inc., 2005.
20. Padma-Nathan H, Stecher VJ, Sweeney M, et al. Minimal time to successful intercourse after sildenafil citrate: results of a randomized, double blind, placebo-controlled trial. Urology 2003; 62:400–403.
21. Gbekor E, Bethell S, Fawcett L, et al. Selectivity of sildenafil and other phosphodiesterase type 5 (PDE5) inhibitors against all human phosphodiesterase families. Eur Urol 2002; 42(suppl 1):63.
22. Levitra-package insert. Bayer Pharmaceuticals Corporation, 2005.
23. Cialis-package insert. Lilly ICOS LLC, 2005.
24. Bischoff E. Potency, selectivity, and consequences of nonselectivity of PDE inhibition. Int J Impot Res 2004; 16(suppl 1):S11–S14.
25. Mann K, Klingler T, Noe S, et al. Effects of yohimbine on sexual experiences and nocturnal penile tumescence and rigidity in erectile dysfunction. Arch Sex Behav 1996; 25:1–16.
26. Brindley GS. Cavernosal α blockade: a new technique for investigating and treating erectile impotence. Impotence. Br J Psychiatry 1983; 143:332–337.
27. Linet OI, Ogrinc FG. Efficacy and safety of intracavernosal alprostadil in men with erectile dysfunction. The Alprostadil study group. NEJM 1996; 334:873–877.
28. Zorgniotti AW, Lefleur RS. Auto-injection of the corpus cavernosum with a vasoactive drug combination for vasculogenic impotence. J Urol 1985; 133:39–41.
29. Krane RJ, Goldstein I, Saenz de Tejada I. Impotence. NEJM 1989; 321:1648–1659.
30. Weiss JN, Badlani GH, Ravalli R, et al. Reasons for high drop-out rate with self-injection therapy for impotence. Int J Impot Res 1994; 6:171–174.
31. Gupta R, Kirschen J, Barrow RC, et al. Predictors of success and risk factors for attrition in the use of intracavernous injection. J Urol 1997; 157:1681–1686.
32. Padma-Nathan H, Hellstrom WJ, Kaiser FE, et al. Treatment of men with erectile dysfunction with transurethral alprostadil. Medicated urethral system for erection (MUSE) study group. NEJM 1997; 336:1–7.
33. Nadig PW, Ware JC, Blumoff R. Noninvasive device to produce and maintain an erection-like state. Urology 1986; 27:126–131.
34. Goldstein I, Krane RJ. Diagnosis and therapy of erectile dysfunction. In: Walsh PC, Gittes RF, Perlmutter A, et al, eds. Campbell's Urology, 6th ed. Philadelphia: WB Saunders, 1993:2591.
35. www.drugstore.com

12 | Care of Older Adults with Diabetes During Hospitalization

Jason L. Gaglia and Martin J. Abrahamson
Joslin Diabetes Center, Department of Medicine, Harvard Medical School, Boston, Massachusetts, U.S.A.

INTRODUCTION

Persons with diabetes are two- to four-fold more likely to require hospitalization than their nondiabetic counterparts. Since older individuals with diabetes often have underlying organ dysfunction and multiple comorbid conditions, providing inpatient care can be quite challenging and complex. When hospitalization is directly related to hyperglycemia, there are often multiple metabolic abnormalities that need to be monitored and corrected. Even when hospitalization is not directly related to diabetes, there is still increased morbidity and mortality in the diabetic population, with higher rates of infection, longer hospital stays, and increased mortality if glycemia is not adequately addressed. Rapid changes in health status can require careful adjustments of diabetes-related medications, many of which have narrow therapeutic windows and can be affected by various medical conditions. In this chapter, we will review presentation and management of older adults hospitalized for severe hyperglycemia, as well as general principles of inpatient care for older individuals with diabetes.

HOSPITALIZATION DUE TO HYPERGLYCEMIC EMERGENCIES
Presentation of Older Patients with Severe Hyperglycemia

The elderly are often a more heterogeneous population than their younger counterparts. The frequency and number of comorbid conditions is greatly increased and the development of diabetes may be insidious in older individuals. In older populations, fasting plasma glucose alone may be inadequate for diagnosis of diabetes, because there is a disproportionate prevalence of postprandial hyperglycemia (1,2). Frequently, the signs and symptoms of new onset diabetes may go unrecognized for an extended period of time, particularly in individuals with confounding comorbid conditions. It is not unusual for older individuals to have diabetes initially noted only in the setting of severe life-threatening hyperglycemia. About 40% of older patients presenting with severe hyperglycemia do not have a known history of diabetes (3,4). Unfortunately, this may lead to delays in hospitalization that can significantly increase mortality (43% mortality vs. 3.4% for younger individuals in one series), with the majority of deaths occurring within 48 hours of admission with frequently no cause other than diabetes being identified (4).

Hyperosmolar hyperglycemic syndrome is more common in older individuals and there is a strong correlation between presenting osmolality and age (5), which may reflect a more prolonged prodromal period of untreated or unrecognized severe hyperglycemia in this population. This effect can even be seen in individuals who are being closely monitored, such as those in nursing homes. Indeed about a third of all patients admitted with hyperosmolality come from nursing homes (3).

Hyperglycemic emergencies are characterized by insulin deficiency relative to insulin demand. Insulin levels are not adequate to maintain normal serum glucose. The metabolic abnormalities associated with this state can further impair insulin secretory capacity and increase insulin resistance, causing a vicious cycle of worsening hyperglycemia and decreasing insulin production (6). In elderly individuals with decreased baseline insulin secretory reserve, this effect may be quite pronounced. The hyperglycemia, in turn, leads to an osmotic diuresis with subsequent dehydration. Although the osmotic contribution of glucose is only 5 mOsm/L for every 90 mg/dL (as opposed to the 2 mOsm/L for each 1 mEq/L increase in serum sodium) even with moderate elevations in glucose, mixed hypertonicity may ensue, with significant free water losses in a relatively hypotonic urine (7).

When hypovolemia becomes severe, the glomerular filtration rate falls, leading to decreased renal losses of glucose and worsening hyperglycemia and hyperosmolality. Insulin deficiency further promotes water losses as insulin itself may enhance reabsorption of water and sodium from the renal tubules (8). If there is insufficient insulin to suppress ketogenesis, the problem may be further compounded because ketones themselves are also osmoticly active and are lost in the urine. To maintain electrical neutrality, cations such as sodium, potassium, calcium, and magnesium are excreted with the ketones. This high solute excretion further impairs water reabsorption (Fig. 1). In older individuals, the propensity for significant dehydration is further enhanced by age-related changes in thirst and a decreased ability to concentrate urine (9). Other factors such as alterations in cognitive and functional status, depression, immobility, and concomitant medications may further exacerbate the situation (10).

The most common precipitant of severe hyperglycemia is infection, which accounts for 20% to 55% of cases, with the most common infections being pneumonia, urinary tract infections, and sepsis. Other acute medical illnesses that may precipitate hyperglycemic emergencies include cerebral vascular accidents, myocardial infarctions, pancreatitis, trauma, and alcohol intoxication (Table 1). Various commonly used medications including diuretics, β-blockers, phenytoin, steroids, pentamidine, sympathomimetic agents, and antipsychotics have all been associated with the development of severe hyperglycemia (Table 2) (11).

The symptoms of uncontrolled diabetes often precede fulminant metabolic decompensation. In older individuals, these symptoms may include malaise, blurred vision, polyuria,

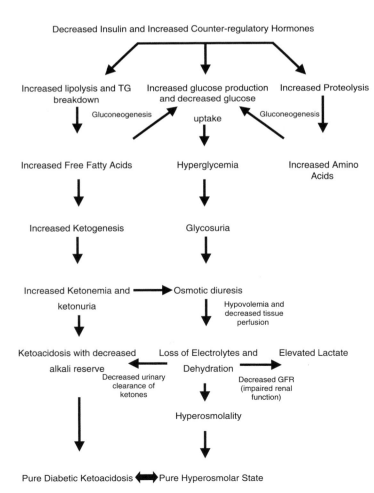

FIGURE 1 Decreased insulin and increased counter-regulatory hormones. *Note*: Relative or absolute insulin deficiency may lead to increased hepatic glucose production, decreased peripheral utilization of glucose, hyperglycemia, osmotic diuresis, and ultimately dehydration. Severe dehydration may lead to lactic acidosis from decreased perfusion and a decreased GFR with worsening hyperglycemia. Ketoacidosis may be found in the setting of more severe insulin deficiency, which augments ketone body production, leading to ketonemia. *Abbreviations*: GFR, glomerular filtration rate; TG, triglycerides.

TABLE 1   Factors Reported to Precipitate Hyperglycemic Crises

Omission of diabetes therapy
  Infections
    Pneumonia
    Urinary tract infection
    Sepsis
    Abscess
  Vascular events
    Cerebral vascular accident
    Myocardial infarction
    Acute pulmonary embolus
    Mesenteric thrombus
Trauma, burns, subdural hematoma
  Heat stroke
  Gastrointestinal events
    Acute pancreatitis
    Acute cholecystitis
    Intestinal obstruction
  Iatrogenic
    Peritoneal dialysis
    Total parenteral nutrition
  Endocrine disorders
    Acromegaly
    Thyrotoxicosis
    Cushing's syndrome
    Pheochromocytoma
    Glucagonoma
  Drugs and medications

polydipsia, weight loss, or delirium. Usually, ketoacidosis evolves fairly rapidly, while hyperosmolarity tends to evolve over a longer period of time. The typical signs of dehydration, including dry mucous membranes, decreased skin turgor, hypotension, and tachycardia, may not be readily apparent in older individuals or masked by medications. There is often blunted cardioacceleration during hypotension in this age group, which may lessen cardiovascular adaptation to dehydration and hinder assessment. A concurrent lactic acidosis may develop due to poor tissue perfusion. As with younger individuals, Kussmaul respirations may be present as a compensatory response to metabolic acidosis and a fruity odor on the breath may reflect exhaled acetone from ketogenesis. Abdominal pain, nausea, and vomiting are more frequent in those with ketosis. Lethargy, obtundation, or coma may develop or focal neurological signs or seizures may be the dominant clinical finding, with the level of consciousness correlating with osmolality rather than acidemia (12).

TABLE 2   Drugs and Medication Reported to Precipitate Hyperglycemic Crises

Steroids
Sympathomimetic agents (dobutamine, terbutaline)
Diuretics (thiazides, ethacrynic acid)
β-blockers (propranolol)
Calcium-channel blockers
H_2 blockers (cimetidine)
Phenytoin
Antipsychotics (chlorpromazine, loxapine, clozapine, olanzapine, risperidone)
α-interferon
Ribavarin
Protease inhibitors
Pentamidine
L-asparagine
FK506
Alcohol

Evaluation of Older Patients with Severe Hyperglycemia

Initial evaluation of older individuals presenting with severe hyperglycemia should include evaluation of plasma glucose, electrolytes, bicarbonate, blood urea nitrogen, creatinine, phosphate, urine and serum ketones, calculation of the anion gap, calculation of serum osmolality, arterial blood gas, complete blood count with differential, urinalysis, and electrocardiogram. Many calculations helpful in the evaluation of severe hyperglycemia are given in Table 3. Measurement of HbA1c may provide useful information about the underlying degree of metabolic control. If clinically indicated, evaluation for a precipitant should be performed. This may include culture of blood, urine, and throat, as well as a chest X ray (with repeat film after hydration), and possibly abdominal or head imaging.

With severe dehydration, central access and invasive monitoring may be necessary during resuscitation. Admission to an intensive care unit allows for increased monitoring. This is especially important if there is hemodynamic instability, decreased level of consciousness and inability to protect the airway, or presence of abdominal distention or succussion splash, or if facilities for an insulin infusion or frequent monitoring are not available in a ward setting. With institution of insulin therapy, the patient requires close monitoring for hypotension, hypoglycemia, and hypokalemia. Glucose should be checked hourly and electrolytes and acid base status checked every two to four hours, as indicated. Venous pH may be utilized if there is no need to measure arterial pO_2 or pCO_2 (venous pH is usually 0.03 units less than the arterial pH). Although useful at the time of presentation, following plasma or urine ketones as measured by the nitroprusside reaction is not helpful in subsequent management of ketoacidosis since the nitroprusside reaction does not measure the principal ketone body, β-hydroxybutyrate. Instead acetoacetate is measured and this may lead to misleading results during the recovery phase as β-hydroxybutyrate is converted to acetoacetate. The bedside measurement of β-hydroxybutyrate, which has recently become available, may prove useful, given the limitation of urine measurements (13).

Leukocytosis with elevated granulocytes is commonly seen and white cell counts of 12,000 to 20,000 are not unusual. Mild leukocytosis by itself does not necessarily indicate infection, but instead may be a response to stress and dehydration. However, white cell counts above 30,000 are highly suggestive of infection. Frequently, hemoglobin and hematocrit are initially elevated by dehydration with a falsely elevated mean corpuscular volume secondary to the relative hypotonicity of cell-counter dilution fluid (339 mOsm/L) compared to the sample.

The serum creatinine at the time of initial presentation is frequently elevated and may indicate intrinsic renal disease or prerenal azotemia in the setting of hypovolemia or may be falsely elevated in the presence of ketonemia. Both acetoacetate and bilirubin interfere with the measurement of creatinine using the alkaline picrate (Jaffe) assay (14). Treatment should lead to resolution of ketosis and restoration of intravascular volume with a decrease in creatinine except in the case of the patient who has intrinsic renal disease. Additional care must be taken in patients with underlying renal disease; if they are oliguric or anuric they may become volume overloaded during treatment and are more prone to life-threatening electrolyte abnormalities. This is especially true in the geriatric population, which has a much higher prevalence

TABLE 3   Commonly Used Calculations in the Evaluation of Severe Hyperglycemia

Calculation of the anion gap
  Gap = [Na] − [Cl + HCO$_3$]
Calculation of serum osmolality
  Osmolality = 2[Na] + (glucose in mg/dL)/18 + (BUN in mg/dL)/2.8 + EtOH/4.6
Calculation of effective serum osmolality
  Effective osmolality = 2[Na] + (glucose in mg/dL)/18
Corrected serum sodium
  Corrected sodium = [Na] + 1.6 (glucose in mg/dL − 100)/100 + 0.002 (triglycerides in mg/dL)
TBW deficit
  TBW deficit (L) = 0.6 × (bodyweight in kg) × (1 − 140/[Na])

Note: Urea is freely permeable and does not contribute to effective osmolality. Some calculations of osmolality include potassium in addition to sodium.
Abbreviations: BUN, blood urea nitrogen; TBW, total body water.

of underlying renal disease. In one series by Malone et al., more than 50% of patients, aged 65 or older, who presented with diabetic ketoacidosis, had underlying renal disease, which is more than twice the rate reported in those less than 65 (15).

Treatment of Patients with Severe Hyperglycemia

The therapeutic goals for the treatment of severe hyperglycemia in older individuals are the same as those in younger individuals. Dehydration is often more pronounced in older individuals and volume resuscitation may be paramount to improve tissue perfusion. Plasma osmolality and electrolyte imbalances must be corrected toward normal and ketogenesis, if present, inhibited. These steps usually lead to correction of acid–base disturbances and hyperglycemia. Finally, it is important to identify and treat any precipitating factors.

Hydration

Fluid replacement lowers the serum glucose independent of insulin, improves insulin sensitivity by reducing the levels of counter-regulatory hormones, and restores intravascular volume. Fluid replacement can decrease serum glucose concentration through dilution (24–36% decline) and improved renal perfusion, increasing glomerular filtration rate, which, in turn, leads to glucosuria (29–76% decline in glucose) (16). The preferred initial fluid is normal saline (0.9% NaCl), which is usually hypotonic relative to the patient's extracellular fluid and remains within the extracellular fluid compartment. Although cardiac output often improves with volume resuscitation, the initial rate of infusion still depends upon the underlying cardiac status and the degree of volume depletion. Normally 15 to 20 mL/kg/hr (1–1.5 L in an average adult) is given in the first hour to rapidly expand the extracellular space (Table 4).

Calculations of total water deficits on the basis of serum sodium concentration must be interpreted with caution because hyperglycemia and hyperlipidemia may cause pseudohyponatremia in the setting of osmotic flux of water from the intracellular to the extracellular compartment. So it is best to use corrected serum sodium, physical examination, and clinical judgment to determine the degree of dehydration. Once the corrected sodium has been normalized, most clinicians change to treatment with half normal saline. The rate of fluid replacement should also take into account ongoing urinary losses with a goal of correcting fluid deficits in about 24 hours and serum osmolality corrected at a rate of approximately 3 mOsm/kg/hr. Once serum glucose has dropped to less than 250 mg/dL, 5% dextrose is frequently added to the fluids and the insulin infusion rate adjusted to maintain blood glucose in the 120 to 180 mg/dL range.

Insulin Therapy

Insulin treatment has multiple beneficial effects including reversal of ketogenesis if present, suppression of lipolysis, inhibition of hepatic gluconeogenesis, and decreasing the effective plasma osmolality by increasing permeability to glucose. However, there are several cautions with insulin therapy in older patients. First, insulin therapy should not be initiated in patients with hypotension and severe hyperglycemia until after volume resuscitation has occurred,

TABLE 4 Suggested Replacement Fluids During Hyperglycemic Emergency

Time	Volume
1st hr	1–1.5 L normal saline
2nd hr	1 L normal saline
3rd hr	500 mL to 1 L normal saline
4th hr	500 mL to 1 L normal or half normal saline
5th hr	500 mL to 1 L normal or half normal saline
Total: first 5 hrs	3.5–5 L
6–12th hr	100–500 mL/hr half normal saline

Note: Administer normal saline or colloid as indicated to maintain hemodynamic stability. Once corrected sodium approaches normal, consider changing to half normal saline (usually about four hours). Change to D5 half normal saline when blood glucose reaches 250 mg/dL. Patients with a prolonged antecedent period may require additional fluid replacement. Use additional caution in patients with known heart disease or impaired renal function.

since the resultant fluid shift from the extracellular to the intracellular compartment, estimated to be as much as 2 to 3 L, may precipitate shock (17). Similarly, since insulin also mediates the re-entry of potassium into the intracellular compartment, insulin administration can lead to life-threatening hypokalemia. So insulin therapy should also be withheld in patients who are hypokalemic at presentation (potassium less than 3.3), until potassium replacement therapy is given (potassium greater than 3.5) (18).

Although there have been several recent studies demonstrating the use of subcutaneous insulin with rapid-acting insulin analogues in the treatment of diabetic ketoacidosis (19,20), these studies have not included older individuals. Since older patients frequently have a greater degree of dehydration with poor tissue perfusion and unreliable subcutaneous absorption of insulin, intravenous administration remains the preferred initial route of administration in this setting. Intravenous administration also offers the advantage of more rapid titration and remains the preferred route of administration pending further study of the rapid-acting insulin analogues.

To start an "insulin drip," the tubing should first be primed with about 50 mL of the insulin/saline solution to minimize subsequent insulin binding to the tubing during therapy. To minimize hypoglycemia, "low dose" insulin therapy has become the standard of care with an initial loading dose of 0.15 U/kg (usually about 10 units) of regular insulin, followed by a continuous infusion at a rate of 0.1 U/kg/hr (usually 5–10 units per hour) (21). At these doses, the serum insulin concentrations are supraphysiological and adequate to overcome insulin resistance associated with the metabolic abnormalities and clinical conditions present. As sensitivity to insulin often decreases with increasing age, it is not unusual for older patients to require titration to larger doses during the acute management of hyperglycemia (15). Once the serum glucose has decreased to less than 250 mg/dL, the rate of infusion may be decreased to 0.05 to 0.1 U/kg/hr. If the serum glucose continues to fall, the insulin infusion should not be discontinued, instead dextrose should be added to the intravenous fluids to maintain a blood glucose level of 120 to 180 mg/dL. A typical protocol is given in Table 5.

Role of Bicarbonate Therapy

Although the use of alkali therapy may seem an attractive method to correct the metabolic acidosis that may be present in severe hyperglycemia, it is usually not necessary because the metabolic acidosis tends to correct with insulin administration as protons are consumed and bicarbonate is regenerated during ketoanion metabolism. Instead, the administration of bicarbonate may lead to rebound alkalosis, worsened hypokalemia, paradoxical central nervous system (CNS) acidosis, worsened intracellular acidosis, and prolongation of ketosis. When studied in a randomized prospective manner, there is no benefit to bicarbonate therapy in patients with a pH between 6.9 and 7.14 (22,23). However, critical studies of patients with pH less than seven have been very small and there have been no prospective randomized studies concerning the use of bicarbonate when the arterial pH is less than 6.9. Severe acidemia has been associated

TABLE 5   Insulin Management Guidelines During Hyperglycemic Emergencies

Regular insulin 10 units IV STAT or 0.1 U/kg/hr
Start regular insulin infusion at 5 U/hr or 0.1 U/kg/hr
Increase by 1 U/hr q 1–2 hr if <10% drop in glucose or no improvement in acid–base status
Decrease insulin by 1–2 U/hr when glucose <250 mg/dL and/or progressive improvement
Do not decrease insulin infusion to <1 U/hr
Add D5 to IV fluids to maintain glucose between 140 and 180 mg/dL
Maintain plasma glucose between 140 and 180 mg/dL
If plasma glucose <60 mg/dL, stop insulin infusion for 30 min to 1 hr and then restart infusion
If plasma glucose is dropping consistently <100 mg/dL, change to IV fluids to D10 to maintain glucose 140–180 mg/dL, while on insulin infusion
Once patient can eat and anion gap is resolving, consider change to subcutaneous insulin
Overlap short-acting (regular) insulin with continuous insulin infusion by at least 30 min
Consider initiation of long-acting insulin at same time, usually easiest at breakfast or dinner
For patients previously managed on insulin: return to prior dose or re-evaluate insulin regimen before returning to prior dose
For new insulin patients: consider a short- or rapid- and long-acting insulin regimen
Avoid transition to oral therapy until acute glucotoxicity has resolved and renal function returned to normal

Abbreviation: IV, intravenous.

with vascular refractoriness to adrenergic action, CNS depression, and impaired myocardial contractility. Therefore, bicarbonate therapy is typically reserved for those individuals with clinical manifestations of acidemia or a pH less than 7.0. Usually one to two ampules of sodium bicarbonate (50–100 mEq) is added to a 1 L of half normal saline to make a nearly isotonic solution, which is administered over a period of one to two hours. If potassium is also low, 10 to 20 mEq of potassium chloride may be added. The venous pH should be rechecked 30 minutes after administration and treatment repeated if the corrected pH remains below 7.0.

Potassium Supplementation

Hypokalemia has been associated with arrhythmias, cardiac arrest, cardiovascular collapse, muscle weakness, and respiratory failure. Potassium is usually an intracellular cation; however, increased extracellular hyperosmolarity secondary to hyperglycemia causes a shift of water and potassium from the intracellular to the extracellular compartment. This potassium shift is further enhanced by insulin deficiency, acidosis, and accelerated breakdown of intracellular proteins. There are usually severe urinary losses of potassium during extreme hyperglycemia due to osmotic diuresis, secondary hyperaldosteronism, and urinary ketoanion excretion in the form of potassium salts. With the administration of fluids and insulin, there is typically a rapid decline in plasma potassium concentration as potassium shifts back into the cells. To prevent hypokalemia, potassium supplementation is begun when the serum potassium concentration is less than 5.5 mEq/L provided the patient does not have acute renal failure or is not oliguric. Usually 20 to 30 mEq/hr of potassium is needed to maintain plasma potassium levels between 4 and 5 (Table 6). Many practitioners utilize potassium chloride alone while others recommend administration of one-third of the potassium replacement as potassium phosphate to avoid excessive chloride administration and to minimize hypophosphatemia (11).

Phosphate Therapy

Like potassium, phosphate shifts from the intracellular to the extracellular compartment with hyperglycemia, and total body phosphate depletion is common even in the setting of initially normal or elevated levels of serum phosphate. The osmotic diuresis accompanying hyperglycemia leads to enhanced urinary phosphate losses and total body depletion. During insulin therapy, phosphate re-enters the intracellular compartment with resultant measured hypophosphatemia. Due to the prolonged unrecognized prodrome and frequent comorbid conditions in many older individuals, phosphate levels are often lower than those typically seen in younger patients. Potential complications of severe hypophosphatemia include decreased cardiac output, respiratory muscle weakness, rhabdomyolysis, CNS depression, seizures and coma, acute renal failure, and hemolytic anemia (24). Interestingly, randomized controlled trials have not demonstrated the clinical benefit of routine phosphate replacement (25,26) but these studies did not look specifically at older individuals.

In theory, phosphate depletion may contribute to decreased concentrations of 2,3-diphosphoglycerate, leading to a shift of the oxygen dissociation curve to the left and decreasing tissue oxygen delivery. Indeed, phosphate replacement has been shown to increase 2,3-diphophoglycerate during treatment, but no effect has been seen on oxygen availability (27). Since intravenous phosphate replacement has not proven beneficial in several studies (25–27) and may cause symptomatic hypocalcemia and hypomagnesemia (28,29), the degree of phosphate replacement and type of phosphate therapy remains controversial. In general, phosphate replacement is usually reserved for those with severe hypophosphatemia of 1.5 mg/dL or less, normal serum calcium concentration, and normal renal function. The use of small amounts of potassium

TABLE 6 Guidelines for Potassium Replacement

Serum K (mEq/L)	Additional K in intravenous fluids
<3.5	40 mEq/L
3.5–4.5	20 mEq/L
4.5–5.5	10 mEq/L
>5.5	Stop K infusion

phosphate intravenously appears to be safe in this setting, with typically 30 to 60 mM potassium phosphate given over 12 to 24 hours. Serum calcium, magnesium, and phosphate levels should all be monitored during phosphate infusion. Oral phosphate replacement remains preferable to intravenous administration and should be implemented as soon as possible.

Closing the Gap

Once the anion gap has closed, the bicarbonate is above 18, and the patient stable and able to eat, the transition to standard subcutaneous insulin should be considered. A frequent mistake is discontinuation of the insulin infusion prematurely before adequate clearance of ketones or without conversion to subcutaneous insulin, leading to rebound acidosis. Since regular insulin administered intravenously only has a half-life of only four to five minutes and subcutaneous insulin requires 30 to 60 minutes for action, short-acting subcutaneous insulin administration should be overlapped by at least 30 minutes to 1 hour with the intravenous infusion. When using rapid-acting insulin analogues, a shorter overlap of at least 15 to 30 minutes may be adequate. Because short-acting insulin may be inadvertently withheld if the patient is euglycemic after transition to a subcutaneous regimen, administration of long-acting insulin at this time to help minimize accidental rebound acidosis is also advocated. For patients in whom total insulin requirements are not known, an initial dose of about 0.5 to 1 U/kg/day is usually given in a mixed regimen including both short- and long-acting insulins. If initiation or reinstitution of oral insulin secretagogues is to be considered, this should not be done until after glucotoxicty and lipotoxicity have resolved.

Complications in Patients with Severe Hyperglycemia

Approximately 10% to 15% of individuals with diabetic ketoacidosis may have evidence of acute pancreatitis by computed tomography (CT) while another 16% to 25% may have nonspecific elevations in amylase and lipase (30,31). The nonspecific hyperamylasemia is thought to be multifactorial, caused by salivary hyperamylasemia, reduced renal clearance of amylase, and increased leakage from the pancreas. Nonspecific hyperlipasemia is less well understood but it is postulated that the reduced glomerular filtration seen with severe hyperglycemia may result in decreased renal clearance and that nonpancreatic lipases may be measured in the current assay generating false-positive results. Acute pancreatitis associated with hyperglycemia is usually seen in the setting of severe hypertriglyceridemia. Insulin deficiency promotes lipolysis, releasing free fatty acids, leading to hypertriglyceridemia. In a recent series by Nair et al., 22% of patients with diabetic ketoacidosis had mild hypertriglyceridemia (greater than 500 mg/dL) and 8% had severe hypertriglyceridemia (greater than 1000 mg/dL). Half of the patients with severe hypertriglyceridemia had evidence of pancreatitis by CT. Acute pancreatitis was more often seen in patients with more severe metabolic acidosis (pH 7.15 vs. 7.31, $P = 0.0001$), and higher serum glucose (934 mg/dL vs. 714 mg/dL $P = 0.02$) at the time of presentation. The hypertriglyceridemia is usually transient, with triglyceride levels decreasing to less than 300 mg/dL with resolution of ketosis (30).

Rhabdomyolysis is an under-recognized feature of hyperglycemic emergencies that results from the destruction of myocytes and leakage of their cellular contents into the plasma. One large series found an incidence of 17%, defined as creatinine kinase levels greater than 1000 IU/L (32). Rhabdomyolysis is usually associated with higher blood glucose levels and serum osmolality and decreased renal function (32,33). Mortality is significantly higher in those who present with rhabdomyolysis and increases with increasing age (32).

During hyperglycemic emergencies, the combination of severe dehydration, increased blood viscosity, low cardiac output, and stimulation of prothrombotic mediators can lead to a hypercoagulable state and thromboembolism. A number of case reports and retrospective reviews from the 1970s suggest an increased incidence of vascular occlusive disease including cerebral infarct, myocardial infarction, pulmonary embolism, mesenteric thrombosis, and disseminated intravascular coagulation with hyperglycemic emergencies (34–36). With the introduction of prophylactic anticoagulation (twice daily low dose heparin) and aggressive early hydration, the incidence of these complications has fallen dramatically in more recent case series (37,38). Although there are no randomized controlled trials demonstrating the safety or efficacy of low-dose or low-molecular-weight heparin in hyperglycemic crises, on the basis of this historic evidence, prophylactic anticoagulation should be considered for all patients without a contraindication to low-level anticoagulation.

Hyperchloremic metabolic acidosis is only present in approximately 10% of patients at the time of admission but develops in most patients with ketoacidosis, four to eight hours after initiation of therapy (39). With ketoacidosis, chloride losses are less than sodium losses because of the excretion of ketoanions as sodium salts and increased chloride reabsorption due to decreased availability of bicarbonate in the proximal tubule (39,40). Since initial replacement fluids usually contain 154 mmol/L of both sodium and chloride (approximately 54 mmol/L in excess of the 100 mmol/L of chloride in the serum) relative hyperchloremia occurs with treatment. This may lead to normalization of the anion gap with a persistent mild reduction in bicarbonate. This is usually of no clinical consequence and gradually corrects over the next 24 to 48 hours by enhanced renal acid excretion.

Acute gastric dilation due to hypertonicity-induced gastroparesis is relatively rare but there is an increased risk of gastrointestinal (GI) bleeding in this setting (41). As the hypertonicity is corrected, this condition should remit, but decompression with a nasogastric tube may be required.

Although rare, adult respiratory distress syndrome (ARDS) may occur during treatment of hyperglycemic emergencies. Relatively hypotonic fluid administration during resuscitation may increase left atrial pressure and decrease osmotic pressure, leading to capillary leak and pulmonary edema. ARDS should be suspected with the development of an increased A-a gradient, dyspnea, hypoxemia, rales, or infiltrates with resuscitation (42). Since crystalloid infusion may be a major factor in the development of respiratory distress, some practitioners favor the addition of colloid administration for treatment of hypotension unresponsive to initial crystalloid replacement (11).

MANAGING DIABETES IN OLDER HOSPITALIZED PATIENTS
Treatment Goals During Hospitalization

In addition to hyperglycemic emergencies, diabetes predisposes to a number of conditions, which may lead to hospitalization, including coronary artery disease, cerebrovascular disease, peripheral vascular disease, nephropathy, and infection. Individuals with diabetes have a two- to four-fold higher hospitalization rate than nondiabetic individuals. Poorly controlled diabetes during hospitalization has been associated with increased infectious complications, delayed wound healing, increased costs, increased length of stay, and increased mortality (43). It is often difficult to predict the effects of illness and hospitalization on glycemia (Table 7), but the tendency in most patients is toward hyperglycemia or frequent fluctuations in glucose concentrations.

The diabetes treatment goals for older individuals in the acute care setting include avoidance of hypo- or hyperglycemia, avoidance of accompanying metabolic abnormalities such as volume depletion or electrolyte abnormalities, meeting nutritional needs, and assessment of patient educational needs. A detailed history including preadmission diabetic medications, home glucose monitoring results, outpatient diet, HbA1c, and presence of diabetic complications will greatly facilitate development of a diabetes care plan to meet these goals. It is now generally recommended that blood glucose be kept between 80 and 110 mg/dL in patients in

TABLE 7   Common Factors Affecting Blood Sugar During Hospitalization

Increased counter-regulatory hormones
Unpredictable oral/enteral/parenteral nutrition
Illness/nausea
NPO for tests
Changing meal times
Cycled tube feedings
Parenteral nutrition, intravenous glucose
Inactivity
Timing of insulin injections
Medications (e.g., corticosteroids, vasopressors)

Abbreviation: NPO, nothing by mouth.

intensive care units. Although controlled studies are lacking in noncritically ill patients, for other (nonpregnant) patients it is recommend that preprandial blood sugars of less than 110 mg/dL and less than 180 mg/dL at all other times be achieved (44,45).

With concomitant increase in infectious complications and poor wound healing in geriatric and diabetic individuals, extra attention must be given to skin and wound care. It is important to take prophylactic measures to prevent the development of pressure ulcers. These may include specialized support surfaces for bedding and wheelchairs to maintain tissue pressure below 30 mmHg.

Nutrition Considerations

Appropriate nutrition can simplify diabetes care and potentially decrease morbidity and mortality. Nutrition needs to be individualized on the basis of body weight, comorbidities, and expected caloric expenditure (typical daily dietary provision of 25–35 kcal/kg body weight). In patients who are eating, avoidance of high glycemic index foods may reduce fluctuations in blood sugar. Consistent carbohydrate meal plans decrease variability in postprandial blood sugars, making it easier to determine appropriate doses of diabetes medications. Particularly in elderly patients it is important to assess for anorexia and weight loss, which is known to increase their risk of morbidity and mortality. It is important to avoid the tendency toward overly restrictive diets in these patients and instead to focus on appropriate mechanical consistency, palatability, and finally glycemic index. A typical meal plan for a noncritically ill patient would provide 1500 to 2000 kcal/day, with about 50% of calories from carbohydrates, 20% from protein, and 30% from fat. More details of nutrition in elderly patients with diabetes are discussed elsewhere, and dietary consultation should be considered for complex cases.

Use of Oral Diabetes Medications

It is important to recognize and prevent drug-related problems in older individuals. It is suggested that an objective criteria such as the Beers criteria be used to identify unsafe medication practices (46). Both new medications being considered during the hospitalization and prior home medications should be reviewed.

For patients with acute myocardial infarction, insulin infusion has been shown to improve outcomes (47), while some sulfonylureas may increase mortality (48). Otherwise, the four primary categories of oral agents—secretagogues, biguanides, thiazolidinediones, and α-glucosidase inhibitors—have not been systematically studied in the hospital setting. In noncardiac patients who were previously well controlled as outpatients and will be eating regularly, it may be reasonable to initially continue many of their outpatient medications with a few caveats. A dose reduction of 25% to 50% should be considered for insulin secretagogues due to a potentially more rigid hospital diet; this might be apparent from the dietary history. Sulfonylureas with primarily renal clearance such as glyburide are generally avoided in the geriatric population. Due to the risk of lactic acidosis, metformin should be immediately discontinued if there is a risk of hemodynamic instability, congestive heart failure (CHF), dehydration, decreased renal perfusion or impaired renal function, or altered hepatic function, perioperative status or radiocontrast studies are planned. Thiazolidinediones may be continued unless there are liver function test abnormalities, concern for new edema, or CHF; in this situation, one should consider holding the thiazolidinediones, given their prolonged effectiveness. α-Glucosidase inhibitors may be continued unless the patient was admitted with a GI illness or develops GI symptoms.

In patients who are not eating or in whom oral intake is in doubt or unpredictable, oral hypoglycemic agents should be discontinued and instead insulin utilized. In this setting, most physicians also discontinue metformin because there are increased concerns of hemodynamic instability and potential radiocontrast studies. One should also discontinue α-glucosidase inhibitors in this setting, because they are only effective when taken with meals.

Insulin Therapy

Multiple controlled studies support the use of insulin and tight glycemic control in critically ill patients (49,50). In this setting, intravenous insulin is the preferred delivery method. It allows for more rapid titration and does not rely upon subcutaneous absorption. Various protocols for intravenous insulin infusion are available (51).

Individuals taking insulin prior to hospitalization should generally have this continued but may require modifications to their regimen. When determining insulin requirements during hospitalization it is important to recognize whether a patient can produce significant endogenous insulin. Several clinical features may be helpful in identifying the degree of insulin deficiency (Table 8). Patients determined to be significantly insulin deficient require basal insulin replacement at all times, even if nil per os (NPO) or normoglycemic, to avoid iatrogenic diabetic ketoacidosis. While fasting, intravenous glucose at 5 to 10 gm/hr is also often given to limit the metabolic effects of starvation.

Insulin treatment can be regarded as having "basal," "nutritional," and "correction" components. When patients are eating discrete meals without other nutritional supplementation such as total parenteral nutrition, enteral feedings, or dextrose infusions, the "nutritional" portion is the same as the standard "prandial" requirement. Insulin requirements may be increased with stress or illness or decreased with prolonged starvation and frequently return to normal with resolution of acute illness.

Basal insulin can be provided via any one of several strategies including continuous subcutaneous insulin infusion or subcutaneous injections of intermediate-acting (including premixed) or long-acting insulin. If not timed appropriately with nutritional intake, peaks exceeding basal requirements particularly from neutral protamine hagedron (NPH) or premixed insulins can result in hypoglycemia.

Prandial insulin is usually administered at mealtime. In patients eating consistent carbohydrate meals, a fixed dose of nutritional insulin may be calculated with a correction for pre-meal blood sugar, which can be easily accomplished in the form of an insulin scale. For patients practicing self-management, "carbohydrate counting" may be employed to allow more flexibility in the meal plan. The rapid-acting insulin analogues are excellent prandial insulins and may even be administered immediately after eating when it is unclear how much food is to be consumed. This is not recommended with regular insulin, which has a rather delayed onset of action. If rapid-acting analogues are utilized and food is not consumed in a timely fashion after administration, severe hypoglycemia may result.

Adjustments in Treatment Regimen for Procedures

If a diabetic patient is to be made NPO for a procedure, it is preferable to schedule the procedure for early morning, because this will greatly facilitate medication adjustments. Blood sugars should be checked every one to two hours before, during, and immediately after procedures. The use of local or regional anesthesia is less likely to perturb glucose levels than general anesthesia.

In patients determined to have severe insulin deficiency, such as individuals with type 1 diabetes, extra care must be taken to avoid iatrogenic ketosis. If subcutaneous insulin is to be continued, one-half to two-third of the usual dose of intermediate-acting (e.g., NPH) insulin is to be given on the morning of the procedure. If the patient uses a "peakless" analogue such as insulin glargine or detemir either full dose or a dose reduction of approximately 20% may be reasonable depending upon dietary history and prior glycemic control. Small doses of regular or rapid-acting insulin may be given if blood glucose is above target, but frequent administration with insulin "stacking" should be avoided. A preferred alternative especially for long and complex procedures is to use intravenous insulin and dextrose infusions adjusted to maintain target blood glucose.

For patients with type 2 diabetes, blood glucose frequently improves when not eating but still may not be normal. Oral medications should be adjusted as described above; generally, all

TABLE 8 Characteristics of Patients with Potential Severe Insulin Deficiency

Known type 1 diabetes
History of diabetic ketoacidosis
History of pancreatectomy or severe pancreatic dysfunction
Extended duration of diabetes (usually disease >10 yr with insulin use >5 yr)
History of metabolic instability with wide fluctuations in blood sugars

oral diabetes medications are held the morning of surgery. If subcutaneous insulin is to be continued, one-half of the intermediate-acting (e.g., NPH) insulin is to be given while NPO. Otherwise, general principles are the same as those described earlier. Postoperatively, when the patient is eating and it is time to reinstate the preoperative diabetes regimen, the patient should again be evaluated for contraindications to the oral medications. Specifically, metformin should not be restarted in patients with renal insufficiency, significant hepatic impairment, or congestive heart failure and secretagogues may need to be adjusted in a stepwise fashion on the basis of oral intake and glycemic control.

Preparing for Discharge

The planned outpatient diabetes regimen is best instituted prior to discharge to ensure adequate glycemic control and avoidance of hypoglycemia. Diabetes "survival skills" and "sick day rules" should be reviewed to ensure the outpatient safety as monitoring often decreases after discharge. Based upon the individual patient's needs, all necessary supportive care such as visiting nurses, physical therapist, and occupational therapist should be in place prior to discharge. It is preferred that patients go home or to rehab with a concrete follow-up plan with medical appointments scheduled ahead of time whenever possible and an emergency contact number provided, in case problems arise.

SUMMARY

Inpatient treatment of older individuals with diabetes can be both challenging and rewarding. During hospitalization, many of the same issues that are seen in older individuals with diabetes in the outpatient setting (and covered elsewhere in this text), including cognitive dysfunction, polypharmacy, increased fall risk, deconditioning, vascular disease, and poor wound healing, may become more apparent. Although many strategies for treating this population have been covered in this chapter, formal diabetes consultation should be considered for any patient with diabetes but particularly those with newly diagnosed diabetes or poorly controlled diabetes as an outpatient, or if glycemic goals are not rapidly met during hospitalization. In addition to inpatient management, consultation can help address educational deficiencies and development of an outpatient diabetes management plan.

Current recommendations regardless of age are for blood sugars in critically ill patients requiring intensive care to be kept between 80 and 110 mg/dL, while other hospitalized patients should ideally have goal blood sugars of less than 110 mg/dL preprandial and less than 180 mg/dL at all other times. Delays in achieving glycemic goals are frequently associated with increased complications, costs, length of stay, and ultimately mortality. This is especially true in the geriatric diabetic population.

REFERENCES

1. Harris MI, Flegal KM, Cowie CC, et al. Prevalence of diabetes, impaired fasting glucose, and impaired glucose tolerance in U.S. adults. The Third National Health and Nutrition Examination Survey, 1988–1994. Diabetes Care 1998; 21(4):518–24.
2. Resnick HE, Harris MI, Brock DB, Harris TB. American Diabetes Association diabetes diagnostic criteria, advancing age, and cardiovascular disease risk profiles: results from the Third National Health and Nutrition Examination Survey. Diabetes Care 2000; 23(2):176–80.
3. Wachtel TJ, Silliman RA, Lamberton P. Predisposing factors for the diabetic hyperosmolar state. Arch Intern Med 1987; 147(3):499–501.
4. Gale EA, Dornan TL, Tattersall RB. Severely uncontrolled diabetes in the over-fifties. Diabetologia 1981; 21(1):25–28.
5. MacIsaac RJ, Lee LY, McNeil KJ, Tsalamandris C, Jerums G. Influence of age on the presentation and outcome of acidotic and hyperosmolar diabetic emergencies. Intern Med J 2002; 32(8):379–385.
6. Rossetti L, Giaccari A, DeFronzo RA. Glucose toxicity. Diabetes Care 1990; 13(6):610–630.
7. Gaglia JL, Wyckoff J, Abrahamson MJ. Acute hyperglycemic crisis in the elderly. Med Clin North Am 2004; 88(4):1063–1084, xii.
8. Skott P, Hother-Nielsen O, Bruun NE, et al. Effects of insulin on kidney function and sodium excretion in healthy subjects. Diabetologia 1989; 32(9):694–699.

9. Phillips PA, Rolls BJ, Ledingham JG, et al. Reduced thirst after water deprivation in healthy elderly men. N Engl J Med 1984; 311(12):753–759.
10. Weinberg AD, Minaker KL. Dehydration. Evaluation and management in older adults. Council on Scientific Affairs, American Medical Association. JAMA 1995; 274(19):1552–1556.
11. Kitabchi AE, Umpierrez GE, Murphy MB, et al. Management of hyperglycemic crises in patients with diabetes. Diabetes Care 2001; 24(1):131–153.
12. Fulop M, Rosenblatt A, Kreitzer SM, Gerstenhaber B. Hyperosmolar nature of diabetic coma. Diabetes 1975; 24(6):594–599.
13. Laffel L. Ketone bodies: a review of physiology, pathophysiology and application of monitoring to diabetes. Diabetes Metab Res Rev 1999; 15(6):412–426.
14. Lolekha PH, Taksinamanee R. Evaluation of serum creatinine measurement by the direct acidification method for errors contributed by noncreatinine chromogens. Clin Chim Acta 1980; 107(1–2):97–104.
15. Malone ML, Gennis V, Goodwin JS. Characteristics of diabetic ketoacidosis in older versus younger adults. J Am Geriatr Soc 1992; 40(11):1100–1104.
16. West ML, Marsden PA, Singer GG, Halperin ML. Quantitative analysis of glucose loss during acute therapy for hyperglycemic hyperosmolar syndrome. Diabetes Care 1986; 9(5):465–471.
17. Metz S. Little risk of hyperosmolar coma following hyperglycemia during cardiopulmonary bypass. Anesthesiology 1991; 75(5):912–913.
18. Abramson E, Arky R. Diabetic acidosis with initial hypokalemia. Therapeutic implications. JAMA 1966; 196(5):401–403.
19. Della Manna T, Steinmetz L, Campos PR, et al. Subcutaneous use of a fast-acting insulin analog: an alternative treatment for pediatric patients with diabetic ketoacidosis. Diabetes Care 2005; 28(8):1856–1861.
20. Umpierrez GE, Cuervo R, Karabell A, Latif K, Freire AX, Kitabchi AE. Treatment of diabetic ketoacidosis with subcutaneous insulin aspart. Diabetes Care 2004; 27(8):1873–1878.
21. Harrower AD. Treatment of diabetic ketoacidosis by direct addition of insulin to intravenous infusion. A comparison of "high dose" and "low dose" techniques. Br J Clin Pract 1979; 33(3):85–86.
22. Gamba G, Oseguera J, Castrejon M, Gomez-Perez FJ. Bicarbonate therapy in severe diabetic ketoacidosis. A double blind, randomized, placebo controlled trial. Rev Invest Clin 1991; 43(3):234–238.
23. Morris LR, Murphy MB, Kitabchi AE. Bicarbonate therapy in severe diabetic ketoacidosis. Ann Intern Med 1986; 105(6):836–840.
24. Knochel JP. Hypophosphatemia. Clin Nephrol 1977; 7(4):131–137.
25. Fisher JN, Kitabchi AE. A randomized study of phosphate therapy in the treatment of diabetic ketoacidosis. J Clin Endocrinol Metab 1983; 57(1):177–180.
26. Wilson HK, Keuer SP, Lea AS, Boyd AE, 3rd, Eknoyan G. Phosphate therapy in diabetic ketoacidosis. Arch Intern Med 1982; 142(3):517–520.
27. Gibby OM, Veale KE, Hayes TM, Jones JG, Wardrop CA. Oxygen availability from the blood and the effect of phosphate replacement on erythrocyte 2,3-diphosphoglycerate and haemoglobin-oxygen affinity in diabetic ketoacidosis. Diabetologia 1978; 15(5):381–385.
28. Winter RJ, Harris CJ, Phillips LS, Green OC. Diabetic ketoacidosis. Induction of hypocalcemia and hypomagnesemia by phosphate therapy. Am J Med 1979; 67(5):897–900.
29. Zipf WB, Bacon GE, Spencer ML, Kelch RP, Hopwood NJ, Hawker CD. Hypocalcemia, hypomagnesemia, and transient hypoparathyroidism during therapy with potassium phosphate in diabetic ketoacidosis. Diabetes Care 1979; 2(3):265–268.
30. Nair S, Yadav D, Pitchumoni CS. Association of diabetic ketoacidosis and acute pancreatitis: observations in 100 consecutive episodes of DKA. Am J Gastroenterol 2000; 95(10):2795–2800.
31. Yadav D, Nair S, Norkus EP, Pitchumoni CS. Nonspecific hyperamylasemia and hyperlipasemia in diabetic ketoacidosis: incidence and correlation with biochemical abnormalities. Am J Gastroenterol 2000; 95(11):3123–3128.
32. Wang LM, Tsai ST, Ho LT, Hu SC, Lee CH. Rhabdomyolysis in diabetic emergencies. Diabetes Res Clin Pract 1994; 26(3):209–214.
33. Moller-Petersen J, Andersen PT, Hjorne N, Ditzel J. Nontraumatic rhabdomyolysis during diabetic ketoacidosis. Diabetologia 1986; 29(4):229–234.
34. Arieff AI, Carroll HJ. Nonketotic hyperosmolar coma with hyperglycemia: clinical features, pathophysiology, renal function, acid-base balance, plasma-cerebrospinal fluid equilibria and the effects of therapy in 37 cases. Medicine (Baltimore) 1972; 51(2):73–94.
35. Tchertkoff V, Nayak SV, Kamath C, Salomon MI. Hyperosmolar nonketotic diabetic coma: vascular complications. J Am Geriatr Soc 1974; 22(10):462–466.
36. Whelton MJ, Walde D, Havard CW. Hyperosmolar non-ketotic diabetic coma: with particular reference to vascular complications. Br Med J 1971; 1(740):85–86.
37. Pinies JA, Cairo G, Gaztambide S, Vazquez JA. Course and prognosis of 132 patients with diabetic non ketotic hyperosmolar state. Diabete Metab 1994; 20(1):43–48.
38. Wachtel TJ, Tetu-Mouradjian LM, Goldman DL, Ellis SE, O'Sullivan PS. Hyperosmolarity and acidosis in diabetes mellitus: a three-year experience in Rhode Island. J Gen Intern Med 1991; 6(6):495–502.

39. Adrogue HJ, Wilson H, Boyd AE 3rd, Suki WN, Eknoyan G. Plasma acid-base patterns in diabetic ketoacidosis. N Engl J Med 1982; 307(26):1603–1610.

40. Oh MS, Banerji MA, Carroll HJ. The mechanism of hyperchloremic acidosis during the recovery phase of diabetic ketoacidosis. Diabetes 1981; 30(4):310–313.

41. Hirsch ML. Gastric hemorrhage in diabetic coma. Diabetes 1960; 9:94–96.

42. Carroll P, Matz R. Adult respiratory distress syndrome complicating severely uncontrolled diabetes mellitus: report of nine cases and a review of the literature. Diabetes Care 1982; 5(6):574–580.

43. Ahmann A. Reduction of hospital costs and length of stay by good control of blood glucose levels. Endocr Pract 2004; 10(suppl 2):53–56.

44. Garber AJ, Moghissi ES, Bransome ED Jr, et al. American College of Endocrinology position statement on inpatient diabetes and metabolic control. Endocr Pract 2004; 10(suppl 2):4–9.

45. Clement S, Braithwaite SS, Magee MF, et al. Management of diabetes and hyperglycemia in hospitals. Diabetes Care 2004; 27(2):553–591.

46. Fick DM, Cooper JW, Wade WE, Waller JL, Maclean JR, Beers MH. Updating the Beers criteria for potentially inappropriate medication use in older adults: results of a US consensus panel of experts. Arch Intern Med 2003; 163(22):2716–2724.

47. Malmberg K. Prospective randomised study of intensive insulin treatment on long-term survival after acute myocardial infarction in patients with diabetes mellitus. DIGAMI (Diabetes Mellitus, Insulin Glucose Infusion in Acute Myocardial Infarction) Study Group. BMJ 1997; 314(7093):1512–1515.

48. Garratt KN, Brady PA, Hassinger NL, Grill DE, Terzic A, Holmes DR Jr. Sulfonylurea drugs increase early mortality in patients with diabetes mellitus after direct angioplasty for acute myocardial infarction. J Am Coll Cardiol 1999; 33(1):119–124.

49. Van den Berghe G, Wilmer A, Hermans G, et al. Intensive insulin therapy in the medical ICU. N Engl J Med 2006; 354(5):449–461.

50. Van den Berghe G, Wouters P, Weekers F, et al. Intensive insulin therapy in the critically ill patients. N Engl J Med 2001; 345(19):1359–1367.

51. Goldberg PA, Siegel MD, Sherwin RS, et al. Implementation of a safe and effective insulin infusion protocol in a medical intensive care unit. Diabetes Care 2004; 27(2):461–467.

13 | Macrovascular Complications of Diabetes in Older Adults

Richard E. Scranton, Jatin K. Dave, and J. Michael Gaziano
Division of Aging, Brigham and Women's Hospital, Harvard Medical School, Boston, Massachusetts, U.S.A.

INTRODUCTION

Diabetes contributes to an astonishing amount of disability, morbidity, and premature death (1). The risk of cardiovascular disease (CVD) is greatly increased among those with diabetes, with a doubling of the risk for individuals over the age of 65 (1). Every indication suggests that the toll from diabetes will continue, making screening and treatment paramount. Coexisting cardiovascular risk factors are prevalent in diabetes and warrant aggressive management including diet, exercise, and usually multiple pharmacologic therapies.

Despite the epidemic of diabetes in older patients, the literature on macrovascular complications of diabetes in older adults is limited. In this chapter, we review the available literature on the epidemiology and pathophysiology of diabetes and insulin resistance among elderly individuals and how it relates to the development of macrovascular disease and the association with other CVD risk factors. We summarize these findings by suggesting screening and treatment approaches while attempting to highlight the differences in approaches to macrovascular complications of diabetes in frail older adults compared to the general population.

INCIDENCE/PREVALENCE

National trends suggest that diabetes incidence is growing for all ages. From 1997 to 2003, the incidence of self-reported diagnosed diabetes increased by 43%; with an even greater magnitude of increase with advancing age (2). Currently, 42% of the diabetic population in the United States is 65 years of age or older; this proportion is projected to increase to 58% by 2050. By the year 2050, cases of diabetes in people aged 75 or older are projected to increase by 300%—the largest increase in diagnosed diabetes of any age group (3).

Diabetes and insulin resistance clearly increases with age. The Rotterdam Study (4), a population cohort study of men and women over the age of 55, reported increasing prevalence rates of diabetes from 5.9% to 19.8% in men and 3.8% to 18.9% in women. In addition, impaired glucose intolerance, as determined by two-hour postglucose challenge, increased from 8.8% to 24.3% for men and 11.0% to 34.7% in women (4). Figure 1 illustrates a greater likelihood of glucose intolerance, insulin resistance, or diabetes with each decade of life.

Nearly 75% of 85-year-olds have some evidence of insulin resistance or frank diabetes. In a study predicting the development of diabetes in the normative aging study cohort, men without diabetes and a fasting glucose of less than 110 mg/dL and those with a marker of insulin resistance—Homeostasis Model Assessment (HOMA) value in the upper tertile (5)—had a fourfold greater risk for developing diabetes compared to men with a HOMA value in the lowest tertile (6). The strongest case for diagnosis and intervention is the apparent exaggerated association with cardiovascular complications.

Comments made are purely the personal opinions of the writers, based in part on experiences which include current and past work in various capacities within the medical industry. For Richard Scranton, these employers include Berlex, Sanofi-Aventis, Pliva, KOS, Pfizer, Merck and Veroscience, J. Michael Gaziano's employers have included Merck, Pfizer, and Bayer.

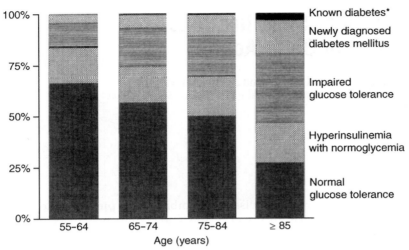

FIGURE 1   Glucose intolerance in subjects who answered "No" to the question "Do you have diabetes mellitus?" among participants in the Rotterdam Study, The Netherlands. *Based on anti-diabetes drug use. *Source*: From Ref. 4.

DIABETES AND THE RISK OF MACROVASCULAR DISEASE

In terms of morbidity and mortality, macrovascular disease represents one of the most significant complications of diabetes mellitus. Macrovascular disease is commonly manifested as coronary heart disease (CHD), cerebrovascular disease (CBVD), and peripheral vascular disease (PVD) (7). CHD is the leading cause of death in older persons, accounting for more than half of deaths; however, almost two-thirds of the deaths are among those with diabetes (8). Diabetes is one of the most important risk factors for CHD and is evident by the fact that age-adjusted CHD death rates have declined significantly except among persons with diabetes (9). Diabetes mellitus also increases the morbidity and mortality following a myocardial infarction (MI) (10).

CBVD is another common cause of morbidity in older persons with diabetes (11–13). The frequency of diabetes among patients aged 65 to 75 years, presenting with stroke, is three times more than that of matched controls (12). Similar to CHD, diabetes affects stroke outcome as well; it increases the risk of stroke-related dementia more than threefold and doubles the risk of recurrence (14,15). Recent studies support the association between diabetes and cognitive impairment or dementia, which may be caused by a combination of macro- and microvascular disease. PVD is another major cause of morbidity in older persons with diabetes, often contributing to the need for lower extremity revascularization or amputations (16). This topic is addressed in detail in the chapter on PVD.

A greater understanding of the pathophysiology of vascular disease among older individuals with diabetes mellitus is critical if we intend to reduce the morbidity and mortality associated with diabetes. Obviously, the paucity of available data among elderly persons is a major limitation when developing conclusions about relative magnitude of the impact of cardiovascular risk factors on coronary disease incidence. This is particularly true when attempting to decide whether to intervene with pharmacological treatments that target glucose control or traditional risk factors associated with diabetes such as dyslipidemia. Often, patients over the age of 70 are included at a lower rate compared to younger subjects in observational studies and from randomized clinical trials involving cardiovascular and diabetes risk factor modification. We must also consider the changing demography of aging. The life expectancy of a 65-year-old is now considered in excess of 20 years (17). In prior cohorts, this was not the case: competing risks for dying (cancer, infections, etc.) may have attenuated the death associated with modifiable cardiovascular risk factors. Also, inaccuracies of causes of death in some observational claims databases likely diminish our ability to assess for a true association. An example of ascertainment bias is illustrated by a compilation of work evaluating exceptional longevity among users of the Veteran Affairs where the authors found significant incongruities in discordant death information between the Veteran Health Affairs Administration records and Medicare records (18).

Observational studies have reported a wide range of coronary and CBVD prevalence among elderly patients with diabetes. The prevalence of any macrovascular disease was 85% in 335 older patients with diabetes (mean age 80 ± 8 years) from a single academic, hospital-based geriatric practice, with the prevalence of CHD, CBVD, and PVD being 44%, 28%, and 26%, respectively (19). In the Cardiovascular Health Study (CHS), in a cohort of 5888 older adults (mean age 73.3 years), 19% were found to have diabetes. Among those with diabetes, the prevalence of any macrovascular disease was 79%, with the prevalence of clinical CHD, CBVD, and PVD being 44.1%, 12.6%, and 7.1%. In addition, the prevalence of subclinical CHD, CBVD, and PVD was 29.3%, 56.0%, and 21.6%, respectively. Thus, four out of five older adults with diabetes have macrovascular disease; about half have CHD, one third have CBVD, and one fifth have PVD. These prevalence rates are about twice that in those without diabetes. Some investigators have suggested that certain cardiovascular risk factors among the elderly do not equal the same risk for adverse consequences compared to those under 65 years of age. This apparent attenuated association was shown between stroke and smoking, hypertension, and previous transient ischemia attacks (20) and between CHD and hypertension (20) (particularly diastolic blood pressure) (21–23), as well as with dyslipidemia (24). A similar argument could be made for the late manifestation of diabetes and subsequent risk for CVD; however, this does not appear to be the case for diabetes.

As a result, the magnitude of an effect of diabetes and other factors on the risk of CVD is less certain in older adults. Subsequent large clinical trials involving the elderly were eventually conducted to assess the benefits of treating hypertension and lipids and some were large enough to evaluate the benefit among subjects with diabetes. Given the risk of diabetes on CHD for younger people, two- to threefold increase for men and threefold increase for women resulting in gender neutralization for risk of cardiovascular death, it is likely the magnitude of risks is consistent in an elderly population as well.

The Finnish study evaluated the association between glycemic control and the risk for CHD (25). They included a cohort of 133 newly diagnosed patients with diabetes mellitus who were aged 45 to 64 years. The second group included 229 newly or previously diagnosed patients with diabetes mellitus, aged 65 to 74, who were followed up for 3.5 years for CHD mortality and coronary disease events. In both cohorts, the degree of hyperglycemic was linearly associated with an increased risk for CHD and cardiovascular events. In the elderly cohort, those with a glycated hemoglobin A1c (HbA1c) in the upper tertile had a threefold greater risk for CHD compared to those in the lowest tertile. In another study, Howard and colleagues addressed the differences between traditional cardiovascular risk factors associated with young subjects and with older subjects. In this study, they compared the Atherosclerosis Risk in Communities, which had an age range of 45 to 64, to the CHS, in which participants were 65 and older. Overall, the traditional risk factors were associated with increased atherosclerosis. They found no differentiation of the association with atherosclerosis for hypertension, low-density lipoprotein (LDL) cholesterol, or body mass index. However, diabetes was not as strongly associated with CHD among white males. In a large clinical trial evaluating the value of treating isolated systolic hypertension in the elderly, baseline factors such as current smoking and the presence of a carotid bruit were associated with a 73% and 113% increased risk of CHD. The presence of diabetes was associated with an even greater risk—121% greater likelihood for CHD (26).

Thus, depending on the cohort, the interplay of other comorbid conditions, cohort selection, access to healthcare, and precision of outcome ascertainment has led to some variability in the interpretation of the association of traditional cardiovascular risk factors and the development of CHD and stroke. However, the majority of the evidence supports a strong increased risk for macrovascular complications among elderly subjects with diabetes. There is also a suggestion that earlier manifestation of insulin resistance is also a forerunner of macrovascular disease.

INSULIN RESISTANCE AND RISK OF CVD

Attempting to assess the association between CVD risk and insulin resistance is limited in part by the by the lack of agreement on what constitutes insulin resistance in the elderly. However, the increased risk for CVD in elderly persons with diabetes is quite convincing and there is growing evidence that earlier manifestations of metabolic derangements may heighten the risk for CVD.

Most of the disagreement concerning the definition of insulin resistance stems from whether a fasting glucose or a two-hour postglucose challenge test is used. In the CHS (27), Smith et al. (28) examined the strength of the association of a fasting versus a two-hour glucose level on predicting cardiovascular events. The CHS is a population-based cohort study of risk factors for CVD in the elderly. In this study's comparison of the relationship between the fasting and two-hour glucose values with the risk of incident CVD, the investigators excluded subjects with a history of myocardial infarction or stroke and those receiving pharmacological treatment for type 2 diabetes. During the 8.5 years of follow-up, 19% of the participants experienced a coronary or cerebrovascular event, of which 27% were fatal. Both fasting and two-hour glucose values were associated with a greater risk of incident cardiovascular events [hazard ratio (HR) 1.66; 95% confidence interval (CI) = 1.39–1.98 for fasting ≥115 mg/dL compared to <115 mg/dL and two-hour glucose level was associated with a linear risk HR of 1.02; (95% CI = 1.00–1.04) per 10 mg/dL (0.6 mmol/L)]. However, in this cohort study of 4014 community-dwelling adults without diabetes, over the age of 65, the two-hour glucose level was a better predictor of incident CHD events. This is similar to the findings in the Diabetes Epidemiology: Collaborative Analysis of Diagnostic Criteria in Europe study (DECODE) (29), which reported a 34% increased risk for cardiovascular events for subjects with two-hour glucose levels in the impaired glucose tolerance range compared to subjects with glucose values in the normal range (30). However, other studies such as the Rancho Bernardo study (31) have failed to find this association. Although in this study they did report that the highest quintile of glycated HbA1c was associated with CVD among women [relative risk of 2.37 for fatal CVD (95% CI = 1.30–4.31, $P = 0.005$) and 2.43 for ischemic heart disease (95% CI = 1.12–5.25, $P = 0.024$)] (31), other studies have found a more pronounced association of hyperglycemia in nondiabetic women (28,32).

Suffice to say, it would appear that the manifestation of CVD is occurring early, prior to glucose elevations in the diabetes range. Once diabetes is established, the risk of developing CVD is doubled compared to those without diabetes. One could then argue that the development of diabetes in the elderly is too late for any meaningful interventions that would provide any benefit from risk factor modification. However, a counter argument would suggest that in order to thwart the advancement of CVD; greater surveillance with appropriate but aggressive intervention is required.

SCREENING AND TREATMENT TO LOWER THE RISK OF CVD

Diabetes treatment strategies directed at the tight control of glucose to prevent macrovascular complications are based on very limited trial data. The approach is therefore based on observational studies. On the other hand, strategies directed at other risk factors among diabetics have clearly been shown to reduce risk.

Screening in the Elderly

As highlighted in American Diabetic Association (ADA) 2006 (33) Standards of Medical Care in Diabetes and American Geriatric Society 2004 guideline for improving the care of older persons with diabetes (34), a personalized strategy with consideration of function, cognition, comorbidities, and life expectancy is recommended. For "highly functional cognitively intact individuals with more than 10 years of life expectancy," the most important strategy for preventing macrovascular complications with diabetes is earlier identification and treatment of those with diabetes and associated risk factors.

To screen for diabetes in addition to annual comprehensive history and physical examination, ADA recommends an fasting plasma glucose test or two-hour oral glucose tolerance test (OGTT) (75 g glucose load) or both, every three years (33). In older adults at high risk for diabetes such as those with first-degree relative with diabetes, those with hypertension or hyperlipidemia, or those with history of vascular disease, more frequent screening is recommended (exact frequency based on the estimated risk). An OGTT is especially helpful in patients with impaired fasting glucose to better define the risk of diabetes; however it would only be warranted if preventive interventions would be readily adopted.

To screen for risk factors in older persons with diabetes, blood pressure measurement at each visit, fasting lipid measurements every two years, and monitoring of A1c at least twice a year (quarterly in patients with changes in therapy or those not meeting the glycemic goals) are recommended. Despite the higher prevalence of CHD in older individuals with diabetes, there is insufficient evidence to recommend early screening for CVD via stress test (35).

For "frail older adults with functional dependency and shorter life expectancy" we recommend an individualized plan based on patient preferences since there is no evidence for benefits or harm of routine screening for diabetes and associated risk factors in such patients. If the patient's primary goal is life prolongation at any cost, then screening would be appropriate. However, if patient's primary goal is to maintain function or to achieve comfort then the aggressive screening in frail older adults with limited life expectancy is not consistent with the patient's goals.

Treatment of Hyperglycemia to Lower Risk of CVD

American Diabetes Association treatment guidelines support an individualized approach to achieve near normoglycemic control and optimize the management of cardiovascular risk factors. The first step is to establish the treatment goals on the basis of careful consideration of risks, benefits, life expectancy, functional status, cognitive status, and patient preferences. Individualized treatment plans based on a particular patient's functional status and preferences are more meaningful than a "one size fits all" approach to management of diabetes in the elderly. Also, additional evidence is needed to firmly establish that glycemic control alone will result in cardiovascular risk modification. The PROactive study (36) was designed to provide supportive evidence to address whether improving glycemic control reduced macrovascular disease. In this secondary prevention study of macrovascular disease in patients with type 2 diabetes, the use of pioglitazone reduced the "principle secondary" composite endpoint of all-cause mortality, nonfatal myocardial infarction and stroke compared to placebo (HR 0.84, 95% CI = 0.72–0.98) (36). However, in his commentary, Skyler (37) points out that the primary composite endpoint of all-cause mortality; nonfatal myocardial infarction; acute coronary syndrome; cardiac intervention, including coronary artery bypass graft, or percutaneous coronary intervention; stroke; major leg amputation (above the ankle); bypass surgery; or revascularization in the leg failed to reach statistical significance. As a consequence, doubts have been raised as to the legitimacy of the study conclusions (38) of a cardiovascular benefit, particularly when 115 additional cases of congestive heart failure occurred in the treated group compared to placebo (39) as well as the fact that the original primary outcome was not found to be significant.

There is however sufficient evidence that the treatment plan should include plans to lower blood pressure and cholesterol as well as to encourage smoking cessation. Although the evidence of efficacy is limited in frail older adults, there are no data to suggest that intervention to control the risk factor causes harm in frail older adults. Considering the absolute risk may be higher in older adults, the intervention may in fact have higher efficacy in high-risk older adults. Careful discussion with patients and their input and commitment are essential, considering the need for a complex regimen including multiple medications and careful monitoring.

Lifestyle Modification
Physical Activity

All guidelines [American Geriatric Society (AGS), ADA, National Cholesterol Education Program (NCEP), and The Seventh Report of the Joint National Committee on Prevention, Detection, Evaluation, and Treatment of High Blood Pressure (JNC 7)] recommend increased physical activity, which has been shown to improve blood glucose control, reduce cardiovascular risk factors, contribute to weight loss, and improve well-being (33,34,40,41). All older patients who are capable of exercising should participate in a regular physical activity program adapted to the presence of complications.

Before beginning the exercise plan, older patients with diabetes should have a detailed medical evaluation with appropriate diagnostic studies. This examination should screen for the presence of macro- and microvascular complications that may be worsened by the physical activity program. Identification of areas of concern may also allow the design of an individualized physical activity plan that can minimize risk to the patient (33,42).

Smoking Cessation

All patients with diabetes should be advised not to smoke and smoking cessation counseling should be a routine component of diabetes care (43).

Diet: Glucose Control by Better Diet

The evidence for lowering glucose with dietary modifications to prevent CVD is lacking; however recent evidence suggests a benefit from reductions in dietary cholesterol in persons with diabetes (44–46).

Antiplatelet Therapy

The 2006 ADA guideline (33) recommends aspirin (75–162 mg/day) in all older adults with diabetes due to their increased risk of CVD. Clopidogrel can be used as an adjunctive therapy in very-high-risk patients or as alternative therapy in aspirin-intolerant patients.

TRADITIONAL CARDIOVASCULAR RISK FACTORS IN THE ELDERLY: HYPERTENSION AND DYSLIPIDEMIA
Hypertension Among the Elderly and Risk for CVD

Isolated systolic hypertension in the elderly was once thought to be a normal consequence of aging and that treatment would potentially lead to adverse consequences. Analysis of observational studies such as the Framingham Heart Study suggested otherwise; the authors found greater survival to the age of 75 among those with a lower systolic blood pressure (47). Subsequently, three large trials revealed that treating hypertension in the elderly reduced morbidity. These included the Systolic Hypertension in Elderly Prevention trial (SHEP) (48), Syst-EUR trial (49), and Systolic Hypertension in China (Syst-China) Trial (50). Each trial enrolled subjects over the age of 60 with systolic blood pressures of $\geq$160 mmHg. In SHEP, the systolic blood pressure was lowered to 143 mmHg, compared to 155 mmHg in the placebo, which resulted in a 36% reduction in incident stroke ($P = 0.0003$), 27% reduction in nonfatal myocardial infarction plus coronary death, and 32% reduction in all cardiovascular events. In the Syst-EUR trial, the primary outcome—incident stroke—was reduced by 42% ($P = 0.003$). In addition, there were reductions in nonfatal strokes (–44%, $P = -0.007$), nonfatal cardiac endpoints (–33%, $P = 0.03$); all fatal and nonfatal cardiac endpoints (–26%, $P = 0.03$), and all cerebrovascular events (–34%, $P = 0.0006$). More recently, the Syst-China Trial (50) enrolled 1253 subjects to active treatment starting with nitrendipine and reported reductions in the incidence of total mortality ($P < 0.01$), fatal and nonfatal stroke ($P < 0.05$), and all cardiovascular endpoints ($P < 0.01$).

In a pooled analysis of these three trials, active treatment compared with placebo reduced all-cause mortality by 17%, cardiovascular mortality by 25%, all cardiovascular endpoints by 32%, total stroke by 37%, and myocardial infarction including sudden death by 25% (51). Staessen et al. performed an additional meta-analysis of eight trials of 15,693 subjects with isolated systolic hypertension and reported that active treatment significantly reduced total mortality by 13% (95% CI = 2–22, $P = 0.02$), cardiovascular mortality by 18%, all cardiovascular complications by 26%, stroke by 30%, and coronary events by 23% (52). The data from these studies and meta-analysis supports the notion that lowering of blood pressure is *essential* in the elderly.

HYPERTENSION AMONG THE ELDERLY WITH DIABETES AND RISK FOR CVD

The SHEP trial was a randomized, double-blinded, placebo-controlled study designed to assess the effect of low-dose, diuretic-based antihypertensive treatment on major cardiovascular event rates in older subjects with and without type 2 diabetes and isolated systolic hypertension (48). The study included 4736 men and women aged 60 years or older, 583 of whom had type 2 diabetes, and they were followed up prospectively for five years. Among subjects with diabetes who received active treatment, systolic blood pressures were lower by 9.8 and 2.2 mmHg on average, respectively. As a result, the active treatment arm experienced a risk reduction in major cardiovascular events (34%), nonfatal and fatal stroke (22%), nonfatal and fatal myocardial infarction (56%), and all-cause mortality (26%).

In a post-hoc analysis of Syst-EUR trial subjects with diabetes, the treated group experienced an overall reduction in mortality of 55%, cardiovascular mortality of 76%, fatal and non-fatal stroke of 73%, and all cardiovascular events of 69% (53). Comparison of the reductions in the same parameters in the nondiabetic subjects, shown in Figure 2, demonstrates a particular benefit of lowering systolic blood pressure in the treated group with diabetes (53).

Also, in the Syst-China trial (50), among a subgroup with diabetes ($n = 98$), there was a consistent trend in the reduction of all endpoints with active treatment. After adjustment for a variety of baseline covariates, active treatment compared to placebo reduced the incidence of total mortality (59%, $P = 0.15$), cardiovascular mortality (57%, $P = 0.22$), all cardiovascular endpoints (74%, $P = 0.03$), and fatal and nonfatal stroke (45%, $P = 0.42$).

The summary of studies in Table 1 supports the notion that lowering blood pressure in persons with diabetes is warranted.

In addition, multiple blood pressure–lowering therapies may be required to treat high-risk individuals in order to reduce the risk of CVD. In the Hypertension Optimal Treatment trial (55), not only did the subjects benefit from treatment of hypertension, but they often required multiple therapies to achieve the study treatment goals. This study included 18,790 subjects, aged 50 to 80, who were randomized to three different diastolic blood pressure goals; 7.9% of the study cohort had diabetes. They found an overall benefit of lowering blood pressure with no apparent threshold of negative effects in the lowest blood pressure target group. In all patients, there was a decline in cardiovascular mortality ($P = 0.005$ for trend), but in the group with diastolic blood pressure ≤80 mmHg (compared with the ≤90 mmHg group), cardiovascular mortality was reduced by 67% ($P = 0.016$). In addition, major cardiovascular events including silent myocardial infarction were reduced by 36% ($P = 0.045$) (55).

Although not all of these studies addressed the question of benefits of the treatment of blood pressure in elderly patients with diabetes, there has been sufficient subanalysis of this population to argue that treatment of hypertension is justified in and may exceed the benefit seen among individuals without diabetes.

LIPID LOWERING IN THE ELDERLY AND CVD RISK

In a review by Mungall (56), the authors raised a similar doubt as seen with hypertension treatment in the elderly with the role of lipid lowering in the elderly. Their negative view seemed justified because a subsequent study, Antihypertensive and Lipid-Lowering Treatment to Prevent Heart Attack Trial (57), failed to find a reduction of either all-cause mortality or CHD in elderly subjects. In the Antihypertensive and Lipid-Lowering Treatment to Prevent Heart

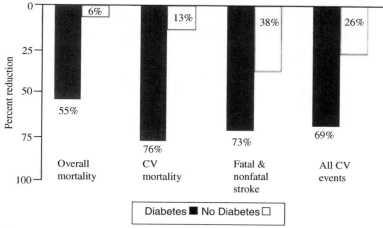

FIGURE 2   Reductions in overall mortality, CV mortality, fatal and nonfatal strokes, and all CV events in the Syst-EUR study in subjects with and without type 2 diabetes. *Abbreviations*: CV, cardiovascular; Syst-EUR, The Systolic Hypertension in Europe (Syst-Eur) Trial. *Source*: From Ref. 53.

TABLE 1 Primary Trials of Hypertension Control Among Those with Diabetes

			Total cardiovascular events	
Trial[a]	Interventions and primary agents	Primary/ subgroup	Relative risk (95% CI)	Absolute risk reduction (95% CI)
SHEP	Thiazide diuretic vs. usual care	Subgroup	0.66 (0.46–0.94)	0.08 (0.01–0.14)
Syst-Eur	Calcium-channel blocker vs. placebo	Subgroup	0.38 (0.20–0.81)	0.08 (0.03–0.13)
HOPE	ACE inhibitor vs. placebo	Subgroup	0.75 (0.64–0.88)	0.05 (0.02–0.07)
RENAAL	Angiotensin II receptor blocker vs. placebo	Primary	0.90[b]	0.02 (−0.03 to 0.07)
HOT	Target diastolic blood pressure <80 or <90 mmHg; multiple agents	Subgroup	0.49 (0.14–0.78)	0.05 (0.02–0.08)
UKPDS	Target blood pressure <180/105 vs. <150/85 mmHg; captopril or atenolol	Primary	0.66[c]	Not reported
ABCD	Target diastolic blood pressure 75 vs. 80–89 mmHg; nisolidipine or enalapril	Primary	No difference	Not reported

[a]Values in parentheses are 95% CIs.
[b]$P > 0.2$.
[c]$P = 0.019$.
Abbreviations: ABCD, appropriate blood pressure control in diabetes; ACE, angiotensin converting enzyme; HOPE, Heart Outcomes and Prevention Evaluation Study; HOT, Hypertension Optimal Treatment Study; IDPM, irbesartan in patients with type 2 diabetes and microalbumin; RENAAL, reduction of endpoints in non insulin dependent diabetes mellitus (NIDDM) with the angiotensin II antagonist losartan; SHEP, Systolic Hypertension in the Elderly Program; Syst-Eur, The Systolic Hypertension in Europe Trail; UKPDS, United Kingdom Prospective Diabetes Study.
Source: From Ref. 54.

Attack study, over half of the participants were over the age of 65 and had well-controlled hypertension and moderately elevated cholesterol. They were randomized to receive either pravastatin or usual care. However, the failure to find a difference in cardiovascular risk is likely explained by the fact that the overall lowering in the cholesterol between the groups only differed by 9.6%. In an observational study conducted by Simons et al. (58), the authors evaluated the association of dyslipidemia in an elderly Australian cohort and raised doubts as to whether treatment is warranted above the age of 70. While CHD and stroke increased with age, the relationship to LDL cholesterol levels did not differentiate the risk for those over the age of 70. Interestingly, low high-density lipoprotein cholesterol and elevated triglycerides were associated with a greater risk for CHD among those over the age of 70. The authors concluded that cholesterol testing for patients up to 70 years is supported by evidence of CHD and stroke prevention through treatment designed to reduce LDL cholesterol in younger-aged groups.

Due to this uncertainty, a clinical trial was designed specifically to determine whether lipid lowering was of benefit to the elderly. The Prospective Study of Pravastatin in the Elderly at Risk (59) addressed whether hyperlipidemic subjects aged 70 to 82 years benefited from the use of a statin. Subjects receiving pravastatin, compared to placebo, experienced a 15% reduction in coronary artery disease (HR 0.85; 95% CI = 0.74–0.97). In a subanalysis of the Long-term Intervention with Pravastatin in Ischemia Disease trial (60), it was found that older subjects (>64 years of age) were at greater risk compared to younger patients (31 to 64 years of age) for the following: death (20.6% vs. 9.8%), myocardial infarction (11.4% vs. 9.5%), unstable angina (26.7% vs. 23.2%), and stroke (6.7% vs. 3.1%) (all $P < 0.001$). The two age groups experienced a similar reduction in cardiovascular risk compared to placebo; subjects aged 65 to 75, who received pravastatin, experienced a reduction in mortality by 21% (CI, 7–32%), death from CHD by 24% (CI, 7–38%), CHD death or nonfatal myocardial infarction by 22% (CI, 9–34%), myocardial infarction by 26% (CI, 9–40%), and stroke by 12% (CI, 215–32%). The numbers-needed-to-treat to prevent a cardiovascular event among older patients were 22 (CI, 17–36) to prevent one death from any cause, 35 (CI, 24–67) to prevent one death from CHD, and 21 (CI, 17–31) to prevent one CHD death or nonfatal myocardial infarction.

Despite the apparent benefit of lipid lowering in the elderly, effective lipid-lowering treatment in the elderly is uncommon. In a retrospective cohort study of 51,559 older nursing home patients with CVD, only 2.6% were prescribed a statin. This is unfortunate because a matched analysis of statin and nonstatin users in the same facility reported a one-year mortality-adjusted HR of 0.69 (95% CI = 0.58–0.81) for statin users. This improved all-cause mortality was achieved for women and men and those over the age of 85 (61). Similar findings were found in a cohort of 396,077 patients over the age of 66, who had a history of CVD or diabetes. In this study, the prescription of statins decreased as the risk for CVD and mortality increased. This treatment-to-risk paradox appears to be common among elderly patients (62).

From this compilation of studies it appears that older patients are at greater risk than younger patients for macrovascular events; therefore, the absolute benefit of treatment is significantly greater. Evidence would also suggest that individuals at high risk for coronary artery disease, even those with "lower" baseline cholesterol levels, should be considered for lipid-lowering treatment (63,64). This is particularly relevant for the elderly, whose cholesterol levels are often lower than those in the younger age groups deemed high-risk for CHD. In theory, the risk for macrovascular complications would be further exaggerated in the elderly who have both diabetes and hyperlipidemia.

LIPID LOWERING AMONG THE ELDERLY WITH DIABETES AND CVD RISK

Unfortunately, large-scale clinical trials of lipid lowering in elderly subjects with diabetes are not available. However, subanalysis of lipid-lowering trials among elderly subjects with diabetes suggests an equal, if not greater, benefit. The Anglo Scandinavian Cardiac Outcomes Trial–Lipid-Lowering Arm (ASCOT–LLA) studied 19,342 hypertensive patients aged 40 to 79, without known CHD, randomized to receive either atorvastatin or placebo in addition to one of two blood-pressure treatment regimens. The study was terminated early because the benefit in the lipid-lowering arm was achieved within one year (reduction in nonfatal myocardial infarction or fatal CHD: HR 0.64, 95% CI = 0.50–0.83) (65). In a subsequent analysis, study subjects with diabetes experienced a similar reduction in events as those without a diagnosis of diabetes (65).

Vijan et al. conducted a meta-analysis (66) of both primary and secondary prevention trials evaluating the value of lipid lowering in diabetes (Table 2). Their findings support the use of lipid-lowering therapy for most subjects with diabetes, including those with a baseline LDL cholesterol levels lower than 115 mg/dL and perhaps even lower than 100 mg/dL.

The Collaborative Atorvastatin Diabetes Study (CARDS) (67), a more recent study, was not included in this analysis because it was terminated early due to a greater benefit in both coronary and stroke reduction among subjects receiving a statin. The CARDS was a multicenter, randomized clinical trial assessing lipid lowering among subjects with diabetes without evidence of coronary artery disease. In CARDS, 2838 patients aged 40 to 75 received either placebo or atorvastatin and were followed up for a mean of 3.9 years. The primary endpoint was the time to an acute CHD event, coronary revascularization, or stroke. Assessed separately, acute CHD events were reduced by 36% (_55 to –9), coronary revascularizations by 31% (–59 to 16), and rate of stroke by 48% (–69 to –11), with the death rate reduced by 27% (–48 to 1, $P = 0.059$) (67). A beneficial risk reduction appeared as early as 18 months after treatment initiation (68).

In a study of the effects of long-term fenofibrate therapy on cardiovascular events in 9795 people with diabetes, aged 50 to 75, with and without CVD [Fenofibrate Intervention and Event Lowering in Diabetes (FIELD) study], a reduction in the primary endpoint of coronary events (CHD death or nonfatal myocardial infarction) was not achieved (69). It is important to note that a greater proportion in the placebo group started lipid-lowering therapy with statins (17% vs. 8%, $P < 0.0001$). Notably, nonfatal myocardial infarction was reduced by 24% (0.76 95%, CI = 0.62–0.94) and cardiovascular revascularization was reduced by 21% (0.79, CI = 0.68–0.93) in the group receiving fenofibrate.

In an additional analysis of the ASCOT–LLA study, the investigators compared outcomes in 4445 subjects 65 years of age or older with those under the age of 65 (5680 subjects). The participants had at least two risk factors including diabetes. In both subgroups the primary endpoint of nonfatal MI and fatal CHD was reduced among the patients receiving atorvastatin compared with placebo (70).

TABLE 2 Summary Statistics of the Effectiveness of Lipid-Lowering Therapy Among Subjects with Diabetes[a]

Study	CHD event rate (control)	CHD event rate (intervention)	Relative risk for CHD event (95% CI)	Absolute risk reduction in CHD (95% CI)	NNT[b]
Primary CVD prevention					
AFCAPS/TexCAPS	6/71	4/84	0.56 (0.17–1.92)	0.04 (−0.04–0.12)	27.1
ALLHAT-LLT	Not reported	Not reported	0.89 (0.71–1.10)	Not reported	Not reported
HHS	8/76	2/59	0.32 (0.07–1.46)	0.07 (−0.01 to 0.15)	14.0
HPS	367/1976	276/2006	0.74 (0.64–0.85)	0.05 (0.03–0.07)	20.8
PROSPER[c]	28/205	32/191	1.23 (0.77–1.95)	−0.03 (−0.10 to 0.04)	−32.3
ASCOT-LLA	46/1274	38/1258	0.84 (0.55–1.29)	0.01 (−0.01 to 0.02)	169.5
Pooled[d]	—	—	0.78 (0.67–0.89)	0.03 (0.01–0.04)	34.5[e]
Secondary CVD prevention					
4s	44/97	24/105	0.50 (0.33–0.76)	0.23 (0.10–0.35)	4.4
CARE	112/304	81/282	0.78 (0.62–0.99)	0.08 (0.01–0.16)	12.3
HPS	381/1009	325/972	0.89 (0.79–1.00)	0.04 (0.00–0.09)	23.1
LIPID	88/386	76/396	0.84 (0.64–1.11)	0.04 (−0.02 to 0.09)	27.7
LIPS	31/82	26/120	0.53 (0.29–0.97)	0.16 (0.03–0.29)	6.2
Post-CABG	14/53	9/63	0.53 (0.18–1.60)	0.12 (−0.03 to 0.27)	8.2
PROSPERc	31/115	38/112	1.26 (0.85–1.87)	−0.07 (−0.19 to 0.05)	−14.3
VA-HIT	116/318	88/309	0.76 (0.57–1.01)	0.08 (0.01–0.15)	12.5
Pooled[d]	—	—	0.76 (0.59–0.93)	0.07 (0.03–0.12)	13.8[e]

[a]From primary and secondary lipid lowering cardiovascular prevention trials.
[b]NNT, numbers needed to treat for benefit.
[c]Shepherd J, Blauw GJ, Murphy MB. Personal Communication.
[d]Pooled estimates generated by using meta-analysis; for primary prevention, there was no heterogeneity between studies, so a fixed-effects model was used; for secondary prevention, there was substantial between-study heterogeneity ($P = 0.026$), so a random-effects model was used.
[e]For primary prevention, the NNT is for 4.3 years; for secondary prevention, the NNT is for 4.9 years.
Abbreviations: 4S, Scandinavian Simvastatin Survival Study; AFCAPS/TexCAPS, Air Force Coronary Atherosclerosis Prevention Study/Texas Coronary Atherosclerosis Prevention Study; ALLHAT-LLT, Antihypertensive and Lipid-Lowering Treatment to Prevent Heart Attack Trial-Lipid-Lowering Trial; ASCOT-LLA, Anglo-Scandinavian Cardiac Outcomes Trial-Lipid-Lowering Arm; CARE, Cholesterol and Recurrence Events Trial; CHD, coronary heart disease; HHS, Helsinki Heart Study; HPS, Heart Protection Study; LIPID, Long-Term Intervention with Pravastatin in Ischemic Disease Trial; LIPS, Lescol Intervention Prevention Study; Post-CABG, Post-Coronary Artery Bypass Graft Trial; PROSPER, Prospective Study of Pravastatin in the Elderly at Risk; VA-HIT, Veterans Administration High-Density Lipoprotein Cholesterol Intervention Trial.
Source: From Ref. 66.

Although not all of these studies addressed the question of benefits of the treatment of lipids in elderly people with diabetes, there has been sufficient subanalysis among this population to argue that treatment of hyperlipidemia is justified and may exceed the benefit seen among individuals without diabetes.

MULTIFACTORIAL INTERVENTION

Based on the evidence presented, a comprehensive approach to risk factor modification is warranted for most elderly persons with diabetes due to the likelihood of comorbid conditions. The Gaede P—multifactorial intervention study (71) was designed to evaluate a multifactorial intervention in type 2 diabetes that included both behavior modification and pharmacologic therapy that targeted hyperglycemia, hypertension, dyslipidemia, and microalbuminuria, along with secondary prevention of CVD with aspirin. The intervention resulted in a 53% lower risk of CVD over seven years. Although the mean age of the study participants was 55 years, the evidence presented throughout this chapter supports a similar approach to modify risk factors in an older population (71).

CONCLUSIONS

Many impediments result in less-than-aggressive management of risk factors for CVD among elderly people with diabetes. Evidence has not been sufficient to dispel concerns about drug-related side effects or questionable benefits in an aged population. In addition, lingering questions about whether the epidemiology of insulin resistance differs in old versus younger individuals and if traditional risk factors for CVD are not sufficient to provide risk predictions in the elderly are often used to justify minimal interventions. Finally, there is the question of whether primary or secondary prevention is justified at such a late manifestation of the disease where life expectancy is already greatly reduced.

Many of these same concerns were initially raised when determining whether to treat dyslipidemia or hypertension in the elderly. However, in both cases, the preponderance of evidence ultimately proved that there was a benefit to treating the elderly. The challenge for addressing this question among the elderly with diabetes is the lack of evidence. The very limited clinical trial information necessitated the reliance on post-hoc analysis or observational studies, which, for the elderly, are subject to many design limitations that may bias the results.

In this chapter, we provided both observational and clinical trial data that support screening for cardiovascular risk factors and a multifactorial approach to risk reduction among the elderly patient with diabetes. We advise an individual approach to disease management that takes into account frailty and risk for adverse drug events. However, we would conclude that ageism should not be the sole reason for withholding treatment. To assure successful aging, appropriate treatment of clinically evident diseases such as diabetes is warranted. Moreover, prevention of subclinical vascular disease is required to increase the quality and the quantity of years in late life (72).

In the ever-increasing older population, aggressive treatment of modifiable risk factors is likely warranted in most of our elderly patients. Future research should include populations of patients over the age of 75, so we may prescribe the ideal combination of therapies to reduce morbidity and mortality.

SUMMARY

Evidence for tight glycemic control to reduce macrovascular risk in the elderly is lacking. However, there is increasing evidence that insulin resistance prior to the diagnosis of diabetes is associated with an increased risk for CVD. Perhaps interventions that maintain euglycemia and reduce insulin resistance will yield greater CVD risk reduction. Hopefully with the advent of new diabetes therapies, clinical trials among elderly individuals with insulin resistance will be able to discern whether the benefit of earlier treatment exceeds the risks and costs of the intervention.

It would appear that lowering both lipids and blood pressure is beneficial among those with diabetes who are 65 years of age or older. Since the current life expectancy at age 65 years is nearly 20 years in most Western countries, secondary prevention may increase the quality of life and the independent lifespan, even if mortality is not delayed. Primary prevention of macrovascular complications is indicated, as the evidence suggests that elderly individuals with diabetes and additional cardiovascular risk factors are at substantial risk for cardiovascular events. Raising the awareness of these findings is critical; it begins with screening and education along with appropriate targeted interventions.

ACKNOWLEDGMENT

The authors would like to thank Susan Nicholl for her thoughtful editorial review of this chapter.

REFERENCES

1. Engelgau MM, Geiss LS, Saaddine JB, et al. The evolving diabetes burden in the United States. Ann Intern Med 2004; 140(11):945–950.
2. Geiss LS, Pan L, Cadwell B, Gregg EW, Benjamin SM, Engelgau MM. Changes in incidence of diabetes in U.S. Adults, 1997–2003. Am J Prev Med 2006; 30(5):371–377.
3. Boyle JP, Honeycutt AA, Narayan KM, et al. Projection of diabetes burden through 2050: impact of changing demography and disease prevalence in the U.S. Diabet Care 2001; 24(11):1936–1940.

4. Stolk RP, Pols HA, Lamberts SW, de Jong PT, Hofman A, Grobbee DE. Diabetes mellitus, impaired glucose tolerance, and hyperinsulinemia in an elderly population. The Rotterdam Study. Am J Epidemiol 1997; 145(1):24–32.

5. Haffner SM, Mykkanen L, Festa A, Burke JP, Stern MP. Insulin-resistant prediabetic subjects have more atherogenic risk factors than insulin-sensitive prediabetic subjects: implications for preventing coronary heart disease during the prediabetic state. Circulation 2000; 101(9):975–980.

6. Lawler EGJ, Scranton RE. Use of HOMA-IR to assess the risk of incident diabetes among men with normal fasting blood sugar in abstract. Diabetologia 2005; 48(suppl 1):A58.

7. Beckman JA, Creager MA, Libby P. Diabetes and atherosclerosis: epidemiology, pathophysiology, and management. JAMA 2002; 287(19):2570–2581.

8. Geiss LS, Herman WH, Smith PJ. Mortality in non-insulin-dependent diabetes. In: Harris MI, Cowie CC, Stern MP, Boyko EJ, Reiber GE, Bennett PH, eds. Diabetes in America. Washington, DC: U.S. Govt. Printing Office, 1995:233–257.

9. Gu K, Cowie CC, Harris MI. Diabetes and decline in heart disease mortality in US adults. JAMA 1999; 281(14):1291–1297.

10. Smith JW, Marcus FI, Serokman R. Prognosis of patients with diabetes mellitus after acute myocardial infarction. Am J Cardiol 1984; 54(7):718–721.

11. Wannamethee SG, Shaper AG, Lennon L. Cardiovascular disease incidence and mortality in older men with diabetes and in men with coronary heart disease. Heart 2004; 90(12):1398–403.

12. Himmelmann A, Hansson L, Svensson A, Harmsen P, Holmgren C, Svanborg A. Predictors of stroke in the elderly. Acta Med Scand 1988; 224(5):439–443.

13. Strachan M. Cognitive decline and the older patient with diabetes. Clin Geriat 2002; 10(6).

14. Luchsinger JA, Tang MX, Stern Y, Shea S, Mayeux R. Diabetes mellitus and risk of Alzheimer's disease and dementia with stroke in a multiethnic cohort. Am J Epidemiol 2001; 154(7):635–641.

15. Hankey GJ, Jamrozik K, Broadhurst RJ, et al. Long-term risk of first recurrent stroke in the Perth Community Stroke Study. Stroke 1998; 29(12):2491–2500.

16. Akbari CM, LoGerfo FW. Diabetes and peripheral vascular disease. J Vasc Surg 1999; 30(2):373–384.

17. NCHS. Health, United States, 2005, with Chartbook on Trends in the Health of Americans with special feature on adults 55–64 years, 2005. NCHS.

18. Lawler. Morbidity, Mortality, and Exceptional Longevity. Boston: Boston University; 2006.

19. Ness J, Nassimiha D, Feria MI, Aronow WS. Diabetes mellitus in older African-Americans, Hispanics, and Whites in an academic hospital-based geriatrics practice. Coron Artery Dis 1999; 10(5):343–346.

20. Insua JT, Sacks HS, Lau TS, et al. Drug treatment of hypertension in the elderly: a meta-analysis. Ann Intern Med 1994; 121(5):355–362.

21. Langer RD, Criqui MH, Barrett-Connor EL, Klauber MR, Ganiats TG. Blood pressure change and survival after age 75. Hypertension 1993; 22(4):551–559.

22. Langer RD, Ganiats TG, Barrett-Connor E. Paradoxical survival of elderly men with high blood pressure. BMJ 1989; 298(6684):1356–1357.

23. Langer RD, Ganiats TG, Barrett-Connor E. Factors associated with paradoxical survival at higher blood pressures in the very old. Am J Epidemiol 1991; 134(1):29–38.

24. Manolio TA, Pearson TA, Wenger NK, Barrett-Connor E, Payne GH, Harlan WR. Cholesterol and heart disease in older persons and women. Review of an NHLBI workshop. Ann Epidemiol 1992; 2(1–2):161–176.

25. Laakso M. Glycemic control and the risk for coronary heart disease in patients with non-insulin-dependent diabetes mellitus. The Finnish studies. Ann Intern Med 1996; 124(1 Pt 2):127–130.

26. Frost PH, Davis BR, Burlando AJ, et al. Coronary heart disease risk factors in men and women aged 60 years and older: findings from the Systolic Hypertension in the Elderly Program. Circulation 1996; 94(1):26–34.

27. Fried LP, Borhani NO, Enright P, et al. The Cardiovascular Health Study: design and rationale. Ann Epidemiol 1991; 1(3):263–276.

28. Smith NL, Barzilay JI, Shaffer D, et al. Fasting and 2-hour postchallenge serum glucose measures and risk of incident cardiovascular events in the elderly: the Cardiovascular Health Study. Arch Intern Med 2002; 162(2):209–216.

29. Balkau B. The DECODE study. Diabetes Epidemiology: Collaborative Analysis of Diagnostic Criteria in Europe. Diabetes Metab 2000; 26(4):282–286.

30. Kuizon D, Gordon SM, Dolmatch BL. Single-lumen subcutaneous ports inserted by interventional radiologists in patients undergoing chemotherapy: incidence of infection and outcome of attempted catheter salvage. Arch Intern Med 2001; 161(3):406–410.

31. Park S, Barrett-Connor E, Wingard DL, Shan J, Edelstein S. GHb is a better predictor of cardiovascular disease than fasting or postchallenge plasma glucose in women without diabetes. The Rancho Bernardo Study. Diabetes Care 1996; 19(5):450–456.

32. Barrett-Connor E, Ferrara A. Isolated postchallenge hyperglycemia and the risk of fatal cardiovascular disease in older women and men. The Rancho Bernardo Study. Diabetes Care 1998; 21(8):1236–1239.

33. Standards of medical care in diabetes—2006. Diabetes Care 2006; 29(suppl 1):S4–S42.
34. Olson DE, Norris SL. Diabetes in older adults. Overview of AGS guidelines for the treatment of diabetes mellitus in geriatric populations. Geriatrics 2004; 59(4):18–24; quiz 5.
35. Young JC. Diagnosis of CAD in patients with diabetes: who to Evaluate. Curr Diab Rep 2003; 3(1): 19–27.
36. Dormandy JA, Charbonnel B, Eckland DJ, et al. Secondary prevention of macrovascular events in patients with type 2 diabetes in the PROactive Study (PROspective Pioglitzone Clinical Trial in Macrovascular Events): a randomised controlled trial. Lancet 2005; 366(9493):1279–1289.
37. Skyler J. PROactive: a sad tale of inappropriate analysis and unjustified interpretation. Clin Diabet 2006; 24(2):63–65.
38. Freemantle N. How well does the evidence on pioglitazone back up researchers' claims for a reduction in macrovascular events? BMJ 2005; 331(7520):836–868.
39. Yki-Jarvinen H. The PROactive study: some answers, many questions. Lancet 2005; 366(9493): 1241–1242.
40. Grundy SM, Cleeman JI, Merz CN, et al. Implications of recent clinical trials for the National Cholesterol Education Program Adult Treatment Panel III guidelines. Circulation 2004; 110(2): 227–239.
41. Chobanian AV, Bakris GL, Black HR, et al. The Seventh Report of the Joint National Committee on Prevention, Detection, Evaluation, and Treatment of High Blood Pressure: the JNC 7 report. JAMA 2003; 289(19):2560–2572.
42. Wei M, Gibbons LW, Mitchell TL, Kampert JB, Lee CD, Blair SN. The association between cardiorespiratory fitness and impaired fasting glucose and type 2 diabetes mellitus in men. Ann Intern Med 1999; 130(2):89–96.
43. Haire-Joshu D, Glasgow RE, Tibbs TL. Smoking and diabetes. Diabetes Care 2004; 27(suppl 1): S74–S75.
44. Harris MI, Eastman RC. Is there a glycemic threshold for mortality risk? Diabet Care 1998; 21(3): 331–333.
45. Kris-Etherton PM. AHA science advisory: monounsaturated fatty acids and risk of cardiovascular disease. J Nutr 1999; 129(12):2280–2284.
46. Hu FB, Stampfer MJ, Rimm EB, et al. A prospective study of egg consumption and risk of cardiovascular disease in men and women. JAMA 1999; 281(15):1387–1394.
47. Goldberg RJ, Larson M, Levy D. Factors associated with survival to 75 years of age in middle-aged men and women. The Framingham Study. Arch Intern Med 1996; 156(5):505–509.
48. Prevention of stroke by antihypertensive drug treatment in older persons with isolated systolic hypertension. Final results of the Systolic Hypertension in the Elderly Program (SHEP). SHEP Cooperative Research Group. JAMA 1991; 265(24):3255–3264.
49. Staessen JA, Fagard R, Thijs L, et al. Randomised double-blind comparison of placebo and active treatment for older patients with isolated systolic hypertension. The Systolic Hypertension in Europe (Syst-Eur) Trial Investigators. Lancet 1997; 350(9080):757–764.
50. Wang JG, Staessen JA, Gong L, Liu L. Chinese trial on isolated systolic hypertension in the elderly. Systolic Hypertension in China (Syst-China) Collaborative Group. Arch Intern Med 2000; 160(2): 211–220.
51. Staessen JA, Wang JG, Thijs L, Fagard R. Overview of the outcome trials in older patients with isolated systolic hypertension. J Jum Hyper 1999; 10:735–742.
52. Staessen JA, Gasowski J, Wang JG, et al. Risks of untreated and treated isolated systolic hypertension in the elderly: meta-analysis of outcome trials. Lancet 2000; 355(9207):865–872.
53. Marks J. Treating hypertension in diabetes: data and perspectives. Clin Diabet 1999; 17.
54. Vijan S, Hayward RA. Treatment of hypertension in type 2 diabetes mellitus: blood pressure goals, choice of agents, and setting priorities in diabetes care. Ann Intern Med 2003; 138:593–602.
55. Hansson L, Zanchetti A, Carruthers SG, et al. Effects of intensive blood-pressure lowering and low-dose aspirin in patients with hypertension: principal results of the Hypertension Optimal Treatment (HOT) randomised trial. HOT Study Group. Lancet 1998; 351(9118):1755–1762.
56. Mungall MM, Gaw A, Shepherd J. Statin therapy in the elderly: does it make good clinical and economic sense? Drugs Aging 2003; 20(4):263–275.
57. Major outcomes in moderately hypercholesterolemic, hypertensive patients randomized to pravastatin vs usual care: the Antihypertensive and Lipid-Lowering Treatment to Prevent Heart Attack Trial (ALLHAT-LLT). JAMA 2002; 288(23):2998–3007.
58. Simons LA, Simons J, Friedlander Y, McCallum J. Cholesterol and other lipids predict coronary heart disease and ischaemic stroke in the elderly, but only in those below 70 years. Atherosclerosis 2001; 159(1):201–208.
59. Shepherd J, Blauw GJ, Murphy MB, et al. The design of a PROspective Study of Pravastatin in the Elderly at Risk (PROSPER). PROSPER Study Group. Am J Cardiol 1999; 84(10):1192–1197.
60. Hunt D, Young P, Simes J, et al. Benefits of pravastatin on cardiovascular events and mortality in older patients with coronary heart disease are equal to or exceed those seen in younger patients: results from the LIPID trial. Ann Intern Med 2001; 134(10):931–940.

61. Eaton CB, Lapane KL, Murphy JB, Hume AL. Effect of statin (HMG-Co-A-reductase inhibitor) use on 1-year mortality and hospitalization rates in older patients with cardiovascular disease living in nursing homes. J Am Geriatr Soc 2002; 50(8):1389–1395.

62. Ko DT, Mamdani M, Alter DA. Lipid-lowering therapy with statins in high-risk elderly patients: the treatment-risk paradox. JAMA 2004; 291(15):1864–1870.

63. Sever PS, Dahlof B, Poulter NR, et al. Prevention of coronary and stroke events with atorvastatin in hypertensive patients who have average or lower-than-average cholesterol concentrations, in the Anglo-Scandinavian Cardiac Outcomes Trial—Lipid Lowering Arm (ASCOT-LLA): a multicentre randomised controlled trial. Lancet 2003; 361(9364):1149–1158.

64. Lewis SJ, Moye LA, Sacks FM, et al. Effect of pravastatin on cardiovascular events in older patients with myocardial infarction and cholesterol levels in the average range. Results of the Cholesterol and Recurrent Events (CARE) trial. Ann Intern Med 1998; 129(9):681–689.

65. Sever PS, Poulter NR, Dahlof B, et al. Reduction in cardiovascular events with atorvastatin in 2532 patients with type 2 diabetes: Anglo-Scandinavian Cardiac Outcomes Trial-Lipid-Lowering Arm (ASCOT-LLA). Diabet Care 2005; 28(5):1151–1157.

66. Vijan S, Hayward RA. Pharmacologic lipid-lowering therapy in type 2 diabetes mellitus: background paper for the American College of Physicians. Ann Intern Med 2004; 140(8):650–658.

67. Colhoun HM, Betteridge DJ, Durrington PN, et al. Primary prevention of cardiovascular disease with atorvastatin in type 2 diabetes in the Collaborative Atorvastatin Diabetes Study (CARDS): multicentre randomised placebo-controlled trial. Lancet 2004; 364(9435):685–696.

68. Colhoun HM, Betteridge DJ, Durrington PN, et al. Rapid emergence of effect of atorvastatin on cardiovascular outcomes in the Collaborative Atorvastatin Diabetes Study (CARDS). Diabetologia 2005; 48(12):2482–2485.

69. Keech A, Simes RJ, Barter P, et al. Effects of long-term fenofibrate therapy on cardiovascular events in 9795 people with type 2 diabetes mellitus (the FIELD study): randomised controlled trial. Lancet 2005; 366(9500):1849–1861.

70. Johnston C. Impact of atorvastatin on cardiovascular events on older patients similiar to benefit in younger patients: presented at ISC. ISC, 2006.

71. Gaede P, Vedel P, Larsen N, Jensen GV, Parving HH, Pedersen O. Multifactorial intervention and cardiovascular disease in patients with type 2 diabetes. N Engl J Med 2003; 348(5):383–393.

72. Newman AB, Arnold AM, Naydeck BL, et al. "Successful aging": effect of subclinical cardiovascular disease. Arch Intern Med 2003; 163(19):2315–2322.

14 | Peripheral Vascular Disease in Older Adults with Diabetes

Gautam V. Shrikhande
Department of Surgery, Beth Israel Deaconess Medical Center, Harvard Medical School, Boston, Massachusetts, U.S.A.

Frank B. Pomposelli
Division of Vascular and Endovascular Surgery, Beth Israel Deaconess Medical Center, Harvard Medical School, Boston, Massachusetts, U.S.A.

INTRODUCTION

Peripheral arterial disease (PAD) is defined as atherosclerosis of the lower extremities and is a marker for atherosclerotic disease in all other blood vessels. The most common symptom of PAD is intermittent claudication, defined as pain, cramping, or aching in the calves, thighs, or buttocks that occurs with walking and is relieved by rest. More extreme presentations of PAD include rest pain, tissue loss, or gangrene. PAD is also a major risk factor for lower extremity amputation, particularly in patients with diabetes. Moreover, even for the asymptomatic patient, PAD is a marker for systemic vascular disease involving coronary, cerebral, and renal vessels, leading to an elevated risk of events such as myocardial infarction, stroke, and death (1). Diabetes and smoking are the strongest risk factors for PAD. Other well-known risk factors are advanced age, hypertension, and hyperlipidemia (2).

In people with diabetes, the risk of PAD is increased by age, duration of diabetes, and presence of peripheral neuropathy. African Americans and Hispanics with diabetes have a higher prevalence of PAD than non-Hispanic whites, even after adjustment for other known risk factors and the excess prevalence of diabetes (1).

Eighty-four percent of patients with diabetes in the U.S. have an element of peripheral vascular disease (3). Diabetes is an important risk factor for the development of lower extremity arterial disease, with the occlusive process affecting the most distal vessels, namely the infrapopliteal arteries (Fig. 1) (4). Other risk factors such as smoking and hypertension tend to affect the aortoiliofemoral arteries. Diabetes accelerates the initiation and propagation of vascular disease, leading to prolonged hospitalizations and elevated risk of infections. Infragenicular smooth muscle cell proliferation stimulated by the inflammatory environment in diabetes is a hallmark of diabetic atherogenesis. It is well known that patients with diabetes have a macroangiopathy similar to atherosclerosis; however, there is a misconception that they have a predilection for "small vessel disease," which implies untreatable, occlusive lesions in the microcirculation (5). It is believed that diabetics do not have a distinctive form of occlusive small artery disease.

CLINICAL EVALUATION

The initial assessment of PAD in patients with diabetes should begin with a thorough medical history and physical examination. Alternative causes of leg pain during exercise include many musculoskeletal disorders. A thorough walking history will elicit classic claudication symptoms. Patients should also be asked if they experience rest pain at night while they are sleeping and whether placing the foot in a dependent position alleviates the symptoms.

On physical examination, dependent rubor, pallor on elevation, absence of hair growth, dystrophic toenails, and cool, dry, fissured skin are signs of vascular insufficiency (Fig. 2). A detailed pulse examination of the carotids, abdominal aorta, femoral, popliteal, and pedal vessels should be performed. If not palpable, a continuous flow Doppler probe can be used to identify flow in the lower extremity vessels. Patients with diabetes are more likely to present

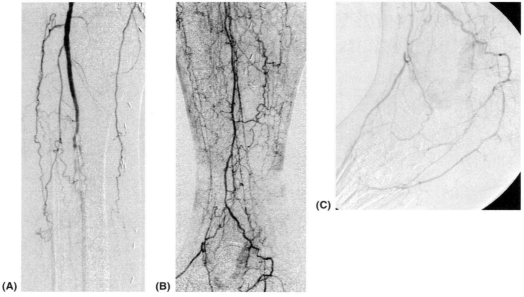

FIGURE 1 (**A**) Patency of the popliteal artery. (**B**) Occlusion of the anterior tibial and posterior tibial arteries with a patent but diseased peroneal artery. (**C**) A patent and non diseased dorsalis pedis artery.

with ulcers or gangrene than claudication and rest pain due to the extensive nature of their disease and lack of normal foot sensation from sensory neuropathy.

Diagnostic studies should include measurement of the ankle-brachial index (ABI), which involves measuring the systolic blood pressures in the ankles (dorsalis pedis and posterior tibial arteries) and arms (brachial artery) using a hand-held Doppler and calculating a ratio.

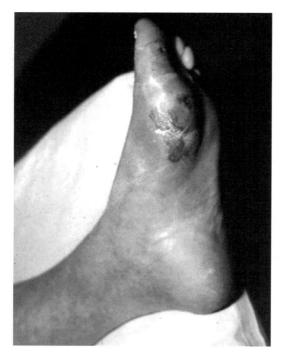

FIGURE 2 Absence of hair growth, dystrophic nails, dry skin, and ulceration can all be seen in a diabetic foot.

This is a noninvasive, quantitative measurement of the patency of the lower extremity arterial system. ABI values greater than 1.0 are seen in normal vessels. A value less than 0.9 is abnormal; claudication can be seen with values of 0.5 to 0.9; rest pain can begin with values of 0.4 or less and tissue loss can be evident when the ABI is less than 0.3. In patients with claudication and palpable pulses, exercise ABIs should be obtained. A reduction in ABI with exercise suggests the presence of significant stenosis. There are some limitations, however, in using the ABI. Calcified, poorly compressible vessels in elderly and some patients with diabetes may artificially elevate values. These issues complicate the evaluation of a patient but are not prevalent enough to detract from the usefulness of the ABI as a noninvasive test to screen for and diagnose PAD in patients with diabetes.

In cases of calcified vessels, pulse volume recordings can be obtained. This study provides a qualitative assessment of blood flow by applying pneumatic cuffs to the upper thigh,

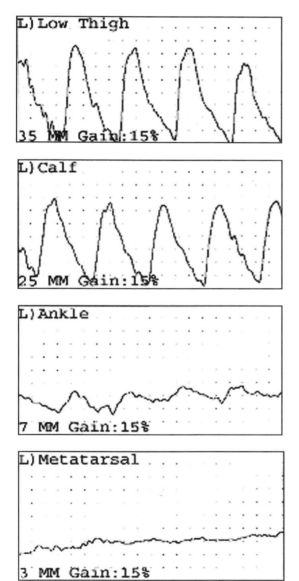

FIGURE 3 Pulse volume recordings showing abnormal measurements on the right.

lower thigh, calf, ankle, and toes and measuring limb volume changes with each beat of the heart. With severe limb disease, poor waveforms with reduced amplitudes are seen (Fig. 3). Furthermore, duplex ultrasound can be used to visualize vessels and identify the location of stenoses or occlusion by measuring the velocity of blood flow. The role of angiography and magnetic resonance angiography (MRA) will be discussed below.

Due to the high prevalence of PAD in patients with diabetes, a screening ABI should be performed in patients over 50 years of age. If normal, the test should be repeated every five years. A screening ABI should be considered in diabetic patients below 50 years of age, who have other PAD risk factors (e.g., smoking, hypertension, hyperlipidemia, or duration of diabetes >10 years) (1).

PREVENTATIVE STRATEGIES

Cigarette smoking is the single most important modifiable risk factor for the development and exacerbation of PAD. In patients with PAD, tobacco use is associated with increased progression of atherosclerosis as well as increased risk of amputation (6). Good glycemic control should be a goal of therapy in all patients with PAD and diabetes in order to prevent microvascular complications. Angiotensin- converting enzyme inhibitors in diabetic patients with and without PAD may reduce the rate of cardiovascular events (7). All patients with diabetes, even if not hypertensive, may benefit from angiotensin-converting enzyme inhibitors. Dyslipidemia with low high-density lipoproteins and elevated low-density lipoproteins (LDL) and triglycerides is associated with diabetes (8). Currently, the use of statins is recommended in patients with PAD, with a goal LDL similar to that recommended in patients with coronary artery disease (1). Clopidogrel has also been shown to reduce cardiovascular events in diabetics (9) and can be considered in patients with severe PAD and diabetes.

MEDICAL TREATMENT OF SYMPTOMATIC PAD

Medical therapy for intermittent claudication currently includes exercise as the most important therapy, as well as the potential use of pharmacologic agents. Exercise therapy has minimal associated morbidity and is likely to improve the cardiovascular risk factor profile. Table 1 outlines an exercise program that we suggest for our patients with claudication. We feel that this regimen is safe but may be difficult for elderly patients who frequently have musculoskeletal pain due to arthritis and may have problems with balance and equilibrium. However, it should be used in any patient who has the capability to ambulate. It is important to stress that this program should be done in consultation with a primary care physician and/or cardiologist. Patients should be instructed that this is not meant to be a leisure activity, but a treatment regimen to be followed closely.

In addition to exercise and smoking cessation, some pharmacologic agents are available for this patient population. Pentoxifylline, a hemorheologic agent, was approved for treating

TABLE 1 Claudication Exercise Program

Pick a time of day where you will not be interrupted (preferably after breakfast). This is not a leisure activity. It needs to become part of your daily life. It should be considered just like a medication that you must take every day

Find a flat area to walk or use a treadmill. Elliptical trainers or Stairmasters are not acceptable alternatives. It can even be walking in a mall

The duration and speed of the walking is not important, just that it be done consistently. Walk at a comfortable pace but do not stroll. Walk until you start to feel the tightness or ache in your muscles. Stop immediately and wait until the discomfort is completely gone. Then, resume walking. Continue this cycle for about 10–15 times each day

Over time, the distance you can walk without pain will increase if this program is followed and you stop smoking. As you improve, you may want to increase the speed of your walk to elicit the symptoms

On the average you should expect to increase your distance by 50–100%. Often this is enough to get you through a normal day without any discomfort. There are also obvious benefits with regard to your heart with this type of exercise

If you experience chest pain, shortness of breath, dizziness or chest tightness, "stop" and bring this to the attention of your cardiologist or primary care doctor

Note: As with any exercise program you should consult with your primary care doctor or cardiologist before starting.

claudication. The results of several trials, however, suggest that it does not increase walking distance to a clinically meaningful extent. Cilostazol, an oral phosphodiesterase type III inhibitor, was also approved for treating intermittent claudication. Significant benefit in increasing maximal walking time has been demonstrated in randomized trials, in addition to improving functional status and health-related quality of life (10). The use of this drug is contraindicated if any degree of heart failure is present, due to concerns about arrhythmias. Cilostazol is the drug of choice if pharmacologic therapy is necessary for the management of PAD in patients with diabetes.

ENDOVASCULAR OPTIONS FOR REVASCULARIZATION

Two general techniques of revascularization exist: open surgical procedures and endovascular interventions. The two approaches are not mutually exclusive and may be combined. Endovascular intervention tends to be more appropriate in patients with focal disease, especially of larger more proximal vessels, and is more commonly performed for claudication. In general, vascular surgeons tend to be more aggressive with endovascular therapy in patients with severe uncorrectable coronary artery disease, poor ventricular function, limited pulmonary reserve, advanced age, renal failure, or hostile abdominal anatomy (such as adhesive disease from prior operations). Thus, even very challenging lesions, which would ideally be treated with open surgery, will be pursued using endovascular techniques in the high-risk, elderly population. It is important to remember that endovascular procedures are not without risk. Complications such as dissection, embolization, pseudoaneurysm formation or thrombosis and the need for repeat interventions do occur.

Endovascular therapeutic options such as percutaneous transluminal angioplasty (PTA) with or without stenting have become the treatment of choice for many lesions involving the common or external iliac artery. With the technological advances of small wires, angioplasty balloons, and other devices, the treatment of smaller-diameter vessels below the inguinal ligament has become more feasible. Stenoses of the superficial femoral artery may be treated with an endovascular approach; however, more durable results appear obtainable with open bypass. The long-term outcome of endovascular management of superficial femoral artery occlusions remains unproven. The efficacy of tibial angioplasty also remains uncertain despite its increased use. Nonetheless, it may provide a means to allow a patient to heal and recover from a limb-threatening situation prior to performing a more definitive procedure.

In diabetic patients with complex multilevel disease in the setting of limb-threatening ischemia, a combination of endovascular and surgical therapy may be an effective treatment option associated with lower morbidity than open bypass alone. One study compared the results of iliac artery PTA performed in conjunction with infrainguinal bypass for limb-threatening ischemia in diabetic and nondiabetic patients. In this study, iliac PTA eliminated the need for a proximal aortic or iliac bypass for the treatment of multilevel occlusive disease and resulted in excellent cumulative patency and limb salvage rates. The presence of diabetes did not alter these favorable results (11).

SURGICAL REVASCULARIZATION

Cardiac risk stratification has been considered an important part of the preoperative assessment of patients undergoing surgery for PAD. The presence of PAD increases the all-cause mortality rate by threefold and the cardiovascular mortality rate by sixfold (12). The incidence of coronary artery disease is increased in diabetic patients compared to nondiabetic patients. The American College of Cardiology and the American Heart Association have addressed the increased risk of adverse cardiac events in diabetic patients undergoing vascular surgery by publishing extensive algorithms to risk-stratify patients having noncardiac surgery (13,14). According to their algorithms, diabetic patients with PAD would warrant a preoperative cardiac evaluation prior to an infrainguinal arterial reconstruction. Although this approach has been widely adopted, its efficacy in reducing adverse perioperative cardiac events is unproven.

At our institution, (Beth Israel Deaconess Medical Center), we evaluated 140 asymptomatic, diabetic patients undergoing infrainguinal arterial reconstructions. Sixty-one of the patients had no cardiac workup and 79 patients underwent some form of cardiac workup. There was no difference in perioperative mortality or in postoperative cardiac morbidity, including myocardial infarction, congestive heart failure, and arrhythmia requiring treatment. Further, there was no difference in survival at 12 and 36 months (15). In another study analyzing 6565 patients (largely diabetic and elderly) undergoing major vascular surgery, there was a lack of association of diabetes with increased postoperative mortality and cardiac morbidity (16). Of the 6565 patients, 62.3% had diabetes and a significant number underwent infrainguinal bypass surgery. Comparing diabetics with nondiabetics, rates of mortality were 0.96% versus 1.46%; myocardial infarction 1.77% versus 1.3%; and congestive heart failure 1.13% versus 1.14%, respectively. The five-year mortality was statistically significantly lower in patients with diabetes. The authors concluded that diabetes alone does not confer a higher mortality or cardiac morbidity rate with vascular procedures. Others have shown that routine cardiac screening or coronary-revascularization strategies before elective vascular surgery are not beneficial (17,18). Thus, with careful perioperative care, routine preoperative cardiac testing in this patient population is not mandatory. Risk stratification is not as important in asymptomatic patients as we once thought.

Successful arterial reconstruction can be determined by an anatomic assessment of the arterial circulation with radiographic imaging. One option is intra-arterial digital subtraction angiography (DSA), which should include the entire arterial circulation from the renal arteries to the base of the toes. Proper imaging of the foot vessels requires views in two planes, usually anteroposterior and lateral, to fully appreciate the quality of the dorsalis pedis artery and its potential use as an outflow target. An alternative to DSA is MRA; the advantage being that it is noninvasive and does not use nephrotoxic contrast. Numerous studies have attempted to compare the effectiveness of DSA to MRA in evaluating lower extremity vessels. Some authors have suggested that MRA is not a substitute for DSA but can serve as a meaningful adjunct in difficult situations such as the detection of distal target vessels in elderly patients with diabetes (19). DSA is superior due to better image resolution, but in some patients with renal insufficiency, MRA is an acceptable alternative.

The goal of arterial reconstructive surgery is to restore adequate blood flow, decrease claudication, decrease rest pain, and heal ulcers. To achieve this, the treatment plan involves bypassing all major occlusions, and with diabetic tissue loss, to restore a palpable pulse. In diabetes, the typical pattern of atherosclerosis in the lower extremities is tibial vessel occlusion with restoration of the foot vessels. Generally, because of the extent of the disease, bypasses are performed to the foot itself. Contraindications to bypass surgery include active angina, recent myocardial infarction, acute renal failure following an arteriogram, sepsis, and recent congestive heart failure. Other patients who may not be appropriate candidates for arterial reconstruction include those with dementia and/or other organic brain syndromes, who are nonambulatory or bedridden and have no likelihood of successful rehabilitation. Similarly, patients with severe flexion contractures of the knee or hip are poor candidates.

In the authors' experience, 40% to 60% of patients with diabetes presenting with ischemic foot complications have an associated infection. Our initial efforts are focused upon controlling the infection by using clinical parameters such as decreased erythema, reduction of fever, return of glycemic control, and normalization of the white blood cell count. Broad-spectrum intravenous antibiotics to cover gram-positive, gram-negative, and anaerobic organisms should be started immediately after cultures are taken, since most infections in diabetics are multimicrobial. Once culture data are available, antibiotics can be appropriately adjusted. We typically wait two to five days prior to surgery; delaying longer can lead to further ischemic tissue damage.

Often, the most efficacious bypass to restore maximal perfusion in diabetes is to the dorsalis pedis artery with an autogenous conduit (20). The inflow source can be any location proximal to which there is no significant stenosis, including the below-knee popliteal artery. One large study spanning a decade reported the results of 1032 bypasses to the dorsalis pedis artery (21). The average age of these patients was 66.8 years, and 91.9% were diabetic. The indications for operation were most commonly nonhealing ulcer and gangrene and, less commonly, rest pain. There was minimal use of prosthetic conduit. There were 10 deaths, 0.97% occurring within the first 30 days of surgery. Thirty-one patients (3%) had cardiac complications including myocardial infarction and congestive heart failure. Significant, limb-threatening postoperative wound infections occurred in 21 limbs (2%), two of which resulted in graft infections and limb loss. The 30-day graft failure rate was 4.2%. Limb salvage was 78.2% and 57.7% at 5 and 10 years, respectively. Patient survival was 48.6% and 23.8% at 5 and 10 years, respectively. The low perioperative mortality seen in the study was attributed to invasive monitoring including pulmonary arterial catheters, β-blockade, judicious intravenous fluid use, and a dedicated vascular nursing unit.

Edema is always seen after arterial reconstruction and may be more prominent in diabetes. Neuropathy and capillary leak of albumin, leading to edema, have a negative impact on wound healing. The anastomosis in dorsalis pedis bypass is covered by minimal subcutaneous tissue. Closure of the wound is designed to minimize tension and obtain accurate approximation of skin edges. If there is cellulitis in the area of the proposed incision, extensive forefoot infection or gangrene, especially where the anastomosis may be performed, a pedal graft should not be done. In the postoperative period, it is helpful to wrap the foot and ankle with an elastic bandage or to keep the foot elevated to minimize swelling and suture line stress. The use of an open toe-healing sandal can be helpful in patients with foot lesions.

Following successful flow of an arterial reconstruction, the patient may need debridement, toe amputation, a split thickness skin graft, a rotational flap, or a free flap (22). In some patients, primary amputation may be proper therapy. This applies to those who have exhausted all available vein conduit or those who have an unsalvageable limb from infection or gangrene, severe contractures, and bedridden status. Patients with terminal cancer and very short life expectancy do poorly with vascular reconstruction and are probably better served by primary amputation. When considering an above-knee verses below-knee amputation, it is important to consider the fact that preservation of the knee joint gives the best chance for rehabilitation.

FUNCTIONAL OUTCOMES IN ELDERLY PATIENTS

It is essential to realize that age alone is not a contraindication to arterial reconstruction. When selecting patients for arterial reconstruction, the functional and physiologic status of the patient is far more important than chronological age. In fact, a limb-salvaging arterial reconstruction may mean the difference for an elderly patient between continued independent living and the need for permanent custodial nursing home care. In addition, lower extremity amputation in elderly patients is associated with considerable mortality and deterioration of functional and residential status (23).

In a frail, elderly patient who is nonambulatory, we would likely use endovascular techniques and perform amputation sooner than in a patient who has fewer comorbidities and is ambulatory. Although most patients are grateful to have their leg saved, little attention is sometimes given to the effect of infrainguinal revascularization on their quality of life. In one study of 156 patients undergoing surgery for PAD, 84% of whom were diabetic with a mean age of 66 years, significantly improved instrumental activities of daily living, mental well-being, and vitality at six months follow-up were reported (24).

In another study, 262 patients, 80 years of age or older, were examined. Sixty-seven percent of the patients had diabetes. The effect of lower extremity arterial reconstruction on ambulatory function and residential status was evaluated. The patient survival rate at five years was 44% and, among living patients, the limb salvage rate at five years was 92%. Residential status and level of ambulatory function were assessed by a scoring system in which one indicated living independently, walking without assistance; two indicated living at home with family, walking with an ambulatory assistive device; three indicated an extended stay in a rehabilitation facility, using a wheelchair; and four indicated requiring permanent nursing home care, bedridden. The mean postoperative residential status and ambulatory function scores were 1.95 and 1.70, respectively. Overall scores remained the same or improved in over three-fourths of the patients. The authors concluded that surgical reconstruction preserves the ability to ambulate and reside at home for most patients while allowing for limb salvage (Fig. 4) (25).

In another study of 88 patients, aged 80 or more, infrainguinal bypass surgery was associated with a perioperative mortality rate of 6%. The one- and three-year limb salvage rates were

Ambulatory Status

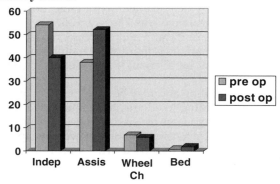

Residence

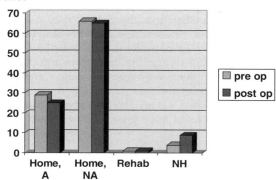

FIGURE 4 Ambulatory status and residential status after lower extremity arterial reconstruction. Preoperative and postoperative values expressed as percentages. Good limb preservation rates were seen in this octogenarian patient population. *Abbreviations*: (Indep-walking independently; Assis-walking with assistance device; Wheel Ch-wheelchair; Bed-bedridden); (Home, A-living alone or with spouse at home; Home, NA-living home, care by family members; Rehab-rehabilitation facility; NH-nursing home). *Source*: From Ref. 25.

94% and 91%, and patient survival rates were 73% and 51%, respectively. One year after operation, 88% of patients were ambulatory, 85% were living at home, and 80% were both living at home and ambulatory. At three years, these results were 86%, 76%, and 71%, respectively. The authors concluded that revascularization for chronic lower extremity ischemia in patients aged 80 or more is appropriate and results in maintenance of independent living in a large majority (26). Morbidity of lower extremity arterial reconstruction is sometimes underestimated in studies that evaluate only clinical outcomes such as limb salvage. However, it is erroneous to conclude that lower extremity arterial surgery impairs functional status.

SUMMARY

PAD is a significant problem in the United States; diabetes and smoking are its greatest risk factors. It usually presents with claudication; however tissue loss, gangrene, and rest pain can be seen with more severe disease. The evaluation relies initially on a thorough history and physical examination as well as noninvasive arterial studies. Screening ABIs should be done in all diabetics over the age of 50, and at a younger age if other risk factors exist. Prevention strategies such as proper glycemic control, statins, hypertension therapy, and antiplatelet agents should all be used. Smoking cessation and exercise are the mainstays of therapy, with cilostazol being a pharmacologic option.

Options for revascularization include open and endovascular techniques. The choice of therapy depends upon disease distribution and the comorbidities of the patients. It is important to properly evaluate these patients with imaging prior to any procedure. In general, elderly, diabetic patients have good results with both open and endovascular techniques, including good limb salvage rates. Functional and ambulatory status can be improved or preserved in a large majority of geriatric patients with diabetes.

REFERENCES

1. American Diabetes Association Consensus Statement. Peripheral arterial disease in people with diabetes. Diabetes Care 2003; 26(12):3333–3341.
2. Criqui MH. Peripheral arterial disease: epidemiological aspects. Vascular Med 2001; 6(suppl 1):3–7.
3. Lucas JW, Schiller JS, Benson V. Summary health statistics for U.S. adults: national health interview survey, 2001. National center for health statistics. Vital Health Stat 2004; 10(218):1–134.
4. Conrad MC. Large and small artery occlusion in diabetics and nondiabetics with severe vascular disease. Circulation 1967; 36:83–91.
5. Akbari CM, Logerfo FW. Diabetes and peripheral vascular disease. J Vasc Surg 1999; 30:373–384.
6. Lassila R, Lepantalo M. Cigarette smoking and the outcome after lower limb arterial surgery. Acta Chir Scand 1988; 154:635–640.
7. Yusuf S, Sleight P, Pogue J, Bosch J, Davies R, Dagenais G. Effects of an angiotensin converting-enzyme inhibitor, ramipril, on cardiovascular events in high-risk patients: the Heart Outcomes Prevention Evaluation Study Investigators. N Engl J Med 2000; 342:145–153.
8. Ford ES, Giles WH, Dietz WH. Prevalence of the metabolic syndrome among US adults: findings from the third national health and nutrition examination survey. JAMA 2002; 287:356–359.
9. Bhatt DL, Marso SP, Hirsch AT, et al. Amplified benefit of clopidogrel versus aspirin in patients with diabetes mellitus. Am J Cardiol 2002; 90:625–628.
10. Regensteiner JG, Ware JE Jr, McCarthy WJ, et al. Effect of cilostazol on treadmill walking, community-based walking ability, and health-related quality of life in patients with intermittent claudication due to peripheral arterial disease: meta-analysis of six randomized controlled trials. J Am Geriatr Soc 2002; 50:1939–1946.
11. Faries PL, Brophy D, Logerfo FW, et al. Combined iliac angioplasty and infrainguinal revascularization surgery are effective in diabetic patients with multilevel arterial disease. Ann Vasc Surg 2001; 15(1):67–72.
12. Mangano DT, Layug EL, Wallace A, et al. Effect of atenolol on mortality and cardiovascular morbidity after noncardiac surgery. N Engl J Med 1996; 335:1713–1720.
13. Eagle KA, Chaitman BR, Ewy GA, et al. Guidelines for perioperative cardiovascular evaluation for noncardiac surgery: report of the American College of Cardiology/American Heart Association Taskforce on Practice Guidelines (Committee on Perioperative Cardiac Evaluation for Noncardiac Surgery). Circulation 1996; 93:1278–1317.
14. Eagle KA, Berger PB, Calkins H, et al. ACC/AHA guideline update for perioperative cardiovascular evaluation for noncardiac surgery. J Am Coll Cardiol 2002; 39:542–553.
15. Monahan TS, Shrikhande GV, Pomposelli FB, et al. Preoperative cardiac evaluation does not improve or predict perioperative or late survival in asymptomatic diabetic patients undergoing elective infrainguinal arterial reconstruction. J Vasc Surg 2005; 41:38–45.
16. Hamdan AD, Saltzberg SS, Sheahan M, et al. Lack of association of diabetes with increased postoperative mortality and cardiac morbidity. Arch Surg 2002; 137:417–421.
17. Mcfalls EO, Ward HB, Moritz TE, et al. Coronary-revascularization before elective major vascular surgery. N Engl J Med 2004; 351:2795–2804.
18. Schueppert MT, Kresowik TF, Corry DC, et al. Selection of patients for cardiac evaluation before peripheral vascular operations. J Vasc Surg 1996; 23:802–809.
19. Dorwiler B, Neufand A, Kreitner K, et al. Magnetic resonance angiography unmasks reliable target vessels for pedal bypass in patients with diabetes mellitus. J Vasc Surg 2002; 35:766–762.
20. Pomposelli FB Jr, Marcaccio EJ, Gibbons GW, et al. Dorsalis pedis arterial bypass: durable limb salvage for foot ischemia in patients with diabetes mellitus. J Vasc Surg 1995; 21:375–384.
21. Pomposelli FB Jr, Kansal N, Hamdan AD, et al. A decade of experience with dorsalis pedis artery bypass: analysis of outcome in more than 1000 cases. J Vasc Surg 2003; 37:307–315.
22. Robenblum BI, Giurini JM, Miller LB, et al. Neuropathic ulcerations plantar to the lateral column in patients with Charcot foot deformity: a flexible approach to limb salvage. J Foot Ankle Surg 1997; 36:360–363.
23. Frykberg RG, Arora S, Pomposelli FB, Logerfo F. Functional outcome in the elderly following lower extremity amputation. J Foot Ankle Surg 1998; 37:181–185.
24. Gibbons GW, Burgess AM, Guadagnoli E, et al. Return to well-being and function after infrainguinal revascularization. J Vasc Surg 1995; 21:35–45.
25. Pomposelli FB, Arora S, Gibbons GW, et al. Lower extremity arterial reconstruction in the very elderly: successful outcome preserves not only the limb but also residential status and ambulatory function. J Vasc Surg 1998; 28:215–225.
26. Nehler MR, Moneta GL, Edwards JM, et al. Surgery for chronic lower extremity ischemia in patients eighty or more years of age: operative results and assessment of postoperative independence. J Vasc Surg 1993; 18:618–626.

15 | Kidney Dysfunction in Older Adults with Diabetes

Mark E. Williams and Robert C. Stanton
Renal Section, Joslin Diabetes Center, Harvard Medical School, Boston, Massachusetts, U.S.A.

INTRODUCTION

Diabetes mellitus is a major health issue affecting an aging U.S. population (1) and is part of a worldwide epidemic of diabetes related to obesity, sedentary lifestyle, poor nutrition (2), aging, and better survival of diabetic patients. Concurrently, elderly individuals represent the fastest growing subgroup of the U.S. general population (3) and one with a large burden of diabetes (4). Death rates from diabetes in the United States have increased by 45% since 1987, and are occurring at older ages (5). The reported incidence of diabetes mellitus in the elderly population is 10% to 17.7% and does not include those who are unaware of their condition (6). The number of elderly persons with diabetes is expected to rapidly grow in the coming decades. Diabetes and age are among the most significant risk factors for chronic kidney disease (CKD) and end-stage renal disease (ESRD) (7). Diabetes is a more powerful determinant of kidney impairment in the elderly than is hypertension (8).

The diabetic kidney disease became the leading cause of CKD and ESRD in the United States in the 1990s, and the elderly individuals comprise the fastest growing subgroup (3). While medicare beneficiaries with diabetes have seen significant improvement with preventative care practices, rates of nephropathy and other long-term complications have risen (1). Prevalence estimates from National Health and Nutrition Examination Survey (NHANES) II and III applied to the U.S. census data indicate that about 30% of older diabetics (2 million individuals) may have microalbuminuria, an early sign of kidney disease. Although NHANES reported depressed kidney function in 16% of individuals over 70 years old, more than twice that many (35%) of elderly diabetics were affected (9,10). Yet, CKD care of older patients with diabetes remains under-recognized and nephrology referrals underutilized (11).

While the natural history of the kidney complication of diabetes has been extensively studied in nonelderly patients with type 1 and type 2 diabetes, much less is known about the disease in the elderly. Nor have interventional studies included significant numbers of elderly patients with diabetes, typically excluding patients over 70 years at entry. Moreover care of elderly patients with diabetic kidney disease appears to be inadequate as studies have shown that American Diabetes Association (ADA) clinical recommendations on kidney care are not being achieved in older patients (12). Clinically, although current guidelines for CKD recommend that all patients with significantly reduced kidney function [glomerular filtration rate (GFR) under 30 mL/min] be referred to a nephrologist (13), older age is associated with delayed referral patterns (14). In addition, elderly individuals with CKD may not be receiving the same recommended general health care as those without CKD (15). Optimal management of the kidney disease in elderly diabetic patients may involve unique risks since diabetes and age are independent predictors of mortality (16). This chapter details the current management and prognosis of CKD and ESRD in elderly patients with diabetic kidney disease.

RENAL FUNCTION IN THE ELDERLY

Accurate assessment of kidney function is fundamental for determining the prevalence and progression of kidney impairment, for morbidity and mortality risk stratification associated with CKD, and for evaluating the impact of new therapies in elderly populations. In an individual patient, an accurate method is essential for analyzing whether kidney function is normal for age, and whether it is stable or worsening. The GFR at birth is 120 to 140 mL/min and gradually declines throughout life. In cross-sectional and longitudinal studies, kidney function as measured by GFR decreases after age 40 years by about 1 mL/min/yr (17) [as renal blood flow diminishes over time, the filtration loss is proportionately less, being reduced by a rise in the filtration fraction (18)]. Functional waning is accompanied by a decrease in kidney weight and volume, mostly due to loss of kidney mass from the outer cortex. In older diabetic patients, histologic changes of diabetic nephropathy are compounded by advanced vascular changes (19). Limited data indicate that the age-related decline in renal function continues at the same rate beyond age 80 years (20). The normal GFR, as measured by insulin clearance for ages 70 to 79 years, is about 89 mL/min/1.73 m², and for ages 80 to 89 years, is about 65 mL/min/1.73 m² (21). The additional effect of disease progress on kidney function therefore must be age adjusted (22). Although no data specific to elderly diabetic patients are available, the decline in kidney function with age is accentuated with comorbidities such as hypertension, atherosclerosis, and heart failure.

It is important to emphasize that serum creatinine level, the most commonly utilized endogenous marker of kidney function, may be deceptive in the elderly. While a rise in serum creatinine nearly always represents a loss in function, the elderly patient may have significant kidney impairment despite a normal serum creatinine level, due to variations in creatinine metabolism (20). The term "concealed renal failure" has been applied to elderly patients with normal serum creatinine but decreasing filtration rate (23). With increasing age, a fall in creatinine clearance is accompanied by a parallel decrease in creatinine excretion, which is reflective of a decreased muscle mass. As a result, the rise in serum creatinine is less (24). In one study, 50% of elderly patients with a normal serum creatinine had a GFR of less than 60 mL/min (20), and the mean creatinine clearance in patients with a normal serum creatinine was only 50 ± 24 mL/min. The increasing recognition of kidney impairment in the elderly may be one reason for the increase in diagnostic kidney biopsies being performed in the elderly (25).

Two alternative methods to estimate GFR in adults are derived equations that are also based upon the serum creatinine level: (*i*) the Cockroft–Gault equation [$(140 - \text{age}) \times \text{wt kg}/72 \times \text{serum creatinine (SCr)} \times 1.73 \text{ m}^2$]; and (*ii*) the modification of diet in renal disease (MDRD) equation [GFR (mL/min/1.73 m²) = $175 \times (\text{SCr})^{-1.154} \times (\text{age})^{-0.203} \times (0.742 \text{ if female}) \times (1.210 \text{ if African American})$ (conventional units)]. The MDRD equation is increasingly used in the United States and has been found to be accurate in diabetic kidney disease (26). A recent study of 160 diabetic patients reported that the MDRD equation has better accuracy in moderate and severe kidney function (27). Neither equation, however, has been validated in the elderly population. Prevalence estimates of decreased kidney function among the elderly vary depending on the equation used (28). Recently, another endogenous marker, plasma cystatin C, has been proposed as a solution to the problem of creatinine-based measurements (29). Serum levels of this low-molecular-weight protein are mainly determined by GFR, independent of muscle mass, gender, or age. However, cystatin C-based GFR estimation was not better than Cockroft-Gault in assessing true GFR in one study (30).

DIAGNOSIS

There have not been studies of the diagnosis of diabetic kidney disease in the elderly. There could be a higher prevalence of unusual presentations of diabetic kidney disease in elderly patients (e.g., decreased GFR without albuminuria), but no studies have addressed this issue. Thus the diagnosis of diabetic nephropathy in the elderly is not different from that in the younger age groups. The classic presentation is albuminuria first, followed by a decline in GFR. The urinalysis is typically unremarkable (i.e., either no or few cells and rare casts). The confounding variables are the expected decline in renal function with aging (on average, 1 mL/min/yr after age 40) and the presence of other factors, primarily hypertension but also long exposure to potentially nephrotoxic medications or preexisting renal disease. A final factor that needs to be considered in the elderly is the existence of renal artery stenosis (RAS). The principal reason for RAS in this age group is atherosclerotic disease.

The approach to diagnosis in the elderly is as follows. First look for the presence of abnormal levels of albumin in the urine as well as decreases in GFR (taking into account expected GFR for age and gender). The National Kidney Foundation has established the following interpretations of kidney disease–based on GFR as follows: stage 1 is a GFR >90 mL/min (with presence of proteinuria or other sign of kidney damage); stage 2 is 60 to 89 mL/min; stage 3 is 30 to 59 mL/min; stage 4 is 16 to 29 mL/min; and stage 5 is <15 mL/min. Stage 3 is moderate disease; and it is important to note that the complications of kidney disease such as anemia and hyperparathyroidism start to occur at this level of GFR (13). Next, through proper history taking, determine the likelihood that hypertension, nephrotoxic medications, or other kidney diseases are present. Then, check the urinalysis. Often a magnetic resonance angiogram (MRA) or Doppler ultrasound to assess renal artery flow is indicated; and a renal ultrasound to assess kidney size is also often indicated (small kidneys suggest CKD). Usually a presumptive diagnosis of diabetic kidney disease can be made after obtaining all of this information. Indications for a renal biopsy include an active urinary sediment (many red blood cells or white blood cells or casts), high quantity of proteinuria (especially greater than 3 g/24 hours), and/or rapidly declining GFR. If kidneys are already atrophied (small in size), a biopsy is not useful as it is unlikely that the approach to treatment would change.

TREATMENT

The hallmark of therapy for diabetic nephropathy is the triad of blood glucose control, blood pressure (BP) control, and administration of angiotensin-converting enzyme inhibitors (ACE-I) or angiotensin-receptor blockers (ARBs). The goals that have been established through many clinical studies are a hemoglobin A1c (HbA1c) of <7%, a BP of <130/80 or 125/75 if proteinuric, and reduction of total urine protein to <500 mg/g of creatinine, or of urine albumin to <300 mg/g of creatinine. Virtually all of these goals have been validated in a young to middle-aged population but not in the elderly population. In this section, we will review what evidence there is for management of diabetic nephropathy in the elderly population.

As with all therapeutic interventions in the elderly, it is essential to make modest changes and allow time for physiologic equilibration before making another change. But it is still important to be persistent in achieving goals, because current approaches to diabetic nephropathy can significantly slow progression of the disease. For example, a study from Scotland by Joss et al. (31) on 90 patients whose mean age was 63 (57% men and 43% women) showed the importance of aggressive intervention. The study was a prospective randomized controlled study. Patients with type 2 diabetes and nephropathy were randomly allocated to an intensive group ($n = 47$) or control group ($n = 43$) and followed for two years. Treatment targets were the same for both groups, but the intensive group was seen as often as required to meet the targets; controls were seen at their normal clinics. Specifically the treatment goals were: systolic BP (SBP) <140 mmHg, diastolic BP (DBP) <80 mmHg, HbA1c < 8%, sodium intake <120 mmol/day, protein intake 0.7 to 1 g/kg of ideal body weight per day, and cholesterol <4 mmol/L or cholesterol:HDL cholesterol ratio <4. The primary end-point was the rate of progression of renal disease in the second year. The results showed that the median rate of progression to renal failure in the intensive group fell from 0.44 mL/min/mo in the creatinine clearance in the first year to 0.14 mL/min/mo in the second year, compared to 0.49 and 0.53 mL/min/mo in the control group ($P = 0.04$ for second year). Considering that mean creatinine clearance at the start of the trial was 55 mL/min, if these results are maintainable, then the onset of dialysis would be delayed by 20 years in the intensive group compared with the control group. Needless to say, reducing the rate of decline in creatinine clearance in the elderly may very well allow the patients to live out the rest of their lives without needing dialysis. In the Joss et al. study, the intensively treated group achieved a rate of decline similar to the nondiabetic, healthy population, which is 1 mL/min/yr or 0.083 mL/min/mo.

Unfortunately, epidemiologic studies suggest that elderly patients are not receiving the care that they should. In the American Journal of Kidney Disease in 2005, Patel et al. reported their study of patients with CKD and diabetes over a three-year period from 2000 to 2002 (11). Clearly this data might not reflect current practice, but considering how slowly doctors change their treatment behaviors, it is likely that the results in this study would be applicable if the study reflects the practice of medicine in 2006. The average age was 66 years and the cohort were mostly men, as the study was done at seven Veterans Administration Hospitals. The authors estimated GFR using the now widely accepted MDRD formula (as previously discussed). The authors found a high prevalence of kidney disease as identified by the previously noted

National Kidney Foundation Criteria (13). In the Patel et al. study of over 10,000 patients, nearly half of the patients had CKD. Of these, only 7.2% were referred to a nephrologist for care; and this referral rate appeared to be age related. As the authors note, a 50-year-old with CKD had a10.5% probability of seeing a nephrologist compared with a 5.6% probability for a 75-year-old. Moreover, as GFR declined, there was a dramatic increase in death rates. For example, diabetics with CKD and stage 4 kidney disease had a death rate more than four times than those without CKD. Thus, slowing down the progressive loss of GFR in the elderly prolongs lives.

Role of Glycemic Control

The goal of an HbA1c of <7 appears to apply for the elderly population as in the younger population. There are no definitive studies on the effects of glycemic control on the progression of kidney disease in the elderly; so no geriatric specific recommendations can be made. What needs to be taken into account though is the effect of the decreased GFR. This has an effect on dosing of both oral hypoglycemic agents and insulin in that there very well may be a decreased drug clearance. Hence, as with drug dosing for many elderly patients, starting with low doses and being very cautious with dose increases is necessary to avoid hypoglycemia.

Role of BP Control

The importance of BP control in slowing the progression of diabetic kidney disease has been established in many studies. There is some debate as to how much the BP should be lowered. The debate centers around the idea that there is a J-shaped curve in mortality. That is, will there be an increase in mortality and worsening of kidney disease when BP goes below a certain level. There are large ongoing clinical studies that should answer that question, but there is evidence in the elderly that accepting BPs higher than what we would accept in a younger population is erroneous (see summary section to find suggestions for referral to nephrologists). The Systolic Hypertension in the Elderly Program evaluated the effects of systolic hypertension. This was a very important study as it evaluated isolated systolic hypertension—the most common hypertensive pattern in elderly patients. Young et al. examined a cohort of 2181 patients who were in the placebo arm of the study to see the relationship between BP and decline in kidney function (32). In general, the SBPs ranged from 160 to 200 and the DBPs ranged from 70 to 90. Only 10% of the patients studied had diabetes, but one could logically extrapolate that the results here would be even more dramatic for patients with diabetes. The results showed that systolic hypertension (and not diastolic hypertension) strongly correlated with declining renal function. From the lowest to the highest SBPs, there was over a twofold increase in risk of progression of kidney disease. This study supports the importance of BP control in the elderly.

How low should the BP be? The diabetic elderly are clearly at higher risk for significant decreases in BP for the following reasons. First, elderly patients tend to have decreased intake of salt and water and higher losses of salt and water through perspiration and via renal and stool losses. Thus, it is important to evaluate salt intake from the standpoint of decreasing BP but also from preventing hypotension. Moreover, the elderly and especially the diabetic elderly patients tend to have some degree of autonomic dysfunction. This would prevent both an increase in heart rate and vasoconstriction at times when this would be required, leading to postural hypotension. Thus, physicians caring for patients with diabetic kidney disease need to be aware of this in order to prescribe drugs appropriately and to determine how low to push the BP. In general, it appears that certainly <140/90 and likely 130/80 are reasonable goals. There is no specific mix of BP medications that are better in the elderly as compared to other groups. But the treatment approaches and the achievement of BP goals must be done slowly and individualized, based on response to medications, medication compliance, and medication cost.

Role of ACE-I and ARB

Another important therapeutic intervention is the use of ACE-I and ARBs in the diabetic elderly. The value of these drugs in slowing the progression of diabetic kidney disease has been established for both type 1 (33) and type 2 (34,35) diabetic patients. The acknowledged current standard of care is to start an ACE-I or ARB in any patient with microalbuminuria or overt proteinuria even if BP is at goal. The physiologic roles of these medicines are not entirely understood, but one action is to reduce glomerular pressure, which may lead to decreased damage to the glomerulus and preservation of renal function. Thus, it is reasonable to use these medicines in elderly diabetic kidney patients. But a recent study by Winkelmayer et al. showed that many elderly patients were not prescribed ACE-Is or ARBs (36). In this study, the authors reviewed Medicare data in the calendar year 2002 on patients in the state of Pennsylvania who were diabetic. They identified 30,750 patients, of whom 21,053 had hypertension and 1243 were identified as having proteinuria or proteinuria and kidney disease. The patients ranged in age from 65 years to over 90, with most of them being between 75 and 84 years. Of the hypertensive-only patients, 50.5% were on an ACE-I or ARB, whereas 40% of the proteinuric patients and 54.7% of the patients with both proteinuria and hypertension were on either an ACE-I or ARB. As the authors note, these percentages are significantly lower when compared to a younger cohort of patients studied by Rosen et al., where "54% of patients with albuminuria, 64% of patients with hypertension, and 74% of patients with both conditions were administered ACE-Is or ARBs in 2000" (37). As Winkelmayer et al. elucidate in the discussion, the possible reasons for the lower percentage of prescriptions of these indicated medicines include concerns over untoward effects of ACE-Is and ARBs in the elderly, such as hyperkalemia and decreased GFR. In addition, there may be an age bias as to the relative value of these medicines in the elderly diabetic. As to the last point, there has been no study focused exclusively on the elderly that has shown that ACE-Is and ARBs are beneficial in this age group. But considering their utility in many other studies, some of which include elderly patients, it is reasonable to prescribe them at this time until further studies are done. The concerns over hyperkalemia or too great a decrease in GFR appear to be misplaced. Both ACE-Is and ARBs will decrease GFR modestly. In general, if the drop is <30% and the GFR remains stable, then the therapeutic benefit is achieved. To monitor significant changes in potassium or GFR, it is routine to check potassium and serum creatinine one week after starting or changing these medicines.

A principal goal of blood sugar control, BP control, and the administration of ACE-Is and ARBs is reduction of proteinuria. Many studies have shown that increases in protein in the urine increase the risk of progressing to renal failure (38). In addition, a large number of studies have shown that microalbuminuria and proteinuria are very strong risk factors for cardiovascular disease (38–40). A recent study by Barzilay et al. explored the association between microalbuminuria and cardiovascular disease in a group of patients with and without hypertension and diabetes, who were 65 years and older (41). They evaluated a wide range of variables including endothelial dysfunction and inflammatory markers in an effort to determine why there is a close association between microalbuminuria and cardiovascular disease. The results showed that there was a close correlation between microalbuminuria and cardiovascular disease with increasing age, inflammatory markers (such as c-reactive protein), and SBP. Interestingly, there was no correlation with endothelial dysfunction. These results underscore the importance of controlling BP and other approaches (blood glucose control and the use of ACE-Is and ARBs) in patients with microalbuminuria to reduce the risk of cardiovascular disease.

A variety of other factors affect the care of the elderly patient with diabetic nephropathy. Anemia has been shown to be an independent risk factor for progression of renal disease (42). Anemia starts to occur with increasing frequency with GFRs of <60 mL/min. Considering the loss of GFR with normal aging, many elderly patients with diabetic nephropathy will have GFRs of <60. Thus routine screening for anemia should be done. If anemia is detected, a standard anemia work-up should ensue and, if necessary, the administration of recombinant erythropoietin should be started. The current recommended range for hemoglobin is 11 to 12.5 g/dL. Thus therapy should be started if hemoglobin is <11 but it should be ensured that it does not go over 13, because much recent data show that there is increased mortality if the erythropoietin-induced increase in hemoglobin is >13. In addition to anemia, hyperparathyroidism is an often undiagnosed complication of kidney disease that increases in frequency with GFR of <60. Considering the high prevalence of osteoporosis in elderly patients, it is very important to measure parathyroid levels. Increased phosphate does not occur usually until stage 4 (GFR <29) or stage 5 (GFR <15) kidney disease. The hyperparathyroidism can be treated with 25-OH vitamin D if the patient's vitamin D level is low. If the level of 25-OH vitamin D is normal, the active form of vitamin D in the form of 1,25,dihydroxyvitamin D should be used for treatment (43). In addition, there are other factors to consider when deciding on medications for treating elderly patients. Elderly patients are likely to have other diseases such as cardiovascular disease. There is a higher risk of volume depletion in the elderly. There is a danger of polypharmacy or confusion in the proper intake of prescribed medications. There may be significant cost limitations for elderly patients due to fixed income or rules of health care insurance coverage. Lastly, there is an increased concern of side effects of medications. Thus all of these factors should be taken into account when deciding on a particular treatment regimen.

END-STAGE RENAL DISEASE

The confluence of general aging of the population and the worldwide epidemic of type 2 diabetes has led to a growing population of elderly diabetic patients with CKD and ESRD. In the United States, the most common etiology of CKD in the elderly population is diabetes. Diabetes and age are among the most significant risk factors for CKD (7), and when added to the World Health Organization global health risks associated with CKD (hypertension, obesity, and hypercholesterolemia), they represent a growing global burden. The management of the elderly patient with diabetes has goals and objectives that are different from those for other patients (44). Nonetheless, little attention has been focused on the elderly diabetic ESRD population, and most available data consider the elderly and diabetic populations separately (45).

Over the past quarter century, the fraction of patients with diabetic renal disease in the total population initiating dialysis in the United States has increased from about one-sixth to almost half, which is related to the epidemic of diabetics and the increased acceptance of diabetic patients into dialysis programs. Patients with diabetes as the primary causes of kidney failure now account for 45% of the incident (i.e., new) ESRD population annually, although the rate has decreased slightly in recent years (45). The rate of ESRD attributed to diabetes rose by 86% between 1993 and 2003, with a median age of 65 years, compared to the prevalent general ESRD population of 58 years. In comparison, the rates of new ESRD due to diabetes appears to be falling in the subgroups of younger white patients and has stabilized in blacks in the age group 20 to 29 years (45). Up to a third of patients with type 2 diabetes will develop ESRD and require renal replacement therapy for survival (46). Globally, Malaysia, Mexico, and the United States have the highest percentage of incident ESRD patients with diabetes. Diabetes is responsible for half of all ESRD cases in New Zealand and Singapore, and is the fastest growing etiology of ESRD in Europe (47).

Over a similar time span, aging trends in the United States have resulted in elderly patients in the general population becoming the fastest growing segment requiring renal replacement therapy (48). The elderly now account for three times more of the prevalent dialysis population than 25 years ago (45). The incidence of ESRD increases with advancing age (49). In the late 1970s, the mean age for the dialysis population was 50.6 years; the average age of the incident-ESRD population in 2003 was nearly 65 years, reflecting a growth rate nearly three times that of the ESRD population as a whole. While the largest proportion of new dialysis patients continues to be in the 45 to 64 year age group, those 75 years or older have surpassed the 65 to 74 year old age group. In a report from Canada, 16% of new dialysis patients were over the age of 75 years (50).

The greatest increase is occurring among the oldest patients according to the latest U.S. Renal Data System report (45). The elderly comprised 27% of new hemodialysis patients in the United States in 2003, and almost a quarter (65,396 patients) of the total on dialysis. In particular, the incidence and prevalence rates for elderly patients with ESRD secondary to diabetes mellitus continues to rise (Fig. 1). This trend for individuals with ESRD, similar to that for diabetic ESRD, is attributed to a growing population of the elderly and a willingness of providers to initiate renal replacement therapy (48).

It follows that the same trends apply when advanced age and diabetes coexist. There was a 35% increase in adults over 75 years of age with diabetes from 1991 to 2000, but it was far surpassed by a 194% increase in new ESRD annually in that population. There are also large numbers of older adults with undiagnosed diabetes. Similar growth has been reported from Europe (51). Diabetes was present in 37% of elderly ESRD patients in Canada (50).

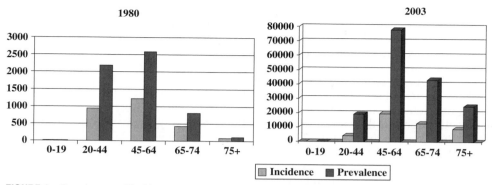

FIGURE 1   Prevalence and incidence of end stage renal disease in patients with diabetes by age group, years 1980 and 2003, in the United States.

   This growing population represents unique challenges in management. Many carry five or more comorbid conditions, including ischemic heart disease, congestive heart failure, and peripheral vascular disease. Cardiovascular disease develops in over 90% of elderly diabetic patients prior to starting dialysis (45). Age and diabetes are risk factors for vascular calcification evident on plain X rays (52). Diabetic ESRD is also associated with increased risk of dementia (53), especially due to vascular disease, leading to adverse outcomes. Patients have hearing and visual disabilities, have coexisting cognitive (54) and psychiatric disorders, frequently require nursing home care or assisted living (55), and may be unwilling or unable to comply with their proposed treatment (56). Elderly hemodialysis patients have a higher incidence of postdialysis hypotension (57), likely made worse by diabetic neuropathy. Both elderly and diabetic patients are less likely to have an arteriovenous fistula, the dialysis access recommended to cause fewer complications (45).
   Achievement of ADA clinical practice recommendations for glycemic control has been far from optimal in the general population (12). Glycemic management is an integral part of medical therapy for the diabetic ESRD patient, but data on the combined goals of optimizing outcomes while minimizing complications are lacking. The geriatric ESRD population may be less likely to benefit from tight control of asymptomatic hyperglycemia, and more likely to suffer adverse effects of hypoglycemia (58). There is broad agreement that symptomatic hyperglycemia should be treated in older patients. However, uncontrolled hyperglycemia in the elderly decreases cognition, functional status, and pain tolerance (55), while increasing injurious falls, nocturia, incontinence, pressure ulcers, and orthostatic hypotension (59). In ESRD, uncontrolled hyperglycemia may produce fluid overload, infection, hyperkalemia, ketoacidosis, may be harmful to endothelial function, and may contribute to atherosclerotic plaque formation directly. Several factors impacting on glycemic management in the presence of ESRD are known to exist, including effects of uremia and the dialysis procedure on insulin and carbohydrate metabolism, pharmacokinetic effects on insulin and oral hypoglycemic agents, and possible effects on the standard laboratory tests for HbA1c (60). Insulin resistance is the dominant effect of uremia on carbohydrate metabolism, unrelated to underlying diabetes, due to a postreceptor defect in insulin action. In addition, insulin secretion is impaired in renal failure, further offsetting the reduced renal insulin clearance. Nonetheless, the need for exogenous insulin may be reduced or sometimes eliminated in the diabetic patient with renal failure. Severe hypoglycemic reactions may occur after treatment with oral hypoglycemic agents, particularly sulfonylureas. Interpretation of glycosylated hemoglobin in kidney failure must take into account the presence of labile changes in blood glucose, the reduced erythrocyte life span in uremia, and false elevations of HbA1c by older techniques using electrical charge to separate hemoglobin fractions (60).
   Monitoring of glycemic control in diabetic ESRD remains far below recommended levels, although specific data on the elderly are not available. While the percent of patients receiving the four HbA1c tests per year, as recommended by ADA guidelines, has increased significantly

from the past decade, fewer than half obtain complete l testing (45). But even though there has been an overall increase in blood glucose monitoring there are still many deficiencies in testing in ESRD patients as follows. Three-quarters of diabetic ESRD patients are not prescribed any diabetic test strips. Over one-third receive no lipid testing at all, and fewer than a quarter receive the minimum goals of one A1c, one lipid test, and one diabetic test strip (45). Nearly two-thirds of diabetic ESRD patients receive insulin therapy, twice that of the non-ESRD population (12). By comparison, the use of secretagogue agents and thiazolidinediones is less common, while metformin, contraindicated in patients with high creatinine levels, is rarely used.

We recently reported the largest analysis of the benefit of glycemic control in diabetic ESRD. Half of type 1 and a third of type 2 ESRD patients were above the ADA glycemic HbA1c goal of 7% (60). Glycohemoglobin levels correlated only roughly with mean random blood glucose measurements, but appeared similar to the Diabetes Control and Complications Trial results. The study found no correlation between HbA1c levels and subsequent 12-month mortality risk. Clinical practice recommendations by the ADA acknowledge individual differences in the risks and benefits of glycemic control. Age, comorbidities, life expectancy, and the risk of hypoglycemia may affect diabetic ESRD glycemic targets. Older persons are at higher risk for drug-associated hypoglycemia (61) and have decreased symptom recognition, worse cognitive impairment, and attenuated physiologic counter-regulatory responses (62). The failure of these data to demonstrate the benefit of tight glycemic control may add to controversy regarding an aggressive glycemic control strategy in elderly diabetic ESRD patients. For those with limited levels of care, that is, reduced life expectancy, and functional and cognitive impairment, incapable of implementing a tight control program, with poor social support or dependent on nursing home care, treatment of symptomatic hyperglycemia may be indicated. Other elderly diabetics with ESRD may merit the more aggressive approach used in younger patients, to further prevent the chronic complications of diabetes.

TRANSPLANTATION

Historically, advanced age has been a relative contraindication for kidney transplantation, because of the limited life expectancy and additional risk of short- and long-term morbidity and mortality (63,64), issues more broadly involving appropriateness of care in the elderly. Since the introduction of transplant cyclosporine, more elderly (>60 years old) patients have undergone successful renal transplantation. The increasing numbers of elderly diabetic patients with ESRD raises significant questions regarding options for renal replacement therapy (49), similar to those raised in the past for diabetic ESRD needing dialysis, and more recently for elderly patients without diabetes seeking transplantation. The number of elderly patients on waiting lists for kidney transplantation began to increase in the 1990s, and transplant outcomes in the elderly improved over a 15-year period (51).

Kidney transplantation is the best treatment for ESRD candidates, including those with diabetes (60) who are now routinely transplanted. However, the percentage of transplanted patients with diabetes is much lower (23%) than that of patients on dialysis who have diabetes. Over the last two decades, renal transplantation for type 1 diabetes has become widely accepted (65). In the United States currently, about half of diabetic recipients now have type 2 diabetes (66). Outcomes remain less favorable for diabetic than for nondiabetic patients (67). Kidney transplantation does not improve other micro- or macrovascular complications of diabetes. Although elderly ESRD patients are not exempted from transplantation, controversy exists because of shorter life expectancy, higher comorbidity rates, and allocation in the context of relative organ shortages (48). Outcome data in the elderly generally refer to those recipients over 60 years old, in whom those selected for transplantation have relatively good short-term graft and patient survival (45). Older recipient age is more commonly associated with death, with a functioning graft (as opposed to failure of the transplant) as the major cause of graft loss (68). Also noted are decreased initial function and delayed graft function (18). Fewer elderly patients receive living-donor kidneys. Specific predictors of poor outcomes in the elderly include higher cardiovascular comorbidity, longer pretransplant dialysis period, and obesity. The number of elderly diabetic recipients has risen steadily (45), with no outcome data separately reported. In Europe, older recipients have less access to kidney transplantation if they are diabetic (69).

No renal transplants were performed in ESRD patients over 75 years old in a single center report from Canada (50). Whether an upper age limit should exist for no longer considering elderly diabetic CKD/ESRD patients as recipient candidates remains uncertain (18).

CARDIOVASCULAR DISEASE IN ESRD

Coronary artery disease (CAD) risk is magnified in both diabetes mellitus and ESRD (70). In ESRD, the relative risk of dying from cardiac causes is higher by a factor of 10 than in the general population. Cardiovascular deaths account for almost three-quarters of deaths in diabetic patients, almost all due to CAD. Diabetic ESRD is the highest-risk group for cardiac death (70). Yet, the increase in cardiovascular events in both diabetes and ESRD appears to derive only partly from conventional risk factors such as hypertension and dyslipidemia (71). Enhanced platelet activity, inflammation, hypercoagulability, and endothelial dysfunction in diabetes, and anemia and disordered mineral metabolism in ESRD have been consistently shown as nontraditional risk factors. Furthermore, diabetes and ESRD are both precursors of accelerated vascular calcification, involving coronary arteries, which may correlate with occlusive coronary disease. ESRD is associated with higher death rates after all types of coronary revascularization. While the number of diabetic ESRD patients at risk for CAD continues to grow, optimal CAD treatment remains uncertain. Both ESRD and diabetes are associated with poorer outcomes from percutaneous coronary interventions as well as coronary bypass surgery. Diabetes roughly doubles the incidence of restenosis after percutaneous angioplasty, rendering the procedure less effective than in the general population. Recent advances in coronary stenting and antiplatelet therapy have led to a growing number of previous percutaneous intervention candidates being treated with stents. The majority of all coronary interventional procedures in the United States now include drug-eluting stents, with sirolimus- or paclitaxel-coated stents. Each agent reduces in-stent stenosis in CAD. However, diabetic patients do remain at relatively high risk, and there is little data on drug-eluting stents in the ESRD population. Advances in adjunctive therapy include the use of more potent antiplatelet therapy and antithrombotic therapy, such as abciximab (a monoclonal antibody against the platelet glycoprotein IIb/IIIa receptor), and clopidrogel, which inhibits ADP-induced platelet aggregation. However, their use poses the potential risk of hemorrhage in elderly ESRD patients. Percutaneous interventions are currently preferred for those with one- or two-vessel disease and preserved left ventricular function. Elderly diabetic ESRD patients will also be at high risk for operative management of left main or multivessel disease, in which case medical therapy might be preferred.

ESRD OUTCOMES

Although diabetic ESRD patients have experienced significant improvement in survival compared to those with other primary diagnoses, they still have the greatest morbidity and lowest survival related to cardiovascular disease, peripheral vascular disease, and infection. The five-year survival rate has risen from 27% to 34% in recent years (45). The highest hospitalization rates are seen in diabetic and older patients. Age is also a powerful predictor of mortality risk. In the elderly, mortality rates worsen with kidney disease more than in other groups. In the general U.S. population, persons aged 75 to 79 have an expected remaining life duration of 10.4 years; for the elderly ESRD patient, it is 2.6 years (45), and in the presence of diabetes, at least 25% less. Some recent studies have reported higher mortality risks for elderly diabetic females on peritoneal dialysis compared to those on hemodialysis. Mortality rates for diabetic and nondiabetic ESRD patients worsen with increasing age (Fig. 2). Cardiac disease remains the single largest cause of mortality. Medicare data indicate a significant effect of diabetes, age, and cardiovascular disease on survival (45). Coronary revascularization procedure rates continue to increase, particularly the use of coronary stents. Older diabetic dialysis patients have a higher incidence of vertebral fracture than nondiabetic ones (72). ESRD costs for diabetic patients exceed those for nondiabetic patients by 15% to 30%, averaging $68,000 annually (45), and total annual medical expenditures are at least 64% higher in diabetic ESRD. Medical costs also rise with advancing age.

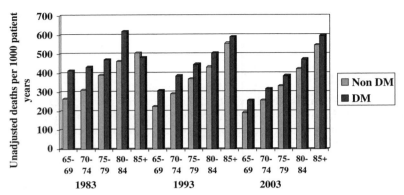

FIGURE 2 Mortality rates for diabetic and nondiabetic patients vary with age.

SCREENING

Screen for the presence of diabetic kidney disease by measuring urine albumin/creatinine ratio and by calculating estimated GFR, using the serum creatinine and the MDRD formula.

1. If urine albumin is elevated, then there is an increased risk of cardiovascular disease and progression of kidney disease. Treat to reduce urine albumin levels by blood glucose control, lowering BP, and by using ACE-Is and/or ARBs.
2. If GFR is lower than expected by aging, then be sure to evaluate for nondiabetic kidney diseases primarily by taking a complete history, evaluating appropriate labs, doing a careful urinalysis, and possibly obtaining radiographic imaging (e.g., renal ultrasound and/or MRI/MRA). A kidney biopsy is rarely needed. If no other kidney diseases are found, then the patient has diabetic kidney disease and more aggressive approaches to management are indicated, such as achieving as low a HbA1c as is reasonable for the patient, lowering BP with a goal of <130/80, and reduction in urine albumin (or total protein level) by adding ACE-Is and/or ARBs.

Remember that the expected GFR is about 100 mL/min/yr at age 40, and the average rate of decline is about 1 mL/min/yr. Thus geriatric patients, depending on age, could well have GFRs <60 due to aging alone. It is very important to remember that whatever the reason for decreased GFR (normal aging or disease), if the GFR is <60, then there is an increased likelihood for having complications of kidney disease such as anemia and hyperparathyroidism.

Guidelines for referral to a nephrologist (from Joslin Guidelines):

1. GFR < 60 mL/min
2. Urine albumin/creatinine ratio > 300 or urine protein/creatinine ratio > 0.5
3. Rapid rise in serum creatinine, abnormal urine sediment, or sudden increase in proteinuria
4. Refinement of renal treatment program needed to prevent further deterioration
5. Problems with ACE-Is or ARBs, difficulties in management of high BP, or hyperkalemia
6. If questioning etiology of kidney failure
7. Anemia
8. Hyperparathyroidism and/or hyperphosphatemia

CONCLUSION

The treatment of diabetic nephropathy in the elderly is based mostly on data from younger age groups. With the population living longer, there is a growing need for studies focused on the elderly population. The assumption that the treatment approaches in the younger age groups applies to the elderly may well be wrong. Nevertheless, until these studies are done, it is prudent to treat the elderly patient with the same approach that one would adopt for a younger patient, tempered by the issues already discussed in the chapter.

REFERENCES

1. Kuo S, et al. Trends in care practices and outcomes among Medicare beneficiaries with diabetes. Am J Prev Med 2005; 29(5):396–403.
2. Zimmet P, Alberti KG, Shaw J. Global and societal implications of the diabetes epidemic. Nature 2001; 414(6865):782–787.
3. Edwards MS, et al. Associations between retinal microvascular abnormalities and declining renal function in the elderly population: the Cardiovascular Health Study. Am J Kid Dis 2005; 46(2): 214–224.
4. Fagot-Campagna A, Bourdel-Marchasson I, Simon D. Burden of diabetes in an aging population: prevalence, incidence, mortality, characteristics and quality of care. Diabetes Metab 2005; 31(2): 5S35–5S52.
5. Jemal A, et al. Trends in the leading causes of death in the United States 1970–2002. JAMA 2005; 294(10):1255–1259.
6. Harris MI, et al. Prevalence of diabetes and impaired glucose tolerance and plasma glucose levels in U.S. population aged 20–74 yr. Diabetes 1987; 36(4):523–534.
7. White SL, et al. Chronic kidney disease in the general population. Adv Chronic Kid Dis 2005; 12(1):5–13.
8. Wasen E, et al. Renal impairment associated with diabetes in the elderly. Diabetes Care 2004; 27(11):2648–2653.
9. Coresh J, et al. Prevalence of chronic kidney disease and decreased kidney function in the adult US population: Third National Health and Nutrition Examination Survey. Am J Kid Dis 2003; 41(1):1–12.
10. Kausz AT. Chronic kidney disease in the older paient. Clin Geriat 2004; 12:39–47.
11. Patel UD, et al. CKD progression and mortality among older patients with diabetes. Am J Kid Dis 2005; 46(3):406–414.
12. Resnick HE, et al. Achievement of American Diabetes Association clinical practice recommendations among U.S. adults with diabetes 1999–2002: the National Health and Nutrition Examination Survey. Diabetes Care 2006; 29(3):531–537.
13. K/DOQI, K/DOQI clinical practice guidelines for chronic kidney disease. Am J Kid Dis 2002; 39(2): S1–S266.
14. Winkelmayer WC, et al. Determinants of delayed nephrologist referral in patients with chronic kidney disease. Am J Kid Dis 2001; 38(6):1178–1184.
15. Kausz AT, et al. General medical care among patients with chronic kidney disease: opportunities for improving outcomes. J Am Soc Nephrol 2005; 16(10):3092–3101.
16. Lee SJ, et al. Development and validation of a prognostic index for 4-year mortality in older adults. JAMA 2006; 295(7):801–808.
17. Rodriguez-Puyol D. The aging kidney. Kid Int 1998; 54(6):2247–2265.
18. Baid-Agrawal S, et al. WCN 2003 satellite symposium on kidney transplantation in the elderly, Weimar, Germany, June 12–14, 2003. Nephrol Dial Transplant 2004; 19(1):43–46.
19. Adler S. Diabetic nephropathy: linking histology, cell biology, and genetics. Kid Int 2004; 66(5): 2095–2106.
20. Rimon E, et al. Can creatinine clearance be accurately predicted by formulae in octogenarian in-patients? QJM 2004; 97(5):281–287.
21. Davies D, Shock N. Age changes in glomerular filtration rate, effective renal plasma flow, and tubular excretory capacity in adult males. J Clin Invest 1950; 29(5):496–507.
22. Premaratne E, et al. Renal hyperfiltration in type 2 diabetes: effect of age-related decline in glomerular filtration rate. Diabetologia 2005; 48(12):2486–2493.
23. Corsonello A, et al. Concealed renal failure and adverse drug reactions in older patients with type 2 diabetes mellitus. J Gerontol A Biol Sci Med Sci 2005; 60(9):1147–1151.
24. Kampmann J, et al. Rapid evaluation of creatinine clearance. Acta Med Scand 1974; 196(6):517–520.
25. Nair R, Bell JM, Walker PD. Renal biopsy in patients aged 80 years and older. Am J Kid Dis 2004; 44(4):618–626.
26. Lewis J, et al. Comparison of cross-sectional renal function measurements in African Americans with hypertensive nephrosclerosis and of primary formulas to estimate glomerular filtration rate. Am J Kid Dis 2001; 38(4):744–753.
27. Rigalleau V, et al. Estimation of glomerular filtration rate in diabetic subjects: Cockcroft formula or modification of Diet in Renal Disease study equation? Diabet Care 2005; 28(4):838–843.

28. Wasen E, et al. Estimation of glomerular filtration rate in the elderly: a comparison of creatinine-based formulae with serum cystatin C. J Intern Med 2004; 256(1):70–78.

29. Knight EL, et al. Factors influencing serum cystatin C levels other than renal function and the impact on renal function measurement. Kid Int 2004; 65(4):1416–1421.

30. Burkhardt H, et al. Creatinine clearance, Cockcroft-Gault formula and cystatin C: estimators of true glomerular filtration rate in the elderly? Gerontology 2002; 48(3):140–146.

31. Joss N, et al. Intensified treatment of patients with type 2 diabetes mellitus and overt nephropathy. Quart J Med 2004; 97(4):219–227.

32. Young J, et al. Blood pressure and decline in kidney function: findings from the systolic hypertension in the elderly program (SHEP). J Am Soc Nephrol 2002; 13(11):2776–2782.

33. Lewis E, et al. The effect of angiotensin-converting-enzyme inhibition on diabetic nephropathy 1993; 329:1456–1462.

34. Brenner B, et al. Effects of losartan on renal and cardiovascular outcomes in patients with type 2 diabetes and nephropathy. N Engl J Med 2001; 345:861–869.

35. Lewis E, et al. Renoprotective effect of the angiotensin-receptor antagonist irbesartan in patients with nephropathy due to type 2 diabetes. N Engl J Med 2001; 345:851–860.

36. Winkelmayer W, et al. Underuse of ACE Inhibitors and angiotensin II receptor blockers in elderly patients with diabetes. Am J Kid Dis 2005; 46(6):1080–1087.

37. Rosen A, et al. Use of angiotensin-converting enzyme inhibitors and angiotensin receptor blockers in high-risk clinical and ethnic groups with diabetes. J Gen Int Med 2004; 19:669–675.

38. Basi S, Lewis J. Microalbuminuria as a target to improve cardiovascular and renal outcomes. Am J Kid Dis 2006; 47(6):927–946.

39. Borch-Johnsen K, et al. Urinary albumin excretion: an independent predictor of ischemic heart disease. Arterioscler Thromb Vasc Biol 1996; 19:1992–1997.

40. Miettinen H, et al. Proteinuria predicts stroke and other atherosclerotic vascular disease events in nondiabetic and non–insulin-dependent diabetic subjects. Stroke 1996; 27:2033–2039.

41. Barzilay J, et al. The relationship of cardiovascular risk factors to microalbuminuria in older adults with or without diabetes mellitus or hypertension: the cardiovascular health study. Am J Kid Dis 2004; 44(1):25–34.

42. Mohanram A, et al. Anemia and end-stage renal disease in patients with type 2 diabetes and nephropathy. Kid Int 2004; 66(3):1131–1138.

43. K/DOQI, K/DOQI clinical practice guidelines for bone metabolism and disease in chronic kidney disease. Am J Kid Dis 2003; 42(suppl 3–4):S1–S201.

44. Chau DL, Shumaker N, Plodkowski A. Complications of type 2 diabetes in the elderly. Geriat Times 2003; 4(2).

45. U.S. Renal Data System, 2005. Annual Data Report 2005. Bethesda, Maryland.

46. Keane WF, Lyle PA. Recent advances in management of type 2 diabetes and nephropathy: lessons from the RENAAL study. Am J Kid Dis 2003; 41(3 suppl 1):S22–S25.

47. Reggenenti P, Schieppati A, Remuzzi G. Progression, remission, regression of chronic renal diseases. Lancet 2001; 357:1601–1608.

48. Hansberry MR, Whittier WL, Krause MW. The elderly patient with chronic kidney disease. Adv Chronic Kid Dis 2005; 12(1):71–77.

49. Nunes P, et al. Do elderly patients deserve a kidney graft? Transplant Proc 2005; 37(6):2737–2742.

50. Letourneau I, et al. Renal replacement in end-stage renal disease patients over 75 years old. Am J Nephrol 2003; 23(2):71–77.

51. Jager KJ, et al. The epidemic of aging in renal replacement therapy: an update on elderly patients and their outcomes. Clin Nephrol 2003; 60(5):352–360.

52. Al Humoud H, et al. Vascular calcification in dialysis patients. Transplant Proc 2005; 37(10): 4183–4186.

53. Kurella M, et al. Chronic kidney disease and cognitive impairment in the elderly: the health, aging, and body composition study. J Am Soc Nephrol 2005; 16(7):2127–2133.

54. Joly D. Dialysis therapy for end stage renal disease in octogenarians. Rev Prat 2005; 55(20): 2255–2262.

55. Mooradian AD, et al. Diabetes mellitus in elderly nursing home patients. A survey of clinical characteristics and management. J Am Geriatr Soc 1988; 36(5):391–396.

56. Halter JB. Geriatric patients. In: Lebovitz HE, ed. Therapy for Diabetes Mellitus and Related Disorders. Alexandria, VA: American Diabetes Association, 1998:234–240.

57. Roberts RG, Kenny RA, Brierley EJ. Are elderly haemodialysis patients at risk of falls and postural hypotension? Int Urol Nephrol 2003; 35(3):415–421.

58. Alam T, Weintraub N, Weinreb J. What is the proper use of hemoglobin A1c monitoring in the elderly? J Am Med Dir Assoc 2006; 7(3 suppl):S60–S4, S59.

59. Morley JE. An overview of diabetes mellitus in older persons. Clin Geriatr Med 1999; 15(2):211–224.

60. Williams ME. Management of the diabetic transplant recipient. Kid Int 1995; 48(5):1660–1674.

61. Shorr RI, et al. Incidence and risk factors for serious hypoglycemia in older persons using insulin or sulfonylureas. Arch Intern Med 1997; 157(15):1681–1686.

62. Matyka K, et al. Altered hierarchy of protective responses against severe hypoglycemia in normal aging in healthy men. Diabet Care 1997; 20(2):135–141.
63. Pirsch J, Stratta R, Armbrust M. Cadaveric renal transplantation with cyclosporine in patients more than 60 years of age. Transplantation 1989; 47:259–261.
64. Stratta R, et al. Cadaveric renal transplantation with quadruple immunosuppression in patients with a positive antiglobulin crossmatch. Transplantation 1989; 47(2):282–286.
65. Fernandez-Fresnedo G, et al. Significance of age in the survival of diabetic patients after kidney transplantation. Int Urol Nephrol 2002; 33(1):173–177.
66. Becker BN, et al. Preemptive transplantation for patients with diabetes-related kidney disease. Arch Intern Med 2006; 166(1):44–48.
67. Wolfe RA, et al. Comparison of mortality in all patients on dialysis, patients on dialysis awaiting transplantation, and recipients of a first cadaveric transplant. N Engl J Med 1999; 341(23):1725–1730.
68. Siddiqi N, McBride MA, Hariharan S. Similar risk profiles for post-transplant renal dysfunction and long-term graft failure: UNOS/OPTN database analysis. Kid Int 2004; 65(5):1906–1913.
69. Van Dijk PC, et al. Renal replacement therapy for diabetic end-stage renal disease: data from 10 registries in Europe (1991–2000). Kid Int 2005; 67(4):1489–1499.
70. Williams M. Coronary revascularization in diabetic chronic kidney disease/endstage renal disease. Clin J Am Soc Nephrol 2006; 1:209–220.
71. Peterson J, Harrington R. Revascularization of coronary atherosclerosis in patients with diabetes mellitus—There is more to it than meets the image intensifier. Am Heart J 2005; 149(190–193).
72. Inaba M, et al. Increased incidence of vertebral fracture in older female hemodialyzed patients with type 2 diabetes mellitus. Calcif Tissue Int 2005; 76(4):256–260.

16 | Diabetic Neuropathy

Peter Novak
Department of Neurology, Boston University Medical Center, Boston, Massachusetts, U.S.A.

Vera Novak
Division of Gerontology, Department of Medicine, Beth Israel Deaconess Medical Center, Harvard Medical School, Boston, Massachusetts, U.S.A.

INTRODUCTION

Diabetic neuropathy is the most common complication of diabetes, but its incidence and prevalence remain unclear. The uncertainty can be in part attributed to differences in methodologies and diagnostic criteria, sensitivity and specificity of diagnostic testing, and lack of systematic prospective studies. Over 60% of people with diabetes are affected with neuropathy and those with pain can become seriously disabled due to lack of effective treatment, which stems from lack of understanding of mechanisms underlying this condition. Diabetic autonomic neuropathy has been associated with increased risk of cardiovascular complications in older adults, and orthostatic hypotension (OH) is an independent predictor of adverse outcomes in elderly people. The prevalence of diabetic autonomic neuropathy varies in the literature, and diagnosis in the geriatric population is often complicated by age-related changes in the autonomic nervous system and multiple comorbidities.

PERIPHERAL AND AUTONOMIC NEUROPATHIES ASSOCIATED WITH DIABETES AND THEIR UNIQUE PRESENTATION IN ELDERLY PEOPLE
Epidemiology

Reports of the prevalence of neuropathy in the American population range from 1.6% up to 80% (1), with an estimated prevalence of 66% for insulin-dependent diabetes (IDDM) and 59% for noninsulin-dependent diabetes (NIDDM) (2). In 1998, a joint committee of the American Diabetes Association and American Academy of Neurology adopted standardized criteria for diagnosis of neuropathy in diabetes (3). Subclinical neuropathy is defined as abnormal electrophysiological testing (decreased nerve conduction velocity and decreased amplitude of evoked muscle and nerve action potentials), quantitative sensory thresholds (for vibration, warming, and cooling), and autonomic function tests (abnormal cardiovascular reflexes, abnormal biochemical responses to hypoglycemia), without clinical symptoms. Clinical neuropathy is defined as a combination of symptomatology and abnormal tests or as symptoms alone plus abnormal test results (4). In the elderly population, the prevalence of peripheral diabetic neuropathy is even more likely to be underestimated due to age-related nerve conduction deficits and distal small- and large-fiber neuropathies. The diagnosis of autonomic neuropathy in the elderly population is also often precluded by multiple comorbidities, age-associated symptoms of autonomic dysfunction, and adverse effects of polypharmacy.

The Rochester Diabetic Neuropathy Study is a population-based, cross-sectional study of diabetic neuropathy with longitudinal follow-up (2,5) that used surveys and quantitative evaluations to diagnose neuropathy and to determine its severity. Of the 380 participants, 26.8% had IDDM and 59% had NIDDM. Neuropathy was found in 60.4% participants, and prevalence was higher in IDDM (66%) than in NIDDM (59%) participants. The most prevalent was distal polyneuropathy (47.3%), followed by carpal tunnel syndrome (31.7%), and autonomic neuropathy (4.8%). Almost all participants were white, reflecting the demographic distribution of Rochester, Minnesota, and thus limiting the study. Elderly people >75 years of age, less-educated people, and those with comorbidities were more likely to be nonparticipants. Age is another important predictor of diabetic neuropathy. Studies in populations >70 years of age, however, remain limited.

The San Luis Valley study that was geographically based in southern Colorado counties was a case–control survey-based study of NIDDM between 1984 and 1986 (6,7). Neuropathy diagnosis was based on bilateral symptoms and bilateral abnormal jerk reflexes and increased cold perception threshold, confirmed by the measurements of an increased vibration threshold. A history of neuropathy accompanied by abnormal jerk reflexes was found in 81%, abnormal reflexes in 10%, and abnormal cold temperature threshold alone in 6% of participants. The prevalence of distal symmetric neuropathy increased significantly with age: 10.3% at 20 to 44 years, 28% at 45 to 64 years, and 32% at 65 to 74 years. The association between impaired glucose tolerance and neuropathy was stronger in young (13%) and middle-aged (14%) groups than in elderly people (5%). Diabetes duration was one of the most important determinants of neuropathy. The prevalence of neuropathy doubled from 16.8% to 33.3% for 10-year disease duration and to 52.6% for those with diabetes duration >25 years.

The 1989 National Health Interview Survey was a population-based interview survey (8) that sampled 2405 subjects with diabetes and compared them with 20,037 subjects without a physician's diagnosis of diabetes. The prevalence of neuropathy was 30.2% for IDDM and 39.7% for NIDDM. In addition to age effect, diabetes duration and history of hypertension increased the risk of neuropathy symptoms by 60%. It is of interest that a recent study of painful nondiabetic small-fiber neuropathy also identified that severity of neuropathy symptoms (small-fiber loss on skin biopsies) and autonomic symptoms (distal loss of sweating and reduced heart-rate variability) were associated with age and that hypertension was the most common comorbidity (9). These findings suggest that an increased prevalence of neuropathy and hypertension with age may share common mechanisms that promote length-dependent cholinergic small-fiber degeneration. The 1999–2002 National Health and Nutrition Survey revisited a previously reported observation that diabetic neuropathy is more prevalent in Hispanic compared to non-Hispanic populations. A survey of 2696 people more than 18 years of age showed that Hispanics with low language acculturation were more likely to have diabetes (odds ratio 1.90, 95% confidence interval 1.02–3.54) and peripheral neuropathy (odds ratio 4.01, 1.40–11.48), after controlling for health insurance and education (10).

Etiology

The pathophysiology of diabetic neuropathy is multifactorial, and a comprehensive theory is still lacking. Chronic hyperglycemia is the most common pathway for diabetic neuropathy and tissue damage. Several factors have been recognized to play a role in the pathogenesis of diabetic neuropathy, such as metabolism, vascular insufficiency, autoimmune destruction of small unmyelinated nerves (C fibers) in a visceral and cutaneous distribution, oxidative stress, and inflammation. The association between the reduction of endogenous concentrations of nerve growth factor and neuropathy has received more attention. The two main features that explain clinical manifestations and complications of diabetic neuropathy are nerve fiber degeneration and microvascular disease. Endothelial cells and neurons are particularly sensitive to the effects of hyperglycemia. Glucose utilization requires metabolism, and ultimately oxidation to carbon dioxide and water to provide adenosine triphosphate and high-energy equivalents (11). Chronic hyperglycemia triggers a cascade of events that leads to accumulation of metabolites of the polyol pathway and a depletion of myoinositol. Signaling of oxidative stress (12,13) in mitochondria and the endoplasmic reticulum triggers an inflammatory response through the release of proinflammatory cytokines including tumor necrosis factor-α, endothelin 1, and interleukins (1–6), and a decreased synthesis of nitric oxide. This cascade leads to the activation of proapoptotic pathways, and ultimately to endothelial cell and neuronal damage and death. Small- and large-nerve fiber impairment seems to develop in parallel with progression of microangiopathy. Impairment of vasomotor and sudomotor functions and lower muscle action potentials appear to coincide with the degree and severity of microangiopathy (14).

Clinical Manifestations

Diabetic neuropathy affects all types of peripheral nerves including somatic (motor and sensory) and autonomic in practically all organ systems. Clinical manifestations can substantially vary from subject to subject. The neuropathy can be progressive or have a monophasic course, can be symmetrical or asymmetrical, and can have positive or negative symptoms. Symptoms can range from none to disabling.

Sensory Symptoms

Sensory symptoms can be positive or negative. Positive symptoms include burning, tingling and itching sensations, hyperesthesia, and pain. Pain may have an insidious onset, with gradual progression, for example, in small-fiber neuropathy, or an abrupt onset of severe pain that is seen in entrapment neuropathies such as carpal tunnel syndrome or diabetic truncal radiculopathy and plexopathies. Symptoms follow the distribution of affected nerves and plexus. Negative symptoms include distal sensory loss and reduced sensation of warm and cold. Distal sensory loss in the feet is a known risk factor for foot ulcers and leg amputations. Visual symptoms that include loss of visual acuity and diminished accommodation and adaptation to dark are important causes of disability in elderly people.

Motor Symptoms

Motor symptoms include muscle weakness distal to nerve injury and may affect signal muscles or muscle groups. Muscle weakness follows pain and the onset may be sudden or may progress over weeks or months. Typical presentations that are dependent on the affected nerves or plexus are described below.

Autonomic Symptoms

Diabetic autonomic neuropathy affects almost all organ systems with numerous presenting symptoms.

Cardiac Autonomic Neuropathy

Cardiac autonomic neuropathy results from the impairment of cardiac–vagal innervation affecting beat-to-beat heart-rate regulation and cardiac reflexes. Heart-rate responses to deep breathing using time-domain and frequency-domain analyses are the most widely used tests for evaluation of cardiac–vagal function. These tests have been validated and normative databases are available (15,16). The next most widely used and validated tests are the heart-rate response to the Valsalva maneuver (Valsalva ratio) and to standing up (30:15 ratio). The sensitivities of heart-rate responses to deep breathing and to the Valsalva maneuver are similar, but the deep breathing test is less dependent on patient cooperation. Reduced heart-rate variability and tachycardia are early presentations of cardiac autonomic neuropathy with diabetes. Other morbid symptoms indicating or resulting from cardiac denervation are sinus tachycardia $\cong 100$ bpm, orthostatic and exercise intolerance, heat intolerance, fainting, and "silent" painless myocardial infarction.

Sudomotor Function

Sympathetically mediated cholinergic small fibers mediate sweating response to heat and emotion. The pre- and postganglionic sudomotor response to a heat stimulus is evaluated by the thermoregulatory sweat test, and the postganglionic response to acetylcholine iontophoresis is evaluated by the quantitative sudomotor axon reflex test. Distal length-dependent loss of sweating is an early feature of diabetic autonomic neuropathy. Distal loss of sweating typically affects the feet and manifests more proximally with progression of neuropathy. Compensatory excessive sweating on the forehead and upper torso are often presenting symptoms of a more widespread sudomotor failure and anhidrosis. Other features include gustatory sweating, impaired skin vasodilatation, and shivering response. "Skin vasoconstrictor reflexes" are often impaired, indicating sympathetic vasoconstrictor failure.

Orthostatic Hypotension

OH is the most severe feature of autonomic neuropathy that develops with adrenergic denervation of mesenteric vascular beds and peripheral vasoconstrictor fibers. Orthostatic blood pressure declines are observed in 5% to 18% of healthy elderly people (17) and in as much as 30% of those over age 75 with multiple pathological conditions, particularly hypertension. Blood pressure fall >20 mmHg systolic or 10 mmHg diastolic within the first minute of standing may occur in up to 50% of elderly people (18). Recently, OH has been recognized as a risk factor for stroke in nursing-home residents (17,19). The true prevalence of OH with diabetic autonomic neuropathy is unknown. It can be as high as 35% to 45% in patients with a history of falls or dizziness (16,20).

It is not known if cerebral vasoregulation is impaired in diabetic autonomic neuropathy with OH. In the upright position, cerebral blood flow is maintained by peripheral vasodilatation. Cerebral hypoperfusion may develop if cerebral vasodilatation fails, or blood pressure falls below the autoregulated range. With impaired vasoregulation, cerebral blood flow declines even with a small change of blood pressure. It is not clear if cerebral vasodilatation is impaired in diabetes and whether it is effective enough to maintain cerebral blood flow. Results of transcranial Doppler studies in patients with OH indicate both normal (21) and abnormal autoregulation (22,23). However, these studies were not focused on diabetes and included different OH etiologies. Presenting symptoms in elderly people are often weakness, cognitive decline, headaches, falls, and, less frequently, dizziness. Postprandial vasodilatation in mesenteric beds aggravates OH, and the degree of mesenteric dilatation correlates with blood pressure decline after a meal (24).

The most prominent "gastrointestinal symptoms" are gastric atony and prolonged emptying, which affect up to 20% to 30% of diabetic patients. Nausea, early satiety, postprandial bloating, and epigastric pain are the most common complaints (25). "Diabetic diarrhea" and fecal incontinence are dramatic symptoms of intestinal neuropathy. Diarrhea is more frequent at nighttime, and can be sudden, explosive, seasonal, poorly controllable, and embarrassing, but it is usually self-limited and does not lead to malnutrition (26).

Impotence

Impotence in diabetic men is common and often the first presenting feature of autonomic neuropathy; partial impotence becomes complete within one to two years, when it usually becomes irreversible. The mechanism includes a combination of impaired neurogenic and sensory innervation to penile smooth muscle and the corpora cavernosa, and impaired endothelium-mediated vasodilatation (27). Retrograde ejaculation is uncommon but may occur in patients with severe autonomic failure. Female sexual dysfunction in diabetes (28) remains poorly understood, but may be mild or associated with infrequent orgasm.

Neurogenic Bladder and Cystopathy

Neurogenic bladder and cystopathy occur more frequently with longer diabetes duration and other complications of diabetes. Atonic bladder has a larger capacity, but lower intravesical pressure; consequently sensational response to bladder filling and urine volume during voluntary voiding are reduced, resulting in larger residual volume (16).

Diagnosis

A diagnosis of diabetic neuropathy should be considered in every patient with diabetes mellitus. It is recommended that all diabetes mellitus patients should be screened for neuropathy at least once a year (29).

Classifications

Several classifications have been suggested for diabetic neuropathy. We adopted the classification of Mendell et al. (30) (Table 1) since it can aid in diagnosis and treatment.

Diabetic Polyneuropathy

Diabetic polyneuropathy is a distal symmetric axonal polyneuropathy. It is the most common form of neuropathy in diabetes and affects sensory, motor, and autonomic nerves. Sensory findings develop in a characteristic stocking-glove distribution. Typical sensory presentation is numbness and tingling affecting the toes and later also the hands. Nerve conduction

TABLE 1 Neuropathy in Diabetes, Classification

Focal and multifocal (asymmetrical)		
Mononeuropathy	Cranial	III, IV, VI, VII nerves
	Truncal	
	Arms	Median, ulnar, radial, typically at entrapment points
	Legs	Peroneal, femoral, typically at entrapment points
Mononeuropathy multiplex	Affects two or more separate nerve areas	
Diabetic thoracolumbar radiculoneuropathy	Truncal neuropathy, abrupt or subacute onset of pain	
Diabetic lumbosacral radiculoplexus neuropathy	"Diabetic amyotrophy"	
Polyneuropathies (symmetrical)		
Diabetic polyneuropathy	Most common	
Acute painful neuropathy	Diabetic neuropathic cachexia	
Insulin neuritis	Painful neuropathy associated with onset of insulin treatment	

abnormalities follow a length-dependent pattern. Muscle weakness is mild and affects distal lower limbs, especially toe extensors and ankle dorsiflexors.

Cranial Neuropathies

Cranial neuropathies usually accompany diabetic polyneuropathy and rarely can be the initial manifestation of diabetic neuropathy. The third nerve palsy (diabetic opthalmoplegia) and the sixth nerve impairment are most frequent, especially in older patients. The seventh nerve is perhaps also frequently affected but differentiation from the common Bell's palsy is difficult. Diabetic opthalmoplegia is associated with a sudden onset of retro-orbital frontal, temporal, or hemicranial pain that within one to several days proceeds to opthalmoplegia that typically spares the pupil. In 50% of patients, the diabetic opthalmoplegia is painless. The pathology is an infarct of the third nerve in the cavernous sinus or small focal brainstem infarcts. Treatment is supportive; the prognosis is excellent, with expected full recovery in three to five months.

Peroneal Neuropathy

Peroneal neuropathy is a relative common form of diabetic mononeuropathy that results in a foot drop and is typically unilateral.

Mononeuropathy Multiplex

Mononeuropathy multiplex involves typically one or more peripheral nerve trunks and has been associated with vasculitis. It has typically a slower step-wise progression and multifocal sensory-motor abnormalities of the lower extremities. It is less common than diabetic polyneuropathy.

Diabetic Thoracolumbar (Truncal) Radiculoneuropathy

The truncal radiculopathy characteristically presents as severe truncal pain that can be unilateral or bilateral with a sudden or insidious onset (over days to weeks).

Diabetic Lumbosacral Radiculoplexus Neuropathy

Diabetic lumbosacral radiculoplexus neuropathy (DLRN) is asymmetrical, lower limb neuropathy that affects people over 50 years of age. The commonly used terms "diabetic amyotrophy" or "femoral neuropathy" are inaccurate, since DLRN affects both proximal and distal muscles. Men are more often affected than women, and there is no relation between DLRN and the duration of diabetes. DLRN presents typically with an abrupt pain in the back, buttocks, and anterior thighs. The pain presentation is an aching, burning, or knife-like sensation. Within days to weeks, the weakness becomes a prominent feature affecting hip, knees, and ankles. In some cases, the other leg becomes affected, beginning with pain that is followed by progressive weakness.

Acute Painful Neuropathy

Acute painful neuropathy, also called diabetic neuropathic cachexia, is a painful neuropathy associated with precipitous and severe weight loss. This entity can be a form of generalized diabetic polyneuropathy.

Insulin Neuritis

Insulin neuritis is a painful neuropathy probably induced by insulin treatment. It is unclear whether this is a separate form of neuropathy or a subset of painful neuropathies associated with diabetes.

Autonomic Neuropathy

Diabetic autonomic neuropathy is a generalized, length-dependent cholinergic and adrenergic neuropathy and may progress to autonomic failure. It affects up to 30% of diabetic patients and is associated with significant morbidity (16).

Painful Neuropathy

Small-fiber neuropathy is the most common cause of painful neuropathies. Although the pain is not the primary presentation of diabetic neuropathy, it can be severe and debilitating when present. The typical presentation of length-dependent small-fiber neuropathy is tactile hypersensitivity, burning, and tingling starting at the feet. Autonomic features that accompany small-fiber neuropathy such as cardiac–vagal impairment, secretory and skin vasomotor signs, hypertension, and impotence overlap with nondiabetic painful small-fiber neuropathies (9).

EFFECTS OF NEUROPATHY ON ACTIVITIES OF DAILY LIVING IN OLDER ADULTS

The duration and severity of chronic hyperglycemia are the most important factors that contribute to development of complications of diabetes in the eye, kidney, and cardiovascular and nervous system. "Diabetic retinopathy" remains the leading cause of "blindness," despite regular ocular exams and increased capabilities for screening. The prevalence of blindness ranges from 0.1% in subjects aged 55 to 64 years to 3.9% in subjects aged 85 years or older; the prevalence of visual impairment ranges from 0.1% to 11.8%. Myopic degeneration and optic neuropathy are the most important causes of impaired vision for patients less than 75 years old. For people older than 75 years, age-related macular degeneration is the major cause of blindness (31).

Lower-Extremity Disease

Lower-extremity disease that includes peripheral arterial disease and neuropathy affects 18.7% of the U.S. population and 30.2% of diabetic patients, and the prevalence increases steeply with age (32). Lower-limb amputations are the ultimate adverse outcomes of vascular disease, foot ulcers, and neuropathy in diabetic patients. Diabetic patients with lower-extremity amputations are older, have more comorbidities, and are more likely to belong to a minority group. Native Americans have the highest risks of amputations [relative risk (RR) 1.74], followed by African Americans (RR 1.41) and Hispanics (RR 1.28) compared to whites. Nephropathy further increases the risk of amputations (33). "Foot ulcers" remain a major challenge for elderly people with diabetes, despite educational programs and overall foot care. Progression of small-fiber neuropathies, in particular impairment of distal vasomotor and sudomotor functions, coincides with the propensity for foot ulcers. Notably, distal loss of sweating seems to be a sensitive indicator of increased risk for foot ulcers (14).

Gait, Balance, and Falls

Poor balance during standing in people with diabetes can be attributed to peripheral neuropathy, muscle weakness, joint stiffness, diminished proprioceptive feedback, and vision loss. The ability to compensate for postural body sway during quiet standing declines with age. People with diabetes have poorer balance when standing in diminished light compared to full light and no light conditions. When the room light was dimmed, sway during standing increased by an average of 25%. There is a significant negative correlation between balance and gait; the worse the balance, the slower and poorer the gait, compared to nondiabetic controls (34). Diabetic peripheral neuropathy has profound effects on gait, affecting both proprioceptive feedback due to sensory loss and motor function due to muscle weakness and pain. Peripheral neuropathy is associated with reduced walking speed, cadence, and step length, and less rhythmic acceleration patterns at the head and pelvis. Compared with controls, diabetics have impaired peripheral sensation, reaction time, and balance (35). Impaired balance and gait become manifest under challenging conditions, such as walking on an uneven surface or in dimmed light.

Falls are the most serious consequence of impaired balance and the leading cause of morbidity in the elderly. A recent prospective study with over 10 months of follow-up (36) has linked diabetes with increased risk of falls in nursing-home residents. Multiple measures that were used to study the association with falls included: clinical diagnoses; medication use; orthostatic changes in blood pressure, gait, or balance; cognitive/mental status; general well being; activities of daily living; affect/behavior; range of motion and/or ambulation; and communication. The incidence of falls was 78% for diabetic and 30% for nondiabetic patients. Common comorbidities such as hypertension, worse balance, multiple medications including angiotensin-converting enzyme inhibitors, and use of assistive device increased the risk of falling, while antidepressants were found to be protective.

MANAGEMENT GUIDELINES FOR DIABETIC NEUROPATHY IN OLDER ADULTS

It is generally accepted that good glycemic control is of utmost importance in symptomatic relief and slowing of progression of diabetic neuropathy. The Diabetes Control Complications Trial (DCCT) (17) demonstrated that tight glycemic control may result in a 60% reduction in the risk of developing clinical neuropathy. The American Diabetes Association (19) has adopted the DCCT-established standards for tight glycemic control in patients with type 1 diabetes, 13 to 39 years of age at initiation of the study: a mean blood glucose level of 155 mg/dL (8.6 mmol/L) and a hemoglobin A1C value of 7.2% (17,19). In patients with type 2 diabetes, the A1C value should be less than 7.0%, and peak postprandial plasma glucose levels should be less than 180 mg/dL (10.0 mmol/L). The American Association of Clinical Endocrinologists (16) recommends an A1C value of less than 6.5% in patients with type 1 or type 2 diabetes.

Management of Pain and Sensory Symptoms

Painful diabetic neuropathy (PDN) can be disabling and debilitating, interfering with activities of daily living, quality of life, and sleep. Diabetic small-fiber neuropathy is typically manifest as burning, shooting, or stabbing pain affecting the distal legs. Symptoms typically worsen at night, often leading to chronic sleep deprivation and depression. Negative motor symptoms, such as muscle weakness and foot drop, may require rehabilitation and assistive devices. DM can lead to a claw foot deformity due to changes in the foot fascia and lower extremity ligaments, ankle stiffness, and loss of fat pad in the foot. Foot numbness can lead to foot ulcerations. All patients need detailed foot care education and should be familiar with foot hygiene that includes feet examination, taking care of calluses, nails, and skin, and wearing proper footwear. Any skin changes including redness, dryness, or skin breakdown should be evaluated and treated by a physician. Patients should be instructed to protect feet from injuries, because even a minor injury can lead to gangrene and amputation.

Pharmacological Management of Pain

Treatment of pain in diabetic neuropathy is an integral part of management that includes glycemic control, foot care, and analgesic medication. Pain in diabetic neuropathy can be disabling, debilitating, and detrimental to quality of life (37,38). In spite of the availability of many pain medications, only a few of them were shown to be effective in high-quality clinical trials. In the ideal case, pain medication should stop the pain. This goal, however, is frequently not realistic, as no medication has been shown to be effective in every patient with PDN (37).

Historically, tricyclic antidepressants (TCAs) have been considered the first line of treatment of PDN. TCAs are effective; however, they are frequently associated with severe side effects. There is a trend to replace TCAs by medications with similar or more increased efficacy and fewer side effects. Only two drugs have received Food and Drug Administration (FDA) approval for treatment of PDN—duloxetine and pregabalin.

Consensus guidelines developed by American Society of Pain Educators (37) divide PDN medications into "first-tier" and "second-tier" categories based on efficacy data from clinical trials. First-tier medications that were shown to be effective in treatment of PDN in at least two randomized controlled trials include duloxetine, oxycodone controlled-release, pregabalin, and all TCAs. The second-tier category includes drugs that provide relief from neuropathic pain, but either the evidence is less strong compared to the first tier of medication or these drugs have not been shown to have efficacy specifically for PDN. These agents include carbamazepine, gabapentin, lamotrigine, tramadol, and venlafaxine ER. There is an additional group of medications with analgesic properties that include topical agents (capsaicin and lidocaine) and citalopram, methadone, paroxetine, phenytoin, and topiramate. These medications might be effective in treatment of PDN but at present the clinical data are limited.

Medications to Avoid

Nonsteroidal anti-inflammatory drugs should be avoided because of questionable effect upon neuropathic pain and increased risk of gastrointestinal bleeding and renal insufficiency. Amitriptyline should not be used for patients older than 60 years. Meperidine, pentazocine, propoxyphene, and vitamin B6 have significant central nervous system toxicity.

General Principles of Pain Management in PDN

It is recommended to set up realistic goals, as 100% suppression of pain might not be achieved (37–39). The choice of medication should be based on the costs, risks, and evidence and not on mechanism of action. A patient should be involved in the process of decision-making regarding use of medications. Patients should be aware that pain medication does not produce instant pain relief. Typically, initial treatment should start with the first-tier mediation. However, first-tier medications and venlafaxine should generally be avoided in the presence of erectile dysfunction. The medication should be titrated to the maximal tolerated dose. Each medication should be given a trial of at least three weeks. Efficacy is considered as a ≥50% reduction in pain. If the response is inadequate, the medication should be switched to either another first-line agent or a second-line agent or adjuvant therapy. The recommendation for initial dosing, titration schedule, and maximal dose is summarized in Table 2.

Tricyclic Antidepressants

TCAs have been used for years in the treatment of a variety of chronic pain syndromes and they are still among the most effective in treatment of neuropathic pain (37). The analgesic effect of TCAs is independent of their antidepressant effect and is probably related to inhibition of serotonin and norepinephrine reuptake. Common and significant side effects limit the use of TCAs, particularly in elderly patients. However, the side effects are fairly predictable. The common effects include dry mouth, dry eyes, drowsiness, confusion, cognitive deficits, and weight gain. TCAs interfere with hepatic, renal, and cardiovascular function and should not be used with monoamine oxidase inhibitors. To reduce side effects, low doses of TCAs, for example 10 mg at bedtime, can be used initially. Although it takes about two weeks to see an antidepressant effect, the pain reduction may start in 2 to 10 days. Failure of one TCA does not preclude trial of another TCA. TCAs are also associated with increased risk of sudden cardiac death, particularly at higher doses. Amitriptyline is a prototype of TCAs. Although it is effective in the treatment of neuropathic pain, it should not be used in the elderly because of its poor side-effect profile. Desipramine has a similar efficacy to amitriptyline, while nortriptyline is slightly less potent but also less sedating (40,41).

TABLE 2 Recommended Medication for Treatment of Painful Diabetic Neuropathy

Drug	Starting dose	Titration	Maximum daily dose	Comments
TCA[a]				
Amitriptyline	10–25 mg QHS	↑10–25 mg q 3–7 days	150 mg	Should not be used in the elderly; consider other TCAs
Nortriptyline	10–25 mg QHS	↑10–25 mg q 3–7 days	150 mg	Less sedating than amitriptyline
Desipramine	10–25 mg QHS	↑10–25 mg q 3–7 days	150 mg	May be as effective as amitriptyline, with fewer side effects
Imipramine	10–25 mg QHS	↑10–25 mg q 3–7 days	150 mg	Probably less effective than amitriptyline
Doxepin	10–25 mg QHS	↑10–25 mg q 3–7 days	150 mg	
Anticonvulsants				
Pregabaline	50 mg t.i.d.	↑50 mg t.i.d. qw	300 mg	FDA approved
Carbamazepine	100 mg b.i.d.	↑100 mg b.i.d. q12h	1200 mg	Similar structure to TCAs, interactions with multiple medications, monitor CBC, LFT's, Na. FDA approved for trigeminal neuralgia
Oxcarbazepine	150 mg b.i.d.	↑75–150 mg b.i.d. qw	1200 mg	Probably equally effective as carbamazepine with fewer side effects
Gabapentin	100–300 mg q.d.-t.i.d.	↑100–300 mg t.i.d.-q.i.d. q 1–7 days	3600 mg	Favorable side-effect profile; reduce if low CrCl; sedation is a limiting factor
Topiramate	25 mg b.i.d.	↑25 mg b.i.d. qw	400 mg	Problems with tolerance, questionable efficacy, weight loss
Zonisamide	25–100 mg q.d.	↑100 mg qw	600 mg	Problems with tolerance
Lamotrigine	25 mg q.d.	↑25–50 mg to b.i.d. q 2 wk	200–400 mg	Needs slow titration, monitor for rash
SNRI				
Duloxetine	20–60 mg q.d.	↑qw	60 mg	FDA approved
Venlafaxine ER	37.5–75 mg q.d.	↑75 mg qw	375 mg	
SSRI				
Fluoxetine	10 mg q.d.	Increase qw	40 mg	Questionable efficacy
Paroxetine	10–40 mg q.d.	Increase qw	40 mg	Less effective than imipramine but fewer side effects
Citalopram	10 mg q.d.	Increase qw	40 mg	
Opioids				
Oxycodone CR	10 mg q.d.	Increase every 3 days by 10 mg with b.i.d. schedule	120 mg	Problems with tolerance and constipation
Tramadol	25–50 mg q.d.-b.i.d.	↑25 mg q3 days with q.i.d. schedule	400 mg	Slow titration may reduce side effects
Methadone	5 mg b.i.d.	Increase to 10 mg b.i.d. in 2–5 days	20 mg	Requires careful titration since it has a very long half-life (24–36 hr)
Atypical antidepressants				
Bupropion SR	100–150 mg q.d.	Increase to b.i.d. in 1 wk	300–400 mg	
Topical agents				
Capsaicin 0.075% cream	t.i.d./q.i.d.			May exacerbate pain initially
Lidocaine patch 5%	1 patch for up 12 hr		3 patches at a time	

Note: The first line medication is highlighted in italics.
[a]Effective but significant side effects.
Abbreviations: ↑, increase; CBC, complete blood count; FDA, Food and Drug Administration; LFTs, liver function tests; QHS, at bedtime q2w; SNRI, serotonin-norepinephrine reuptake inhibitors; SSRI, serotonin reuptake inhibitors; TCA, tricyclic antidepressants.

Anticonvulsants

Anticonvulsants are as effective as TCAs (37). The maximal dose for pain management is in general lower than the maximal dose used for epilepsy treatment.

Pregabalin binds to the α_2-δ subunit of presynaptic calcium channels in the central nervous system. Pregabalin was found to be effective and safe in the treatment of diabetic pain in three randomized, double-blind, placebo-controlled trials (42–45), and it was approved by FDA in 2004 for treating PDN and postherpetic neuralgia. The most common side effects include dizziness, somnolence, and peripheral edema. The dose should be adjusted in patients with renal impairment.

Carbamazpine and its 10-keto analog oxcarbamazepine reduce high-frequency neuronal spiking by modulating sodium and calcium channels. Carbamazepine was approved by FDA for trigeminal neuralgia and is effective for reducing diabetic pain (46,47). It has a similar structure to TCAs; however, it can cause aplastic anemia, agranulocytosis, and hyponatremia; hence cell count, liver functions, and sodium level should be monitored. In addition, carbamazepine interacts with multiple medications, further limiting its utility. Oxcarbamazepine seems to have a better side-effect profile but hyponatremia can occur (48,49).

Gabapentin is widely used in pain management. It was approved for management of postherpetic neuralgia in 2002. The mechanism of action remains unclear. Gabapentin is probably effective in the treatment of PDN (37,50); it is generally well tolerated, and the most common side effects include dizziness and somnolence. The side effects are typically mild, occur early during treatment, are dose dependent, and usually resolve upon slowing down the titration schedule. A more bothersome side effect is peripheral edema, which can prompt discontinuation of the drug.

Lamotrigine blocks voltage-dependent sodium channels and modulates both calcium and potassium channels. Lamotrigine is probably effective; it is well tolerated by most patients if titrated slowly (51). The common side effects include dizziness, nausea, headaches, and somnolence. Lamotrigine is however associated with a skin rash in 9% to 10% of patients and Stevens–Johnson syndrome in 0.3%. Patients should monitor skin changes and the drug should be discontinued if a skin rash is present.

Topiramate enhances GABA-activated chloride channels and blocks kainate and AMPA receptors. Topiramate is modestly effective; however side effects are common and may limit its utility (52–54). Side effects include diarrhea, loss of appetite, somnolence, and weight loss.

Zonisamide (55) has multiple mechanisms of actions that include blockade of sodium and calcium channels, modulation of dopaminergic and GABAergic systems, facilitation of dopaminergic and serotonergic transmission, and weak inhibition of carbonic anhydrase. Zonisamide has long a half-life (63 hours), enabling once-a-day dosing. Side effects are frequent and include dizziness, restlessness, insomnia, headaches, and irritability. The main limitation of zonisamide is its poor tolerability.

Serotonin-Norepinephrine Reuptake Inhibitors

Duloxetine is a selective serotonin- and norepinephrine-reuptake inhibitor. Duloxetine was found to be effective for pain relief in PDN in two randomized, double-blind, placebo-controlled trials and it is the first medication approved by FDA for PDN treatment (56–58). No significant changes in dosing are required in the geriatric population. Common side effects include nausea, tiredness, dizziness, constipation, dry mouth, and increased sweating and muscle weakness. Most side effects occur early in treatment and diminish over time.

Venlafaxine ER is a dual serotonin- and norepinephrine-reuptake inhibitor. Norepinephrine modulation is more prominent at higher doses and is probably responsible for its analgesic effect. Venlafaxine ER appears to be effective for diabetic neuropathic pain (37,59,60), with advantageous once-daily dosing. Somnolence and nausea are common.

Serotonin-reuptake inhibitors have weak analgesic potency, are weaker than TCAs, and in general should not be used for monotherapy of neuropathic pain (39). Paroxetine (61) and citalopram (62) were found to be mildly effective while fluoxetine was found to be effective only in depressed patients (40).

Atypical Antidepressants

Bupropion is a novel, nonsedating antidepressant that presumably modulates central norad-renergic and dopaminergic systems and has limited effects upon the serotinergic system. In one double-blind randomized trial, bupropion SR was found to be effective for treating neuropathic pain (63). The role of bupropion in the treatment of diabetic pain remains to be established.

Opioids

Oxycodon blocks μ-opioid receptors. Oxycodone (controlled release) is effective in the treatment of PDN (64,65) and is among the first-tier medications. Although the side effects are frequent (constipation, sedation, dizziness, and dry mouth), they are considered mild to moderate. As with any other opioids, patients should be evaluated for signs of possible abuse.

Tramadol is a weak opioid and mixed serotonin–norepinephrine-reuptake inhibitor. Tramadol is an effective analgesic (66), but frequent occurrence of tiredness, dizziness, nausea, and constipation may limit its utility in geriatric patients. Another disadvantage of tramadol is its potential to provoke seizures, the need for four-times-a-day dosing, and concerns about dependence.

Other opioids that have been tried for pain control in PDN include morphine, methadone, levorphanol, and hydromorphone; however, their use in the treatment of diabetic pain remains controversial. These drugs are usually reserved for patients who fail nonopioid therapy (37,67–69).

Topical Agents

Capsaicin cream depletes substance P in nerves and causes epidermal denervation. Capsaicin is effective; however, it may temporarily increase the pain by producing a burning sensation that dissipates with prolonged use (70,71). Common side effects (10% of patients) are cough, skin irritation, and rash. Disadvantages of capsaicin are that it must be applied three or four times a day and may take several weeks to have an effect.

Lidocaine patch (5%) is a local anesthetic agent that appears to be effective, with minimal side effects (72). Lidocaine patch was approved for treatment of postherpetic neuralgia in 1999.

Nonpharmacological Management of Pain

Limited evidence exists with respect to the effectiveness of nondrug treatment (37). Acupuncture may relieve neuropathic pain or reduce the need for pain medications and is associated with minimal risk. Acupuncture may be tried in selected patients. There is limited evidence that spinal cord stimulation and electromagnetic neural stimulation may be helpful. There is no good evidence about the effectiveness of transcutaneous electrical nerve stimulation or magnetic insoles in the treatment of pain in PDN.

Management of Autonomic Dysfunction

OH is the most disabling complication of diabetic autonomic neuropathy (73). Treatment of OH should start with dietary modifications and physical measures. Diet adjustment aims to increase intravascular volume and to prevent postprandial hypotension. Expansion of the blood volume can be achieved by adequate hydration and increased sodium intake. The recommended daily water intake is 2 to 2.5 L and up to 10 to 20 g of sodium. Water is very effective for acute elevation of the blood pressure. For example, 450 mL of water can temporarily raise the mean blood pressure by as much as 40 mmHg.

Postprandial hypotension can be minimized or prevented by taking small, frequent meals with reduced carbohydrate content and drinking caffeinated coffee. Caffeine blocks adenosine-mediated postprandial splanchnic vasodilatation. To prevent tachyphylaxis, only one to two cups of coffee (200–250 mg of caffeine) should be consumed in the morning. Alcohol should be avoided since it precipitates vasodilatation.

Physical maneuvers increase orthostatic tolerance and may reduce dizziness while standing. Squatting is effective in preventing loss of consciousness in presyncope. Leg-crossing while standing is also effective, if the patient is able to maintain balance. Waist-high elastic stockings and a corset prevent venous pooling and improve orthostatic blood pressure.

Another nonpharmacologic intervention is to raise the head of the bed by 10° to 20°. This can help prevent supine hypertension and the nocturnal diuresis that occurs while sleeping in patients with autonomic neuropathy.

Medical treatment of OH should be considered if the dietary adjustments and physical measures fail. Fludrocortisone and proamatine are first-line treatments of OH. Both drugs can induce supine hypertension with the potential for end-organ damage, therefore baseline renal (creatinine) and cardiac (ejection fraction) functions should be obtained when treating elderly patients.

Fludrocortisone is a potent synthetic mineralocorticoid that at small doses sensitizes vessels to norepinephrine; at larger doses, it retains sodium and expands blood volume. Dosing starts at 0.1 mg q.d. or b.i.d.; the maximal dose is 1 mg/day. It takes up to two weeks to develop a full pressor effect. The expected weight gain is 2 to 5 lb, and patients may develop benign pedal edema. Side effects include supine hypertension, congestive heart failure, peripheral edema, hypokalemia (in up 50% of patients if potassium is not supplemented), and headache.

Proamatine is an α_1-adrenoreceptor agonist that is metabolized to the active compound desglymidodrine with a half-life of four hours. The starting dose is 2.5 mg (breakfast and lunch; the last dose should not be later than 6 P.M.) with dose escalations of 2.5 mg increments every week if necessary. The maximum recommended daily dose is 30 mg. Side effects are common and include sensation of goose flesh (chills), paraesthesia of the scalp, pruritus, urinary retention, and supine hypertension.

Epoetin α is a recombinant human erythropoetin that increases the hematocrit in two to six weeks. Epoetin α is usually reserved for patients with severe autonomic failure complicated by anemia and for patients who do not respond to or cannot tolerate fludrocortisone and proamatine. Epoetin α is given by intravenous or subcutaneous injection; the initial dose is 25 to 75 U/kg three times weekly, Once the hematocrit is normalized, the maintenance dose is 25 U/kg three times weekly. Epoetin α also can cause supine hypertension.

REFERENCES

1. Vinik AI, Holland MT, La Beau JM, Liuzzi FJ, Stansberry KB, Colen LB. Diabetic neuropathies. Diabet Care 1992; 15:1926–1975.
2. Dyck PJ, Kratz KM, Karnes JL, et al. The prevalence by staged severity of various types of diabetic neuropathy, retinopathy, and nephropathy in a population-based cohort: the Rochester Diabetic Neuropathy Study. Neurology 1993; 43:817–824.
3. American Diabetes Association. Standards of medical care in diabetes. Diabet Care 2006; 29(suppl 1): S4–S42.
4. Eastman RC. Neuropathy in diabetes. Diabetes in America. 2nd ed. National Diabetes Data Group, National Institute of Health, 339–348.
5. Dyck PJ, Litchy WJ, Lehman KA, Hokanson JL, Low PA, O'Brien PC. Variables influencing neuropathic endpoints: the Rochester Diabetic Neuropathy Study of Healthy Subjects. Neurology 1995; 45:1115–1121.
6. Hamman RE, Marshall JA, Baxter J, et al. Methods and prevalence of non-insulin dependent diabetes mellitus: the San Luis Valley Diabetes Study in biethnic Colorado population. Am J Epidemiol 1990; 129:295–311.
7. Franklin GM, Kahn LB, Baxter J, Marshall JA, Hamman RF. Sensory neuropathy in non-insulin-dependent diabetes mellitus: the San Luis Valley Diabetes Study. Am J Epidemiol 1990; 131: 633–643.
8. National Center for Health Statistics. Current estimates from the National Health Interview Survey. 1989 Vital and Health Statistics Series 10(176), 1990.
9. Novak V, Freimer ML, Kissel JT, et al. Autonomic impairment in painful neuropathy. Neurology 2001; 56:861–868.
10. Mainous AG 3rd, Majeed A, Koopman RJ, et al. Acculturation and diabetes among Hispanics: evidence from the 1999–2002 National Health and Nutrition Examination Survey. Public Heatlh Rep 2006; 121:60–66.
11. McCall AL. Cerebral glucose metabolism in diabetes mellitus. Eur J Pharmacol 2004; 490:147–158.
12. Yu T, Robotham JL, Yoon Y. Increased production of reactive oxygen species in hyperglycemic conditions requires dynamic change of mitochondrial morphology. Proc Natl Acad Sci 2006; 21(103): 2653–2658.

13. Monnier L, Mas E, Ginet C, et al. Activation of oxidative stress by acute glucose fluctuations compared with sustained chronic hyperglycemia in patients with type 2 diabetes. JAMA 2006; 295: 1681–1687.
14. Ogawa K, Sasaki H, Yamasaki H, et al. Peripheral nerve functions may deteriorate parallel to progression of microangiopathy in diabetic patients. Arch Phys Med Rehabil 2004; 85:245–252.
15. Low PA. Laboratory evaluation of autonomic function. In: Low PA, ed. Clinical Autonomic Disorders. 2nd ed. Lippincott-Raven, 1997:179–208.
16. Maser RE, Mitchel BD, Vinik AI, Freeman R. The association between cardiovascular autonomic neuropathy and mortality in individuals with diabetes: a meta-analysis. Diabet Care 2003; 6: 1895–1901.
17. Rutan GH, Hermanson B, Bild DE, Kittner SJ, LaBaw F, Tell GS. Orthostatic hypotension in older adults. The Cardiovascular Health Study. CHS Collaborative Research Group. Hypertension 1992; 19:508–519.
18. Chokroverty S, Barron KD, Katz FH, Del Greco F, Sharp JT. The syndrome of primary orthostatic hypotension. Brain 1969; 92:743–768.
19. Hussain M, Ooi WL, Lipsitz LA. Intra-individual postural blood pressure variability and stroke in elderly nursing home residents. J Clin Epidemiol 2001; 54:488–494.
20. Low PA, Walsh JC, Huang CY, McLeod JG. The sympathetic nervous system in diabetic neuropathy: a clinical and pathological study. Brain 1975; 98:341–356.
21. Bondar RL, Dunphy PT, Moradshahi P, et al. Cerebrovascular and cardiovascular responses to graded tilt in patients with autonomic failure. Stroke 1997; 28(9):1677–1685.
22. Lagi A, Bacalli S, Cencetti S, Paggetti C, Colzi L. Cerebral autoregulation in orthostatic hypotension. A Transcranial Doppler Study. Stroke 1994; 25:1771–1775.
23. Novak V, Novak P, Spies JM, Low PA. Autoregulation of cerebral blood flow in orthostatic hypotension. Stroke 1998; 29(1):104–111.
24. Fujimura J, Camilleri M, Low PA, Novak V, Novak P, Opfer-Gehrking TL. Effect of perturbations and a meal on superior mesenteric artery flow in patients with orthostatic hypotension. J Auton Nerv Syst 1997; 67:15–23.
25. Kassander P. Asymptomatic gastric retenion in diabetes (gastroparesis diabeticorum) Ann intern Med 1958; 48:797–812.
26. Barnet JL, Vinik AI. Gastrointestinal disturbances. In: Lebowitz AE, ed. Therapy for Diabetes Mellitus and Related Disorders. Alexandria, VA: American Diabetes Association, 1991:279–287.
27. Ellenberg M. Impotence in diabetes: the neurogenic factor. Ann Intern Med 1971; 75:213–219.
28. Ellenberg M. Sexual aspects of female diabetic patients. Mt. Sinai J. Med 1977; 44:495–500.
29. American Diabetes Association. Standards of Medical care in diabetes. Diabet Care 2006; 29 (suppl 1): S4–S42.
30. Mendell JR. Diagnosis and management of peripheral nerve disorders. In: Mendell JR, Kissel JT, Cornblath DR, eds. Diabetic Neuropathies. New York: Oxford University Press, 2001:373–390.
31. Klaver CCW, Wolfs RC, Vingerling JR, Hofman A, de Jong PTVM. Age-specific prevalence and causes of blindness and visual impairment in an older population. The Rotterdam Study. Arch Ophthalmol 1998; 116:653–658.
32. Gregg EW, Sorlie P, Paulose-Ram R, et al. 1999–2000 National health and nutrition examination survey. Diabet Care 2004; 27:1591–1997.
33. Young BA, Maynard C, Reiber G, Bouko EJ. Effects of ethnicity and nephropathy on lower-extremity amputation risk among diabetic veterans. Diabet Care 2003; 26:495–501.
34. Petrovsky JS, Cuneo M, Lee S, Johnson E, Lohman E III. Correlations between gait and balance in people with and without type 2 diabetes I normal and subdued light. Med Sci Monit 2006; 12(7): CR273–CR281 [Epub 2006 Jun 28].
35. Menz HB, Lord SR, St. George R, Fitzpatrick RC. Walking stability and sensorimotor function in older people with diabetic peripheral neuropathy. Arch Phys Med Rehabil 2004; 85:245–252.
36. Maurer MS, Burcham J, Cheng H. Diabetes mellitus is associated with increase risk for falls in elderly residents of a long-term facility. J Gerontol A Biol Sci Med Sci 2005; 60:1145–1146.
37. Argoff CE, Backonja MM, Belgrade MJ, et al. Consensus guidelines: treatment planning and options. Diabetic peripheral neuropathic pain. Mayo Clin Proc 2006; 81(4 suppl):S12–S25. [Review. Erratum in: Mayo Clin Proc 2006; 81(6):854].
38. Dworkin RH, Backonja M, Rowbotham MC, et al. Advances in neuropathic pain: diagnosis, mechanisms, and treatment recommendations. Arch Neurol 2003; 60(11):1520–1534.
39. Mendell JR, Sahenk Z. Clinical practice. Painful sensory neuropathy. N Engl J Med 2003; 348(13): 1243–1255.
40. Max MB, Lynch SA, Muir J, Shoaf SE, Smoller B, Dubner R. Effects of desipramine, amitriptyline, and fluoxetine on pain in diabetic neuropathy. N Engl J Med 1992; 326(19):1250–1256.
41. McQuay HJ, Tramer M, Nye BA, Carroll D, Wiffen PJ, Moore RA. A systematic review of antidepressants in neuropathic pain. Pain 1996; 68(2–3):217–227.
42. Lesser H, Sharma U, LaMoreaux L, Poole RM. Pregabalin relieves symptoms of painful diabetic neuropathy: a randomized controlled trial. Neurology 2004; 63:2104–2110.

43. Richter RW, Portenoy R, Sharma U, Lamoreaux L, Bockbrader H, Knapp LE. Relief of painful diabetic peripheral neuropathy with pregabalin: a randomized, placebo-controlled trial. J Pain 2005; 6:253–260.
44. Rosenstock J, Tuchman M, LaMoreaux L, Sharma U. Pregabalin for the treatment of painful diabetic peripheral neuropathy: a double-blind, placebo-controlled trial. Pain 2004; 110:628–638.
45. Lyrica [package insert]. New York, NY: Pfizer Inc, 2005.
46. Rull JA, Quibrera R, Gonzalez-Millan H, Lozano Castaneda O. Symptomatic treatment of peripheral diabetic neuropathy with carbamazepine (Tegretol): double blind crossover trial. Diabetologia 1969; 5:215–218.
47. Wilton TD. Tegretol in the treatment of diabetic neuropathy. S Afr Med J 1974; 48:869–872.
48. Dogra S, Beydoun S, Mazzola J, Hopwood M, Wan Y. Oxcarbazepine in painful diabetic neuropathy: a randomized, placebo-controlled study. Eur J Pain 2005; (5):543–554.
49. Grosskopf J, Mazzola J, Wan Y, Hopwood M. A randomized, placebo-controlled study of oxcarbazepine in painful diabetic neuropathy. Acta Neurol Scand 2006; 114(3):177–180.
50. Backonja M, Beydoun A, Edwards KR, et al. Gabapentin for the symptomatic treatment of painful neuropathy in patients with diabetes mellitus: a randomized controlled trial. JAMA 1998; 280: 1831–1836.
51. Eisenberg E, Lurie Y, Braker C, et al. Lamotrigine reduces painful diabetic neuropathy: a randomized, controlled study. Neurology 2001; 57:505–509.
52. Raskin P, Donofrio PD, Rosenthal NR, et al. Topiramate vs. placebo in painful diabetic neuropathy: analgesic and metabolic effects. Neurology 2004; 63:865–873.
53. The Topiramate Diabetic Neuropathic Pain Study Group. Topiramate in painful diabetic polyneuropathy: findings from three double-blind placebo-controlled trials. Acta Neurol Scand 2004; 110:221–231.
54. Carroll DG, Kline KM, Malnar KF. Role of topiramate for the treatment of painful diabetic peripheral neuropathy. Pharmacotherapy 2004; 24(9):1186–1193.
55. Atli A, Dogra S. Zonisamide in the treatment of painful diabetic neuropathy: a randomized, double-blind, placebo-controlled pilot study. Pain Med 2005; 6(3):225–234.
56. Goldstein DJ, Lu Y, Detke MJ, Lee TC, Iyengar S. Duloxetine vs. placebo in patients with painful diabetic neuropathy. Pain 2005; 116:109–118.
57. Raskin J, Pritchett YL, Wang F, et al. A double-blind, randomized multicenter trial comparing duloxetine with placebo in the management of diabetic peripheral neuropathic pain. Pain Med 2005; 6:346–356.
58. Cymbalta [package insert]. Indianapolis, Ind: Eli Lilly and Company; 2005.
59. Rowbotham MC, Goli V, Kunz NR, Lei D. Venlafaxine extended release in the treatment of painful diabetic neuropathy: a double-blind, placebo-controlled study. Pain 2004; 110:697–706. [published correction appears in Pain 2005; L13:248].
60. Sindrup SH, Bach FW, Madsen C, Gram LF, Jensen TS. Venlafaxine versus imipramine in painful polyneuropathy: a randomized, controlled trial. Neurology 2003; 60:1284–1289.
61. Sindrup SH, Gram LF, Brosen K, Eshoj O, Mogensen EF. The selective serotonin reuptake inhibitor paroxetine is effective in the treatment of diabetic neuropathy symptoms. Pain 1990; 42(2):135–144.
62. Sindrup SH, Bjerre U, Dejgaard A, Brosen K, Aaes-Jorgensen T, Gram LF. The selective serotonin reuptake inhibitor citalopram relieves the symptoms of diabetic neuropathy. Clin Pharmacol Therapeut 1992; 52(5):547–552.
63. Semenchuk MR, Sherman S, Davis B. Double-blind, randomized trial of bupropion SR for the treatment of neuropathic pain. Neurology 2001; 57(9):1583–1588.
64. Gimbel JS, Richards P, Portenoy RK. Controlled-release oxycodone for pain in diabetic neuropathy: a randomized controlled trial. Neurology 2003; 60:927–934.
65. Watson CP, Moulin D, Watt-Watson J, Gordon A, Eisenhoffer J. Controlled-release oxycodone relieves neuropathic pain: a randomized controlled trial in painful diabetic neuropathy. Pain 2003; 105:71–78.
66. Harati Y, Gooch C, Swenson M, et al. Double-blind randomized trial of tramadol for the treatment of the pain of diabetic neuropathy. Neurology 1998; 50:1842–1846.
67. Hays L, Reid C, Doran M, Geary K. Use of methadone for the treatment of diabetic neuropathy. Diabet Care 2005; 28(2):485–487.
68. Morley JS, Bridson J, Nash TP, Miles JB, White S, Makin MK. Low-dose methadone has an analgesic effect in neuropathic pain: a double-blind randomized controlled crossover trial. Palliat Med 2003; 17:576–587.
69. Nelson KA, Park KM, Robinovitz E, Tsigos C, Max MB. High-dose oral dextromethorphan versus placebo in painful diabetic neuropathy and postherpetic neuralgia. Neurology 1997; 48:1212–1218.
70. Capsaicin Study Group. Treatment of painful diabetic neuropathy with topical capsaicin: a multicenter, double-blind, vehicle-controlled study. Arch Intern Med 1991; 151:2225–2229.
71. Tandan R, Lewis GA, Krusinski PB, Badger GB, Fries TJ. Topical capsaicin in painful diabetic neuropathy: controlled study with long-term follow-up. Diabet Care 1992; 15:8–14.
72. Meier T, Wasner G, Faust M, et al. Efficacy of lidocaine patch 5% in the treatment of focal peripheral neuropathic pain syndromes: a randomized, double-blind, placebo-controlled study. Pain 2003; 106: 151–158.
73. Low PA, ed. Clinical Autonomic Disorders. Philadelphia: Lippincott-Raven, 1997.

17 | Ophthalmic Complications in Older Adults with Diabetes

Jerry D. Cavallerano, Deborah K. Schlossman, Rola N. Hamam, and Lloyd Paul Aiello
Beetham Eye Institute, Joslin Diabetes Center and Department of Ophthalmology, Harvard Medical School, Boston, Massachusetts, U.S.A.

INTRODUCTION

The elderly population is often beset by a unique set of medical risks and social challenges. These problems include, among others, higher risks of depression, cognitive impairment, injurious falls, pharmacologic use, and potentially more severe effects from hypotension and hypoglycemia as a result of aggressive blood glucose or blood pressure control in patients with diabetes. In addition, the elderly often experience additional barriers to complying with the repetitive routine lifelong follow-up necessary for optimum diabetic eye care. Although there are relatively few ocular diseases that are unique to the elderly patient population, it is well documented that failing eyesight limits quality of life and independence and often leads to depression and isolation in the elderly (1,2). Visual impairment increases the risk of depression and falls and makes it more likely that an older person will be admitted to a hospital or die at an earlier age. Diabetic retinopathy (DR) remains the leading cause of new-onset blindness in the United States and most developed countries, and diabetes prevalence and its associated complications increase with age. The aging of the overall population in the United States not only results in significant increases in numbers of elderly patients with type 2 disease, but with advances in medical care, there are many more elderly patients surviving with type 1 disease. In diabetic patients, glycemic and blood pressure control are mainstays of clinical care for reducing the risks of eye disease and other microvascular and macrovascular complications; however, in the elderly, the medical approach and optimum targets must often be adjusted.

In this chapter, the ophthalmic complications of diabetes will be discussed, with an emphasis on those that have particular relevance to the elderly population. Details of the pathogenesis, clinical findings, characterization, and care of diabetic eye disease have been extensively described elsewhere (3,4) and will be summarized only in abbreviated form here.

BACKGROUND AND EPIDEMIOLOGY

According to the Centers for Disease Control and Prevention, 19% of persons 70 years of age and older have some degree of visual impairment, which is defined as vision loss that cannot be corrected by glasses or contact lenses alone (5). In the year 2000, approximately 937,000 Americans (0.78%) were considered legally blind (best-corrected visual acuity of 20/200 or worse in the better-seeing eye), and an additional 2.4 million Americans (1.98%) had visual impairment. The leading causes of blindness in white, black, and Hispanic Americans aged 40 years or older were, respectively, age-related macular degeneration (AMD) (54.4%, 4.4%, 14.3%), cataract (8.7%, 36.8%, 14.3%), glaucoma (6.4%, 26.0%, 28.6%), DR (5.4%, 7.3%, 14.3%), and other causes (25.0%, 25.6%, 28.6%) (6).

Vision loss in the elderly is projected to rise rapidly as the American population ages. Although DR is an important cause of visual impairment in the general population, it is not clearly directly related to age, as are cataracts and AMD. While almost half of all AMD patients are 70 years or older, only one-quarter of patients with DR are over age 70 (5). However, the duration of diabetes is closely associated with the onset and severity of DR and thus indirectly associated with age.

Of the 20.8 million Americans with diabetes mellitus, 10.3 million are 60 years of age or older, representing nearly 21% of this age group. This diabetic population includes those with type 1 diabetes, usually of long duration, type 2 diabetes, and those who have diabetes but are not aware of their condition. In 2005, approximately 750,000 new cases of diagnosed diabetes occurred in the 40- to 59-year-old age group, and 600,000 new cases of diagnosed diabetes occurred in the 60 years or older age group (7).

Nearly all patients with type 1 diabetes and more than 60% of patients with type 2 diabetes develop some degree of retinopathy after 20 years (7–9). In the U.S. reports of patients with type 2 diabetes, approximately 20% had retinopathy at the time of diabetes diagnosis (9) and most had some degree of retinopathy over subsequent decades. In the United Kingdom Prospective Diabetes Study (UKPDS), nearly 40% of the subjects enrolled in the study, all of whom had type 2 diabetes, had some level of DR at the time of enrollment (10). Approximately 4.1 million Americans 40 years of age and older have some evidence of DR, and 1 in 12 with diabetes in this age group has advanced, sight-threatening eye disease (7).

Indeed, DR remains the leading cause of new cases of legal blindness among Americans between the ages of 20 and 74 years and the leading cause of severe (worse than 5/200 in both eyes) and moderate visual loss (doubling of the visual angle, e.g., 20/20 reduced to 20/40) in working age Americans (11). There is a higher risk of more frequent and severe ocular complications in type 1 diabetes (12). Approximately 25% of patients with type 1 diabetes have retinopathy after five years, with this figure increasing to 60% and 80% after 10 and 15 years, respectively. Because type 2 diabetes accounts for 90% to 95% of the diabetic population in the United States, type 2 disease represents a higher proportion of patients with visual loss. These patients tend to be older and thus represent the majority of the elderly population at risk of diabetic ocular complications.

Proliferative diabetic retinopathy (PDR) is the most threatening form of retinopathy and is present in approximately 25% of type 1 patients with diabetes of 15 years' duration (8). An estimated 700,000 persons have PDR, 130,000 with high-risk PDR, 500,000 with macular edema, and 325,000 with clinically significant macular edema (CSME) in the United States (13–17). An estimated 63,000 cases of PDR, 29,000 high-risk PDR, 80,000 macular edema, 56,000 CSME, and 12,000 to 24,000 new cases of legal blindness occur each year as a result of DR (13,17,18). Blindness has been estimated to be 25 times more common in persons with diabetes than in those without the disease (19,20). Computer-simulated estimates of the medical and economic impact of retinopathy-associated morbidity predict that in the absence of good glycemic control, 72% of patients with type 1 diabetes will develop PDR requiring scatter (panretinal) photocoagulation over their lifetime and that 42% will develop macular edema (14–17,21–27). Since current estimates are that only 60% of patients in need of retinopathy treatment are receiving appropriate ophthalmic care (28), as of 1990 more than $620 million and 173,540 person-years of sight would be realized annually if all patients with both type 1 and type 2 diabetes were to receive care according to currently suggested guidelines (15,16).

DR—PATHOPHYSIOLOGY AND CLINICAL FINDINGS

DR, a well-characterized, sight-threatening, chronic microvascular complication that eventually afflicts virtually all patients with diabetes mellitus, is common in both type 1 and type 2 diabetes (7). DR is characterized by gradually progressive alterations in the retinal microvasculature, leading to areas of retinal nonperfusion, increased vasopermeability, and pathologic intraocular proliferation of retinal vessels. The complications associated with the increased vasopermeability, termed *macular edema,* and uncontrolled neovascularization, termed *PDR,* can result in severe and permanent visual loss. With appropriate medical and ophthalmologic care, more than 90% of visual loss resulting from PDR can be prevented (29). Nevertheless, DR remains the leading cause of new-onset blindness in working-aged persons in most developed countries of the world (7). Thus, the primary clinical care emphasis for the prevention of vision loss is directed at the early identification, accurate classification, and timely treatment of retinopathy.

Chronic hyperglycemia is the central initiating factor of diabetic microvascular disease in the eye and elsewhere in the body. Both the duration and the magnitude of hyperglycemia are strongly correlated with the extent and rate of progression of diabetic microvascular disease. Prior to clinically evident retinopathy, physiologic changes already exist, including increased retinal vascular permeability, loss of retinal vascular pericytes (supporting cells for retinal endothelial cells), thickening of vascular endothelium basement membrane, and alterations in retinal blood flow (30–38). With increasing loss of retinal pericytes, the retinal vessel wall develops outpouchings *(microaneurysms)*, which are often the initial clinical sign of retinopathy. The vessels also become fragile and are prone to bleed or leak. Rheologic changes occur in DR as a result of increased platelet aggregation, integrin-mediated leukocyte adhesion, and endothelial damage (39–41). Disruption of the blood retinal barrier may ensue, with increased vascular permeability (42,43), leakage of blood and serum from the retinal vessels into the retina, and resulting retinal hemorrhages, retinal edema, and hard exudates. Moderate visual loss follows if the fovea is affected by the leakage (27).

With advancing retinopathy, there is decreased vascular perfusion, often leading to obliteration of the capillaries and small vessels. The resulting retinal ischemia is a potent inducer of angiogenic growth factors such as insulin-like growth factors, basic fibroblast growth factor, hepatocyte growth factor, and vascular endothelial growth factor (VEGF) (44–47). These factors promote the development of new vessel growth (PDR) and retinal vascular permeability (diabetic macular edema) (48–52). This mechanistic understanding has provided new targets against which novel therapies have been devised. These novel therapies such as VEGF inhibitors, corticosteroids, and protein kinase C (PKC)-β inhibitors (53–61) have entered clinical trials, with promising initial results, and are likely to increase therapeutic options for patients with diabetic eye disease in the near future. It remains unknown at this time, however, how effective such new therapies in the elderly population will be and what side effects may result.

Proliferating new vessels in DR are fragile and have a tendency to bleed, resulting in preretinal and vitreous hemorrhages. These intraocular hemorrhages often cause prolonged visual loss by blocking the visual axis. Membranes on the retinal surface can be induced by blood. These membranes may contract and result in distortion of the retina with subsequent visual distortion. Although all retinal neovascularization eventually becomes quiescent, as with most scarring processes there is progressive fibrosis of the new vessels associated with contraction. In the eye, such forces may exert traction on the retina, leading to tractional retinal detachment and retinal tears potentially resulting in severe and permanent visual loss if left untreated. When the retina is severely ischemic, the concentration of angiogenic growth factors may reach sufficient concentration in the anterior chamber to cause abnormal new vessel proliferation on the iris and the anterior chamber angle (46,62). If this anterior segment neovascularization causes blockage of aqueous outflow through the trabecular meshwork, neovascular glaucoma may result (63).

In short, causes of visual loss from complications of diabetes mellitus include retinal ischemia involving the fovea, macular edema at or near the fovea, preretinal or vitreous hemorrhages, retinal detachment, and neovascular glaucoma. Visual loss may also result from a predilection of diabetic patients for other conditions such as retinal vessel occlusion, accelerated atherosclerotic disease, and embolic phenomena—all conditions also more common in the elderly population.

CLINICAL CLASSIFICATION OF DR

DR is broadly classified into nonproliferative diabetic retinopathy (NPDR) and PDR categories (64–67). Macular edema may coexist with either group and is not used in the classification of level of retinopathy. The historical terms *background retinopathy* and *preproliferative diabetic retinopathy* have been replaced by defined levels of NPDR, which are more specific and prognostically important. Generally, DR progresses from no retinopathy, through mild, moderate, severe, and very severe NPDR and eventually on to PDR. The level of NPDR is determined by the extent and location of clinical manifestations of retinopathy. The level of NPDR establishes the risk of progression to sight-threatening retinopathy and dictates appropriate clinical management and follow-up.

PDR is characterized by vasoproliferation of the retina and its complications, including new vessels on the optic disc, new vessels elsewhere on the retina, preretinal hemorrhage (PRH), vitreous hemorrhage, and fibrous tissue proliferation. On the basis of the extent and location of these lesions, PDR is classified as *early PDR* or *high-risk PDR*. Larger areas of these complications as well as new vessels that are on or near the optic disc are associated with greater risks of visual loss. Patients with severe NPDR and PDR should be considered for treatment with laser photocoagulation.

Diabetic macular edema can be present with any level of DR. When edema involves or threatens the center of the macula, it is called CSME (64,68,69). CSME is a clinical diagnosis that is not dependent on visual acuity or results of ancillary testing such as fluorescein angiography and can be present even when vision is 20/20 or better.

OCULAR TREATMENT OF DR

The mainstays of current clinical management of DR have been defined by five major, randomized, multicentered clinical trials: the Diabetic Retinopathy Study (DRS) (70–83), the Early Treatment Diabetic Retinopathy Study (ETDRS) (84–103), the Diabetic Retinopathy Vitrectomy Study (DRVS) (104–108), the Diabetes Control and Complications Trial (DCCT) (109–114), and the UKPDS (115). These studies have elucidated delivery and proper timing for laser photocoagulation surgery for the treatment of both DR and diabetic macular edema. They have also established guidelines for vitrectomy surgery, aspirin use, and blood pressure control.

Without photocoagulation, eyes with high-risk PDR have a 28% risk of severe visual loss within two years (23). Severe visual loss is defined as best-corrected acuity of 5/200 that lasts at least four months—thus the degree of vision loss is substantially worse than the 20/200 level, which defines legal blindness. The DRS demonstrated that scatter (panretinal) laser photocoagulation was effective in reducing the risk of severe vision loss from PDR by 50% or more. In scatter laser photocoagulation, 1200 to 1800 laser burns are applied to the peripheral retinal tissue, focused at the level of the retinal pigment epithelium. Large vessels are avoided, as are areas of preretinal hemorrhage. The total treatment is usually applied in two or three sessions, spaced one to two weeks apart.

Untreated CSME is associated with an approximate 25% chance of moderate visual loss after three years (defined as at least doubling the visual angle, e.g., 20/40 reduced to 20/80) (27). The ETDRS demonstrated that focal laser photocoagulation for CSME reduced the five-year risk of moderate vision loss from nearly 30% to less than 15% (69). Focal laser photocoagulation places 50 to 100 μm diameter mild intensity laser burns in the central retina 500 to 3000 μm from the center of the macula to reduce retinal edema. Eyes with CSME are generally considered for focal laser photocoagulation and/or novel antipermeability approaches. If macular edema is present, patients with severe or very severe NPDR should be considered for focal treatment of macular edema whether or not the macular edema is clinically significant, because they are likely to require scatter laser photocoagulation in the near future, and scatter photocoagulation, while beneficial for PDR, may exacerbate existing macular edema. Novel therapeutic approaches such as anti-VEGF therapies are now being used in some clinical settings to treat diabetic macular edema (57,59). These therapies are becoming more commonly employed in cases where focal/grid laser entails an inadequate response or cannot be performed. Definitive multicenter, randomized, controlled clinical trials are currently underway to define the true efficacy and safety profile of these new approaches.

The ETDRS also demonstrated that scatter laser photocoagulation applied when an eye approaches or just reaches high-risk PDR reduces the risk of severe vision loss to less than 4%. The ETDRS clarified the natural history of DR and the risk of progression of retinopathy based on the baseline level of retinopathy (94–97). In addition, elevated total cholesterol, low-density lipoprotein (LDL) cholesterol, and triglyceride levels were found to be associated with faster development of hard exudates (116) and the risk of moderate visual loss (117). Finally, the ETDRS identified specific lesions that placed an eye at high risk for visual loss (96).

Consequently, proper diagnosis of the level of retinopathy determines appropriate timing of follow-up evaluation and when to initiate laser photocoagulation. It is therefore essential that these patients receive routine lifelong ophthalmic evaluation as a critical component of care for patients with diabetes. As will be discussed below, this is of additional importance for elderly patients who have additional risks and treatment limitations.

Eyes with high-risk PDR should receive prompt scatter laser photocoagulation. Eyes with severe NPDR or worse may be considered for scatter laser photocoagulation. Treatment prior to high-risk PDR is more commonly considered in the elderly population due to their predominance of type 2 diabetes where laser surgery of DR prior to the development of high-risk PDR reduces the risk of severe visual loss and the need for pars plana vitrectomy by 50% as compared to waiting for high-risk PDR to develop, especially when macular edema is present (113).

The DRVS demonstrated that early surgery within the eye called vitrectomy was useful in restoring vision and preventing worsening of vision for some persons who have severe vision loss due to vitreous hemorrhage or severe fibrovascular proliferation. Although the treatment benefits demonstrated in the DRVS, which was completed in 1989, are not totally applicable today due to dramatic advances in surgical techniques and the advent of laser endophotocoagulation that have occurred in the intervening years, vitrectomy surgery is a key approach to preserving or improving vision in diabetic patients with severe complications of retinopathy. Since vitrectomy surgery generally requires sedation or occasionally general anesthesia, and since elderly individuals are at greater risk for surgical and anesthetic complications, halting the disease prior to the need for surgery in this population is of further importance.

DR and diabetic macular edema are usually most amenable to laser surgery before any vision has been lost. Consequently, it is imperative that health-care providers educate their patients regarding the natural course and effectiveness of treatment so as to motivate patients to seek regular eye examinations even in the absence of symptoms. This is particularly true in the elderly population where access to care, physical limitations, recognition of visual changes, and financial consideration may serve as impediments to routine ophthalmologic follow-up.

Major advances in our understanding of the basic mechanisms underlying the progression of DR have been made over the past decade. This knowledge has made possible the identification of new therapeutic targets and development of novel therapeutic agents directed against the progression of NPDR, PDR, and diabetic macular edema. Since the mainstay of DR treatment is laser photocoagulation surgery, which is an inherently destructive technique resulting in focal destruction of areas of the retina, a noninvasive and nondestructive therapy would be of great clinical importance. Current clinical studies include agents that effect oxidative stress (antioxidants) (114,115), cyclooxygenase 2 (COX-2) inhibitors (23,69), corticosteroids (118,119) and numerous growth factors such as VEGF (120–122), PKC (49,123,124). In addition, surgical intervention trials and trials of novel biochemical compounds are planned for future investigation. The efficacy, applicability, and safety profile of all these new agents await the results of these and future clinical trials. Whether these novel therapies will require special consideration in the elderly population, and the elderly diabetic population in particular, is unknown.

COMPREHENSIVE EYE EXAMINATION

As indicated earlier, an accurate ocular examination detailing the extent and location of retinopathy-associated findings is critical for determining the severity of DR and subsequently undertaking monitoring and treatment decisions in patients with diabetes. Even in the non-elderly population, many diabetic patients do not receive adequate eye care (28,125). In one study, 55% of patients with high-risk PDR or CSME had never had laser photocoagulation (28). In fact, 11% of type 1 and 7% of type 2 patients with high-risk PDR necessitating prompt treatment had not been examined by an ophthalmologist within the past two years (125).

The comprehensive eye examination is the mainstay of such evaluation and is necessary on a repetitive, lifelong basis for patients with diabetes (64,126). Dilated ophthalmic examination is superior to undilated evaluation because only 50% of eyes are correctly classified with respect to the presence and severity of retinopathy through undilated pupils (127,128). Because of the complexities of the diagnosis and treatment of PDR and CSME, ophthalmologists with specialized knowledge and experience in the management of DR are required to determine and provide appropriate surgical intervention (129). Thus, it is recommended that all patients with diabetes should have dilated ocular examinations by an experienced eye care provider (ophthalmologist or optometrist), and diabetic patients should be under the direct or consulting care of an ophthalmologist experienced in the management of DR at least by the time severe NPDR or diabetic macular edema is present (64). Effort must be made to help the elderly patient overcome their additional barriers to acquiring timely and consistent quality eye care.

INITIAL OPHTHALMIC EVALUATION

The recommendation for initial ocular examination in persons with diabetes is based on prevalence rates of retinopathy. Approximately 80% of type 1 patients have retinopathy after 15 years of disease, but only about 25% have any retinopathy after five years (8). The prevalence of PDR is less than 2% at five years and 25% by 15 years. The onset of vision-threatening retinopathy is rare in children prior to puberty, regardless of the duration of diabetes (9,130–133); however, significant retinopathy may arise within six years of diabetes onset when diagnosed between the ages of 10 and 30 years (128). Thus, in patients older than 10 years of age, initial ophthalmic examination is recommended beginning five years after the diagnosis of type 1 diabetes mellitus (3,64,130).

However, of importance in elderly patients, when type 2 diabetes is present, the onset date of diabetes is frequently unknown, and more severe disease can be observed at diagnosis. Up to 3% of patients first diagnosed after age 30 (type 2) can have CSME or high-risk PDR at the time of initial diagnosis of diabetes (134). Thus, initial ophthalmic examination in adult patients with type 2 diabetes should occur shortly after diagnosis (3,64,130).

FOLLOW-UP OPHTHALMIC EXAMINATION

Since risk of retinopathy progression is well correlated with severity of NPDR, follow-up ocular examination is primarily determined from the extent of retinopathy observed at each visit (64). Significant sight-threatening retinopathy can initially occur with no or minimal symptoms; thus, even patients with no clinically evident DR and no known ocular problems require annual comprehensive ophthalmic examinations even if they are totally asymptomatic. The importance of timely follow-up is particularly important to stress in elderly patients where initial symptoms may be masked by vision loss from other conditions, cognitive abilities, or communication constraints.

SYSTEMIC CONSIDERATIONS IN ELDERLY DIABETIC PATIENTS
Blood Glucose Control

The DCCT conclusively demonstrated that both the risk of development of any retinopathy and the rate of retinopathy progression once it was present were significantly reduced after three years of intensive insulin therapy for patients with type 1 diabetes (135). The effect of reducing the HbA(1c) in this group from 9.1% for conventional treatment to the 7.3% for intensive treatment resulted in a benefit maintained through seven years of follow-up, even though the difference in mean HbA(1c) levels of the two former randomized treatment groups was only 0.4% at one year ($P < 0.001$), continued to narrow and became statistically insignificant by five years (8.1% vs. 8.2%, $P = 0.09$). The further rate of progression of complications from their levels at the end of the DCCT remains less in the former intensive treatment group. Thus, the benefits of 6.5 years of intensive treatment extend well beyond the period of its most intensive implementation (113,136–138).

Although there are no clinical data on the ocular microvascular complications of diabetes in relation to glycemic control specifically in elder adults, the UKPDS did evaluate late middle-aged persons with new-onset type 2 diabetes and minimal comorbid conditions. In these patients, a 1% reduction in A1C was associated with declines in microvascular complications and any diabetes-related end point of 37% and 21%, respectively. Thus, elderly diabetic patient should benefit significantly from appropriate glycemic control.

Although the American Diabetes Association (ADA) guidelines generally suggest lowering A1C in younger persons (<~65 years) to 7.0% or less, this level of control is often not possible. Issues in goal setting in older patients with diabetes are discussed in detail in Chapter 20. Intensive glycemic control is associated with a threefold increase in severe hypoglycemic episodes. In the elderly, frequent and/or severe hypoglycemic episodes impart additional risk of falls and cognitive impairment. In frail elderly patients where such risks are substantial, a less stringent A1C target may be more appropriate (139,140).

Blood Pressure Control

Similar results were identified in the UKPDS when evaluating the effect of tight blood pressure control on various aspects of DR (141). Within 4.5 years after randomization, those under tight blood pressure control had a highly significant reduction in findings associated with retinopathy, less photocoagulation, and reduced blindness. Furthermore, high blood pressure was identified as an independent risk factor for progression of DR, and tight blood pressure control with either a β-blocker or an ACE-inhibitor reduced the risk of clinical complications from diabetic eye disease.

It is clear from these and other studies that hypertension increases the progression of DR and its associated risks. The Appropriate Blood Pressure Control in Diabetes (ABCD) Study demonstrated that reduction of blood pressure even in those normotensive at baseline had an effect on reducing retinopathy complications (142). Tight blood pressure control is a key component of appropriate eye care in diabetic patients. Elderly patients, however, have reduced tolerance for blood pressure reduction and severe hypotensive episodes can lead to injuries and associated morbidity and mortality. Thus, blood pressure targets in elderly diabetic patients need to be tailored to be as optimal as is safe and tolerated for each individual.

Aspirin and Anticoagulation

Aspirin use has been clearly associated with a reduction in acute myocardial infarction, other cardiovascular events, and cardiovascular mortality in older adults and those with diabetes (143–147). It has been recommended that older adults with diabetes who are not on other anticoagulation therapy and who do not have contraindications for aspirin therapy should be offered 81 to 325 mg/day aspirin. The question thus commonly arises as to whether such anticoagulation therapy is contraindicated in persons with diabetic eye disease. The ETDRS specifically evaluated the use of 650 mg of aspirin in patients with diabetes (92). The study conclusively demonstrated that the use of aspirin did not alter the course of DR and determined that aspirin use was not associated with increased risk of vitreous hemorrhage or PRH or stroke. Similar results have been observed with other anticoagulants. There is one case report of vitreous hemorrhage associated with retinopathy after thrombolysis (148); however, approximately 90,000 patients have been involved in clinical trials of thrombolytic agents in myocardial infarction, of which 10% had diabetes mellitus without any reports of ocular complications (149–152).

Thus, elderly patients who require the use of aspirin or anticoagulants for optimum medical care should not be discontinued from treatment due to the presence of DR alone.

Trauma from Falling

Older persons with diabetes have increased risks of falls and associated injury (153–155). Visual impairment is one of the numerous risk factors for falls in diabetic individuals (155,156). It is also well documented that trauma from falls in older adults is associated with high morbidity and mortality (157–159). Thus, maintenance of vision in the elderly diabetic population is important not only for sighted functions of daily life, but also to reduce added morbidity and mortality should the vision limitation contribute to a fall injury. Chapter 7 has a detailed discussion on falls in elderly patients with diabetes.

Cognitive Impairment and Depression

Patients with type 2 diabetes are at risk for decreased cognitive function (160–168). Functions such as memory, learning, and verbal skills may be affected. Depression is also more common in persons with diabetes (169–171). Indeed, symptoms can be severe enough to impede appropriate diabetes self-management (172). In addition, visual impairment is associated with higher rates of depression. In the general population, approximately 5% of adults suffer from depressive disorders; however, in those with vision impairment, nearly one-third of participants in most studies were classified as depressed. Vision impairment is associated with as much as a

2.3 times greater risk of depression than found in persons without a vision problem (134,173–176). Indeed, visual loss is one of three conditions independently associated with depression when demographical factors, social support, and all other health conditions are accounted for (177,178). Cognitive dysfunction and depression in elderly patients with diabetes are discussed in detail in Chapter 6.

OCULAR CONDITIONS IN ELDERLY DIABETIC PATIENTS

Most persons who have had diabetes for 15 or more years will have some evidence of retinopathy. Although the vast majority of people with extended durations of diabetes will have some degree of ocular disease, it is possible to have diabetes for 50 or more years with no or minimal clinical abnormalities. In a study at the Joslin Diabetes Center evaluating 98 patients with type 1 diabetes of 50 or more years, severity of DR did not correlate with duration of diabetes, age of onset of diabetes, current A1c levels, lipid levels, body-mass index, or C-peptide levels—in direct contrast to patients with less-extensive duration of disease. In the study, 8% of patients had no DR, 48% had no or mild NPDR, and 43% had severe NPDR or PDR in the eye with more severe disease (179).

Diabetes can affect all structures of the eye. While cataracts, dry eye syndrome, glaucoma, and arterial and venous occlusions are more likely to occur in an elderly population, diabetes is an added risk factor for each of these conditions. People with diabetes are more susceptible to corneal drying and erosions, cataracts, glaucoma, arterial and venous occlusions, and retinopathy.

Glaucoma is an irreversible damage to the optic nerve, usually caused by increased intraocular pressure. It is a slowly progressive disease that can cause blindness if untreated. It is estimated that half of the people who have glaucoma are asymptomatic and unaware that they have it. Glaucoma is more prevalent in older blacks than older whites (180). Open-angle glaucoma is 1.4 times more common in the diabetic population than in the nondiabetic population (181). The prevalence of glaucoma increases with age and duration of diabetes. In a study of 76,318 women enrolled in the Nurses' Health Study, Pasquale and coworkers found that type 2 diabetes mellitus is associated with an increased risk of primary open-angle glaucoma in women (182).

Cataracts, or opacities in the lens of the eye, are the leading treatable cause of visual impairment in the elderly. They account for 50% of blindness worldwide (180). According to the National Eye Institute, over half of all Americans aged 65 years and older have cataracts. Diabetes can result in transitory refractive changes (119), alterations in accommodative ability (183), and cataracts, which occur earlier in life and progress more rapidly than in patients without diabetes (183,184). Diabetes increases the risk of cataracts by 60% (183,184). Patients with later-onset diabetes have unique risk factors associated with cataract development including age of the patient, lower intraocular pressure, smoking, and lower diastolic blood pressure (185,186). These are in addition to the risks observed for earlier-onset diabetic patients, which include duration of diabetes, retinopathy status, diuretic use, and elevated glycosylated hemoglobin (185).

Both phacoemulsification and extracapsular cataract extraction with intraocular lens implantation are appropriate surgical therapies. The primary prognosticators of postoperative vision and progression of retinopathy are preoperative presence of diabetic macular edema and level of NPDR (186–189). Patients with active PDR should be treated with full scatter (panretinal) laser treatment prior to cataract surgery, and patients with type 2 diabetes and severe NPDR should also be strongly considered for preoperative scatter laser photocoagulation (190). Similarly, clinically significant diabetic macular edema or macular edema threatening vision should be treated four to six months prior to cataract surgery.

AMD is the leading cause of irreversible visual impairment in the elderly. The incidence of AMD increases sharply with age, affecting 25% of people 70 years and older (5). Some believe that severe AMD and severe DR occur together less frequently than might be expected. Nevertheless, AMD can be diagnostically confused with DR especially when accompanied by severe macular edema, and elderly patients commonly confuse the different conditions of diabetic macular edema and AMD.

Even with optimal ocular and systemic care, vision loss from diabetes can still occur. In those diabetic elderly patients who experience severe vision loss, visual rehabilitation with low-vision aids can be of significant benefit.

OTHER SYSTEMIC CONSIDERATIONS

DR is affected by several conditions that are more common in the elderly population. These include hypertension, renal disease, dyslipidemia, and anemia. Patients with type 1 diabetes have a 17% prevalence of hypertension at baseline and a 25% incidence after 10 years (191). There is a 38% to 68% prevalence of hypertension in type 2 diabetes (192–194). Diabetic patients with hypertension are more likely to develop retinopathy, diffuse macular edema, and more severe levels of retinopathy (195–197) and have more rapid progression of retinopathy when compared with diabetic patients without hypertension (198–200). The 1148 patient-randomized, prospective UKPDS in persons with type 2 diabetes showed a 34% ($P = 0.0004$) and 47% ($P = 0.004$) reduction in risk of DR progression and moderate visual acuity loss, respectively, in patients assigned to intensive blood pressure control (201).

Renal disease has been associated in several ways with DR. Proteinuria or microalbuminuria is associated with retinopathy (202–214) and the presence and severity of DR are indicators of the risk of gross proteinuria (206,215). Conversely, proteinuria predicts PDR (204,207,216). Half of all patients with type 1 diabetes mellitus with PDR and 10 or more years of diabetes have concomitant proteinuria (202). In type 1 diabetes mellitus, the prevalence of PDR increases from 7% at onset of microalbuminuria to 29% four years after onset of albuminuria as compared with 3% and 8%, respectively, in patients without persistent microalbuminuria (205). The ABCD Trial found that both the severity and progression of retinopathy were associated with overt albuminuria (142,217,218). The presence of gross proteinuria at baseline is associated with 95% increased risk of developing macular edema among patients with type 1 diabetes mellitus (195), and dialysis may improve macular edema in diabetic patients with renal failure (218).

With regard to dyslipidemia, in 2709 ETDRS patients in whom serum levels were measured, elevated total cholesterol, LDL cholesterol, and triglyceride levels were associated with faster development of hard exudates. In addition, the risk of moderate visual loss was associated with the extent of exudate (117).

In the ETDRS, baseline low hematocrit was an independent risk factor for development of high-risk PDR and of severe visual loss (219). A cross-sectional study involving 1691 patients revealed a twofold increased risk of any retinopathy in patients with a hemoglobin level of less than 12 g/dL as compared to those with a higher hemoglobin concentration using multivariate analyses controlling for serum creatinine, proteinuria, and other factors (220). In patients with retinopathy, those with low hemoglobin levels have a fivefold increased risk of severe retinopathy compared with those with higher hemoglobin levels. There have been limited reports of resolution of macular edema and hard exudate with improvement or stabilization of visual acuity in erythropoietin-treated patients after an increase in mean hematocrit (221).

SUMMARY: OPTIMIZING THE EYE CARE OF THE ELDERLY DIABETIC PATIENT

The optimal ophthalmic care of a patient with diabetes necessitates a team approach that includes patient identification, routine lifelong follow-up, accurate disease severity assessment, timely therapeutic intervention, and comprehensive optimization of glycemic, blood pressure, and lipid control. The elderly diabetic patient has additional risks in terms of disease progression as well as limitations and side effects associated with treatment. In the elderly, particular care is indicated in setting targets for glycemic control, blood pressure, blood lipids, renal disease, cardiovascular intervention, and anemia. Such targets should be as close to the general recommended guidelines as possible taking into account the unique limitations of age and the individual patient. In addition, the risks of retinopathy, macular edema, and numerous other ocular conditions are increased in the elderly, further emphasizing the need for regular, lifelong ophthalmic evaluation by eye care providers experienced in the care of patients with diabetes (222–224).

GLOSSARY AND ABBREVIATIONS PERTINENT TO DIABETIC EYE DISEASE

Background diabetic retinopathy (BDR)   An outdated term referring to some stages of nonproliferative diabetic retinopathy. Because this terminology is not closely associated with disease progression, it has been replaced by the various levels of nonproliferative diabetic retinopathy.

Clinically significant macular edema (CSME) Thickening of the retina in the macular region of sufficient extent and location to threaten central visual function.

Cotton wool spot A gray or white area lesion in the nerve fiber layer of the retina resulting from stasis of axoplasmic flow as a result of microinfarcts of the retinal nerve fiber layer.

Diabetes Control and Complications Trial (DCCT) A multicenter, randomized clinical trial designed to address whether intensive insulin therapy could prevent or slow the progression of systemic complications of diabetes mellitus.

Diabetic retinopathy (DR) Retinal pathology related to the underlying systemic disease of diabetes mellitus.

Diabetic Retinopathy Study (DRS) The first multicenter, randomized clinical trial to demonstrate the value of scatter (panretinal) photocoagulation in reducing the risk of visual loss among patients with all levels of diabetic retinopathy.

Diabetic Retinopathy Vitrectomy Study (DRVS) A multicenter clinical trial evaluating early vitrectomy for patients with very advanced diabetic retinopathy or nonresolving vitreous hemorrhage.

Early Treatment Diabetic Retinopathy Study (ETDRS) A multicenter, randomized clinical trial that addressed at what stage of retinopathy scatter (panretinal) photocoagulation was indicated, whether focal photocoagulation was effective for preventing moderate visual loss from clinically significant macular edema, and whether aspirin therapy altered the progression of diabetic retinopathy.

Focal or grid laser photocoagulation A type of laser treatment whose main goal is to reduce vascular leakage either by focal treatment of leaking retinal microaneurysms or by application of therapy in a grid-like pattern for patients with clinically significant macular edema.

Hard exudate Lipid accumulation within the retina as a result of increased vasopermeability.

High-risk-characteristic proliferative diabetic retinopathy (HRC-PDR) Proliferative diabetic retinopathy of a defined extent, location, and/or clinical findings that is particularly associated with severe visual loss.

Microaneurysm (Ma) An early vascular abnormality consisting of an outpouching of the retinal microvasculature.

Neovascular glaucoma (NVG) Elevation of intraocular pressure caused by the development of neovascularization in the anterior segment of the eye.

Neovascularization at the disc (NVD) Retina neovascularization occurring at or within 1500 μm of the optic disc.

Neovascularization elsewhere (NVE) Retinal neovascularization that is located more than 1500 μm away from the optic disc.

Neovascularization of the iris (NVI) Neovascularization occurring on the iris (*rubeosis iridis*), usually as a result of extensive retinal ischemia.

No light perception (NLP) The inability to perceive light.

Nonproliferative diabetic retinopathy (NPDR) Severities of clinically evident diabetic retinopathy that precede the development of proliferative diabetic retinopathy.

Preproliferative diabetic retinopathy (PPDR) An outdated term referring to more advanced levels of nonproliferative diabetic retinopathy. Because this terminology is not closely associated with disease progression, it has been replaced by the various levels of nonproliferative diabetic retinopathy.

Proliferative diabetic retinopathy (PDR) An advanced level of diabetic retinopathy, where proliferation of new vessels or fibrous tissue occurs on or within the retina.

Rubeosis iridis See Neovascularization of the Iris (NVI).

ACKNOWLEDGMENT

The authors thank Ms. Rita Botti for her exceptional technical assistance in the preparation of this chapter.

REFERENCES

1. Newman SC, Hassan AI. Antidepressant use in the elderly population in Canada. Results from a national survey. J Gerontol A Biol Sci Med Sci 1999; 54A:M527–M530.
2. Dalberto MJ, Seeman T, McAvay GL, et al. Factors related to current and subsequent psychotropic drug use in an elderly cohort. J Clin Epidemiol 1997; 50:357–364.
3. Aiello LP et al. Diabetic retinopathy: technical review. Diabetes Care 1998; 21:143–156.
4. Aiello LP et al. Complications of diabetes mellitus. Brownlee et al. In Press.
5. Center for Disease Control. Available from http://www.cdc.gov/nchs/data/ahcd/agingtrends/02vision.pdf
6. The Eye Disease Prevalence Research Group. Causes and prevalence of visual impairment among adults in the United States. Arch Ophthalmol 2004; 122:477–485.
7. National Diabetes Data Group. Diabetes in America, 2nd ed. Washington, DC: US Government Printing Office, 1995.
8. Klein R, Klein BE, Moss SE, et al. The Wisconsin Epidemiologic Study of diabetic retinopathy: II. Prevalence and risk of diabetic retinopathy when age at diagnosis is less than 30 years. Arch Ophthalmol 1984; 102:520–536.
9. Klein R, Klein BE, Moss SE, et al. The Wisconsin Epidemiologic Study of diabetic retinopathy: III. Prevalence and risk of diabetic retinopathy when age at diagnosis is 30 or more years. Arch Ophthalmol 1984; 102:527–532.
10. Kohner EM, Aldington SJ, Stratton IM, et al. United Kingdom Prospective Diabetes Study, 30: diabetic retinopathy at diagnosis of non-insulin-dependent diabetes mellitus and associated risk factors. Arch Ophthalmol 1998; 116:297–303.
11. National Society to Prevent Blindness: Data Analysis. Vision Problems in the United States: Facts and Figures, 1980. (National Society to Prevent Blindness, 500 E. Remington Road, Schaumburg, IL 60173.)
12. Klein R, Klein BE, Moss SE. Visual impairment in diabetes. Ophthalmology 1984; 91:1–9.
13. Klein R, Klein BE, Moss SE, Cruickshanks KJ. The Wisconsin Epidemiologic Study Of diabetic retinopathy: XV. The long-term incidence of macular edema. Ophthalmology 1995; 102:7–16.
14. Javitt JC, Canner JK, Sommer A. Cost effectiveness of current approaches to the control of retinopathy in type 1 diabetics. Ophthalmology 1989; 96:255–264.
15. Javitt JC, Aiello LP, Bassi LJ, et al. Detecting and treating retinopathy in patients with type I diabetes mellitus: savings associated with improved implementation of current guidelines. American academy of ophthalmology. Ophthalmology 1991; 98:1565–1573.
16. Javitt JC, Aiello LP, Chiang Y, et al. Preventive eye care in people with diabetes is cost-saving to the federal government: implications for health-care reform. Diabetes Care 1994; 17:909–917.
17. Javitt JC, Aiello LP. Cost-effectiveness of detecting and treating diabetic retinopathy [see comments]. Ann Intern Med 1996; 124(1 Pt 2):164–169.
18. Center for Disease Control. National Diabetes Fact Sheet. National Estimates on Diabetes. Available at http://www.cdc.gov/diabetes/pubs/estimates.htm. Oct 12, 2006.
19. Kahn HA, Hiller R. Blindness caused by diabetic retinopathy. Am J Ophthalmol 1974; 78:58–67.
20. Palmberg PF. Diabetic retinopathy. Diabetes 1977; 26:703–709.
21. Dasbach EJ, Fryback DG, Newcomb PA, et al. Cost-effectiveness of strategies for detecting diabetic retinopathy. Med Care 1991; 29:20–39.
22. The Diabetic Retinopathy Study Research Group. Diabetic Retinopathy Study Report No. 6: design, methods, and baseline results. Invest Ophthalmol Vis Sci 1981; 21(1 Pt 2):149–209.
23. The Diabetic Retinopathy Study Research Group. Indications for photocoagulation treatment of diabetic retinopathy: Diabetic Retinopathy Study Report No. 14. Int Ophthalmol Clin 1987; 27: 239–253.
24. The Diabetic Retinopathy Study Research Group. Photocoagulation treatment of proliferative diabetic retinopathy: the second report of diabetic retinopathy study findings. Ophthalmology 1978; 85:82–106.
25. The Early Treatment Diabetic Retinopathy Study Research Group. Photocoagulation for diabetic macular edema: Early Treatment Diabetic Retinopathy Study Report No. 1. Arch Ophthalmol 1985; 103:1796–1806.
26. The Early Treatment Diabetic Retinopathy Study Research Group. Techniques for scatter and local photocoagulation treatment of diabetic retinopathy: Early Treatment Diabetic Retinopathy Study Report No. 3. Int Ophthalmol Clin 1987; 27:254–264.

27. The Early Treatment Diabetic Retinopathy Study Research Group. Early photocoagulation for diabetic retinopathy. ETDRS report no. 9. Ophthalmology 1991; 98(5 suppl):766–785.

28. Klein R, Klein BE, Moss SE, et al. The Wisconsin Epidemiologic Study of diabetic retinopathy: VI. Retinal photocoagulation. Ophthalmology 1987; 94:747–753.

29. Ferris FL. How effective are treatments for diabetic retinopathy? JAMA 1993; 269:1290–1291.

30. Shore AC, Tooke JE. Microvascular function and haemodynamic disturbances in diabetes mellitus and its complications. In: Pickup J, Williams G, eds. Textbook of Diabetes. Vol. 1. Oxford, England: Blackwell Scientific, 1997:1–13, Chapter 43.

31. Kihara M, Schmelzer JD, Poduslo JF, et al. Aminoguanidine effects on nerve blood flow, vascular permeability, electrophysiology, and oxygen free radicals. Proc Natl Acad Sci USA 1991; 88:6107–6111.

32. Engerman RL, Kern TS. Progression of incipient diabetic retinopathy during good glycemic control. Diabetes 1987; 36:808–812.

33. Cogan DG, Toussaint D, Kuwabara T. Retinal vascular patterns: IV. Diabetic retinopathy. Arch Ophthalmol 1961; 66:366–378.

34. Konno S, Feke GT, Yoshida A, et al. Retinal blood flow changes in type I diabetes: a long-term follow-up study. Invest Ophthalmol Vis Sci 1996; 37:1140–1148.

35. Grunwald JE, Riva CE, Sinclair SH, et al. Laser Doppler Velocimetry Study of retinal circulation in diabetes mellitus. Arch Ophthalmol 1986; 104:991–996.

36. Bursell SE, Clermont AC, Kinsley BT, et al. Retinal blood flow changes in patients with insulin-dependent diabetes mellitus and no diabetic retinopathy. Am J Physiol 1996; 270(1 Pt 2): R61–R70.

37. Sosula L, Beaumont P, Hollows FC, Jonson KM. Dilatation and endothelial proliferation of retinal capillaries in streptozotocin-diabetic rats: quantitative electron microscopy. Invest Ophthalmol 1972; 11:926–935.

38. Speiser P, Gittelsohn AM, Patz A. Studies on diabetic retinopathy: III. Influence of diabetes on intramural pericytes. Arch Ophthalmol 1968; 80:332–337.

39. Barouch FC, Miyamoto K, Allport JR, et al. Integrin-mediated neutrophil adhesion and retinal leukostasis in diabetes. Invest Ophthalmol Vis Sci 2000; 41:1153–1158.

40. Miyamoto K, Khosrof S, Bursell SE, et al. Vascular endothelial growth factor (VEGF)-induced retinal vascular permeability is mediated by intercellular adhesion molecule-1 (ICAM-1). Am J Pathol 2000; 156:1733–1739.

41. Miyamoto K, Khosrof S, Bursell SE, et al. Prevention of leukostasis and vascular leakage in streptozotocin-induced diabetic retinopathy via intercellular adhesion molecule-1 inhibition. Proc Natl Acad Sci USA 1999; 96:10836–10841.

42. Stitt AW, Gardiner TA, Archer DB. Histological and ultrastructural investigation of retinal microaneurysm development in diabetic patients. Br J Ophthalmol 1995; 79:362–367.

43. Cunha-Vaz J, Faria DA Jr, Campos AJ. Early breakdown of the blood-retinal barrier in diabetes. Br J Ophthalmol 1975; 59:649–656.

44. Meyer-Schwickerath R, Pfeiffer A, Blum WF, et al. Vitreous levels of the insulin-like growth factors I and II, and the insulin-like growth factor–binding proteins 2 and 3, increase in neovascular eye disease: studies in nondiabetic and diabetic subjects. J Clin Invest 1993; 92:2620–2625.

45. Nishimura M, Ikeda T, Ushiyama M, et al. Increased vitreous concentrations of human hepatocyte growth factor in proliferative diabetic retinopathy. J Clin Endocrinol Metab 1999; 84:659–662.

46. Aiello LP, Avery RL, Arrigg PG, et al. Vascular endothelial growth factor in ocular fluid of patients with diabetic retinopathy and other retinal disorders [see comments]. N Engl J Med 1994; 331:1480–1487.

47. Adamis AP, Miller JW, Bernal MT, et al. Increased vascular endothelial growth factor levels in the vitreous of eyes with proliferative diabetic retinopathy. Am J Ophthalmol 1994; 118:445–450.

48. Aiello LP, Hata Y. Molecular mechanisms of growth factor action in diabetic retinopathy. Curr Opin Endocrinol Diabetes 1999; 6:146–156.

49. Aiello LP, Bursell SE, Clermont A, et al. Vascular endothelial growth factor–induced retinal permeability is mediated by protein kinase C in vivo and suppressed by an orally effective β isoform–selective inhibitor. Diabetes 1997; 46:1473–1480.

50. Miller JW, Adamis AP, Aiello LP. Vascular endothelial growth factor in ocular neovascularization and proliferative diabetic retinopathy. Diabetes Metab Rev 1997; 13:37–50.

51. Okamoto N, Tobe T, Hackett SF, et al. Transgenic mice with increased expression of vascular endothelial growth factor in the retina: a new model of intraretinal and subretinal neovascularization [see comments]. Am J Pathol 1997; 151:281–291.

52. Ozaki H, Hayashi H, Vinores SA, et al. Intravitreal sustained release of VEGF causes retinal neovascularization in rabbits and breakdown of the blood-retinal barrier in rabbits and primates. Exp Eye Res 1997; 64:505–517.

53. The PKC-DRS Study Group. Manuscript Writing & Study Executive Committee: Aiello LP, Davis MD, Milton RC, Sheetz MJ, Arora V, Vignati L. The effect of ruboxistaurin on visual loss in patients with moderately severe to very severe nonproliferative diabetic retinopathy: initial results of the PKC-DRS multicenter randomized clinical trial. Diabetes 2005; 54:2188–2197.

54. Strøm C, Sander B, Klemp K, Aiello LP, Lund-Andersen H, Larsen M. Effect of ruboxistaurin on blood-retinal barrier permeability in relation to severity of leakage in diabetic macular edema. Invest Ophthalmol Vis Sci 2005; 46(10):3855–3858.
55. Aiello LP, Clermont A, Arora V, Davis MD, Sheetz MJ, Bursell SE. Inhibition of PKC-β by oral administration of ruboxistaurin (ly333531) mesylate is well-tolerated and ameliorates diabetes-induced retinal hemodynamic abnormalities in patients. Invest Ophthalmol Vis Sci 2005; 47(1):86–92.
56. The PKC-DMES Study Group. Manuscript Writing & Study Executive Committee: Aiello LP, Davis MD, Milton RC, Sheetz MJ. Effect of Ruboxistaurin, in Patients with Diabetic Macular Edema: 30-month results of the randomized PKC-DMES clinical trial. Arch Ophthalmol 2007; 125:318–324.
57. The PKC-DRS2 Study Group. Manuscript Writing & Study Executive Committee: Aiello LP, Davis MD, Girach A, Kles KA, Milton RC, Sheetz MJ, Vignati L, Zhi X. Effect of ruboxistaurin on visual loss in patients with diabetic retinopathy. Ophthalmol 2006; 113:2221–2230.
58. Tuttle KR, Bakris GL, Toto RD, McGill JB, Hu K, Anderson PW. The effect of ruboxistaurin on nephropathy in type 2 diabetes. Diabetes Care 2005; 28(11):2686–2690.
59. Cunningham ET, Adamis AP, Altaweel M, et al. and the Macugen Diabetic Retinopathy Study Group. A phase II randomized double-masked trial of pegaptanib, an anti-vascular endothelial growth factor aptamer, for diabetic macular edema. Ophthalmol 2005; 46:3855–3858.
60. Chun DW, Heier JS, Topping TM, Duker JS, Bankert JM. A pilot study of multiple intravitreal injections of ranibizumab in patients with center-involving clinically significant diabetic macular edema. Ophthalmology 2006; 113(10):1706–1712.
61. Jager RD, Aiello LP, Patel SC, Cunningham ET. Risks of intravitreal injection: a comprehensive review. RETINA 2004; 24(5):676–698.
62. Tripathi RC, Li J, Tripathi BJ, et al. Increased level of vascular endothelial growth factor in aqueous humor of patients with neovascular glaucoma. Ophthalmology 1998; 105:232–237.
63. Tolentino MJ, Miller JW, Gragoudas ES, et al. Vascular endothelial growth factor is sufficient to produce iris neovascularization and neovascular glaucoma in a nonhuman primate. Arch Ophthalmol 1996; 114:964–970.
64. Aiello LP, Gardner TW, King GL, et al. Diabetic retinopathy: technical review. Diabetes Care 1998; 21:143–156.
65. The Diabetic Retinopathy Study Research Group. Four risk factors for severe visual loss in diabetic retinopathy. The third report from the Diabetic Retinopathy Study. Arch Ophthalmol 1979; 97:654–655.
66. Wilkinson CP, Ferris FL III, Klein RE, et al. Proposed international clinical diabetic retinopathy and diabetic macular edema disease severity scales. Ophthalmology 2003; 110(9):1677–1682; Chew EY. A simplified diabetic retinopathy scale. Ophthalmology 2003; 110(9):1677–1682.
67. Chew EY. A simplified diabetic retinopathy scale. Ophthalmology 2003; 110(9):1675–1676.
68. The Early Treatment Diabetic Retinopathy Study Research Group. Treatment techniques and clinical guidelines for photocoagulation of diabetic macular edema. Early Treatment Diabetic Retinopathy Study Report No. 2. Ophthalmology 1987; 94:761–774.
69. The Early Treatment Diabetic Retinopathy Study Research Group. Photocoagulation for diabetic macular edema: Early Treatment Diabetic Retinopathy Study Report No. 4. Int Ophthalmol Clin 1987; 27:265–272.
70. Diabetic Retinopathy Study Research Group. Preliminary report on effects of photocoagulation therapy. DRS Report No. 1. Am J Ophthalmol 1976; 81:1–14.
71. Diabetic Retinopathy Study Research Group. Photocoagulation treatment of proliferative diabetic retinopathy. DRS Report No. 2. Ophthalmology 1978; 85:82–106.
72. Diabetic Retinopathy Study Research Group. Four risk factors for severe visual loss in diabetic retinopathy. DRS Report No. 3. Arch Ophthalmol 1979; 97:654–655.
73. Diabetic Retinopathy Study Research Group. A short report of long-term results. DRS Report No. 4. Proc 10th Congr Int Diabetes Fed Vienna, Sept 9–14, 1979. North Holland: Excerpta Medica, 1980:789–94.
74. Diabetic Retinopathy Study Research Group. Photocoagulation treatment of proliferative diabetic retinopathy: relationship of adverse treatment effects to retinopathy severity. DRS Report No. 5. Dev Ophthalmol 1981; 2:248–261.
75. Diabetic Retinopathy Study Research Group. Design methods and baseline results. DRS Report No. 6. Invest Ophthalmol 1981; 21(1 Pt 2):149–209.
76. Diabetic Retinopathy Study Research Group. A modification of the airlie house classification of diabetic retinopathy. DRS Report No. 7. Invest Ophthalmol 1981; 21(1 Pt 2):210–226.
77. Diabetic Retinopathy Study Research Group. Photocoagulation treatment of proliferative diabetic retinopathy. Clinical applications of diabetic retinopathy study (DRS) findings. DRS Report No. 8. Ophthalmology 1981; 88:583–600.
78. Ederer F, Podgor MJ, DRS Research Group. Assessing possible late treatment effects in stopping a clinical trial early: a case study. DRS Report No. 9. Cont Clin Trial 1984; 5:373–381.
79. Rand LI, Prud'homme GJ, Ederer F, Canner PL, DRS Research Group. Factors influencing the development of visual loss in advanced diabetic retinopathy. DRS Report No. 10. Invest Ophthalmol 1985; 26:983–991.

80. Kaufman SC, Ferris F, Swartz M, DRS Research Group. Intraocular pressure following panretinal photocoagulation for diabetic retinopathy. DRS Report No. 11. Arch Ophthalmol 1987; 102:807–809.
81. Diabetic Retinopathy Study Research Group. Macular edema in diabetic retinopathy study patients. DRS Report No. 12. Ophthalmology 1987; 94:754–760.
82. Diabetic Retinopathy Study Report No. 13: factors associated with visual outcome after photocoagulation for diabetic retinopathy. Invest Ophthalmol 1989; 30:23–28.
83. Diabetic Retinopathy Study Research Group. Indications for photocoagulation treatment of diabetic retinopathy. DRS Report No. 14. Int Ophthalmol Clin 1987; 27:239–253.
84. Early Treatment Diabetic Retinopathy Study Research Group. Photocoagulation for diabetic macular edema. ETDRS Report No. 1. Arch Ophthalmol 1985; 103:1796–1806.
85. Early Treatment Diabetic Retinopathy Study Research Group. Treatment techniques and clinical guidelines for photocoagulation of diabetic macular edema. ETDRS Report No. 2. Ophthalmology 1987; 96:761–774.
86. Early Treatment Diabetic Retinopathy Study Research Group. Techniques for scatter and local photocoagulation treatment of diabetic retinopathy. ETDRS Report No. 3. Int Ophthalmol Clin 1987; 27:254–264.
87. Early Treatment Diabetic Retinopathy Study Research Group. Photocoagulation for diabetic macular edema. ETDRS Report No. 4. Int Ophthalmol Clin 1987; 27:265–272.
88. Early Treatment Diabetic Retinopathy Study Research Group. Case reports to accompany early treatment diabetic retinopathy study reports No. 3 and 4. Int Ophthalmol Clin 1987; 27:273–333.
89. Early Treatment Diabetic Retinopathy Study Research Group. Detection of diabetic macular edema: ophthalmoscopy versus photography. ETDRS Report No. 5. Ophthalmology 1989; 96:746–751.
90. Early Treatment Diabetic Retinopathy Study Research Group. C-peptide and the classification of diabetes patients in the early treatment diabetic retinopathy study. ETDRS Report No. 6. Ann Epidemiol 1993; 3:9–17.
91. Early Treatment Diabetic Retinopathy Study Research Group. Design and baseline patient characteristics. ETDRS Report No. 7. Ophthalmology 1991; 98:741–756.
92. Early Treatment Diabetic Retinopathy Study Research Group. Effects of aspirin treatment on diabetic retinopathy. ETDRS Report No. 8. Ophthalmology 1991; 98:757–765.
93. Early Treatment Diabetic Retinopathy Study Research Group. Early photocoagulation for diabetic retinopathy. ETDRS Report No. 9. Ophthalmology 1991; 98:766–785.
94. Early Treatment Diabetic Retinopathy Study Research Group. Grading diabetic retinopathy from stereoscopic color fundus photographs: an extension of the modified airlie house classification. ETDRS Report No. 10. Ophthalmology 1991; 98:786–806.
95. Early Treatment Diabetic Retinopathy Study Research Group. Classification of diabetic retinopathy from fluorescein angiograms. ETDRS Report No. 11. Ophthalmology 1991; 98:807–822.
96. Early Treatment Diabetic Retinopathy Study Research Group. Fundus photographic risk factors for progression of diabetic retinopathy. ETDRS Report No. 12. Ophthalmology 1991; 98:823–833.
97. Early Treatment Diabetic Retinopathy Study Research Group. Fluorescein angiographic risk factors for progression of diabetic retinopathy. ETDRS Report No. 13. Ophthalmology 1991; 98:834–840.
98. Early Treatment Diabetic Retinopathy Study Research Group. Aspirin effects on mortality and morbidity in patients with diabetes mellitus. ETDRS Report No. 14. JAMA 1992; 268:1292–1300.
99. Early Treatment Diabetic Retinopathy Study Research Group. Aspirin effects on the development of cataracts in patients with diabetes mellitus. ETDRS Report No. 16. Arch Ophthalmol 1992; 110:339–342.
100. Early Treatment Diabetic Retinopathy Study Research Group. Pars plana vitrectomy in the early treatment diabetic retinopathy study. ETDRS Report No. 17. Ophthalmology 1992; 99:1351–1357.
101. Early Treatment Diabetic Retinopathy Study Report No. 19. Focal photocoagulation treatment of diabetic macular edema: relationship of treatment effect to fluorescein angiographic and other retinal characteristics at baseline. Arch Ophthalmol 1995; 113:1144–1155.
102. Chew EY, Klein ML, Murphy RP, Remaley NA, Ferris FL III, ETDRS Research Group. Early Treatment Diabetic Retinopathy Study Report No. 20. Effects of aspirin on vitreous/preretinal hemorrhage in patients with diabetes mellitus. Arch Ophthalmol 1995; 13:52–55.
103. Chew EY, Klein ML, Ferris FL III, et al. ETDRS Research Group. Early Treatment Diabetic Retinopathy Study Report No. 22. Association of elevated serum lipid levels with retinal hard exudates in diabetic retinopathy. Arch Ophthalmol 1996; 114:1079–1084.
104. Diabetic Retinopathy Vitrectomy Study Research Group. Two–year course of visual acuity in severe proliferative diabetic retinopathy with conventional management. DRVS Report No. 1. Ophthalmology 1985; 92:492–502.
105. Diabetic Retinopathy Vitrectomy Study Research Group. Early vitrectomy for severe vitreous hemorrhage in diabetic retinopathy. Two year results of a randomized trial. DRVS Report No. 2. Arch Ophthalmol 1985; 103:1644–1652.
106. Diabetic Retinopathy Vitrectomy Study Research Group. Early vitrectomy for severe proliferative diabetic retinopathy in eyes with useful vision. Results of a randomized trial. DRVS Report No. 3. Ophthalmology 1988; 95:1307–1320.

107. Diabetic Retinopathy Vitrectomy Study Research Group. Early vitrectomy for severe proliferative diabetic retinopathy in eyes with useful vision. DRVS Report No. 4. Ophthalmology 1988; 95:1321–1334.

108. Diabetic Retinopathy Vitrectomy Study Report No. 5: early vitrectomy for severe vitreous hemorrhage in diabetic retinopathy. Four-year results of a randomized trial. Arch Ophthalmol 1990; 108:958–964.

109. Diabetes Control and Complications Trial Research Group. Are continuing studies of metabolic control and microvascular complications in insulin-dependent diabetes mellitus justified? N Engl J Med 1988; 318:246–250.

110. The Diabetes Control and Complications Trial Research Group. The relationship of glycemic exposure (HbA$_{1c}$) to the risk of development and progression of retinopathy in the Diabetes control and complications trial. Diabetes 1995; 44:968–983.

111. The Diabetes Control and Complications Trial Research Group. Progression of retinopathy with intensive versus conventional treatment in the diabetes control and complications trial. Ophthalmology 1995; 102:647–661.

112. The Diabetes Control and Complications Trial Research Group. Hypoglycemia in the diabetes control and complications trial. Diabetes 1997; 46:271–286.

113. The Diabetes Control and Complications Trial Research Group. Lifetime benefits and costs of intensive therapy as practiced in the diabetes control and complications trial. JAMA 1996; 276: 1409–1415.

114. The Diabetes Control and Complications Trial Research Group. The effect of intensive treatment of diabetes on the development and progression of long term complications in insulin dependent diabetes mellitus. N Engl J Med 1993; 329:977–986.

115. UK Prospective Diabetes Study (UKPDS) Group. Intensive blood-glucose control with sulphonylureas or insulin compared with conventional treatment and risk of complications in patients with type 2 diabetes (UKPDS 33). Lancet 1998; 352(9131):837–853. Erratum in: Lancet 1999; 354(9178):602.

116. Ferris FL, Chew EY, Hoogwerf BJ. Serum lipids and diabetic retinopathy. Early treatment diabetic retinopathy study research group. Diabetes Care 1996; 19:1291–1293.

117. Chew EY, Klein ML, Ferris FL, et al. Association of elevated serum lipid levels with retinal hard exudates in diabetic retinopathy. Early treatment diabetic retinopathy study (ETDRS) Report No. 22. Arch Ophthalmol 1996; 114:1079–1084.

118. Martidis A, Duker JS, Greenberg PB, et al. Intravitreal triamcinolone for refractory diabetic macular edema. Ophthalmology 2002; 109:920–927.

119. Massin P, Audren F, Haouchine B, et al. Intravitreal triamcinolone acetonide for diabetic diffuse macular edema, preliminary results of a prospective controlled trial. Ophthalmology 2004; 111:218–225.

120. Aiello LP, Pierce EA, Foley ED, et al. Suppression of retinal neovascularization in vivo by inhibition of vascular endothelial growth factor (VEGF) using soluble VEGF-receptor chimeric proteins. Proc Natl Acad Sci USA. 1995; 92:10457–10461.

121. Robinson GS, Pierce EA, Rook SL, Foley E, Webb R, Smith LE. Oligodeoxynucleotides inhibit retinal neovascularization in a murine model of proliferative retinopathy. Proc Natl Acad Sci USA. 1996; 93:4851–4856.

122. Adamis AP, Shima DT, Tolentino MJ, et al. Inhibition of vascular endothelial growth factor prevents retinal ischemia-associated iris neovascularization in a nonhuman primate. Arch Ophthalmol 1996; 114:66–71.

123. Xia P, Aiello LP, Ishii H, et al. Characterization of vascular endothelial growth factor's effect on the activation of protein kinase C, its isoforms, and endothelial cell growth. J Clin Invest 1996; 98: 2018–2026.

124. Ishii H, Jirousek MR, Koya D, et al. Amelioration of vascular dysfunctions in diabetic rats by an oral PKC β inhibitor. Science 1996; 272:728–731.

125. Witkin SR, Klein R. Ophthalmologic care for persons with diabetes. JAMA 1984; 251:2534–2537.

126. Comprehensive Adult Eye Evaluation: Preferred Practice Pattern, 1989. San Francisco: American Academy of Ophthalmology, 1989.

127. Klein R, Klein BE, Neider MW, et al. Diabetic retinopathy as detected using ophthalmoscopy, a nonmydriatic camera, and a standard fundus camera. Ophthalmology 1985; 92:485–491.

128. Moss SE, Klein R, Kessler SD, Richie KA. Comparison between ophthalmoscopy and fundus photography in determining severity of diabetic retinopathy. Ophthalmology 1985; 92:62–67.

129. Sussman EJ, Tsiaras WG, Soper KA. Diagnosis of diabetic eye disease. JAMA 1982; 247:3231–3234.

130. Klein R, Klein BE, Moss SE, et al. Retinopathy in young-onset diabetic patients. Diabetes Care 1985; 8:311–315.

131. Krolewski AS, Warram JH, Rand LI, et al. Risk of proliferative diabetic retinopathy in juvenile-onset type I diabetes: a 40-year follow-up study. Diabetes Care 1986; 9:443–452.

132. Klein BE, Moss SE, Klein R. Is menarche associated with diabetic retinopathy? Diabetes Care 1990; 13:1034–1038.

133. Kostraba JN, Klein R, Dorman JS, et al. The epidemiology of diabetes complications study: IV. Correlates of diabetic background and proliferative retinopathy. Am J Epidemiol 1991; 133: 381–391.
134. Branch LG, Horowitz A, Carr C. The implications for everyday life of incident self-reported visual decline among people over age 65 living in the community. Gerontologist 1989; 19:259–365.
135. The DCCT Research Group. The Diabetes Control and Complications Trial (DCCT). Design and methodologic considerations for the feasibility phase. Diabetes 1986; 25:530–545.
136. The Diabetes Control Complications Trail Research Group. The Kroc Collaborative Study Group. Blood glucose control and the evolution of diabetic retinopathy and albuminuria. N Engl J Med 1984; 311:365–372.
137. The Diabetes Control Complications Trial Research Group. The relationship of glycemic exposure (HbA1c) to the risk of development and progression of retinopathy in the diabetes control and complications trial. Diabetes 1995; 44:968–983.
138. Writing Team for the Diabetes Control and Complications Trial/Epidemiology of Diabetes Interventions and Complications Research Group. Effect of intensive therapy on the microvascular complications of type 1 diabetes mellitus. JAMA 2002; 287(19):2563–2569.
139. American Diabetes Association. Standards of medical care for patients with diabetes mellitus. Diabetes Care 2003; 26(suppl 1):S33–S50.
140. California Healthcare Foundation/American Geriatrics Society Panel on Improving Care for Elders with Diabetes. Guidelines for improving the care of the older person with diabetes mellitus. JAGS 2003; 51:S265–S280.
141. Matthews DR, Stratton IM, Aldington SJ, Holman RR, Kohner EM: UK Prospective Diabetes Study Group. Risks of progression of retinopathy and vision loss related to tight blood pressure control in type 2 diabetes mellitus: UKPDS 69. Arch Ophthalmol 2004; 122(11):1631–1640.
142. Villarosa IP, Bakris GL. The appropriate blood pressure control in diabetes (ABCD) trial. J Hum Hypertens 1998; 12:653–655.
143. Harpaz D, Gottlieb S, Graff E, et al. Effects of aspirin treatment on survival in non-insulin-dependent diabetic patients with coronary artery disease. Israeli bezafibrate infarction prevention study group. Am J Med 1998; 105:494–499.
144. Johnson ES, Lanes SF, Wentworth CE III, et al. A metaregression analysis of the dose-response effect of aspirin on stroke. Arch Intern Med 1999; 159:1248–1253.
145. de Gaetano G. Low-dose aspirin and vitamin E in people at cardiovascular risk: a randomized trial in general practice. Collaborative group of the primary prevention project. Lancet 2001; 357: 89–95.
146. Herbert PR, Hennekens CH. An overview of the 4 randomized trials of aspirin therapy in the primary prevention of vascular disease. Arch Intern Med 2000; 160:3123–3127.
147. Antiplatelet Trialists' Collaboration. Collaborative overview of randomized trials of antiplatelet therapy-I. Prevention of death, myocardial infarction, and stroke by prolonged antiplatelet therapy in various categories of patients. BMJ 1994; 308:81–106.
148. Caramelli B, Tranchesi B Jr, Gebara OC, et al. Retinal haemorrhage after thrombolytic therapy (letter). Lancet 1991; 337:1356–1357.
149. Barbash GI, White HD, Modan M, Van de WF. Significance of diabetes mellitus in patients with acute myocardial infarction receiving thrombolytic therapy. Investigators of the international tissue plasminogen activator/streptokinase mortality trial. J Am Coll Cardiol 1993; 22:707–713.
150. ISIS-2 (Second International Study of Infarct Survival) Collaborative Group. Randomized trial of intravenous streptokinase, oral aspirin, both, or neither among 17,187 cases of suspected acute myocardial infarction: ISIS-2. [see comments]. Lancet 1988; 2:349–360.
151. ISIS-3 (Third International Study of Infarct Survival) Collaborative Group. ISIS-3: a randomised comparison of streptokinase versus tissue plasminogen activator versus anistreplase and of aspirin plus heparin versus aspirin alone among 41,299 cases of suspected acute myocardial infarction. [see comments]. Lancet 1992; 339:753–770.
152. Gruppo Italiano per lo Studio della Sopravvivenza nell'Infarto Miocardico GISSI-2: a factorial randomised trial of alteplase versus streptokinase and heparin versus no heparin among 12,490 patients with acute myocardial infarction. [see comments]. Lancet 1990; 336:65–71.
153. Kelsey JL, Browner WS, Seeley DG, et al. Risk factors for fractures of the distal forearm and proximal humerus. The study of osteoporotic fractures research group. Am J Epidemiol 1992; 135:477–489.
154. Schwartz AV, Sellmeyer DE, Ensrud KE, et al. Older women with diabetes have an increased risk of fracture: a prospective study. J Clin Endocrinol Metab 2001; 86:32–38.
155. Cummings SR, Nevitt MC, Browner WS, et al. Risk factors for hip fracture in white women. Study of osteoporotic fractures research group. N Engl J Med 1995; 332:878–773.
156. Gregg EW, Mangione CM, Cauley JA, et al. Diabetes and incidence of functional disability in older women. Diabetes Care 2002; 25:61–67.
157. Tinetti ME, Williams TF, Mayewski R. Fall risk index for elderly patients based on number of chronic disabilities. Am J Med 1986; 80:429–434.

158. Robbins AS, Rubenstein LZ, Josephson KR, et al. Predictors of falls among elderly people. Results of two population-based studies. Arch Intern Med 1989; 149:1628–1633.

159. American Geriatrics Society British Geriatrics Society, American Academy of Orthopedic Surgeons Panel on Falls Prevention. Guideline for the prevention of falls in older persons. J Am Geriatr Soc 2001; 49:664–672.

160. Gregg EW, Yaffe K, Cauley JA, et al. Is diabetes associated with cognitive impairment and cognitive decline among older women? Study of osteoporotic fractures research group. Arch Intern Med 2000; 160:174–180.

161. U'Ren RC, Riddle MC, Lezak MD, et al. The mental efficiency of the elderly person with type II diabetes mellitus. J Am Geriatr Soc 1990; 38:505–510.

162. Worrall G, Moulton N, Briffert E. Effect of type II diabetes mellitus on cognitive function. J Fam Pract 1993; 36:639–643.

163. Ott A, Stolk RP, Hofman A, et al. Association of diabetes mellitus and dementia. The Rotterdam study. Diabetologia 1996; 39:1392–1397.

164. Strachan MW, Deary IJ, Ewing FM, et al. Is type II diabetes associated with an increased risk of cognitive dysfunction? A critical review of published studies. Diabetes Care 1997; 20:438–445.

165. Stewart R, Liolitsa D. Type 2 diabetes mellitus, cognitive impairment and dementia. Diabet Med 1999; 16:93–112.

166. Bent N, Rabbitt P, Metcalfe D. Diabetes mellitus and the rate of cognitive ageing. Br J Clin Psychol 2000; 39:349–362.

167. Ryan CM, Geckle M. Why is learning and memory dysfunction in type 2 diabetes limited to older adults? Diabetes Metab Res Rev 2000; 16:308–315.

168. Sinclair AJ, Girling AJ, Bayer AJ. Cognitive dysfunction in older subjects with diabetes mellitus. Impact on diabetes self-management and use of care services. All Wales Research into Elderly (AWARE) Study. Diabetes Res Clin Prac 2000; 50:203–212.

169. Peyrot M, Rubin RR. Levels and risks of depression and anxiety symptomatology among diabetic adults. Diabetes Care 1997; 20:585–590.

170. Anderson RJ, Freedland KE, Clouise RE, et al. The prevalence of comorbid depression in adults with diabetes: a meta-analysis. Diabetes Care 2001; 24:1069–1078.

171. Ciechanowski PS, Katon WJ, Russo JE. Depression and diabetes: impact of depressive symptoms on adherence, function, and costs. Arch Intern Med 2000; 160:3278–3285.

172. Lynes JM, Niculescu A, Tu X, Reynolds CF III, Caine ED. The relationship of medical comorbidity and depression in older, primary care patients. Psychosomatics 2006; 47(5):435–439.

173. Campbell VA, Crews JE, Moriarty DG, Zack MM, Blackman DK. Surveillance for sensory impairment, activity limitation, and health-related quality of life among older adults—United States, 1993–1997. MMWR 1999; 48(SS–8):131–157.

174. Caraballese C, Appollonio I, Rozzini R, et al. Sensory impairment and quality of life in a community elderly population. J Am Geriatr Soc 1993; 41(4):401–407.

175. Wahl H-W, Oswald F, Zimprich D. Everyday competence in visually impaired older adults: a case for person-environment perspectives. Gerontologist 1999; 39(2):140–149.

176. Wahl H-W, Schilling O, Oswald F, Heyl V. Psychosocial consequences of age-related visual impairment: comparison with mobility-impaired older adults and long-term outcome. J Gerontol Psychosoc Sci 1999; 54B(5):304–316.

177. Bazargan M, Hamm-Baugh VP. The relationship between chronic illness and depression in a community of urban black elderly persons. J Gerontol B Psychol Sci Soc Sci 1995; 50(2):S119–S127.

178. Verbrugge LM, Patrick DL. "Seven chronic conditions: their impact on us adults' activity levels and use of medical services." Am J Public Health 1995; (85):173–182.

179. Sun JK, Keenan HA, Cavallerano JD, Aiello LP, King GL. Ocular characteristics and retinopathy risk factors in patients with 50 years or more of type 1 diabetes mellitus. ARVO 2006 Annual Meeting, Fort Lauderdale, FL.

180. Javitt JC, Wang F, West SK. Blindness due to cataract: epidemiology and prevention. Ann Rev Public Health 1996; 17:159–177.

181. Klein BE, Klein R, Moss SE. Intraocular pressure in diabetic persons. Ophthalmology 1984; 91:1356–1360.

182. Marmor MF. Transient accommodative paralysis and hyperopia in diabetes. Arch Ophthalmol 1973; 89:419–421.

183. Klein BE, Klein R, Moss SE. Prevalence of cataracts in a population-based study of persons with diabetes mellitus. Ophthalmology 1985; 92:1191–1196.

184. Ederer F, Hiller R, Taylor HR. Senile lens changes and diabetes in two population studies. Am J Ophthalmol 1981; 91:381–395.

185. Bursell SE, Baker RS, Weiss JN, et al. Clinical photon correlation spectroscopy evaluation of human diabetic lenses. Exp Eye Res 1989; 49:241–258.

186. Dowler JG, Hykin PG, Hamilton AM. Phacoemulsification versus extracapsular cataract extraction in patients with diabetes. Ophthalmology 2000; 107:457–462.

187. Borrillo JL, Mittra RA, Dev S, et al. Retinopathy progression and visual outcomes after phacoemulsification in patients with diabetes mellitus. Trans Am Ophthalmol Soc 1999; 97:435–445. Am J Ophthalmol 2000; 129:832.

188. Kato S, Fukada Y, Hori S, et al. Influence of phacoemulsification and intraocular lens implantation on the course of diabetic retinopathy. J Cataract Refract Surg 1999; 25:788–793.

189. Chung J, Kim M, Kim H, et al. Effect of cataract surgery on the progression of diabetic retinopathy. J Cataract Refract Surg 2002; 25:626–630.

190. Ferris F. Early photocoagulation in patients with either type 1 or type II diabetes. Tr Am Ophth Soc 1996; XCIV:505–537.

191. Klein R, Klein BE, Lee KE, et al. The incidence of hypertension in insulin-dependent diabetes. Arch Intern Med 1996; 156:622–727.

192. Thai Multicenter Research Group on Diabetes Mellitus. Vascular complications in non-insulin-dependent diabetics in Thailand. Diabetes Res Clin Pract 1994; 25:61–69.

193. Klein R, Klein BE, Moss SE, DeMets DL. Blood pressure and hypertension in diabetes. Am J Epidemiol 1985; 122:75–89.

194. Fujimoto WY, Leonetti DL, Kinyoun JL, et al. Prevalence of complications among second-generation Japanese-American men with diabetes, impaired glucose tolerance, or normal glucose tolerance. Diabetes 1987; 36:730–739.

195. Klein R, Klein BE, Moss SE, Cruickshanks KJ. The Wisconsin Epidemiologic Study of diabetic retinopathy: XVII. The 14-year incidence and progression of diabetic retinopathy and associated risk factors in type 1 diabetes [see comments]. Ophthalmology 1998; 105:1801–1815.

196. Zander E, Heinke P, Herfurth S, et al. Relations between diabetic retinopathy and cardiovascular neuropathy: a cross-sectional study in IDDM and NIDDM patients. Exp Clin Endocrinol Diabetes 1997; 105:319–326.

197. Diabetes Drafting Group. Prevalence of small vessel and large vessel disease in diabetic patients from 14 centres: the World Health Organization multinational study of vascular disease in diabetics. Diabetologia 1985; 28:615–640.

198. Agradh CD, Agradh E, Torffvit O. The association between retinopathy, nephropathy, cardiovascular disease, and long-term metabolic control in type 1 diabetes mellitus: a 5-year follow-up study of 442 adult patients in routine care. Diabetes Res Clin Pract 1997; 35:113–121.

199. Lopes de Faria JM, Jalkh AE, Trempe CL, McMeel JW. Diabetic macular edema: risk factors and concomitants. Acta Ophthalmol Scand 1999; 77:170–175.

200. Marshall G, Garg SK, Jackson WE, et al. Factors influencing the onset and progression of diabetic retinopathy in subjects with insulin-dependent diabetes mellitus. Ophthalmology 1993; 100: 1133–1139.

201. UK Prospective Diabetes Study Group. Tight blood pressure control and risk of macrovascular and microvascular complications in type 2 diabetes: UKPDS 38. [see comments]. BMJ 1998; 317:703–713. Erratum in: BMJ 1999; 318:29.

202. Klein R, Klein BE, Moss SE, et al. The Wisconsin epidemiology study of diabetic retinopathy: V. Proteinuria and retinopathy in a population of diabetic persons diagnosed prior to 30 years of age. In: Friedman EA, L'Esperance FA Jr, eds. Diabetic Renal-Retinal Syndrome. 3rd ed. Orlando: Grune & Stratton, 1986:245–264.

203. Kullberg CE, Arnqvist HJ. Elevated long-term glycated haemoglobin precedes proliferative retinopathy and nephropathy in type 1 (insulin-dependent) diabetic patients. Diabetologia 1993; 36: 961–965.

204. Klein R, Moss SE, Klein BE. Is gross proteinuria a risk factor for the incidence of proliferative diabetic retinopathy? Ophthalmology 1993; 100:1140–1146.

205. Mathiesen ER, Ronn B, Storm B, et al. The natural course of microalbuminuria in insulin-dependent diabetes: a 10-year prospective study. Diabet Med 1995; 12:482–487.

206 Park JY, Kim HK, Chung YE, et al. Incidence and determinants of microalbuminuria in Koreans with type 2 diabetes. Diabetes Care 1998; 21:530–534.

207. Hasslacher C, Bostedt-Kiesel A, Kempe HP, Wahl P. Effect of metabolic factors and blood pressure on kidney function in proteinuric type 2 (non–insulin-dependent) diabetic patients. Diabetologia 1993; 36:1051–1056.

208. Collins VR, Dowse GK, Plehwe WE, et al. High prevalence of diabetic retinopathy and nephropathy in Polynesians of Western Samoa. Diabetes Care 1995; 18:1140–1149.

209. Lee ET, Lee VS, Kingsley RM, et al. Diabetic retinopathy in Oklahoma Indians with NIDDM: incidence and risk factors. Diabetes Care 1992; 15:1620–1627.

210. Esmatjes E, Castell C, Gonzalez T, et al. Epidemiology of renal involvement in type II diabetics (NIDDM) in Catalonia. The Catalan diabetic nephropathy study group. Diabetes Res Clin Pract 1996; 32:157–163.

211. Savage S, Estacio RO, Jeffers B, Schrier RW. Urinary albumin excretion as a predictor of diabetic retinopathy, neuropathy, and cardiovascular disease in NIDDM. Diabetes Care 1996; 19:1243–1248.

212. Fujisawa T, Ikegami H, Yamato E, et al. Association of plasma fibrinogen level and blood pressure with diabetic retinopathy, and renal complications associated with proliferative diabetic retinopathy, in type 2 diabetes mellitus. Diabet Med 1999; 16:522–526.

213. Cruickshanks KJ, Ritter LL, Klein R, Moss SE. The association of microalbuminuria with diabetic retinopathy. The Wisconsin Epidemiologic Study of diabetic retinopathy. Ophthalmology 1993; 100:862–867.
214. Roy MS. Diabetic retinopathy in African Americans with type 1 diabetes—the New Jersey 725: II. Risk factors. Arch Ophthalmol 2000; 118:105–115.
215. Klein R, Klein BE, Moss SE, Cruickshanks KJ. Ten-year incidence of gross proteinuria in people with diabetes. Diabetes 1995; 44:916–923.
216. Mogensen CE, Chachati A, Christensen CK, et al. Microalbuminuria: an early marker of renal involvement in diabetes. Uremia Invest 1985; 9:85–95.
217. Nelson RG, Knowler WC, Pettitt DJ, et al. Incidence and determinants of elevated urinary albumin excretion in Pima Indians with NIDDM. Diabetes Care 1995; 18:182–187.
218. Gomes MB, Lucchetti MR, Gazzola H, et al. Microalbuminuria and associated clinical features among Brazilians with insulin-dependent diabetes mellitus. Diabetes Res Clin Pract 1997; 35:143–147.
219. Davis MD, Fisher MR, Gangnon RE, et al. Risk factors for high-risk proliferative diabetic retinopathy and severe visual loss: Early Treatment Diabetic Retinopathy Study Report No. 18. Invest Ophthalmol Vis Sci 1998; 39:233–252.
220. Qiao Q, Keinanen-Kiukaanniemi S, Laara E. The relationship between hemoglobin levels and diabetic retinopathy. J Clin Epidemiol 1997; 50:153–158.
221. Friedman EA, Brown CD, Berman DH. Erythropoietin in diabetic macular edema and renal insufficiency. Am J Kidney Dis 1995; 26:202–208.
222. Morley JE. The elderly type 2 diabetic patient: special considerations. Diabet Med 1998; 1(suppl 4): S41–S46.
223. Klein BE, Klein R, Moss SE. Incidence of cataract surgery in the Wisconsin Epidemiologic Study of diabetic retinopathy. Am J Ophthalmol 1995; 119:295–300.
224. Klein BE, Klein R, Wang Q, Moss SE. Older-onset diabetes and lens opacities: The Beaver Dam Eye Study. Ophthalmic Epidemiol 1995; 2:49–55.

18 | Foot Care in Older Adults with Diabetes Mellitus

Aristidis Veves
Joslin-Beth Israel Deaconess Foot Center and Microcirculation Laboratory, Harvard Medical School, Boston, Massachusetts, U.S.A.

Thomas E. Lyons
Division of Podiatry, Beth Israel Deaconess Medical Center, Harvard Medical School, Boston, Massachusetts, U.S.A.

INTRODUCTION

Complications involving the foot in patients with diabetes mellitus are common and yet carry with them potentially serious consequences. Conditions affecting the foot range from simple conditions affecting the skin and toenails to the more severe and potentially limb-threatening conditions such as ulcerations and infections. Despite adequate therapy, these more serious conditions may result in prolonged hospitalizations. In fact, foot pathology remains the leading diabetic complication requiring hospitalization (1). The incidence of diabetes in the general population is expected to rise and therefore we can expect the prevalence of diabetic foot complications will increase as well. This represents a great public health challenge, which will continue to burden the health-care system. Nonetheless, a great deal of progress has been made in our understanding of how diabetic foot complications arise and the best ways to prevent and treat them and ultimately reduce amputation. This is an important goal because we must strive to maintain the mobility of the aged as this will allow them to maintain their health and independence.

EPIDEMIOLOGY

The focus of discussion of diabetic foot complications centers mainly around lower extremity ulceration, infection, and amputation. A large part of health-care resources and expenditures for diabetes is utilized in treating these entities, which themselves contribute significant morbidity and mortality to diabetic patients.

Diabetic foot ulcerations are characterized by a delay in healing. There are a number of factors responsible for the development of ulcerations and essentially center around the pathophysiologic effects of diabetes, structural changes in the architecture of the diabetic foot, and environmental factors. Annually, 2% of all diabetic patients will develop a foot ulcer (2), while 15% will ulcerate over a lifetime (2,3). The prevalence of diabetic foot ulcers has been reported to range from 5.3% to 10.5% (2,4–6). When ulceration does develop, the cost of treatment may be fairly low for simple interventions. However, for more extensive and complex ulcerations, the cost of treatment may be in the range of several thousands of dollars (7). It is therefore important to intervene as early and as effectively as possible to minimize the need for more costly interventions such as hospitalization and amputation, the cost of which is often many times that of the cost of effective ulcer treatment (8). The importance of successful ulcer management becomes even more clear when one considers that 85% of amputations arise from ulcerations (9,10). Another disturbing statistic is that 15% of all foot ulcers will ultimately require amputation, representing the major risk factor for amputation (2). Other risk factors for amputation include increased duration of diabetes, poor glycemic control, peripheral neuropathy, peripheral vascular disease (PVD), and history of foot ulcers, previous amputations, retinopathy, and nephropathy (11–16).

In the United States, approximately one-half of all amputations are performed on patients with diabetes (17). Amputation rates also vary with both gender and ethnicity. Being male,

African-American, or Hispanic has been associated with greater risk for amputation (18,19). The reasons for this appear to be due to lack of access to education and routine preventative care. When programs designed to prevent and promote awareness of diabetic foot complications were instituted in high-risk populations, the rate of amputations was decreased by nearly 50% (20,21).

Lower extremity amputations in the diabetic population are estimated at 60,000 cases annually with an estimated expense of $30,000 to $60,000 per case (22). More disturbingly, the incidence of lower extremity amputations continues to escalate despite greater awareness levels and promotion of preventative care. Since 1990, the rate of lower extremity amputation in patients with diabetes increased by a staggering 26%.

As evidenced by the statistics, diabetic foot complications can be an overwhelming burden to patients, their families, and health-care professionals. The total cost of diabetic foot complications in the United States has been estimated to approach four billion dollars annually, as extrapolated from the costs of ulcer care and amputations (23). Continued efforts to identify high-risk patients, ensure adequate availability of preventative care, and prompt treatment remain the best means of reducing the destructive consequences of amputations and death.

DIABETIC FOOT ULCERATION
The Pathway to Foot Ulceration

The risk factors for diabetic foot ulceration can be categorized into three distinct groups: pathophysiologic changes, anatomic deformities, and environmental influences. Pathophysiologic changes at the biomolecular level lead to peripheral sensory neuropathy, PVD, and a compromised immune system with alteration in wound-healing capabilities. Motor neuropathy and Charcot neuroarthropathy are the major contributors to foot deformity. Finally, external factors in the form of acute or chronic trauma often precipitate the initiation of ulceration.

It is important to note that there is interplay between these risk factors that triggers a pathway leading to ulceration. The causal pathway to foot ulceration can consist of a number of component causes such as peripheral neuropathy, foot trauma, foot deformity, lower limb ischemia, foot edema, and callus formation. However, a critical triad of neuropathy, minor foot trauma, and foot deformity was found in greater than 63% of foot ulcers in one study (24).

As shown in Figure 1, in the vast majority of diabetic foot ulceration, the first major component is the development of sensory neuropathy that causes pain insensitivity or reduced

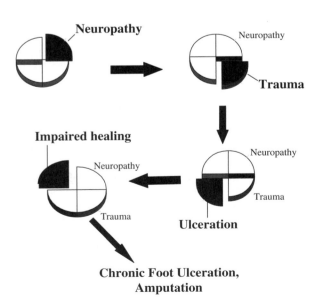

FIGURE 1 The pathway to foot ulceration. Sensory neuropathy, associated with pain insensitivity, is the first component of the pathway. However, the development of ulceration also requires the existence of trauma, usually related to the plantar tissue stress and injury that results from the development of high foot pressures during walking. The presence of the third component, impaired wound healing due to reduced blood flow in the ulcer area and aberrant expression of growth factors and cytokines, prevents the wound closure and leads to the development of chronic ulceration an, in some cases, amputation. *Source*: From Ref. 10.

sensitivity (10). The next component is the development of trauma, usually related to the foot pressures that develop under the foot during walking that are often elevated in patients with diabetes mellitus. The third major component is the impaired wound healing, related to reduced blood supply at the wound area and abnormal expression of growth factors and other cytokines that are involved in the healing process. It is usually the combination of these three major components that leads to the development of chronic ulceration and, in a substantial number of cases, amputation of the lower extremity.

Peripheral Sensory Neuropathy

Reported in approximately 30% to 50% of all diabetic patients, peripheral sensory neuropathy has been found to be the most common and sensitive predictor for foot ulceration in the diabetic patient (25,26). In a study that specifically studied casual pathways of diabetic foot ulceration, the presence of neuropathy was reported in 78% of cases (24). In the elderly over the age of 70, peripheral neuropathies may be present not only from diabetes but also from a variety of conditions (27).

The presence of peripheral sensory neuropathy initiates a series of events that eventually results in foot ulceration. With an inability to detect the pain signals that warn of impending tissue trauma and encourage rest or at least gait modification, a patient may continue to walk on a foot that is sustaining damage leading to ulceration. The propagation of this vicious cycle, of increased forces coupled with impaired protective sensation, may cause this site of injury to progress to the development of an ulcer.

Autonomic and Motor Neuropathy

Autonomic neuropathy is a common finding in patients with long-standing diabetes. In the lower extremity, autonomic neuropathy can cause arteriovenous shunting, resulting in a vasodilatory condition in the small arteries (28). The resultant distension of the foot veins is not diminished even with foot elevation. Consequently, a neuropathic edema recalcitrant to diuretic therapy is observed. This is in addition to the edema seen with other entities in the elderly. In addition to swelling, the neuropathic foot is also noted to be warm as a result of arteriovenous shunting (29). Abnormalities in autonomic neuropathy are also responsible for the decreased activity of the sweat glands of the feet. These changes in the diabetic foot can result in skin that is prone to dryness and fissuring, predisposing the patient to the risk of infection (30).

Motor neuropathy in the foot causes weakness and wasting of the small intrinsic muscles, classically termed the "intrinsic minus" foot (Fig. 2). This leads to muscular imbalance with a characteristic clawing of the toes and plantar flexion of the metatarsal heads. The fat pad on the plantar aspect of the forefoot may disrupt or shifts anteriorly. Atrophy of the intrinsic muscles within the arch reduces the bulk of the arch area for weight bearing. The result is prominent metatarsophalangeal joints, which serve as areas of focal pressures with possible irritation from footwear. Coupled with sensory neuropathy, these prominences clinically demonstrate the equation for ulcer genesis—elevated plantar foot pressures in the setting of sensory loss.

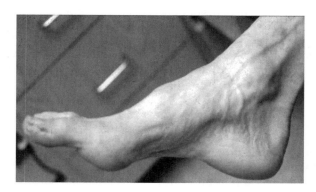

FIGURE 2 Changes related to motor neuropathy (minor foot). There is extensive wasting of the intrinsic muscles of the foot that results to clawing of the toes and prominence of the metatarsal heads.

Peak Plantar Pressures

Diabetic ulcers can occur on any part of the foot, but they are clinically observed most frequently on the plantar surfaces. The predilection of diabetic foot ulcers to the plantar surfaces is related to the trauma that develops in these areas due to the increased peak plantar pressures during walking (31).

Under normal conditions, the foot has the ability to distribute high forces that are applied on the plantar surface and therefore avoid the development of high foot pressures. This ability is greatly impaired in diabetes and is mainly related to the foot changes that are related to motor neuropathy (described above) and to the restriction of joint mobility (see below). As a result of this, the pressures under certain areas of the diabetic foot can be considerably high and lead to tissue injury even after walking short distances. In the presence of sensory neuropathy, the patient is unaware of initial warning signs of this injury, such as pain, and continues to walk until tissue integrity is compromised and foot ulceration occurs.

Numerous studies have shown that foot pressures are high in diabetic neuropathic patients (32–35). The high pressures tend to aggregate in the forefoot area or sites with bony prominence in the case of patients with Charcot neuroarthropathy. Usually, most ulcers develop under these areas of high foot pressures, but the development of ulceration in other foot areas can also occur.

The development of high foot pressures starts in the early stages of diabetic neuropathy, even in the subclinical phase of the disease. One of the first steps is the transfer of high peak pressures from the heel area to the forefoot area, in the absence of any clinically detectable neuropathy (34). As neuropathy worsens and the clawing of the toes develops, there is further transfer of peak pressures from the toes to the forefoot area. In cases of severe neuropathy, the forefoot pressures are so high that the ratio between forefoot and rear foot pressures is increased and can be used as an alternative of foot pressure measurement in identifying the at-risk patient for foot ulceration (36).

There is ample evidence, either from cross-sectional or from prospective clinical studies, that high foot pressures can predict foot ulceration (32,33,37,38). However, foot pressure measurements are characterized by a relatively low sensitivity and are not recommended as a screening tool (31). However, as they also have a satisfactory specificity, they can be employed in selected cases of at-risk patients to guide for the provision of proper foot wear that reduces high pressures and therefore decreases the risk of foot ulceration (39).

Limited Joint Mobility

Restriction of joint mobility is well documented in diabetes and is related mainly to collagen glycosylation that results in increased cross-linking of collagen fibers and thickening of the periarticular structures such as tendons, ligaments, and joint capsules (40,41). At the foot level, the subtalar and metatarsophalangeal joints are most commonly involved. The involvement of the subtalar joint seems critical as it impairs the ability of the foot to adapt to the ground surface and absorb the shock that develops when the heel makes contact with the ground during walking. As a result of this, high foot pressures develop, mainly in the forefoot area, and are believed to further contribute to the development of foot ulceration (35,42–44). Interestingly, limited joint mobility appears to vary with racial differences, with patients of Caucasian background having significantly less joint mobility compared to black patients (45).

Collagen glycosylation is also implicated in shortening and decreasing the resiliency of the Achilles tendon in diabetic patients, which can result in an equinus deformity with a further shift of plantar forces to the forefoot region (46). Surgical lengthening of the Achilles tendon has been found to effectively distribute plantar pressures more uniformly, decreasing the peak forces at the metatarsal region (47).

Peripheral Vascular Disease

Macrocirculation

PVD in not uncommon in diabetic foot ulceration and can be present in 30% of this population (25). Ischemia by itself is not a big risk factor for development of a foot ulcer. However, it is a big risk factor for delayed healing and amputation after an ulcer has already developed. PVD in diabetes is characterized by impairment at both the microcirculation and the macrocirculation level. Although histologically similar to disease in nondiabetic subjects, atherosclerosis in the patient with diabetes has certain clinically relevant differences. From the vascular surgeons' perspective, the most important difference in lower extremity atherosclerosis in diabetes is the location of atherosclerotic occlusive lesions in the artery supplying the leg and the foot. In patients without diabetes, atherosclerosis most commonly involves the infrarenal aorta, iliac arteries, and superficial femoral artery, with relative sparing of the more distal arteries. In patients with diabetes, however, the most significant occlusive lesion occurs in the crural arteries distal to the knee, the anterior tibial artery, peroneal artery, or posterior tibial artery, but with sparing of the arteries of the foot (7). Moreover, diabetic patient who smoke may have a combination of both patterns of disease, making successful revascularization more complex.

Microcirculation

There has been the notion that patients with diabetes have "small vessel disease." This was because of an article by Goldenberg in 1959, demonstrating periodic acid Schiff-positive material occluding arterioles in amputated limbs, and that explained in part the impaired wound healing (48). It was therefore thought that restoring circulation to the diabetic foot was hopeless for a many years. It seems that after years of trying to dispel the myth of "small vessel disease," we have now redirected our attention back to the impairments in the microcirculation. While there are no occlusive lesions in the diabetic microcirculation, structural changes do exist, most notably, thickening of the basement membrane. However, this does not result in narrowing of the capillary lumen (49). Instead, these changes decrease the elastic properties of the capillary vessel walls and therefore limit vasodilatation capacity. The basement membrane thickening may also act as a barrier to the normal exchange of nutrients and cellular migration, decreasing the ability of the diabetic foot to fight infection (50).

Despite these structural changes, it is currently understood that the most important changes in the microcirculation are functional. More specifically, over the last decade, it has been realized that these changes are related mainly to the dysfunction of the endothelial cell and vascular smooth muscle cell of the arterioles and the impairment of the nerve-axon reflex.

The endothelium, one cell layer in thickness, forms the luminal surface of all blood vessels. Normally, the endothelium synthesizes and releases substances such as nitric oxide, endothelin, and prostaglandins that are vital in regulating vasoconstriction and vasodilation and, therefore, in maintaining vascular tone and regulating blood flow (51). The main action of the vasomodulators is directed at the vascular smooth muscle cells that are adjacent to the endothelial cells. It should also be emphasized that, in contrast to large vessels, no atherosclerotic changes such as monocyte migration or foam cell formation are observed in the microcirculation. In addition, endothelial cells are involved in the angiogenesis, an important factor of the wound-healing process.

Recent work over the last decade has shown that there is reduced vasodilatory capacity in patients with diabetes and prediabetes and may be present in both patients with large vessel disease and those with adequate perfusion (52–55).

Another important factor that affects the neuropathic foot microcirculation is the impairment of the nerve-axon reflex. Under normal conditions, stimulation of the C-nociceptive fibers leads to retrograde stimulation of adjacent fibers, which secrete a number of vasomodulators, such as substance P, calcitonin gene–related peptide, histamine, and so on, and produce vasodilation (also known as Lewis triple flare response) (Fig. 3). This response is equal to one-third of the maximal vasodilatory capacity and is responsible for the hyperemia that is observed in areas that are close to injury.

As it would be expected, the nerve-axon reflex-related vasodilation is almost absent in diabetic naturopathic patients. This response remains absent even after successful bypass surgery to the pedal arteries that establishes satisfactory blood flow in the foot large vessels (56). This is probably the main reason that hyperemia, a major sign of inflammation, is absent in diabetic patients with infection of the foot. Thus, even the presence of neuropathy alone can lead to impaired blood flow under conditions of stress (57–59).

At the molecular level, the reduction of endothelium-dependent vasodilation seems to be related to the reduced expression of endothelial nitric oxide synthase (eNOS) by the endothelial

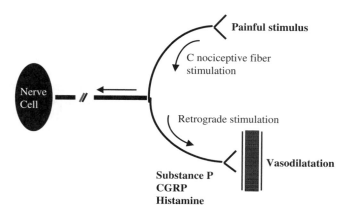

FIGURE 3 The nerve-axon reflex. Stimulation of the C-nociceptive fibers causes retrograde stimulation of adjacent fibers that release active vasodilators such as histamine, substance P, and calcitonin gene–related peptide. The final result is hyperemia during injury or inflammation. Due to the presence of peripheral neuropathy, this response (also known in physiology as Lewis triple flare response) is absent in diabetic patients. *Abbreviation:* CGRP, calcitonin-gene-related peptide.

cells of the microvasculature that is located in the skin of neuropathic foot (52). Whether this reduction is also related to the development of neuropathy is not clear. However, the expression of eNOS by endothelial cells at the forearm level is not affected by diabetes. Other mechanisms that contribute to the observed functional changes include reduced poly (adenosine diphosphate-ribose) polymerase activity and increased nitrotyrosine formation (55).

Despite the lack of complete understanding of the involved mechanisms, the main understanding from work that was conducted over the last decade is that the microcirculation of diabetic neuropathic foot fails to maximally vasodilate under conditions of stress. Thus, even in the absence of any peripheral disease and in the presence of good blood flow in the large vessels, the skin blood flow is impaired when injury occurs and this is one of the major factors that is related to impaired wound healing. Therefore, the neuropathic diabetic foot should be considered functionally ischemic regardless of the presence or absence of vascular disease. In addition, lack of hyperemia should not be interpreted as lack of inflammation or infection.

Impaired Wound Healing

As shown in Figure 1, impaired wound healing is a major factor that contributes to the development of chronic foot ulceration and amputation. Initially it was thought that failure to heal a diabetic ulcer was related to continuous walking on the injured foot, mainly due to the pain insensitivity, and the existence of peripheral arterial disease. However, it is currently realized that two other major factors contribute to this impairment, namely the functional changes in the microcirculation and changes in cellular activity and the expression of the various growth factors and cytokines that is normally involved in tissue repair and wound healing.

The normal wound-healing process entails a complex interplay between connective tissue formation, cellular activity, and growth factor activation (60). In diabetes, there are major abnormalities an all the above mechanisms. Thus, collagen synthesis is markedly decreased, at the collagen peptide production level as well as the post-translational modification of collagen degradation (40). In addition, hyperglycemia can potentially mitigate the cellular activity in the inflammatory process. More specifically, the morphological characteristics of macrophages are transformed in such a manner that impairs their function (61). Furthermore, inhibition of skin keratinocyte proliferation in the presence of increased cellular differentiation leads to an imbalance in keratinocyte production, an essential step in the wound-healing process (62). Finally, the expression of various growth factors such as platelet-derived growth factor and vascular endothelial growth factor is reduced, while the expression of matrix metalloproteinases (MMPs) is increased. The upgraded expression of the MMPs results in increased proteolytic activity and inactivation of the growth factors that are necessary for proper wound healing (63).

The final result of the above changes is that the diabetic ulcers do not progress out of the inflammatory phase of the wound-healing process. Under normal circumstances, during this phase that lasts only two to three days, the wound is cleaned by bacteria and is covered by an eschar that is devoid of any tensile strength. The inflammatory phase is followed by the proliferative phase that is characterized by angiogenesis, expression of numerous growth factors, cell migration, and collagen production and results in complete wound closure. It is currently believed that aberrant expression of growth factors and cytokines is the main reason that the diabetic foot ulcers fails to progress to the proliferative phase and remains in a chronic inflammatory state. Further understanding of this process will help in the development of new treatments in the future (64,65).

Additional Risk Factors

Other risk factors for the development of diabetic foot ulcers include long duration of diabetes, prior foot ulcer, and prior amputation. Duration of diabetes for greater than 20 years has been found to increase the risk of ulceration sixfold when compared to patients with a history of diabetes of less than nine years (66). A number of studies have demonstrated that a prior history of ulceration or amputation significantly increases the likelihood of a subsequent ulcer (5,67).

Changes in the Foot with Aging

Diabetes as we have come to appreciate can have profound effects on the body's systems at all levels. At the same time, there are significant changes that occur with the foot during the aging process. PVD may affect the foot during the aging process as well as with diabetes. There may be some common characteristics of PVD due to aging or with diabetes depending on the patient and duration of diabetes. Whatever the level involved, we may see diminished or absent pulses, cooler skin temperature, atrophied skin, and loss of hair. The nails may become brittle and thick. And with severe forms of PVD, dependent rubor and pallor with elevation are frequently seen (68).

As mentioned previously, peripheral nerve dysfunction occurs in the elderly especially as people age into their eighth decade. Symptoms of neuropathy may be present in approximately 50% of elderly patients with diabetes as well as approximately 10% of those without diabetes and include tingling sensations, numbness, or altered sensation, a feeling of tightness (common as people approach 80 years and beyond). Burning may be experienced and is not uncommon (69–71).

A number of dermatological changes occur in the feet of elderly patients. The stratum corneum contains less moisture and thus thicker skin tends to be drier, brittle, less elastic, and prone to cracking and fissuring. Turnover time for the stratum corneum is increased significantly often necessitating a longer period of treatment for some skin conditions. The epidermal rete ridges flatten resulting in a decreased area of contact between the dermis and epidermis. This may help to explain why the elderly are more prone to epidermal tears. This is also the reason to advise caution to the elderly when using adhesive corn pads that can tear the skin upon removal. Other dermatologic changes that occur are those of the nails, which often become thick and dystrophic often due to fungal invasion, damage to the nail root or matrix, and changes associated with PVD (72).

The subcutaneous tissue, which is the body's intrinsic cushion, tends to atrophy with age. This means that there is less protection with those areas of the foot that are weight bearing. For an individual who is barefoot, this area is the plantar aspect of the foot. For those with shoes, this includes the plantar aspect of the foot as well as any point of the foot that comes in to contact with the shoe especially at sites of bony prominences. Dense fibroadipose tissue contained within fibrous septa on the plantar aspect of the forefoot and heel may rupture displacing this material resulting in less cushion. For patients with normal sensation, less cushion on the plantar aspect of the foot may result in pain especially in areas of pressure such as under the heel and ball of the foot. For those with diabetes and neuropathy, this represents the perfect scenario for ulcer formation (73).

Musculoskeletal changes with age also occur. Atrophy of muscles occurs, which can result in reduced bulk of the intrinsic muscles of the foot resulting in a more prominent arch and metatarsophalangeal joints. Interestingly, the arch of the foot has a tendency to flatten or progressively pronate. If this does not occur, then a prominent arch may result in elderly patients who have diabetic neuropathy. If the arch does flatten, then atrophy of the intrinsic muscles of the foot occurs with the result being a flatter foot that may have plantar bony prominences less well protected with a soft-tissue cushion that is devoid of bulk from the intrinsic muscle atrophy. The joints of the ball of the foot may become less flexible and stiffen. This may be due to changes in the connective tissues or the result of foot deformities with inherent restricted range of motion. This occurs with hallux limitus where there is reduced range of motion at the great toe joint often associated with degenerative joint disease. Also with this condition, a dorsal bunion may form and is a site of pressure exerted by a shoe is susceptible to breakdown. Bunion deformities associated with hallux valgus are very common and can progress to a rigid deformity with time. The prominence with hallux valgus over the medial aspect of the first metatarsal phalangeal (MTP) is prone to breakdown with shoe pressure. The same is true with hammertoe deformities, which are toes that have contractures at the interphalangeal joints and they too may become rigid after a period of time. As hammertoes form, the interphalangeal joints may rub against the shoe forming a hyperkeratosis, which has the potential for ulceration. Hammertoes also may exert a retrograde force on the metatarsal heads that results in the lesser metatarsophalangeal joints becoming more prominent with a callus often forming as a result of this repetitive loading with pressure during walking. Calluses themselves may act to increase foot pressures focally under the MTPs as the callus thickens increasing the risk of ulceration in the setting of neuropathy (74). Any prominence on the foot whether from an osteophyte or from a deformity predisposes our elderly patients with diabetes to ulceration especially if any or all of the aforementioned changes occur.

Clinical Examination and Screening Techniques to Identify the Patient at Risk of Foot Ulceration

Prevention remains the best means of averting the potentially devastating results of diabetic foot complications. It has been estimated that up to 80% of diabetic foot ulcers are preventable (75). To that end, screening for risk factors by way of clinical examination of the diabetic foot has been recommended on a routine basis (76). Routine examination of the "at-risk" diabetic foot should include clinical inspection, neurologic examination, and vascular assessment.

Clinical evaluation of the diabetic foot should begin with a history of previous ulceration or amputation. A past history of ulceration or amputation increases the risk for future ulceration, infection, and amputation. It has been demonstrated that 60% of diabetic patients with a history of a foot ulcer will develop another ulcer within a year following wound healing (77). This is due to three distinct factors. First, the risk factors that were necessary to cause the previous ulceration remain present. Secondly, the skin over the previous ulcer site may be weakened and, therefore, more prone to subsequent breakdown. Finally, areas of previous amputation may demonstrate deformity and more importantly, since the foot is a dynamic structure, any change effected by an amputation may result in biomechanical imbalances that create areas of high pressure at other sites allowing for resultant ulcerations elsewhere.

The history of symptoms of neuropathy should also be elicited. More specifically, the patient should be asked for the existence of numbness in his/her feet or legs and painful symptoms such as described elsewhere in this textbook. However, it should be emphasized that the absence of neuropathic symptoms is not equated to the absence of neuropathy as the process of the development of neuropathy is insidious and that a large number of patients develop neuropathic ulceration without having ever noticed any symptoms.

Clinical examination usually starts with the inspection for foot deformities and limitation of joint mobility. Both of these entities increase foot pressures that lead to ulceration. Osseous prominences can be observed secondary to Charcot neuroarthropathy, motor neuropathy, and common foot deformities such as hallux abductovalgus, hallux limitus, and hammertoes, not limited to the diabetic foot. In addition, the examiner should look for callus formation and areas of erythema due to irritation from shoe wear. In the past, the presence of calluses was speculated to be a protective mechanism with debridement of these lesions not recommended. However, it is now well known that calluses are actually focal areas of increased pressure and can serve as sites of potential ulceration (74). So, should calluses be debrided? Yes, if the callus is thick with a deep core and especially if it is associated with discomfort or perhaps intraepidermal bleeding. There are some situations where the callus should not be debrided. Some calluses are broad and flat and if trimmed, pared, or debrided may be thinned to the extent that

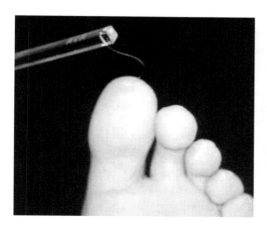

FIGURE 4 The 5.07 Semmes-Weinstein monofilament. The filaments is flexed when 10 g of pressure is applied on the skin. Failure to feel a 5.07 monofilament strongly indicates that the patient is at risk of developing foot ulceration.

the protection afforded by the callus is no longer present making the skin susceptible to breakdown. Any areas of erythema secondary to shoe wear irritation should be protected with padding or appropriate accommodative shoe wear dispensed to alleviate the pressure.

The next step in screening should involve neurologic testing for identification of the foot with loss of protective sensation. The perception of pain, touch, and vibration can be easily tested using simple standard equipment such as a pinprick, cotton wool, and a tuning fork. The main feature the clinician should look for is a sensory level below which the above modalities are reduced. The examination should be completed by testing the ability of the patient to feel a 5.07 Semmes–Weinstein Monofilament (SWM) at the great toe or the metatarsal heads (Fig. 4). Inability to feel the 5.07 SWM and/or the presence of a sensory level can identify 99% of all diabetic patients who are at risk of foot ulceration (78,79). As both these techniques are simple, not time-consuming, and not require any expensive equipment, they should be performed at least once a year in all diabetic patients. Patients with abnormality in any of these two tests should be considered at risk of ulceration and should be provided preventive care as described below in this chapter (75,79,80).

The final part of the examination should involve the vascular assessment. PVD is the cause in roughly 25% of foot ulcers and can contribute to the nonhealing of foot ulcers (81). One could then speculate that the incidence of PVD in older diabetic patients would be higher. The vascular evaluation in this population is even more important especially when an open wound is present. Vascular assessment includes a brief history for the existence of claudication and the palpation of all lower extremity pulses. The absence of palpable foot pulses or the existence of a nonhealing ulceration should prompt noninvasive vascular examination along with consultation with a vascular surgeon. The importance and value of a vascular clinician with the necessary expertise to evaluate and intervene in a timely fashion to increase blood flow cannot be understated. It is only when pulsatile blood flow is established that we, as foot surgeons, can then perform limb salvage procedures on the foot with an improved chance of obtaining a healed foot that is functional and ulcer-free.

Classification of Diabetic Foot Ulcers

There have been numerous classification schemes proposed for describing diabetic foot ulcers. The most commonly used and most often referred to is the Wagner system (82). The Wagner system classifies diabetic foot ulcers into five distinct grades, based on anatomical location, depth, and presence of ischemia. Wagner grade 0 describes a preulcerative or postulcerative lesion. There is no break in skin, but risk factors such as calluses and foot deformities are present. Wagner grade 1 ulcerations are superficial, full thickness ulcers with penetration past the epidermis. Grade 1 lesions are indicative of the presence of peripheral sensory neuropathy along with at least one other risk factor for ulceration. Continued weight bearing on grade 1 ulcerations will cause deepening of foot ulcers past the dermis with involvement of deeper structures such as tendons, ligaments, joint capsules, and neurovascular structures. Ulcers to this depth are considered Wagner grade 2 lesions. Grade 2 lesions do not probe to bone and osteomyelitis is not present. Wagner grade 3 ulcerations are characterized by the presence of deep infection with bone involvement. Abscess formations or osteomyelitis is commonly present in these deep ulcerations. Wagner grade 4 ulcers present with partial gangrene of the foot. Grade 4 ulcers demonstrate extensive vascular insufficiency, sepsis, and tissue necrosis that will necessitate aggressive management by a limb salvage team in order to limit tissue loss and possible amputation. Grade 5 ulcers are characterized by extensive necrosis and gangrene, which is usually best addressed with primary amputation.

The Wagner classification system for diabetic foot ulcers has withstood the test of time due to its simplicity, ease of use, and universal ability to be communicated among various medical personnel. However, for the most part, we only use Wagner grades 0 through 3 with any regularity and rarely does anyone use grades 4 or 5 to describe a patient's condition. In addition, the Wagner classification system fails to gauge the degree of ischemia in grades 1 through 3 and its inability to address the combination of infection and ischemia. Additionally, it does not provide predictions on healing and outcomes. In response, other classification systems have been proposed to address these deficiencies.

Other classification systems proposed include one described by Brodsky and Lavery that aims to be more inclusive if all types of neuropathic foot lesions in addition to providing predictors of outcomes and response to therapy (83). The San Antonio wound classification system mirrors the Wagner classification, but instead incorporates the presence or absence of infection and/or ischemia within each grade (84). This classification scheme has the added benefit of predicting outcomes, with results deteriorating with increasing stage and grade. While these newer classifications are more inclusive, the comprehensiveness makes them difficult to remember and use in the clinical setting.

As a result of the lack of a universally accepted classification system, there continues to be some confusion as to the best classification system. However, classification systems are useful as long as they are reasonably simple to remember. Instead of worrying about classifications, it is important to remember three parameters when describing a wound. First, describe as to whether the wound is superficial or deep. Superficial wounds for the most part are external wounds with no connections to the inner compartments of the foot. A deep wound on the other hand is one, which connects with the inner part of the foot and therefore carries with it a greater chance of abscess formation or extension to osseous structures with resultant osteomyelitis. As long as a wound remains superficial, the chance of deeper more serious involvement remains slim. Second, note the presence or absence of infection. An infectious process that is associated with an ulcer carries with it a greater sense of urgency in terms of resolution of the infection. This is especially true with deeper wounds that may have an associated abscess that needs to be urgently drained. Comparing this scenario with that of a superficial wound without infection, one can appreciate the difference in seriousness associated with these two situations. Incidentally, most infected superficial wounds associated with infection have a cellulitis that is easily treated. Third, evaluate and describe the vascular status of a patient with an ulcer. A patient with adequate perfusion has a better prognosis than a patient with poor blood supply, that is, ischemia. One can appreciate that depth, presence of infection, and presence of ischemia are the terms to describe an ulceration and they also provide a clue as to the patients' prognosis. Positive prognostic indicators are ulcers that are superficial, in a patient well perfused and without infection, while negative prognostic indicators are deep ulcers, presence of infection, and poor perfusion. Until a useful classification is devised that is easy to remember, these three parameters will more than adequately describe and characterize ulcerations in a clinical setting.

TREATMENT PRINCIPLES OF FOOT ULCERATION

Treatment of diabetic foot ulcers varies greatly depending on the severity of the ulceration as well as the presence of ischemia. However, the cornerstones of treatment for full thickness ulcers should consist of adequate debridement, off-loading of pressure, treatment of infection, and local wound care.

Debridement

The goal of wound debridement is the complete removal of all necrotic, dysvascular, and nonviable tissue in order to achieve a red, granular wound bed. Debridement of a wound achieves several goals including the removal of necrotic and nonviable tissue. This in turn will help to reduce the bacterial load of the wound and allow for a more adequate visualization of the wound. In addition, any bleeding incurred will help with the release of growth factors from platelets into the wound. Sharp surgical debridement using sharp instruments such as a scalpel blade is considered the treatment of choice (Fig. 5) (85). Using this technique, all nonviable tissue can be removed, until a healthy bleeding ulcer bed is produced with saucerization of the wound edges. This procedure can be performed in the office setting, except in the rare cases when extensive debridement is required or sensation to the foot intact and the use of the operating room may be required. In addition, in the event that ischemia is suspected, aggressive debridement should be delayed until vascular examination and revascularization is achieved.

Other debridement techniques are also available, but none has gained universal acceptance. Autolytic debridement refers to the body's own mechanism of removing devitalized tissue with the use of special dressings. This process is primarily undertaken by macrophages, which release proteolytic enzymes to degrade nonviable tissue (86). However, this method requires adequate arterial perfusion as well as wound hydration and can be slow and tedious. Enzymatic debridement involves the use of topical agents with the ability to degrade necrotic tissue via proteolytic enzymes as in the case of eschars or ulcerations with a fibrous base (87). Finally, mechanical debridement gently loosens and removes slough from the wound bed. The simplest form of this technique is the commonly applied wet-to-dry saline gauze. Upon removable of this dressing, the dried gauze will be slightly adhered to the wound bed, thereby removing the very superficial tissue. While this is an inexpensive and relatively easy technique, it can remove both viable and nonviable tissue and can cause pain in the sensate foot. It is useful in a wound requiring debridement. However, once a wound with a base of red granulation tissue ready to begin epithelializing is achieved, consideration must be given to switch to a nonadherent dressing so as not to pull off the epithelializing tissues from the periphery of the wound.

Pressure Off-Loading

Reduction of pressures is essential in the healing of plantar foot ulcers. As discussed previously, ulcerations occur in high-pressure areas of the insensate foot. There are a number of methods employed for the reduction of foot pressures, with varying success rates. The most popular methods include total contact casting, half-shoes, short leg walkers, and felted foam dressings.

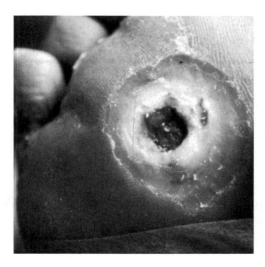

FIGURE 5 A grade 2 ulcer after surgical debridement. Adequate debridement is achieved when all exuberant callous tissue and necrotic tissue have been removed and a clean granular base is revealed.

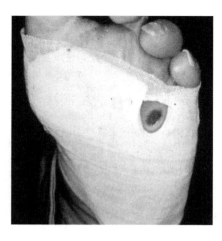

FIGURE 6 The felted foam dressing is an effective pressure off-loading modality for patients with Wagner 1 and 2 foot ulcers. The felted foam can stay in place for one week while wound care and wound assessment can be performed through the aperture portion.

Total contact casting has been considered the most effective means of off-loading diabetic foot ulcers as measured by wound-healing rate (88). Described by Paul Brand, total contact casting involves the use of a well-molded minimally padded plaster cast to distribute pressures evenly to the entire limb. It allows for patient mobility during treatment and has been found to help control edema linked to impairment of healing (89). The main advantage and likely effectiveness of total contact casting however is the forced patient compliance due to the inability to remove the apparatus. Disadvantages include the considerable skill and time required for application, the possibility of secondary skin lesions due to cast irritation especially in the elderly, and the inability to assess the wound daily. It is rarely used in elderly patients who might be frail and prone to falls.

Due to the considerable disadvantages associated with the total contact cast, few clinicians use it as the technique of choice in regular clinical practice. Instead, commercially available off-the-shelf devices such as the half-shoe and short leg walker are more commonly used. Both these devices are relatively inexpensive, easy to use, and readily accepted by the patient. However, pressure reduction is significantly less compared to total contact casting and patient compliance cannot be assured due to the removable nature of the devices (90).

Felted foam dressings are accommodative off-loading devices fashioned from a felt-foam pad with an aperture corresponding to the ulceration for customized pressure relief. The pad is generally attached by tape or rubber cement directly to the patient's skin, preventing migration of the pad and ensuring a degree of patient compliance (Fig. 6). Wound care and wound assessment can be performed through the aperture portion. The felted foam is often used in conjunction with a surgical shoe or half-shoe and must be changed every 10 to 14 days to ensure integrity of the dressing. Felted foam dressings in combination with a surgical shoe or half-shoe were found to be more effective in pressure reduction when compared to a short leg walker or a half-shoe alone (91).

Treatment of Infection

A diabetic foot ulcer serves as a portal of entry for bacteria with subsequent infection. Diagnosis of infection is primarily based on clinical appearance, relying on clinical signs such as erythema, edema, pain, tenderness, and warmth. The severity of the infection can range from a superficial cellulitis to a deep abscess or necrotizing fasciitis with systemic toxicity. Care must be taken to diagnose and treat infections sufficiently as mild cellulitis can rapidly progress to a limb-threatening infection if left untreated.

The diagnosis and course of treatment can be facilitated with diagnostic tools such as cultures, radiographs, and more advanced imaging techniques. When clinical infection of an ulcer is suspected, cultures of the wound will aid in directing subsequent antibiotic therapy. It should be noted that clinically uninfected ulcers should not be cultured, as the organisms recovered will only consist of colonizing flora. Empirical antibiotic therapy should be started, with revision of therapy following culture results.

Radiographic imaging of the infected foot can demonstrate increased density and thickening of the subcutaneous fat along with blurring of the usually visible fat planes (92). Presence of osseous changes such as periosteal reaction, cortical bone destruction, and focal osteopenia may suggest a diagnosis of osteomyelitis. However, these changes only become evident after osteomyelitis has been present for 10 to 14 days and require up to 50% bone loss before becoming recognizable (93). Advanced imaging techniques such as magnetic resonance imaging and computed tomography may aid in the accurate diagnosis of osteomyelitis as well as in the demonstration of abscess formations.

Treatment of infection involves debridement of all necrotic tissue and drainage of purulent collections along with antibiotic therapy. Antibiotic selection should take into account the likely causative organisms while bearing in mind the potential toxicity of the agents. In the diabetic foot, the bacteria most likely responsible for non–limb-threatening infections are staphylococcus and streptococci, while limb-threatening infections are generally the consequence of a polymicrobial infection (94).

Empiric antibiotic selection should be based on the suspected bacterial pathogens along with modifications to address anticipated resistant pathogens that may have been selected during prior hospitalizations. Antibiotic selection should minimize toxicity and be cost-effective. Broad-spectrum antimicrobial therapy should be begun empirically with reassessment following the results of culture and sensitivities. Treatment regimens should then be simplified based on the culture data. The main antibiotic regimens for initial empiric therapy that are employed in our unit are shown in Table 1 (95).

The duration of antimicrobial therapy for severe soft-tissue infections of the foot is based on response to the antibiotics and wound care. Two weeks of therapy is the usual guideline; however, recalcitrant infections may require longer courses. Even if the ulcer has not fully healed, antibiotics can be discontinued when evidence of infection has resolved. Continuation of antibiotics beyond this duration has not demonstrated any effect on wound healing (96,97).

Wound Care

The effective use of dressings is essential to ensure the optimal management of diabetic foot ulcers. In recent years, the concept of a clean, moist wound-healing environment has been widely accepted. Benefits to this approach include prevention of tissue dehydration and cell death, acceleration of angiogenesis, and facilitating the interaction of growth factors with the

TABLE 1 Selected Antibiotic Regimens for Initial Empiric Therapy of Foot Infections in Patients with Diabetes Mellitus[a]

Infection	Antimicrobial regimen[a]
Non–limb threatening	Cephalexin 500 mg p.o. q 6 hr
	Clindamycin 300 mg p.o. q 8 hr
	Amoxicillin-clavulanate (875/125 mg) one q 12 hr
	Dicloxacillin 500 mg p.o. q 6 hr
	Levofloxacin 500–750 mg p.o. q day
Limb threatening	Ceftriaxone[b] 1 g IV daily plus clindamycin 450–600 mg IV q 8 hr
	Ciprofloxacin 400 mg IV q 12 hr plus clindamycin 450–600 mg IV q 8 hr
	Ampicillin/sulbactam 3 g IV q 6 hr
	Ticarcillin/clavulanate 3.1 g IV q 4–6 hr
	Piperacillin/tazobactam 3.375 g IV q 4 hr or 4.5 g IV q 6 hr
	Fluoroquinolone[c] IV plus metronidazole 500 mg IV q 6 hr
Life threatening	Imipenem-cilastatin 500 mg IV q 6 hr
	Piperacillin/tazobactam 4.5 g IV q 6 hr plus gentamicin[d] 1.5 mg/kg IV q 8 hr
	Vancomycin 1 g IV q 12 hr plus gentamicin plus metronidazole

[a]Doses for patients with normal renal function.
[b]An alternative is cefotaxime 2 g IV q 8 hr.
[c]Fluoroquinolone with increased activity against gram-positive cocci, for example, levofloxacin 500 to 750 mg IV q day.
[d]Can be given as single daily dose 5.1 mg/kg/day.
Abbreviations: IV, intravenously; p.o., periorally.
Source: From Ref. 89.

target cells (98). In addition, patients have reported less discomfort with moist wound dressings. The notion that a moist wound environment increases the risk of developing an infection appears to be unfounded. There are a multitude of wound-care products available on the market that promotes moist wound healing; however, wet-to-dry normal saline gauze remains the standard of care.

Treatment by Ulcer Severity

Treatment of the diabetic foot ulcer should be individually tailored according to the size, depth, location, and presence/absence of infection or ischemia. Location of the ulcer will give clues as to the etiology of the wound, whether it is due to shoe pressure or an osseous prominence. Size and depth play a key role in determining the length of time required for wound healing. The presence of infection should be addressed with appropriate antibiotic therapy or surgical incision and drainage when required. Ischemic ulcers demand revascularization techniques in order for wound healing to proceed.

The treatment of ulcers based on grade, as delineated by the Wagner classification, will be presented here. It is important to note that as a general rule, Wagner grades 0 and 1 and the vast majority of grade 2 ulcers are largely managed on an outpatient basis while Wagner grades 3, 4, and 5 may require hospitalization. Table 2 describes the management of specific Wagner classified foot ulcers based on treatment rendered and medical personnel involved.

Wagner Grade 0

As mentioned earlier, all patients identified as being at risk of developing foot ulceration should be classified as grade 0. The management of the grade 0 foot consists primarily of patient education and regular foot care in an effort to prevent the development of foot ulceration. Regarding education, the patients should be informed of the risks associated with the neuropathic foot along with the early signs and symptoms of infection. In addition, the need of regular foot care by a specialist and the avoidance of self-care should be emphasized. Finally the daily inspection of the foot by the patient or a member of his/her close environment should be arranged. Literature with simple and easily understood guidelines is available worldwide by various sources and all patients should have access to this information.

Regular visits for podiatric care should be part of the patient's health-care management. Clinical inspection of the feet should be performed with evaluation of vascular perfusion to the foot. Hyperkeratotic lesions such as corns and calluses should be debrided at these visits. Shoe and sock modifications may be necessary to accommodate and pad any foot deformities. Extra-depth diabetic shoes and custom-molded inserts both serve to protect osseous prominences and also effectively reduce plantar foot pressures (99). High foot pressures can also be alleviated with the use of padded hosiery, which are locally available at shoe and sport stores (100).

TABLE 2 Principles of Treatment and Medical Personnel Involved in Diabetic Foot Ulcers Based on the Wagner Classification

	Principles of treatment	Provider involved
Wagner 0	Patient education, outpatient routine preventative foot care, and protective shoe wear	Diabetes educator, podiatrist, pedorthotist
Wagner 1	Outpatient ulcer care with debridement and off-loading	Podiatrist
Wagner 2	Outpatient ulcer care with debridement, off-loading, and wound care. Treatment of infection as warranted	Podiatrist
Wagner 3	Outpatient/inpatient ulcer care consisting of bedside or surgical debridement with off-loading and wound care. Treatment of infection as necessary	Podiatrist, surgeon, infectious disease specialist
Wagner 4	Inpatient care consisting of surgical debridement and antibiotic therapy. Revascularization may be required with possible amputation	Podiatrist, vascular surgeon, infectious disease specialist, orthopedic surgeon
Wagner 5	Inpatient care consisting of revascularization if possible and probable amputation	Vascular surgeon, orthopedic surgeon, rehabilitation therapist

Wagner Grade 1

Grade 1 ulceration is defined as one that has penetrated beyond the epidermis. The presence of sensory neuropathy and at least one other risk factor is assured. The ulcer should be evaluated for size, depth, location, and any signs of infection. The presence of drainage as well as the type of drainage should be noted.

The hallmark of treatment in these ulcers is debridement of all nonviable tissue, local wound care, off-loading of pressures, and antibiotic therapy if warranted. Sharp debridement of the ulcer should be performed as previously discussed in this chapter. Following debridement, the foot must be off-loaded to eliminate all pressure from the site of ulceration to promote epithelialization. The authors commonly use the felted foam dressing for off-loading. This method is easy to perform, relatively inexpensive and reproducible. Wound care can be performed through the window of the felted foam dressing.

Ulcerations that recur may warrant surgical correction of any underlying structural deformity. Surgical procedures such as digital arthroplasties, metatarsal osteotomies, metatarsal head resections, and midfoot and hindfoot exostectomies have all proved useful in the prevention of recurrent ulcerations (101–105).

Wagner Grade 2

Grade 2 is a full thickness ulcer that penetrates beyond the dermis with involvement of deeper structures such as tendons, ligaments, or joint capsules. The management of such ulcers is usually based on an outpatient basis, although hospitalization can be considered in deep wounds that expose tendons and complications such as PVD and infection is suspected.

Outpatient care for the full thickness ulcer that has a noninfected granulating basis is similar to that of the grade 1 ulceration described above. Broad-spectrum antibiotics may be added in case infection is suspected and dressing changes may be performed more often in cases of heavy exudates. Advanced wound-care products may be considered for patients who are not exhibiting a satisfactory progress using the criteria previously described.

Involvement of deep structures to the base of the ulcer should be managed with aggressive debridement, complete bed rest, empiric use of broad-spectrum antibiotics, and occasionally hospitalization (106). The foot may require surgical debridement in order to remove all necrotic and nonviable tissue that may impede granulation tissue. Debridement should be carried out until there is evidence of healthy, red, granulation tissue to the base. Additionally, all sinus tracts should be explored and drained. Intraoperative deep cultures should be taken for identification of the pathogen responsible for infection.

In the event that vascular insufficiency is suspected, incision and drainage of the infected foot should not be delayed. Adequate drainage of the infected foot is paramount to limb salvage. Delaying of surgical drainage may lead to further tissue loss as well as potential limb loss (107). Instead, vascular consultation should be initiated as soon as possible, even if it occurs after surgical drainage.

Wagner Grade 3

Grade 3 ulcerations are characterized by the presence of deep infection with bone involvement and abscess collections. Grade 3 ulcers are usually the result of grade 2 ulcers that fail to respond aggressive bacterial infections or puncture wounds resulting in direct inoculation of bone. Due to the depth of these ulcers and the presence of purulent collections and bone infection, these ulcers require hospitalization with adequate drainage of all infection and debridement of all infected bone. Prolonged antibiotic therapy may be required.

Adequate drainage of infection is key in managing grade 3 ulcerations. All sinus tracts must be explored and all necrotic and nonviable tissue debrided. In cases of severe infection, open amputations of digits or rays may be required to prevent the spread of infection. Once the infection has cleared and granulation of the wound bed observed, thought can be given to coverage of the wound. In instances where soft-tissue coverage is adequate, delayed primary closure can be undertaken. However, more often than not in these extensive wounds, significant soft-tissue defects may be present, requiring osseous remodeling in addition to tissue flaps or skin grafts to provide wound coverage (108). No single technique can be applied universally. Instead, a flexible approach will maximize limb salvage.

Wagner Grade 4

Grade 4 ulcerations demonstrate partial foot gangrene. These ulcers are usually complicated by ischemia, osteomyelitis, and sepsis. A team approach is required in order to minimize the extent of tissue loss and prevent amputation. Consultations with vascular surgeons, podiatrists, infectious disease specialists, and plastic surgeons are essential for limb salvage. The primary goal in the management of these ulcers is to limit the extent of tissue loss.

Gangrenous changes can result from minor trauma in the face of severe arterial insufficiency or when overwhelming infection results in occlusion of digital arterial branches (10,109). Initial treatment of gangrene secondary to severe arterial insufficiency should begin with vascular assessment followed by revascularization when possible (103). In severe infections resulting in local ischemia, aggressive drainage along with appropriate antibiotic therapy should be instituted to limit tissue loss.

Wagner Grade 5

Grade 5 ulcerations demonstrate extensive necrosis of the entire foot as a direct result of arterial insufficiency. Primary amputation is the only treatment for extensive gangrene. However, vascular assessment and revascularization should always be attempted to allow for amputation at the most distal level of the foot.

SUMMARY

The treatment of diabetic foot complications in elderly patients is a challenge when one considers the effects of diabetes and the aging process together. Every body system is affected as is the foot. Since the elderly tolerate deconditioning far less than younger patients, prompt recognition of potential problems combined with education to affect behavior modification is important to avoid the development of these complications. When prevention has failed and a complication arises, prompt and efficient treatment in the earliest stage is highly preferable. This is easy to understand when one considers the importance of mobility in maintaining optimal health overall, as well as for our patients with diabetes. Maintaining the best glycemic control possible decreases the chance for long-term complications including foot complications. This in turn allows our patients to maintain their mobility, which is such a vital part of their diabetes treatment program.

REFERENCES

1. Gibbons G, Eliopolos G. Infection of the diabetic foot. In: Kozak G, Hoar CJ, Rowbotham J, Wheelock F, Gibbons G, Campbell DR, eds. Management of Diabetic Foot Problems. Philadelphia: Saunders, 1984: 97–102.
2. Ramsey SD, Newton K, Blough D, et al. Incidence, outcomes, and cost of foot ulcers in patients with diabetes. Diabetes Care 1999; 22:382–387.
3. Palumbo PJ, Melton LJ. Peripheral vascular disease and diabetes. In: Harris MI, Hamman RF, eds. Diabetes in America. Washington, DC: US Govt. Printing Office, 1985:XV, 1–21.
4. Borssen B, Bergenheim T, Lithner F. The epidemiology of foot lesions in diabetic patients aged 15–50 years. Diabet Med 1999; 7:438–444.
5. Kumar S, Asche HA, Fernando DJS. The prevalence of foot ulceration and its correlates in type 2 diabetic patients: a population-based study. Diabet Med 1994; 11:480–484.
6. Moss SE, Klein R, Klein BEK. The prevalence and incidence of lower extremity amputation in a diabetic population. Arch Intern Med 1992; 152:610–616.
7. Harrington C, Zagari MJ, Corea J, Klitenic J. A cost analysis of diabetic lower extremity ulcers. Diabetes Care 2000; 23:1333–1338.
8. Apelqvist J, Ragnarson-Tennvall G, Persson U, Larson J. Diabetic foot ulcers in a multi-disciplinary setting: an economic analysis of primary healing and healing with amputation. J Intern Med 1994; 235:463–471.
9. Reiber GE, Boyko E, Smith DG. Lower extremity ulcers and amputations in individuals with diabetes. In: Boyko EJ, Reiber GE, Bennett PH, eds. Diabetes in America. Washington, DC: US Govt. Printing Office, 1995:409–427.
10. Pecoraro RE, Reiber GE, Burgess EM. Pathways to diabetic limb amputation: basis for prevention. Diabetes Care 1990; 13:513–521.
11. Reiber GE, Pecorraro RE, Koepsell TD. Risk factors for amputation in patients with diabetes mellitus: a case-control study. Ann Intern Med 1992; 117:97–105.

12. Lehto S, Pyorala K, Ronnemaa T, Laakso M. Risk factors predicting lower extremity amputations in patients with NIDDM. Diabetes Care 1996; 19:607–612.
13. Nelson RG, Gohdes DM, Everhart JE, et al. Lower extremity amputations in NIDDM: 12 yr follow-up study in Pima Indians. Diabetes Care 1988; 11:8–16.
14. Sittonen OL, Niskanen LK, Laakso M, Tiitonen J, Pyorala K. Lower extremity amputations in diabetic and nondiabetic patients. Diabetes Care 1988; 11:8–16.
15. Resnick HE, Valsania P, Phillips CL. Diabetes mellitus and nontraumatic lower extremity amputation in black and white Americans: the national health and nutrition examination survey epidemiologic follow-up study, 1971–1992. Arch Intern Med 1999; 159:2470–2475.
16. Wrobel JS, Mayfield JA, Reiber GE. Geographic variation of lower-extremity major amputation in individuals with and without diabetes in the Medicare population. Diabetes Care 2001; 24:1–5.
17. Most RS, Sinnock P. The epidemiology of lower extremity amputations in diabetic individuals. Diabetes Care 1983; 6:87–91.
18. Flegal KM, Ezzati TM, Harris M, et al. Prevalence of diabetes in Mexican Americans, Cubans and Puerto Ricans from the Hispanic health and nutrition examination survey, 1982–1984. Diabetes Care 1991; 14:628–638.
19. Roseman JM. Diabetes in black Americans. In: Diabetes in America. Washington, DC: US Govt. Printing Office, 1985.
20. Edmonds ME, Blundell MP, Morris ME, Thomas EM, Cotton LT, Watkins PJ. Improved survival of the diabetic foot: the role of a specialized foot clinic. J Med 1986; 60:763–771.
21. Lippmann HI. Must loss of a limb be a consequence of diabetes mellitus? Diabetes Care 1979; 2:432–436.
22. Reiber GE. Diabetic foot care: guidelines and financial implications. Diabetes Care 1992; 15:29–31.
23. Apelqvist J, Bakker K, van Houtum WH, Nabuurs-Franssen MH, Schaper NC. International consensus and practical guidelines on the management and the prevention of the diabetic foot. International Working Group on the Diabetic Foot. Diabetes Metab Res Rev 2000; 16(suppl 1):S84–S92.
24. Reiber GE, Vileikyte L, Boyko EJ, et al. Causal pathways for incident lower-extremity ulcers in patients with diabetes from two settings. Diabetes Care 1999; 22:157–162.
25. Young MJ, Breddy JL, Veves A, Boulton AJM. The prediction of diabetic neuropathic foot ulceration using vibration perception thresholds. A prospective study. Diabetes Care 1994; 17:557–560.
26. Adler AI, Boyko EJ, Ahroni JH, Stensel V, Forsberg RC, Smith DG. Risk factors for diabetic peripheral sensory neuropathy. Results of the Seattle prospective diabetic foot study. Diabetes Care 1997; 96:223–228.
27. Taylor R, Bradley WG. Peripheral neuropathies. In: Hazzard WR, Andres R, Bierman E, Blass JP, eds. Principles of Geriatric Medicine and Gerontology. New York: McGraw-Hill, 1990:977–982.
28. Ward JD, Simms JM, Knight G, Boulton AJM, Sandler DA. Venous distension in the diabetic neuropathic foot. J R Soc Med 1983; 76:1011–1014.
29. Boulton AJM, Scarpello JHB, Ward JD. Venous oxygenation in the diabetic neuropathic foot: evidence of arteriovenous shunting? Diabetologia 1982; 22:6–8.
30. Tegner R. The effect of skin temperature on vibratory sensitivity in polyneuropathy. J Neurol Neurosurg Psychiatry 1985; 48:176–178.
31. Boulton AJ, Hardisty CA, Betts RP, et al. Dynamic foot pressure and other studies as diagnostic and management aids in diabetic neuropathy. Diabetes Care 1983; 1:26–33.
32. Stokes IA, Furis IB, Hutton WC. The neuropathic ulcer and loads on the foot in diabetic patients. Acta Orthop Scand 1975; 46:839–847.
33. Ctercteko G, Dhanendran M, Hutton WC, et al. Vertical forces acting on the feet of diabetic patients with neuropathic ulceration. Br J Surg 1981; 68:608–614.
34. Veves A, Fernando DJ, Walewski P, et al. A study of plantar pressures in a diabetic clinic population. Foot 1991; 2:89–92.
35. Fernando DJ, Masson EA, Veves A, Boulton AJ. Relationship of limited joint mobility to abnormal foot pressures and diabetic foot ulceration. Diabetes Care 1991; 14(1):8–11.
36. Caselli A, Pham HT, Giurini JM, Armstrong DG, Veves A. The forefoot-to-rearfoot plantar pressure ratio is increased in severe diabetic neuropathy and can predict foot ulceration. Diabetes Care 2002; 25:1066–1071.
37. Veves A, Murray HJ, Young MJ, et al. The risk of foot ulceration in diabetic patients with high foot pressure: a prospective study. Diabetologia 1992; 35:660–663.
38. Kelly PJ, Coventry MB. Neurotrophic ulcers of the feet: review of 47 cases. JAMA 1958; 168:388.
39. Sarnow MR, Veves A, Giurini JM, et al. In-shoe foot pressure measurements in diabetic patients with at-risk feet and in healthy subjects. Diabetes Care 1994; 17:1002–1006.
40. Crisp AJ, Heathcote JG. Connective tissue abnormalities in diabetes mellitus. J R Coll Phys 1984; 18:132–141.
41. Vlassara H, Brownlee M, Cerami A. Nonenzymatic glycosylation: rose in the pathogenesis of diabetic complications. Clin Chem 1986; 32:B37–B41.
42. Delbridge L, Perry P, Marr S, et al. Limited joint mobility in the diabetic foot: relationship to neuropathic ulceration. Diabet Med 1988; 5:333–337.

43. Mueller MJ, Diamond JE, Delitto A, Sinacore DR. Insensitivity, limited joint mobility, and plantar ulcers in patients with diabetes mellitus. Phys Ther 1989; 69:453–462.
44. Birke JA, Franks BD, Foto JG. First ray joint limitation, pressure, and ulceration of the first metatarsal head in diabetes mellitus. Foot Ankle 1995; 16:277–284.
45. Veves A, Sarnow MR, Giurini JM, et al. Differences in joint mobility and foot pressures between black and white diabetic patients. Diabet Med 1995; 12:585–589.
46. Grant WP, Sullivan R, Soenshine DE, et al. Electron microscopic investigation of the effects of diabetes mellitus on the Achilles tendon. J Foot Ankle Surg 1997; 36:272–278.
47. Armstrong DG, Stacpoole-Shea S, Nguyen HC, Harkless LB. Lengthening of the Achilles tendon in diabetic patients who are at high risk for ulceration of the foot. J Bone Joint Surg 1999; 81A:535–538.
48. Goldenberg SG, Alex M, Joshi RA, Blumenthal MT. Nonatheromatous peripheral vascular disease of the lower extremity in diabetes mellitus. Diabetes 1959; 8:261–273.
49. Parving HH, Viberti GC, Keen H, Christiansen JS, Lassen NA. Hemodynamic factors in the genesis of diabetic microangiopathy. Metabolism 1983; 32:943–949.
50. Rayman G, Williams SA, Spencer PD, et al. Impaired microvascular hyperaemic response to minor skin trauma in type I diabetes. BMJ 1986; 292:1295–1298.
51. Vane JR, Anggard EE, Botting RM. Regulatory functions of the vascular endothelium. N Engl J Med 1990; 323:27–36.
52. Veves A, Akbari CM, Primavera J, et al. Endothelial dysfunction and the expression of endothelial nitric oxide synthetase in diabetic neuropathy, vascular disease, and foot ulceration. Diabetes 1998; 47:457–463.
53. Arora S, Smakowski P, Frykberg RG, Freeman R, LoGerfo FW, Veves A. Differences in foot and forearm skin microcirculation in diabetic patients with and without neuropathy. Diabetes Care 1998; 21:1339–1344.
54. Caballero AE, Arora S, Saouaf R, et al. Microvascular and macrovascular reactivity is reduced in subjects at risk for type 2 diabetes. Diabetes 1999; 48:1856–1862.
55. Szabo C, Zanchi A, Komjati K, et al. Poly (ADP-Ribose) polymerase is activated in subjects at risk of developing type 2 diabetes and is associated with impaired vascular reactivity. Circulation 2002; 106:2680–2686.
56. Arora S, Pomposelli F, LoGerfo FW, Veves A. Cutaneous microcirculation in the neuropathic diabetic foot improves significantly but not completely after successful lower extremity revascularization. J Vasc Surg 2002; 35:501–505.
57. Caselli A, Rich J, Hanane T, Uccioli L, Veves A. Role of C-nociceptive fibers in the nerve axon reflex-related vasodilation in diabetes. Neurology 2003; 60:297–300.
58. Hamdy O, Abou-Elenin K, LoGerfo FW, Horton ES, Veves A. Contribution of nerve-axon reflex-related vasodilation to the total skin vasodilation in diabetic patients with and without neuropathy. Diabetes Care 2001; 24:344–349.
59. Parkhouse N, LeQueen PM. Impaired neurogenic vascular response in patients with diabetes and neuropathic foot lesions. N Engl J Med 1988; 318:1306–1309.
60. Schilling JA. Wound healing. Physiol Rev 1968; 48:374–423.
61. Zykova SN, Jenssen TG, Berdal M, et al. Altered cytokine and nitric oxide secretion in vitro by macrophages from diabetic type II-like db/db mice. Diabetes 2000; 40:1451–1458.
62. Spravchikov N, Sizyakov G, Gartsbein M, et al. Glucose effects on skin keratinocytes. Diabetes 2001; 50:1627–1635.
63. Cooper DM, Yu EZ, Hennesey P, et al. Determination of endogenous cytokines in chronic wounds. Ann Surg 1994; 219:688–692.
64. Jude EB, Boulton AJ, Ferguson MW, Appleton I. The role of nitric oxide synthase isoforms and arginase in the pathogenesis of diabetic foot ulcers: possible modulatory effects by transforming growth factor β 1. Diabetologia 1999; 42:748–757.
65. Loots MA, Lamme EN, Zeegelaar J, Mekkes JR, Bos JD, Middelkoop E. Differences in cellular infiltrate and extracellular matrix of chronic diabetic and venous ulcers versus acute wounds. J Invest Dermatol 1998; 111:850–857.
66. Rith-Najarian SJ, Stolusky T, Gohdes DM. Identifying diabetic patients at high risk for lower-extremity amputation in a primary health care setting. Diabetes Care 1992; 22:1036–1042.
67. Boyko E, Ahroni JH, Stensel V, et al. A prospective study of risk factors for diabetic foot ulcer: the Seattle diabetic foot study. Diabetes Care 1999; 22:1036–1042.
68. Woolley DC. Peripheral vascular disease. In: Ham RJ, Sloane PD, eds. Primary Care Geriatrics: A Case-Based Approach. 2nd ed. St. Louis: Mosby-yearbook, 1992:578–583.
69. Richardson JK, Ashton-Millere JA. Peripheral neuropathy, an often overlooked cause of falls in the elderly. Postgrad Med 1996; 99:161–172.
70. Belmin J, Valensi P. Diabetic neuropathy in elderly patients. What can be done? Drugs Aging 1996; 8:416–429.
71. Richardson JK, Ashton-Miller JA, Lee SG, Jacobs K. Moderate peripheral neuropathy impairs weight transfer and unipedal balance in the elderly. Arch Phys Med Rehabil 1996; 77:1152–1156.

72. Gilchrest BA. Aging of the human skin. In: Hazzard WR, Blass JP, Ettinger WH, Halter JB, Ouslander JG, eds. Principles of Geriatric Medicine and Gerontology. New York: McGraw-Hill, 1998: 573–590.
73. Sarafian SK, ed. Topographic anatomy. In: Anatomy of the Foot and Ankle. 1st ed. Philadelphia: JB Lippincott, 1983:350–356.
74. Young MJ, Cavanagh PR, Thomas G, Johnson MM, Murray H, Boulton AJM. The effect of callus removal on dynamic plantar pressures in diabetic patients. Diabet Med 1992; 9:55–57.
75. Mayfield JA, Reiber GE, Sanders LJ, et al. Preventative foot care in people with diabetes. Diabetes Care 1998; 21:2161–2177.
76. Boulton AJM, Gries FA, Jervell J. Guidelines for the diagnosis and outpatient management of diabetic peripheral neuropathy. Diabet Med 1998; 15:508–514.
77. Helm PA, Walker SC, Pulliam GF. Recurrence of neuropathic ulcerations following healing in a total contact cast. Arch Phys Med Rehabil 1991; 72:967–970.
78. Kumar S, Fernando DJ, Veves A, Knowles EA, Young MJ, Boulton AJ. Semmes-Weinstein monofilaments: a simple, effective and inexpensive screening device for identifying diabetic patients at risk of foot ulceration. Diabetes Res Clin Pract 1991; 13:63–67.
79. Pham H, Armstrong DG, Harvey C, Harkless LB, Giurini JM, Veves A. Screening techniques to identify people at high risk for diabetic foot ulceration. Diabetes Care 2000; 23:606–611.
80. McNeely MJ, Boyko E, Ahroni JH. The independent contributions of diabetic neuropathy and vasculopathy in foot ulceration: how great are the risks? Diabetes Care 1995; 18:216–219.
81. Thompson FJ, Veves A, Ashe H, et al. A team approach to diabetic foot care—the Manchester experience. Foot 1991; 1:75–82.
82. Wagner FW. The dysvascular foot: a system for diagnosis and treatment. Foot Ankle 1981; 2:64.
83. Lavery LA, Armstrong DG, Harkless LB. Classification of diabetic foot wounds. J Foot Ankle Surg 1996; 36:528–531.
84. Armstrong DG, Lavery L, Harkless LB. Validation of a diabetic wound classification system. Diabet Med 1998; 21:855–859.
85. Steed DL, Donohoe D, Wbster MW, Lindsley L. Diabetic Ulcer Study Group. Effect of extensive debridement and treatment on the healing of diabetic foot ulcers. J Am Coll Surg 1996; 183:61–64.
86. Clark RAF. Mechanisms of cutaneous wound repair. In: Fitzpatrick TB et al., eds. Hematology in General Medicine. New York: McGraw-Hill, 1993.
87. Bale S. A guide to wound debridement. J Wound Care 1997; 6:179–182.
88. Armstrong DG, Nguyen HC, Lavery LA, et al. Offloading the diabetic foot wound: a randomized clinical trial. Diabetes Care 2001; 24:1019–1022.
89. Mueller MJ, Diamond JE, Sinacore DR, et al. Total contact casting in treatment of diabetic plantar ulcers. Diabetes Care 1989; 12:364–387.
90. Lavery LA, Vela SA, Lavery DC, et al. Reducing dynamic foot pressures in high-risk diabetics with foot ulcerations: a comparison of treatments. Diabetes Care 1996; 19:818–821.
91. Birke JA, Fred B, Krieger LA, Sliman K. The effectiveness of an accommodative dressing in offloading pressure over areas of previous metatarsal head ulceration. Wounds 2003; 15:33–39.
92. Cheung Y, Hochman M, Brophy DP. Radiographic changes in the diabetic foot. In: Veves A, Giurini JM, Logerfo FW, eds. The Diabetic Foot. Totawa: Humana Press, 2002:179–205.
93. Bonakdar-Pour A, Gaines VD. The radiology of osteomyelitis. Orthop Clin North Am 1983; 14: 21–37.
94. Lipsky BA, Pecoraro RE, Wheat LJ. The diabetic foot: soft tissue and bone infection. Infect Dis Clin North Am 1990; 4:409–432.
95. Karchmer AW. Microbiology and treatment of diabetic foot infections. In: Veves A, Giurini JM, LoGerfo FW, eds. The Diabetic Foot. Medical and Surgical Management. Totawa, NJ: Humana Press, 2002:207–220.
96. Lipsky BA, Pecoraro RE, Larson SA, Hanley ME, Ahroni JH. Outpatient management of uncomplicated lower-extremity infections in diabetic patients. Arch Intern Med 1990; 150:790–797.
97. Jones EW, Edwards R, Finch R, Jaffcoate WJ. A microbiologic study of diabetic foot lesions. Diabet Med 1984; 2:213–215.
98. Field FK, Kerstein MD. Overview of wound healing in a moist environment. Am J Surg 1994; 167(1A):2S–6S.
99. Chanteleau E, Kushner T, Spraul M. How effective is cushioned therapeutic footwear in protecting diabetic feet. Diabet Med 1990; 7:355–359.
100. Veves A, Masson EA, Fernando DJS, Boulton AIM. Studies of experimental padded hosiery to reduce foot pressures in diabetic neuropathy. Diabetes Care 1989; 12:653–655.
101. Gudas CJ. Prophylactic surgery in the diabetic foot. Clin Podiatr Med Surg 1987; 4:445–458.
102. Tillo TH, Giurini JM, Habershaw GM, Chrzan JS, Rowbotham JL. Review of metatarsal osteotomies for the treatment of neuropathic ulcerations. J Am Podiatr Med Assoc 1990; 80:211–217.
103. Giurini JM, Basile P, Chrzan JS, Habershaw GM, Rosenblum BI. Panmetatarsal head resection: a viable alternative to the transmetatarsal amputation. J Am Podiatr Med Assoc 1993; 83:101–107.

104. Giurini JM, Rosenblum BI. The role of foot surgery in patients with diabetes. Clin Podiatr Med Surg 1995; 12:119–127.

105. Rosenblum BI, Giurini JM, Chrzan JS, Habershaw GM. Preventing loss of the great toe with the hallux interphalangeal joint arthroplasty. J Foot Ankle Surg 1994; 33:557–560.

106. Gibbons GW. The diabetic foot: amputations and drainage of infection. J Vasc Surg 1987; 5:791–793.

107. Taylor LM, Porter JM. The clinical course of diabetic patients who require emergent foot surgery because of infection or ischemia. J Vasc Surg 1987; 6:454–459.

108. Attinger CE. Use of soft tissue techniques for the salvage of the diabetic foot. In: Kominsky SJ, ed. Medical and Surgical Management of the Diabetic Foot. Boston: Mosby-Year Book, 1994.

109. Edmonds M, Foster A, Oreenhill M, et al. Acute septic vasculitis not diabetic micro angiopathy leads to digital necrosis in the neuropathic foot. Diabet Med 1992; 9(suppl):P85.

19 | Infections in Older Adults with Diabetes

Suzanne F. Bradley

Geriatric Research Education and Clinical Center, Veterans Affairs Ann Arbor Healthcare Center, and Divisions of Geriatric Medicine and Infectious Diseases, Department of Internal Medicine, University of Michigan Medical School, Ann Arbor, Michigan, U.S.A.

INTRODUCTION

Numerous reports in the clinical literature describe an increased risk of infection in patients with diabetes mellitus (1). The relationship between increased infection risk and diabetes mellitus is very complex. Increased risk has been ascribed directly to metabolic effects such as hyperglycemia, ketoacidosis, and dyslipidemia on host defenses. In addition, indirect effects of the complications of diabetes, such as neuropathy and vascular disease, can impair host resistance to infection. Despite alterations in host defenses, only some infections seem to occur with increasing frequency in the diabetic patient (1–3).

Similarly, aging has been associated with increased susceptibility to some infections. Older adults also represent an ever-increasing proportion of patients with diabetes mellitus, particularly those due to type II or insulin resistance. How the process of aging and the effects of diabetes might interact to increase infection risk among older adults is incompletely understood (4). In the older adult, host resistance to infection may be diminished due to effects of aging itself, diabetes, and other common comorbid illnesses, and treatment of some of those conditions (Table 1). Increased risk of postsurgical wound infection has been independently associated with increasing age and poor long-term preoperative glycemic control (5). The effect of ketoacidosis on infection risk has not been rigorously assessed in the older adults because that metabolic condition is uncommon. The impact of hyperlipidemia and renal and vascular disease on infection in the aging diabetic has similarly not been evaluated in controlled studies. It is just as conceivable that age and diabetes mellitus are markers for more frequent hospitalization, medical procedures, and exposure to the health-care system leading to contact with more virulent microorganisms that are more likely to cause disease.

PATHOPHYSIOLOGY OF INCREASED INFECTION RISK IN OLDER DIABETICS
The Immune System, Diabetes Mellitus, and Age

What effects might diabetes mellitus have on the immune system that might account for increased risk of infection? The immune system is conceptually divided into two systems based on different mechanisms to differentiate self from nonself. The innate or nonspecific immune system is the most primitive, differentiating self from nonself through the activities of phagocytic cells, the complement system, and natural killer (NK) cells. The acquired or adaptive immune system specifically recognizes new antigens via antigen-presenting cells (macrophages, B lymphocytes, and dendritic cells) with resulting proliferation of specific T-helper cells that remember the antigen, generation of cytotoxic T-cells, and production of specific antibody by B lymphocytes.

The innate immune system and neutrophil functions have been studied most commonly in the diabetic; few controlled for age, duration of disease, or glycemic control, and cohorts typically included patients with type I as well as type II diabetes mellitus. Defects in chemotaxis, adherence, phagocytosis, oxidative burst, and killing have been described in some studies of neutrophils from diabetic patients when compared with controls. The monocyte/macrophage system has been studied less often and may be impaired as well. Defects in complement and the adaptive immune system, such as declines in the proportion of CD4+ lymphocytes, defects in memory cells, and impaired NK cell functions, are found primarily in patients with type I diabetes (3,6,7).

TABLE 1   Factors that Alter Host Defenses and Risk for Infection in Older Patients with Diabetes Mellitus

Host defense	Alterations	Contributing factors
Innate immune system	Decline in neutrophil functions, e.g., chemotaxis, adherence, phagocytosis, oxidative burst, and microbicidal killing	Hyperglycemia, dyslipidemia, Ketoacidosis, comorbid conditions, e.g., myeloproliferative diseases, medications
Adaptive immune system	Changes in lymphocyte responses, e.g., increase memory T-cells, increase abnormal antibody production, impaired lymphocyte responses to new antigens	Aging alone, comorbid conditions, e.g., malnutrition, medications, lymphoproliferative disease, autoimmune disease
	Impairment CD4+ lymphocytes, memory cells, NK cells	Diabetes (type I only)
Nonspecific defenses	Disruption of cutaneous barriers	Peripheral neuropathy, immobility, devices
	Increased tissue necrosis	Vascular disease
	Reduction in normal flora	Antibiotic use
Limit exposure	Acquisition antibiotic-resistant or virulent pathogens	Health-care facility stay, procedures

Abbreviation: NK, natural killer.

The most consistent and dramatic changes in cellular functions are found most often in the setting of high glucose levels, and some improvement is seen with improvement in glycemic control (6,7). In type I diabetics, ketoacidosis has been associated with impaired neutrophil functions. Other metabolic consequences associated with poor glycemic control, such as hyperlipidemia and low zinc levels, also may modulate the immune response (3,7).

In contrast with the diabetic patient, older adults have defects primarily in the adaptive rather than the innate immune system. With aging, there is a reduction in the ability of the acquired immune system to proliferate in response to new antigens, and the proportion of CD4+ T-helper lymphocytes shifts from naïve CD45RA+ cells toward an increase in memory CD45+R0+ cells. Even among some subpopulations of memory cells, the ability to respond to old stimuli with expression of interleukin-2 (IL-2) and IL-2 receptors is reduced.

Similarly with aging, there is a shift among B lymphocytes toward differentiated marrow plasma cells with increased production of autoantibodies. B-cells may proliferate less well and produce less antibody, or antibody may be less specific for an infection and functionally less protective. Overall, the sum of age-related changes in the T- and B-lymphocytes of the acquired immune system primarily results in lower levels of functional antibody (4,8).

Neutrophil functions appear to be intact in healthy older adults. There is, however, some suggestion that once phagocytosis of an organism occurs, older neutrophils become more susceptible to programmed cell death or apoptosis. Increased death among aged neutrophils may be due to increased susceptibility to cytokines that promote apoptosis (4,8).

Other Nonspecific Host Defenses

Nonspecific host defenses against infectious diseases may also be compromised in diabetics and older adults. Diabetes has been shown to accelerate peripheral vascular changes seen with increasing age, and reduced blood flow and higher risks of tissue necrosis, secondary infection, and amputation are seen (9–11). When controlled for age and gender, diabetics have a four- to sixfold greater risk of vascular disease than nondiabetics (9). Furthermore, older diabetics have an eightfold increased risk of amputation compared with younger diabetics (10). Joslin observed that the time from the diagnosis of diabetes to development of gangrene was much shorter in the older adult (11).

Cutaneous and mucosal trauma is also a major risk factor for the development of infection. In addition to the sensory neuropathy of diabetes, there are conditions commonly seen in older adults that can alter the ability to perceive, interpret, or respond to pressure or painful stimuli. Cognitive impairment and immobility can result in breaches of cutaneous barriers with potential introduction of infecting pathogens. Some skin trauma in the older adults occurs out of medical necessity due to invasive procedures, use of devices, or injectable medications. Most of the evidence suggests that older adults with diabetes and associated vascular or neuropathic complications are at increased risk of infection.

INDIVIDUAL PATHOGENS ASSOCIATED WITH INFECTION IN OLDER DIABETICS
Staphylococcus aureus

The prevalence of *S. aureus* infection is greatest among persons who carry the organism chronically in their anterior nares or on their skin (Table 2). *S. aureus* carriage is found primarily when skin or mucosal barriers are disrupted by dermatologic conditions, percutaneous devices, surgical procedures, and chronic wounds. Insulin-dependent diabetics and those with neuropathic or vascular ulcers have high rates of *S. aureus* colonization and, therefore, increased risk of staphylococcal infection. Illnesses requiring the chronic use of needles, including diabetes mellitus, are associated with increased *S. aureus* colonization and infection risk (2,3,12). Healthy aging alone has not been associated with increased risk of staphylococcal colonization or infection (12).

Whether the increased prevalence of diabetes with increasing age accounts for increased rates of *S. aureus* infection seen in the elderly remains controversial (12). Cluff et al. found increased rates of *S. aureus* bacteremia in the very young and in the elderly (13). Diabetes was the second most common comorbidity and was found most often in the older adults. In other studies, diabetes appeared to be common in hospitalized, nursing home, and community-dwelling elderly with *S. aureus* bacteremia; however, it was not a risk for older adults with *S. aureus* pneumonia who required intensive care (12). In nursing home studies, diabetes and peripheral vascular disease were independent risk factors for infection as well as colonization with methicillin-resistant *S. aureus* (MRSA) (12).

S. aureus is a highly virulent pathogen that can cause localized infection of the skin and soft tissues or become invasive causing bacteremia and metastatic infection of virtually every organ system. Antimicrobial susceptibilities are no longer predictable based on whether the infection was acquired at home or in a health-care setting. Community-acquired MRSA is becoming an increasing problem worldwide. Cultures of abscess material, blood, sputum, bone, and cerebrospinal fluid should be obtained and sent for culture and antimicrobial susceptibilities if serious *S. aureus* infection is suspected or if the patient is not responsive to empiric treatment of a localized infection (Table 3). Endocarditis may complicate up to 30% of cases of *S. aureus* bacteremia; the diagnosis must be excluded by echocardiography in any patient regardless of the number of blood cultures positive and even if the physical examination if unimpressive for clinical findings suggestive of the diagnosis. Prevention of *S. aureus* infection primarily consists of good wound care with the use of clean dressings and bandages to prevent contamination, and frequent cleansing. Strategies to eradicate *S. aureus* carriage and prevent infection are still experimental (12).

Group B β-Hemolytic Streptococcal Infection

Diabetes is a major risk factor for severe group B streptococcal infection. When controlled for age, diabetes, and related conditions such as peripheral and cerebrovascular disease, renal failure, and wounds, poorly controlled diabetes may play a role in increased group B streptococcal colonization and infection rates as hyperglycemia is associated with a decline in neutrophil superoxide production.

TABLE 2 Infectious Diseases Associated with Diabetes Mellitus and Increasing Age: Individual Pathogens

Individual pathogens	Primary sources	Major predisposing risk factors
Staphylococcus aureus	Humans	DM, health-care exposures, colonization, devices, abnormal skin
Group B streptococci	Humans	Aging, DM, perineal colonization, ulceration, urinary obstruction
Listeria monocytogenes	Food, environment	Aging, DM, achlorhydria, abnormal adaptive immunity
Salmonellosis	Humans, animals, food, water	Aging, DM, achlorhydria, antacids, PVOD, abnormal adaptive immunity, cholelithiasis, urinary abnormalities, prostheses
Tuberculosis	Humans	Aging, DM
Zygomycosis	Environment	DM, ketoacidosis, neutrophil dysfunction
Candidiasis	Humans	Aging, DM, increased debility, poor oral hygiene, xerostomia, colonization, antibiotics

Abbreviations: DM, diabetes mellitus; PVOD, peripheral vascular occlusive disease.

TABLE 3 Treatment and Prevention of Infection in Older Adults with Diabetes Mellitus

Individual pathogens	Preferred antibiotic treatment[a]	Prevention
Staphylococcus aureus[b] Methicillin-resistant		Good wound care, experimental— decolonization, vaccine
IV indicated	Vancomycin[a], daptomycin, linezolid, trimethoprim-sulfamethoxazole, tigecycline	
PO indicated	Sulfamethoxazole[a], doxycycline	
Methicillin-susceptible	Antistaphylococcal penicillins (PO/IV)[a] First-generation cephalosporins (PO/IV) Vancomycin (IV only)	
Group B streptococci	Penicillin/ampicillin (PO/IV)[a], cephalosporins (PO/IV), vancomycin (IV only)	Wound care, relief urinary stasis, aspiration precautions, experimental—vaccine
Listeria monocytogenes	Ampicillin + gentamicin (IV)[a], trimethoprim-sulfamethoxazole (IV)	Cook processed foods, avoid unpasteur- ized dairy products, avoid unnecessary acid blockers
Salmonellosis	Ciprofloxacin (PO/IV), ceftriaxone (IV)	Avoid contaminated water, cook food thoroughly
Tuberculosis	See guideline[c]	Isoniazid 300 mg daily PO + pyridoxine for 9 mo; rifampin 300 mg bid PO for 4 mo
Zygomycosis	Liposomal amphotericin B (IV), surgical debridement, control ketoacidosis/ hyperglycemia, experimental—posaconazole	Control hyperglycemia, prevent ketoacidosis
Candidiasis	Remove urinary, IV devices, azoles (topical, PO, IV)[d], alternatives— caspofungin (IV), amphotericin (IV, intravesicular)	Improve oral hygiene, denture repair, avoid steroids and antibiotics, avoid device use

Clinical syndromes	Initial empiric treatment	Prevention
Emphysematous	Broad-spectrum penicillin (IV); third- generation cephalosporin + metroni- dazole or clindamycin (IV); emergent surgical consultation	
Cholecystitis		None
Pyelonephritis		None
Necrotizing fasciitis	Broad-spectrum penicillin; third- generation cephalosporin + clindamy- cin (IV); emergent surgical consultation; emergent infectious diseases consultation	None
Diabetic foot, ulcers/ osteomyelitis	Broad-spectrum penicillin (IV); penicillin/ampicillin + β-lactamase inhibitor (IV); third-generation cephalosporin (IV) + clindamycin or metronidazole (PO/IV); quinolone (PO/IV) + clindamycin or metronida- zole (PO/IV)	Daily foot inspection, no walking barefoot, proper footwear, orthotics, good wound care, assess for treatable vascular disease
Malignant otitis externa	Antipseudomonal penicillin (IV), Antipseudomonal cephalosporin (IV), ciprofloxacin (IV)	Early assessment of ear pain, avoid maceration of ear canal

[a]The choice of antimicrobial route should be based on the clinical syndrome present, the severity of illness, and history of allergies or drug intolerances. Many of the clinical syndromes listed here are uncommon and can be quite severe. Early consultation with a physician expert in the management of these infections is recommended.

[b]In general, β-lactam antibiotics are the preferred treatment for *S. aureus* infections unless the bacteria are methicillin-resistant or the patient has allergies to those drugs. In severe life-threatening infections, empiric vancomycin IV is appropriate until antimicrobial susceptibilities are available.

[c]From Ref. 14.

[d]*Candida albicans* is susceptible to all antifungal agents. If the patient has a known infection with *Candida glabrata* or *Candida kruseii*, then a nonazole antifungal agent can be considered.

Abbreviations: IV, intravenous; PO, per os.

Aging alone is probably a less important risk factor than debility and comorbid disease for infection with this organism. Group B streptococci frequently colonize the gastrointestinal, urogenital, and oropharyngeal mucosa; rates have not been shown to increase with aging. It is thought that skin ulceration and aspiration facilitate invasion by colonizing bacteria. Overall, studies of group B streptococcal antibodies in healthy older adults without diabetes suggest that neutrophil and humoral functions are normal (15).

However, most deaths (50%) and a significant proportion of severe group B streptococcal infections (>40%) do occur in the elderly (15). There is no evidence that differences in strain virulence account for the increased incidence of disease in this population. Rates of severe group B streptococcal disease are highest among old frail, nursing home residents. When risk factors for group B streptococcal infection were compared in young versus older adults, nursing home residence and severe debility were the most important predisposing conditions.

The manifestations of group B streptococcal infection include skin and soft tissue infection, osteomyelitis, septic arthritis, urinary tract infection (UTI), pneumonia, bacteremia, meningitis, and endocarditis. Appropriate cultures should be obtained. Patients with symptoms of severe systemic illness should have blood cultures done to exclude more invasive disease that might require more prolonged intravenous antibiotic therapy. Most of these infections will respond to treatment with β-lactam antibiotics (Table 3). Prevention of group B streptococcal disease should focus on prevention of aspiration, wound care, and relief of urinary stasis. Vaccines for group B streptococcal infection for older adults are under development (15).

Listeriosis

Listeria is ubiquitous in the environment and frequently ingested with contaminated food, particularly cold meats and unpasteurized cheeses (16). Stomach acid and cell-mediated immunity, which can be impaired in older adults, play an important role in preventing intracellular invasion by this organism (16). Most nonpregnancy-associated infections with *Listeria monocytogenes* occur in older adults, particularly those with underlying medical conditions; diabetes is frequently cited as a risk factor (16,17). Meningitis, brain abscess, endocarditis, febrile gastroenteritis, and bacteremia are some of the more common manifestations of this uncommonly diagnosed infection (16). Blood cultures, imaging of the central nervous system, lumbar puncture, and echocardiography should be considered during evaluation of infection with this organism. Prolonged intravenous treatment may be required and effective antibiotic choices are limited (Table 3). To prevent Listeria infection, food should be thoroughly cooked and unnecessary acid blockers avoided. Delicatessen foods, although precooked, often become contaminated and grow even under refrigerator conditions.

Salmonellosis

In the developed world, Salmonella are acquired through animal contact, the ingestion of contaminated food, and food products, and occasionally from fomites. Gastric acid is a major defense against this organism. Older adults with achlorhydria or use of acid-blocking medications are at increased risk of acquiring intestinal infection with dissemination to distant sites. Vascular disease, cholelithiasis, nephrolithiasis, prosthetic devices, or other anatomic abnormalities also predispose to salmonella infection. Diabetes, autoimmune disease, malignancy, immunosuppressive drugs, and others have also been associated with increased risk of infection (18).

Clinical manifestations of salmonellosis range from localized gastrointestinal disease to bacteremia with dissemination to blood vessels, bone, or soft tissues where abscesses may form. Salmonellae are increasingly resistant to antibiotics and appropriate specimens should be collected for culture and antimicrobial susceptibilities. Routine treatment of salmonella gastroenteritis is recommended in older adults who are more likely to have transient bacteremia and increased risk of metastatic infection. Quinolones are currently the most reliable oral agent to treat gastroenteritis. For more invasive disease, prolonged intravenous therapy with ceftriaxone should be considered (Table 3). To prevent salmonellosis, hands should be cleansed following animal contact and prior to meals. Water that is possibly contaminated should be avoided and alternative sources of clean water sought. Foods at risk of contamination should be thoroughly cooked (18).

Tuberculosis

In the preantimicrobial era, tuberculosis (TB) was most common and often fatal in young patients with severe diabetes (19,20). Today, TB is commonly seen in older adults who develop disease due to waning adaptive immunity and reactivation of latent infection acquired while young (21).

Diabetes is common in patients with TB disease; it has been suggested that diabetes might predispose patients to reactivation of latent infection (20). For that reason, a positive tuberculin skin test of ≥10 mm induration in a diabetic is a moderate-risk indication for treatment of latent TB infection (LTBI) (21). In two large studies of TB disease from China, reactivation of prior infection was more common among older diabetics when compared with younger diabetics (22,23).

Diagnosis of TB disease is based on likelihood of exposure, results of two-step tuberculin skin testing presence of suggestive symptoms and findings on chest roentgenography, and presence of granulomas on histopathology, and acid fast bacilli on smear and culture (21), Unfortunately, in older adults, the time to diagnosis and treatment can be significantly delayed due to atypical presentation, lack of suspicion, and lack of typical findings on diagnostic tests. In one series, tuberculin skin tests were falsely negative in 38% of the elderly versus 20% of the young with TB disease. In this population, cavitation and upper lobe disease may be less common with mass-like lesions or lower lobe infiltrates more typically seen on chest roentgenograph or computerized tomography (CT) (21–23).

The treatment of TB disease is beyond the scope of this paper and the reader should refer to in-depth guidelines written on the subject (Table 3) (21). In the presence of exposure by history and positive tuberculin skin test ≥10 mm, but in the absence of clinical symptoms and signs of disease, treatment for LTBI should be offered to diabetics regardless of age. Single drug therapy, typically with isoniazid or rifampin, is safe in older adults with appropriate monitoring (Table 3) (21).

Zygomycosis (Mucormycosis)

The zygomycetes are prevalent in the environment and are readily inhaled. Inhalation of spores leads to invasion of sinuses or pulmonary infection with local spread or distant dissemination to the central nervous system or other organs. Diabetes is a leading predisposing risk factor for the development of zygomycosis in addition to malignancy, transplantation, and renal failure (1–4,24). Zygomycosis has been associated in particular with ketoacidosis; neutrophils are primarily required for the containment and killing of these hyphal invaders (25). The typical patient with zygomycosis is young with type I insulin-dependent diabetes, hyperglycemia, and ketoacidosis. However, in one large series of 929 cases, 80% of patients with zygomycosis had type II diabetes and 34% had ketoacidosis suggesting that the typical older diabetic with uncontrolled diabetes could be at risk (24).

Infections with zygomycetes may present as rhinosinusitis with extension into the central nervous system, pulmonary infection, or dissemination to other organs. Zygomycetes rapidly invade blood vessels causing severe facial or pleuritic pain in a severely ill patient. Necrosis may involve the nasal turbinates and extend to the palate and periorbital tissues. Biopsy of necrotic areas yields characteristic hyphae. These hyphae are fragile and may not grow if crushed during preparation of the tissue culture. Imaging by CT or magnetic resonance imaging (MRI) should be done to delineate the extent of the infection especially if surgery is contemplated. Treatment includes correction of the hyperglycemia and ketoacidosis, surgical debridement of necrotic tissue if possible, and use of antifungal agents. Currently, prolonged intravenous treatment with liposomal amphotericin B is the only antifungal treatment available (Table 3). Mortality can approach 17% even with optimal medical and surgical management. Oral posaconazole is experimental and in phase 3 trials (4). Prevention should focus on control of glycemia and ketoacidosis (1–4,24,25).

Candidiasis

There is evidence that mucosal colonization with *Candida* spp. increases with increasing age even in healthy older dentate adults (26). Oropharyngeal colonization may increase with debility as a consequence of poor oral hygiene, ill fitting denture use, age-related xerostomia, and that related to use of anticholinergic medications, antibiotic use, diabetes, corticosteroid use, and other factors (26,27). Similarly, presence of funguria has been reported most commonly in patients with abnormal urinary tracts, those who use bladder catheters, women, older adults, and diabetics (2,3,4,28). It has been reported that oropharyngeal, vaginal, and urinary colonization with yeast occur in approximately 50% of subjects in a geriatric hospital (29).

Manifestations of candidiasis in older adults with diabetes include mucosal infection such as thrush, denture stomatitis, chelitis, and genitourinary tract infection (2–4). Mucosal infection likely reflects waning T-cell–mediated immunity with increasing age and overgrowth due to factors related above. Systemic candidiasis or fungemia is rarely seen unless pyelonephritis or an indwelling intravenous catheter is present (30).

For most oral or vaginal infections with *Candida albicans*, treatment with a topical agent or an azole such as fluconazole for 14 days is sufficient (Table 3). Symptomatic candiduria should be treated with fluconazole and removal of an indwelling urethral catheter if present (30). If treatment fails, speciation of the yeast may be necessary to determine if resistance to azoles is an issue (30). Improvement in oral hygiene, denture care, and fit, and avoidance of steroid and antibiotic use may help prevent relapses of infection (27).

INFECTIOUS SYNDROMES ASSOCIATED WITH DIABETES AND AGING
Infections of Soft Tissue and Bone
Necrotizing Soft Tissue Infections

Secondary polymicrobial infection of devitalized necrotic tissue compromised by the effects of pressure and vascular insufficiency is the hallmark of the diabetic skin and soft tissue infection. Infection may be confined to superficial layers of the skin (cellulitis), fascia (fasciitis), muscle (myositis or gangrene), or bone (osteomyelitis) (Table 4) (1–3,5,28).

The severity of the infection may be directly proportional to the virulence of the pathogen and depth of the infection. Gas or crepitance on examination reflects the presence of obligate or facultative anaerobes and not necessarily the severity of the disease. For example, gas formation can be prominent in a more superficial nonclostridial anaerobic cellulitis and less impressive in a much more invasive infection, an entity referred to as necrotizing fasciitis type I or synergistic necrotizing cellulitis. Regardless of the name used, this polymicrobial infection can extend to muscle.

The fasciitis typically associated with diabetes is categorized as type I (polymicrobial, mixed anaerobic/aerobic infection) rather than the more notorious type II form also referred to as group A streptococcal gangrene (monomicrobial, with occasional *S. aureus* coinfection). Polymicrobial fasciitis involving the perineum in males has been referred to as Fournier's gangrene (1–4,28).

In the severely ill patient, urgent surgical exploration for deeper infection due to fasciitis or myositis should be considered, especially if the severity of illness, pain, and laboratory

TABLE 4   Infectious Diseases Associated with Diabetes Mellitus and Increasing Age: Clinical Syndromes

Clinical syndromes	Major predisposing risk factors
Necrotizing fasciitis, type I	DM, obesity, prior wound or trauma, PVOD
Fournier's gangrene	DM, trauma/surgery, male genitals
Cellulitis, synergistic necrotizing	DM, age, cardiorenal disease, trauma of lower extremities/perineum
Diabetic foot ulcer/osteomyelitis	DM, prior trauma or wounds, peripheral neuropathy, PVOD
Malignant otitis externa	DM, hearing aids, antibiotics, maceration (swimming, otic drops)
Emphysematous pyelonephritis	DM, aging, obstruction, hyperglycemia, vascular insufficiency, neutrophil defects
Emphysematous cholecystitis	DM, aging, male gender, gallstones, PVOD

Abbreviations: DM, diabetes mellitus; PVOD, peripheral vascular occlusive disease.

abnormalities is out of proportion with physical findings on examination. In those instances, surgical debridement of devitalized tissue is required in addition to antimicrobial therapy. Especially in cases of type II fasciitis, it is essential that surgery not be delayed to obtain imaging studies, delay can be fatal. Empiric intravenous antibiotic treatment directed against *S. aureus*, streptococci, obligate anaerobes (Clostridia and Bacteroides fragilis), and gram-negative bacilli should be given until culture and susceptibility of surgical specimens are known (Table 3) (1–4,28).

Diabetic Foot Infections

For less severely infected deep neuropathic ulcers, a less urgent approach may be taken. Exploration of the ulcer with a blunt sterile probe should be undertaken to assess depth and presence of palpable bone. MRI and bone scan are helpful, if clearly diagnostic for acute osteomyelitis. MRI can be particularly useful to evaluate the extent of the infection if surgery is considered, determine the acuity of the osteomyelitis if prior studies are indeterminate, and evaluate other causes of positive studies such as Charcot joints. Culture of deep tissue or bone obtained can be useful to guide antimicrobial treatment. Prevention of skin and soft tissue infection should focus on daily foot inspection, proper footwear, and foot care. Early ulcers should be aggressively treated with reduction in pressure at affected areas using appropriate orthotics, local wound care, and assessment for revascularization (1,9).

Malignant Otitis Externa (Invasive Otitis Externa)

Malignant otitis externa is an uncommon infection that predominantly affects older diabetics (1–4,28). Moisture and irritation of the ear canal following swimming, use of otic drops, antibiotics, and hearing aids provide a hospitable niche for replication of microorganisms, most commonly *Pseudomonas aeruginosa*.

Invasion of local tissues results in an external otitis, which presents with pain (75–100%), purulent drainage (50–80%), and swelling of the ear canal. Spread down the crypts of Santorini leads to a painful swollen mastoid process and compresses the seventh nerve as it leaves the styloid foramen resulting in a Bell's palsy (33%). Travel between the cartilaginous and bony ear to the base of the skull leads to swelling and compression of cranial nerves IX–XII with impairment of the tongue and gag reflexes (25%). Osteomyelitis of the temporal bone and the base of the skull, meningitis, and death may ensue in 20% of patients (2–4,28).

Diagnosis is based on clinical findings of external otitis, isolation of a causative organism from the ear canal, and mastoiditis by radiograph or evidence of osteomyelitis, meningeal enhancement, or other intracranial complications by CT or MRI. The cornerstone of treatment is aggressive and prolonged intravenous antibiotic treatment with antipseudomonal agents for four to eight weeks (Table 3). Relapse may occur in up to one-third of patients within three to six months; therefore, close follow-up is warranted. To prevent severe infectious complications, all ear pain in a diabetic should be evaluated with referral to an otolaryngologist if it does not rapidly improve with conservative management (2–4,28).

Complicated UTIs

The prevalence of asymptomatic bacteriuria is increased in older adults and patients with diabetes. Treatment of asymptomatic bacteriuria in both groups has not led to a reduction in symptomatic infection, complications of UTI, morbidity, or mortality. Nephrolithiasis and development of neurogenic bladder can predispose the elderly patient to upper UTI. Pyelonephritis involves 80% of UTI in diabetics; poor response to treatment should suggest perinephric abscess or papillary necrosis (1–4).

Emphysematous pyelonephritis is found almost exclusively in older adults with diabetes mellitus. Risk factors include presence of gas forming bacteria, vascular compromise, hyperglycemia, and impairment of the innate immune system. The hallmark of this disease is the presence of gas in the upper urinary tract due to polymicrobial infection involving facultative anaerobes *Escherichia coli* and *Klebsiella* spp and other bacteria. Infection may involve renal parenchyma (emphysematous pyelonephritis), the collecting system (emphysematous pyelitis), and bladder (emphysematous cystitis) or extend to the perinephric space. Diagnosis is made by clinical suspicion of UTI, symptoms of pyelonephritis if present, and imaging to demonstrate gas in the genitourinary system. Appropriate treatment includes intravenous antibiotic therapy based on culture results, relief of obstruction if present, and nephrectomy for extensive disease (Table 3) (1–4,28,31).

Gastrointestinal Infections
Emphysematous Cholecystitis
Biliary infections are common in older adults due to increased rates of cholelithiasis and vascular disease. While gallstones are most common in women, infectious complications such as empyema, gangrene, and perforation occur most commonly in older men. Diabetics account for more than one-third of cases of emphysematous cholecystitis found predominantly in elderly males. Emphysematous cholecystitis may follow acalculous cholecystitis; gallstones may be present only 50% of the time. Arterial insufficiency of the cystic artery leads to necrosis of the gallbladder wall. Normal gastrointestinal flora thrives in that low oxygen tension environment resulting in secondary infection with obligate and facultative anaerobes. *Clostridia perfringens* and other gas-producing bacteria such as *E. coli* and *S. aureus* may be isolated singly or as part of a polymicrobial infection. Patients are severely ill. Hallmarks of the diagnosis are right upper quadrant crepitus on examination and gas in the gall bladder wall on imaging. Mortality is high; early suspicion, diagnosis, and emergency surgical intervention are essential in addition to broad-spectrum antimicrobial therapy (Table 3) (1–4,28).

SUMMARY

Both aging and diabetes mellitus increase the risk for infection, but the mechanisms underlying this risk are different. Infections in diabetics primarily reflect alterations in the innate immune system associated with poor glycemic control. As a result, infections associated with neutrophil defects such as staphylococcal streptococcal, pseudomonal, and zygomycoses infections have been seen with increased frequency in the diabetic. In the older adult, defects in the acquired immune system dominate with increased frequency of listeriosis, mucocutaneous candidiasis, and reactivation of TB.

Overlap between the kinds of infections seen in diabetics and the elderly does occur. Some risk factors are increased in both diabetics and the older adult, such as vascular disease and alterations in skin integrity. The presence of vascular disease contributes to infection with anaerobes and Salmonella in both groups. The nature of the immune defect also varies with the type of diabetes; type I diabetics do have defects in the acquired immune system that could account for some of this overlap. Young insulin-dependent diabetics are also at risk of reactivation TB and mucocutaneous candidiasis as a result. Neutrophil defects can occur in the older adult with underlying illness or as a consequence of medications. Whether the presence of diabetes in the older host leads to an additive risk of infection is still the subject of debate.

Some infections in the diabetic are quite uncommon and life-threatening. Infections present atypically in the older adult with delay in diagnosis and treatment. As the prevalence of diabetes continues to climb among a world population that is rapidly aging, we will see more of these unusual and severe infections. Until we can develop better methods to prevent and treat many of these infections, optimizing diabetic control remains our best strategy.

REFERENCES

1. Joshi M, Caputo GM, Weitekamp MR, et al. Infections in patients with diabetes mellitus. N Engl J Med 1999; 341(25):1906–1912.
2. Wheat LJ. Infection and diabetes mellitus. Diabetes Care 1980; 3(1):187–197.
3. Deresinski S. Infections in the diabetic patient: strategies for the clinician. Pract J Diagn Treat 1995; 1(1):1–12.
4. Rajagopalan S. Serious infections in elderly patients with diabetes mellitus. Clin Infect Dis 2005; 40(7):990–996.
5. Dronge AS, Perkal MF, Kancir S, Concato J, Aslan M, Rosenthal RA. Long-term glycemic control and postoperative infectious complications. Arch Surg 2006; 141(4):375–380.

6. Geerlings SE, Hoepelman AIM. Immune dysfunction in patients with diabetes mellitus (DM). FEMS Immunol Med Microbiol 1999; 26(3–4):259–265.
7. Moutschen MP, Scheen AJ, Lefebvre PJ. Impaired immune responses in diabetes mellitus: analysis of the factors and mechanisms involved. Relevance to the increased susceptibility of diabetic patients to specific infections. Diabete et Metabolisme 1992; 18(3):187–201.
8. Castle SC. Clinical relevance of age-related immune dysfunction. Clin Infect Dis 2000; 31(2): 578–585.
9. Lipsky BA, Pecoraro RE, Ahroni JH. Foot ulceration and infection in elderly diabetics. Clin Geriatr Med 1990; 6(4):747–769.
10. Minaker KL. Aging and diabetes mellitus as risk factors for vascular disease. Am J Med 1987; 82(1B):47–53.
11. Joslin EP. The menace of diabetic gangrene. N Engl J Med 1934; 211(1):16–20.
12. Bradley SF. *Staphylococcus aureus* infections and antibiotic resistance in older adults. Clin Infect Dis 2002; 34(2):211–216.
13. Cluff LE, Reynolds RC, Page DL, Breckenridge JL. Staphylococcal bacteremia and altered host resistance. Ann Intern Med 1968; 69(5):859–873.
14. American Thoracic Society, Centers for Disease Control, Infectious Diseases Society of America. Treatment of tuberculosis. MMWR 2003; 52(RR11):1–77.
15. Edwards MS, Baker CJ. Group B streptococcal infections in elderly adults. Clin Infect Dis 2005; 41(6):839–847.
16. Lorber B. Listeriosis. Clin Infect Dis 1997; 24(1):1–11.
17. Goulet V, Marchetti P. Listeriosis in 225 non-pregnant patients in 1992: clinical aspects and outcome in relation to predisposing conditions. Scan J Infect Dis 1996; 28(4):367–374.
18. Hohmann EL. Nontyphoidal salmonellosis. Clin Infect Dis 2001; 32 (2):263–269.
19. Boucot KR, Dillon ES, Cooper DA, Meier P. Tuberculosis among diabetics: the Philadelphia Survey. Am Rev Tuberc 1952; 65(6S):1–5.
20. Zack MB, Fulkerson LL, Stein E. Glucose intolerance in pulmonary tuberculosis. Am Rev Resp Dis 1973; 108(5):1164–1169.
21. Thrupp L, Bradley S, Smith P, Simor A, Gantz N, Society for Healthcare Epidemiology of America Committee on Long-Term Care. Tuberculosis prevention and control in long-term-care facilities for the older adult. Infect Control Hosp Epidemiol 2004; 25(12):1097–1108.
22. Leung CC, Yew WW, Chan CK, et al. Tuberculosis in older people: a retrospective and comparative study from Hong Kong. J Am Geriatr Soc 2002; 50(7):1219–1226.
23. Liaw Y-S, Yang P-C, Yu C-J, et al. Clinical spectrum of tuberculosis in older persons. J Am Geriatr Soc 1995; 43(3):256–260.
24. Roden MM, Zaoutis TE, Buchanan WL, et al. Epidemiology and outcome of zygomycosis: a review of 929 reported cases. Clin Infect Dis 2005; 41(5):634–653.
25. Ribes JA, Vanover-Sams CL, Baker DJ. Zygomycetes in human disease. Clin Microbiol Rev 2000; 13(2):236–301.
26. Kleinegger CL, Lockhart SR, Vargas K, Soll DR. Frequency, intensity, species, and strains of oral *Candida* vary as a function of host age. J Clin Microbiol 1996; 34(9):2246–2254.
27. Shay K, Ship JA. The importance of oral health in the older patient. J Am Geriatr Soc 1995; 43(12):1414–1422.
28. Smitherman KO, Peacock JE. Infectious emergencies in patients with diabetes mellitus. Med Clin N Amer 1995; 79(1):53–77.
29. Narhi TO, Ainamo A, Meurman JH. Salivary yeasts, saliva, and oral mucosa in the elderly. J Dent Res 1993; 72(6):1009–1014.
30. Kauffman CA. Candiduria. Clin Infect Dis 2005; 41(S6):371–376.
31. Huang J-J, Tseng C-C. Emphysematous pyelonephritis: clinicoradiological classification, management, prognosis, and pathogenesis. Arch Intern Med 2000; 160(6):797–805.

20 | Goal Setting in Older Adults with Diabetes

Elbert S. Huang
Department of Medicine, The University of Chicago, Chicago, Illinois, U.S.A.

GENERAL POPULATION GOALS OF DIABETES CARE

Diabetes increases a patient's risk of developing microvascular and cardiovascular complications over his/her lifetime (1–3). Fortunately, this risk can be substantially reduced with modern diabetes care, which is an amalgam of medications designed to modify the various risk factors, namely serum glucose, blood pressure, and serum cholesterol levels, that are classically associated with these complications. Self-care behaviors such as diet, exercise, and self-glucose monitoring are also important adjuncts to achieving optimal risk factor levels and preventing complications. In the past decade, the benefits of the individual components of modern diabetes care as well as the benefits of comprehensive diabetes care have been clearly illustrated in the United Kingdom Prospective Diabetes Study (UKPDS), the Kumamoto Study, Steno-2 Study, and subgroup analyses of larger blood pressure and cholesterol-lowering studies (4–8).

The results from these trials have provided support for the risk factor goals of diabetes care promulgated in clinical practice guidelines (Table 1). The common theme of these recommendations is that patients with diabetes should strive for near-normal levels of all risk factors including serum glucose, blood pressure, and cholesterol. For blood glucose control, the target glycosylated hemoglobin (HbA_{1c}) has remained at less than 7% over the past 10 years (12). For blood pressure control, the target blood pressure changed from less than 130/85 mmHg to less than 130/80 mmHg in 2000. The Joint National Committee on Prevention, Detection, Evaluation, and Treatment of High Blood Pressure released a report in November of 1997 strongly recommending the intensive control of blood pressure in patients with diabetes (13,14). For serum cholesterol control, the recommended low-density lipoprotein (LDL) cholesterol target changed in 1999 from less than 130 mg/dL in patients without heart disease and less than 100 mg/dL in patients with heart disease to less than 100 mg/dL in all patients (15). More recently, recommendations for lowering cholesterol levels even further to less than 70 mg/dL have emerged (16). In the next several years, the results of the Action to Control Cardiovascular Risk in Diabetes (ACCORD) may actually lead to even lower risk factor goals.

The evolution of risk factor goals has important implications for the growing population of older patients who live with diabetes today. The chief question for patients and their health-care providers is whether or not the risk factor goals set forth in clinical practices guidelines should be the diabetes care goals for an individual patient. When striving for these intensive risk factor goals, providers are assuming that a patient's primary health-care goal is to optimally prevent microvascular and cardiovascular complications. For some older patients, prevention of all complications is indeed the primary goal of diabetes care while for other older patients, the overall context of their health may alter the balance of risks and benefits related to achieving intensive glucose, blood pressure, and cholesterol control. In order to successfully individualize the care of older diabetes patients, providers and patients must consider the data from available clinical studies, the characteristics of the individual patient, and the goals and preferences of the individual patient in order to arrive at treatment decisions that will be best for the patient.

In this chapter, we will introduce the general concept of goal setting in health care, describe an approach to individualizing diabetes care in older patients, and provide practical examples of how to approach goal setting with older patients.

GOAL SETTING IN HEALTH CARE

It is important for patients and providers to be reminded of the fact that the risk factor goals of diabetes care exist within a hierarchy of health-care goals that range from the most general

TABLE 1   Risk Factor Goals for Diabetes Care

	American Association of Clinical Endocrinologists (2002)	ADA General Population Goals (2004)	California Healthcare Foundation/ American Geriatrics Society Guidelines (2003)	
Glycosylated hemoglobin target	≤6.5%	<7%	Nonfrail patient	<7%
			Frail patient	<8%
Preprandial glucose	<110 mg/dL	90–130 mg/dL	—	
Postprandial glucose	<140 mg/dL	<180 mg/dL	—	
Systolic blood pressure target	—	<130 mmHg	Nonfrail patient	140 mmHg
			Frail patient	130 mmHg
Diastolic blood pressure target	—	<80 mmHg	<80 mmHg	

Abbreviation: ADA, American Diabetes Association.
Source: From Refs. 9–11.

goals to specific goals (17). Failing to recognize this hierarchy of goals can lead one to focus almost entirely on treatment-specific goals that may not contribute to a patient's ability to achieve his/her general health-care goals. General health-care goals address the broader question of why we pursue health-care treatments in the first place. For most providers and public health officials, the traditional goal of health care has been the prevention of morbidity and mortality. In the fields of aging and geriatrics research, the proposed goal of health care for older patients has been more specifically conceived as achieving compressed morbidity (18). When asked about their health-care goals, older patients, including those living with diabetes, have been found to focus almost entirely on their functional status and their independence (17,19). The language of patients is distinct from the biomedical language of health-care providers but in meaning, the goals of patients are highly related to the ideas of compressed morbidity as well as the idea of enhanced quality-of-life. Specific health-care goals include the prevention of disease-specific complications, the provision of appropriate medications, and the achievement of specific risk factor goals. When treating a patient, it is always important to review the potential benefit that may be accrued from achieving a specific health-care goal and determine whether or not it will truly contribute to the overall well-being of the patient.

This review process is particularly important in the setting of diabetes where the various components of diabetes care provide distinct health benefits. Glucose control definitively prevents microvascular complications such as diabetic retinopathy, neuropathy, and nephropathy (4,5). Glucose control may also prevent cardiovascular complications. For type 2 diabetes patients, the cardiovascular benefits of intensive glucose control have been recently illustrated in the long-term follow-up study of type 1 diabetes patients enrolled in the Diabetes Complication and Control Study (20). For type 2 diabetes patients, observational studies have illustrated a continuous relationship between glucose levels and the probability of cardiovascular events (21), but trial results have not yet been definitive (5). Blood pressure control has been found to prevent a wide range of microvascular and cardiovascular complications, including coronary heart disease and stroke (7). Cholesterol control acts to specifically prevent coronary heart disease but has less clear benefits for stroke prevention (22). Because blood pressure control has such wide-ranging benefits, it has been deemed by some experts as the highest priority among the various components of diabetes care (23). This conclusion may change if even more intensive control of glucose levels is found to prevent cardiovascular events in the ACCORD trial.

GOALS FOR OLDER PATIENTS WITH DIABETES

For older diabetes patients, the specific risk factor goals of diabetes care should be based on consideration for the balance of benefits and risks of different levels of risk factor control as well as the overall health-care goals of the individual patient. While diabetes practice guidelines have always acknowledged the importance of individualizing diabetes care, the first major clinical guideline to formally advocate an individualized approach to identifying risk factors goals of diabetes care for older patients was published in 2003 by the California Healthcare Foundation/American Geriatrics Society (CHF/AGS) panel (Table 1). The guideline provides a valuable framework for approaching diabetes care goals in older patients.

The CHF/AGS guideline panel distinguishes between older patients who are relatively healthy and functionally stable from older patients who are frail, have significant comorbid illnesses, and have a limited life expectancy (less than five years) (Table 1). The first group of healthy older patients is advised to strive for the same risk factor goals as those promoted for general population. The second group of frail patients is believed to have an unfavorable risk-benefit ratio for both intensive glucose and blood pressure control. In the case of intensive glucose control, frail patients are felt to be unlikely to benefit from intensive control and are, simultaneously, at high risk for experiencing hypoglycemia and polypharmacy (11). As a result, the panel recommends that these patients strive for less-intensive HbA_{1C} such as 8%. In the case of blood pressure control, frail patients are felt to be at particularly high risk for orthostasis and falls. In order to address this concern, the panel calls for a less-intensive systolic blood pressure goal of 140 mmHg for frail patients. The guideline does not recommend any significant differentiation with regard to cholesterol control goals and aspirin prophylaxis. This effectively identifies cardiovascular prevention as a top priority for all older patients living with diabetes. In 2004, the American Diabetes Association incorporated these recommendations into their care guidelines and reiterated that it was reasonable to set less-aggressive target glycemic goals for older patients with advanced diabetes complications and life-limiting comorbid illnesses (10).

The primary aims of these guidelines have been to help older patients avoid the complications of diabetes that are most likely to occur for the individual and to minimize the daily burden and side effects of medications. These guidelines also have a broader intention of refocusing the attention of the provider from purely focusing on risk factor control of diabetes to also considering the presence of geriatric syndromes. The term, geriatric syndromes, refers to one symptom or a complex of symptoms with high prevalence in frail older patients, resulting from multiple diseases and multiple risk factors. Geriatric syndromes can have a devastating effect on quality of life of older patients. Specific syndromes such as falls (24) and polypharmacy (25) have some direct implications for how intensely providers may actually manage diabetes-related risk factors. Other geriatric syndromes such as depression (26), cognitive impairment (27), urinary incontinence (28), and chronic pain (29) are more common among older patients with diabetes and may be of great importance to the patient. Providers, unfortunately, have limited time and attention during clinical encounters with older patients and so reminding providers to screen for these syndromes may ultimately help patients address complaints that significantly affect their quality-of-life. Addressing these geriatric syndromes in addition to reconsidering the risk factor goals of diabetes care will, in effect, move the attention of providers from disease-specific goals to the overall health-care goals of patients. All of these considerations encourage a holistic approach to care for an older patient for whom diabetes may in fact not be his/her most important concern.

Clinical Criteria for Individualizing Goals of Diabetes Care

Despite the development of new geriatric-specific diabetes care guidelines, there is yet no consensus on the ideal approach to individualizing diabetes care goals among older patients. A variety of different clinical characteristics have been proposed as criteria. Each characteristic has relative strengths and weaknesses and consideration for multiple characteristics will be necessary when making actual treatment decisions.

Life expectancy is considered to be a primary method for distinguishing between older diabetes patients who will or will not benefit from intensive risk factor control. This is clearly an important consideration for intensive glucose control but less so for blood pressure and cholesterol control. For intensive glucose control, the UKPDS illustrated that at least nine years of ongoing intensive glucose control was required before evidence of treatment benefit was achieved in middle-aged patients with new-onset diabetes. This time to treatment effect was most likely due to the fact that the microvascular complications of diabetes take many years to develop. Because UKPDS began with patients with new-onset diabetes, the development of complications was prolonged and hence the observed benefits of intensive glucose control were delayed. Based on this result, it is suspected that older patients should have at least five years of life expectancy in order to benefit from intensive lowering of glucose levels. On the other hand, this same concern for limited life expectancy does not exist when treating hypertension (30), using 3-hydroxy-3-methyl-glutaryl-CoA (HMG-CoA) reductase inhibitors (statins) (8), or using angiotensin converting enzyme inhibitors (31) where the benefits of treatments have been accrued as early as two to three years in clinical trials. Many of these trials have in fact been conducted in older populations who were at high risk of developing cardiovascular complications.

Age is, in and of itself, the most powerful predictor of life expectancy and should be an important first factor to consider. From disease simulation studies, we know that the benefits of intensive glucose control steadily decline as the age of onset increases because of changing background mortality (32,33). Beyond age, we can differentiate between patients with and without significant comorbid illness. We know from studies of comorbidity indices that they have predictive power for mortality (34). In addition to comorbidity, functional status is known as an independent predictor of mortality among older patients (35). Very recently, a prognostic index for four-year mortality that combines age, comorbidity, and functional status has been developed and may be of use in stratifying diabetes patients (Table 2) (36).

Another way to distinguish among older patients is to identify those older patients who will be at greatest risk for suffering from the adverse effects of treatments such as hypoglycemia as well as classic geriatric syndromes such as falls and polypharmacy. Many of the same characteristics that will likely limit the benefits of intensive risk factor control are also the characteristics that increase the risk for side effects and geriatric syndromes. The risk of hypoglycemia is highest among patients who are over the age of 80 (RR 1.8, 95% CI 1.4–2.3) and use five or more concomitant medications (RR 2.0, 95% CI, 1.7–2.4) (37). The risk of falls in older patients is highest among patients with orthostasis, depressive symptoms, impairments in cognition, vision, balance, gait, or muscle strength, and the use of four or more prescription medications (24). Polypharmacy itself is recognized as a geriatric syndrome. Polypharmacy can not only increase the risk of hypoglycemia and falls but is also associated with cognitive deficits and depression. Unfortunately, comprehensive diabetes care is intimately linked to a standard form of polypharmacy that worsens as the duration of diabetes progresses (38). Concerns regarding polypharmacy raise questions regarding the possible harms of routinely prescribing drugs such as statins or aspirin that may be reducing the risk of cardiovascular disease but adding to the complexity of a patient's medication regimen.

The concept of geriatric syndromes overlaps to some extent with the concept of frailty, which has its own body of literature. Frail patients are at risk for various geriatric syndromes, hospitalization, and mortality all of which may limit their likelihood of benefiting from intensive risk factor control. Frailty has previously been equated with disability, comorbidity, or advanced old age but is in fact a distinct clinical concept. Recent efforts have been made to redefine frailty as a biologic syndrome where patients develop a decreased resilience to external stress that is the result of repeated insults to multiple organ systems (39). Efforts to characterize the phenotype of frailty have involved defining a clinical syndrome of three or more of the following criteria: unintentional weight loss, self-reported exhaustion, weakness, slow walking speed, and low physical activity. Other investigators have attempted to identify older patients at risk for functional decline or death using tools that may be more easily applied in health services research (40). The Vulnerable Elder Survey was developed using the 1993 and 1995 Medicare Current Beneficiary Survey and has been used in the development of the assessing care of vulnerable elders (ACOVE) measures (Table 3). These efforts to develop comprehensive measures of frailty (39,40) may eventually lead to useful tools for clinical practice but they are currently used primarily for research and health services purposes.

Apart from these clinical characteristics, some older patient may have sentinel conditions that may dictate whether or not intensive risk factor control can be practically pursued. Dementia or cognitive impairment is a sentinel condition for diabetes because it not only affects background more mortality but also alters the ability of patients to fully participate in the self-care (41). Patients who have already developed end-stage complications

TABLE 2 Prognostic Index for Four-Year Mortality in Older Adults

Risk factor	Assigned score
Age	
60–64	1
65–69	2
70–74	3
75–79	4
80–84	5
≥85	7
Male sex	2
Comorbidities	
Diabetes mellitus	1
Cancer	2
Lung disease	2
Heart failure	2
BMI < 25	1
Current smoker	2
Functional measures	
Bathing	2
Managing finances	2
Walking several blocks	2
Pushing/pulling heavy objects	1

Total score	Percentage with score who die in 4 years
0	1
1	2
2	2
3	3
4	6
5	8
6	9
7	15
8	20
9	20
10	28
11	45
12	44
13	59
≥14	64

Abbreviation: BMI, body mass index.
Source: From Ref. 36.

of diabetes such as blindness or end-stage renal disease also pose unique challenges for providers. Like the demented, blind patients may have particular difficulties in adhering to complex treatments without special assistance. Patients with end-stage renal disease will typically require wholesale revision of their glucose-lowering regimens because their inability to clear insulin.

While there are clinical characteristics that may limit a patient's likelihood of benefiting from intensive risk factor control, there are also clinical characteristics that may increase a patient's likelihood of developing the traditional complications of diabetes and, as a result, the likelihood of benefiting from intensive risk factor control. A remarkably important clinical characteristic to consider is the patient's duration of diabetes. Much of the discussion in the literature regarding limited life expectancy and diabetes is most applicable to older patients who have new-onset diabetes. However, it is known that 75% of older diabetes patients have actually lived with diabetes for over five years and that the mean duration of diabetes increases with age (42). These observations are crucial because increasing duration of diabetes is independently associated with higher risk of multiple microvascular complications of diabetes. Unlike

TABLE 3   Vulnerable Elder Survey-13

Risk factor	Assigned score
Age	1 point for age 75–84 3 points for age ≥85
In general, compared to other people of your age, would you say that your health is (poor, fair, good, very good, excellent)	1 point for Poor or Fair
How difficult, on average do have with the following physical activities (No difficulty, A little Difficulty, Some Difficulty, A lot of Difficulty, Unable to do): Stooping, crouching, or kneeling Lifting or carrying objects as heavy as 10 pounds Reaching or extending arms above shoulder level Writing, or handling and grasping small objects Walking a quarter of a mile Heavy housework such as scrubbing floors or washing windows	1 point for A lot of Difficulty or Unable to do

Because of your health or physical condition, do you have any difficulty:
Shopping for personal items (like toilet items or medicines) (Yes, No, Do not do):
  If Yes, do you get help with shopping? (Yes, No)
  If Do not do, is that because of your health? (Yes, No)
Managing money (like keeping track of expenses or paying bills) (Yes, No, Do not do):
  If Yes, do you get help with managing money? (Yes, No)
  If Do not do, is that because of your health? (Yes, No)
Walking across the room (use of cane or walker is OK) (Yes, No, Do not do):
  If Yes, do you get help with walking? (Yes, No)
  If Do not do, is that because of your health? (Yes, No)
Doing light housework (like washing dishes, straightening up, or light cleaning) (Yes, No, Do not do):
  If Yes, do you get help with light housework? (Yes, No)
  If Do not do, is that because of your health? (Yes, No)
Bathing or showering (Yes, No, Do not do):
  If Yes, do you get help with bathing or showering? (Yes, No)
  If Do not do, is that because of your health? (Yes, No)
	4 points for one or more Yes responses 4a through 4e

Total score	Percentage with score who decline or die in 2 years
0	6.1
1	14.2
2	24.3
3	36.9
4	54.9

Source: From Ref. 40.

analyses of patients with new-onset diabetes, disease simulation studies of diabetes complications have found that intensive glucose control in patients with prevalent diabetes is highly effective and cost-effective as duration of diabetes increases (43). In addition to duration of diabetes, older patients who already have developed early stages of microvascular complications are in fact at significant risk for going on to develop end-stage complications of their disease. This increased risk again enhances the benefits of intensive glucose control. So a major consideration for providers and patients is whether or not the decision to intensify glucose control is occurring in new-onset diabetes versus prevalent diabetes with early stage complications.

All of these clinical factors are important to consider and, at present, there is no formal guidance on how to simultaneously consider all of these factors across multiple components of diabetes care. It is fairly clear that the older patient who falls into the category of individuals who will likely benefit from intensive risk factor goals and will not experience adverse side effects or geriatric syndromes as a result of intensive therapy should pursue it (Table 4). At the same time, patients who are unlikely to benefit from intensive therapy and are at high risk of

TABLE 4 Distribution of Older Diabetes Patients by Benefits and Risks of Intensive Risk Factor Control

	Low likelihood of benefiting from intensive risk factor control of diabetes[a]	High likelihood of benefiting from intensive risk factor control of diabetes[b]
Low likelihood of experiencing side effects or geriatric syndromes[c]	A	B
High likelihood of experiencing side effects or geriatric syndromes[d]	C	D

[a]For example, new-onset diabetes, limited life expectancy, advanced age, multiple comorbid illnesses, and poor functional status.
[b]For example, extended duration of diabetes, prior intermediate complications of diabetes, and prior cardiovascular events.
[c]For example, younger age, no comorbid illnesses, and good functional status.
[d]For example, advanced age, multiple comorbid illnesses, multiple prescription drugs, and poor functional status.

adverse events and geriatric syndromes should avoid intensive risk factor control. The problem is that the majority of older diabetes patients likely fall into the other subcategories where the risks and benefits of intensive risk factor control are not as clear. Table 5 provides case examples of patients who may fit within these various categories.

Communication About Goal Setting with Older Patients

Communicating about the goals of diabetes care is a challenge regardless of the age of the patient. The terms used by patients and providers are oftentimes confused and some times deserve special educational effort on the part of health-care professionals. A particular challenge in the setting of diabetes is that the risk factor goals of diabetes are not consistently related to any tangible symptoms and may not have a definite relationship with the actual treatments that a patient receives in order to achieve those specific risk factor goals. Patients and providers may never have explicit discussion regarding general health-care goals or the more specific risk factor goals. Providers may simply assume that the lowest achievable risk factor levels are the risk factor goals for a patient. Without specific education, patients may not be aware of their current risk factor levels or what those levels are associated with. They will however be very familiar with their daily treatments and what is entailed in performing these daily tasks.

Establishing the general health-care goals of a patient is an important initial discussion that should occur because it accomplishes several important benefits for the patient–provider relationship. An open-ended discussion regarding the overall health-care goals and general conceptions of health and illness of the patient may prove to be a particularly effective way of understanding a patient's preferences and help a provider determine the tone of subsequent clinical encounters. The process of involving older patients is likely to be invaluable in identifying appropriate treatment goals and plans for the individual patient. It is important to emphasize to older patients that the overall purpose of the discussion and derivation of an individualized treatment plan is to help them achieve their overall health-care goals. Without this emphasis, any discussion of modified treatment goals will suggest to the patients that the provider is doing less for them or suggesting that their prognosis is poor.

The second component of communication about goals involves eliciting and incorporating patients' specific preferences regarding risk factor goals and treatments. Such discussions may be extremely difficult with some older patients who may not have an understanding of the

TABLE 5 Case Examples of Older Diabetes Patients

Patient category	Patient description
A	75-yr-old woman with new-onset diabetes, no comorbid illnesses, no functional impairments
B	70-yr-old woman with 20 yr history of diabetes, early diabetic retinopathy, hypertension, hypercholesterolemia, no comorbid illnesses, no functional impairments
C	68-yr-old man with 3–4 yr history of diabetes, no prior diabetic complications, severe dilated cardiomyopathy, ventricular tachycardia, on 13 medications, unable to walk across home
D	72-yr-old man with 18 yr history of diabetes, recurrent foot ulcers, diabetic retinopathy, multiple episodes of hypoglycemia, and cognitive deficits

significance of specific risk factor levels or the value of risk reduction. Thus, to even begin a discussion regarding diabetes risk factor goals, providers must first educate patients and their families about the role of diabetes-related risk factors in increasing the risk of complications and then proceed to talk about the risks and benefits of achieving different risk factor goals over time. Equally important is to have a discussion with an older patient regarding the actual medications that may be needed to bring about risk factor goals. Treatments are highly concrete for patients and they are likely to have strong preferences regarding the use of pills and insulin. We have found that patient treatment preferences regarding specific treatments vary widely and that treatment preferences are essential preferences to consider in treatment decisions in diabetes (44). Patient attitudes regarding complications, on the other hand, are almost uniformly negative and we have found that they do not significantly influence decision analytic results.

An important consideration in communicating about health-care goals in older patients is that many older patients rely on family members or friends to help them with their treatment decisions. Family members or friends are important to consider because they may in fact be responsible for implementing daily treatments for many older patients. In addition, in the case of the older person with cognitive deficits, the family member or friend may in fact be serving as a surrogate decision maker. In most cases, it is preferable to rely on the patient whenever possible. Prior studies of the treatment preferences of older cognitively intact patients have shown that surrogate decision makers oftentimes report preferences for the patient that have little correlation with the patient's views (45).

AN OVERALL APPROACH TO GOAL SETTING AND INDIVIDUALIZING DIABETES CARE IN OLDER PATIENTS

The accompanying figure helps to organize the concepts discussed in this chapter regarding goal setting for older diabetes patients (Fig. 1). The process of geriatric patient assessment,

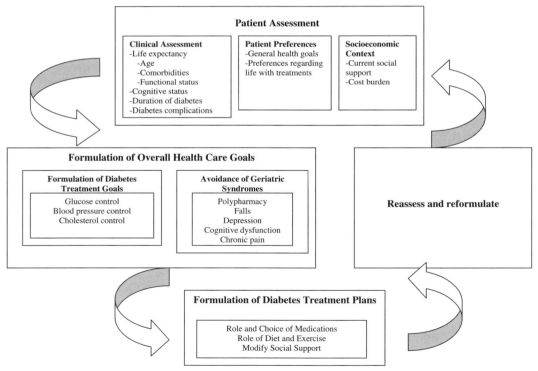

FIGURE 1   An approach to individualizing diabetes care in older people.

formulation of health-care goals, and development of treatment plans is meant to be a process that should be revisited throughout the life of an older patient. The process should begin with a clinical assessment, elicitation of patient preferences, and determination of the social context of the patient. The clinical assessment should include consideration of the patients overall life expectancy, which can be estimated by age, comorbidities, and functional status. The presence of specific sentinel conditions such as dementia should be determined. These factors are important for determining the likelihood of benefit from intensive treatments but also may be predictors of geriatric syndromes. Duration of diabetes and the presence of diabetes complications are also important to consider as they can help the providers understand the baseline risk of developing complications. Equally important are considerations for the patient's goals for care and his/her preferences regarding how to achieve them. Since an older patient's quality-of-life may be significantly influenced by their daily experience with medications, considerations regarding how an older patient perceives his/her quality-of-life with certain treatments may be as important as their perceptions regarding the significance of potential complications of diabetes. The socioeconomic context of the patient is also important to ascertain as the lack of social support and financial resources may increase the burden of intensive treatments.

Following this initial assessment of the older patient, the overall health-care goals and diabetes treatment goals are formulated. For example, is the overall health-care goal to prevent all possible complications related to diabetes at all costs? Is the overall goal for the patient to avoid medications? The answers to these questions will help the patient and provider formulate the specific goals of diabetes care. These goals help to determine the risk factor goals that will be appropriate for the patient. In addition, detection and management of geriatric syndromes will also deserve specific attention as they may also be part of the patients' overall goals for health care. These geriatric syndromes may in fact affect decisions regarding the intensity of lowering risk factor goals.

The final step in the process is the development of the actual treatment plan, which should be highly associated with the initial patient assessment and establishment of diabetes treatment goals.

FUTURE DIRECTIONS

The ideas introduced in recent geriatric diabetes care guidelines and in this chapter may make intuitive sense to providers but they should be viewed with some caution. Many of the ideas related to goal setting and individualizing care in older diabetes patients have yet to be evaluated in clinical trials.

There is particular uncertainty around how to identify patients who will benefit or be harmed by intensive risk factor control related to diabetes. The clinical characteristics that have been promoted as criteria for stratifying patients have face validity and may provide clear decisions for some older patients. However, it is very likely that many older patients will have clinical characteristics that are predictive of increased risk of complications related to diabetes as well as increased risk of geriatric syndromes related to diabetes therapies.

Another important unresolved aspect of goal setting among older diabetes patients is how to respond to dynamic changes in the health status of older patients. Older patients may move into and out of states of illness and functional impairment on a regular basis. We now know that the functional impairment in older patients actually comes and goes and is not fixed (46). The problem with dynamic health states is that we may begin with goals consistent with intensive diabetes care in a given patient but be forced to modify treatment goals as illnesses develop. Lessons from clinical trials would suggest that we should continue intensive treatments for a series of years to ensure that their benefits are realized. On the other hand, data on comorbidities and functional status would tell us that the benefits of continuing intensive treatments are minimal. These issues related to altering therapies in the midst of an older patient's history with diabetes are complex and should be studied in greater depth.

REFERENCES

1. Nathan DM, Singer DE, Godine JE, Perlmuter LC. Non-insulin-dependent diabetes in older patients: complications and risk factors. Am J Med 1986; 81:837–842.
2. Nathan DM, Meigs JB, Singer DE. The epidemiology of cardiovascular disease in type 2 diabetes mellitus: how sweet it is…or is it? Lancet 1997; 350(suppl 1):S14–S19.
3. Kuller LH. Stroke and diabetes. In: Harris MI, ed. Diabetes in America. 2nd ed. Bethesda: National Institutes of Health, 1995:449–456.
4. Ohkubo Y, Kishikawa H, Araki E, et al. Intensive insulin therapy prevents the progression of diabetic microvascular complications in Japanese patients with non-insulin-dependent diabetes mellitus: a randomized prospective 6-year study. Diabetes Research and Clinical Practice 1995; 28:103–117.
5. U.K. Prospective Diabetes Study Group. Intensive blood-glucose control with sulphonylureas or insulin compared with conventional treatment and risk of complications in patients with type 2 diabetes (UKPDS 33). Lancet 1998; 352(9131):837–853.
6. Gaede P, Vedel P, Larsen N, Jensen GV, Parving HH, Pedersen O. Multifactorial intervention and cardiovascular disease in patients with type 2 diabetes. N Eng'l J Med 2003; 348(5):383–393.
7. U.K. Prospective Diabetes Study Group. Tight blood pressure control and risk of macrovascular and microvascular complications in type 2 diabetes: UKPDS 38. Br Med J 1998; 317:703–713.
8. Heart Protection Study Collaborative Group. MRC/BHF Heart Protection Study of cholesterol lowering with simvastatin in 20536 high–risk individuals: a randomised placebo-controlled trial. Lancet 2002; 360:7–22.
9. The American Association of Clinical Endocrinologists Medical Guidelines for the Management of Diabetes Mellitus: the AACE System of Intensive Diabetes Self-Management—2002 Update. Endocr Pract 2002; 9(suppl 1):41–82.
10. American Diabetes Association. Standards of medical care in diabetes. Diabetes Care 2004; 27(suppl 1):S15–S35.
11. Brown AF, Mangione CM, Saliba D, Sarkisian CA, California Healthcare Foundation/American Geriatrics Society Panel on Improving Care for Elders with Diabetes. Guidelines for improving the care of the older person with diabetes mellitus. J Am Geriatr Soc 2003; 51(suppl 5 Guidelines): S265–S280.
12. American Diabetes Association. Standards of medical care for patients with diabetes mellitus. Diabetes Care 1997; 20(suppl 1):S5–S13.
13. Joint National Committee on Prevention D, Evaluation, and Treatment of High Blood Pressure and the National High Blood Pressure Education Program Coordinating Committee. The sixth report of the joint national committee on prevention, detection, evaluation, and treatment of high blood pressure. Arch Intern Med 1997; 157(21):2413–2446.
14. Chobanian AV, Bakris GL, Black HR, et al. The seventh report of the joint national committee on prevention, detection, evaluation, and treatment of high blood pressure: the JNC 7 report. JAMA 2003; 289(19):2560–2572.
15. American Diabetes Association. Standards of medical care for patients with diabetes mellitus. Diabetes Care 1999; 22(suppl 1):S32–S41.
16. Grundy SM, Cleeman JI, Merz CNB, et al. Implications of recent clinical trials for the National Cholesterol Education Program Adult Treatment Panel III Guidelines. Circulation 2004; 110:227–239.
17. Bradley EH, Bogardus ST Jr, Tinetti ME, Inouye SK. Goal-setting in clinical medicine. Soc Sci Med 1999; 49(2):267–278.
18. Fries JF. Aging, natural death, and the compression of morbidity. N Engl J Med 1980; 303:130–135.
19. Huang ES, Gorawara-Bhat R, Chin MH. Self-reported goals of older patients with type 2 diabetes mellitus. J Am Geriatr Soc 2005; 53:306–311.
20. The Diabetes Control and Complication Trial/Epidemiology of Diabetes Interventions and Complications (DCCT/EDIC) Study Research Group. Intensive diabetes treatment and cardiovascular disease in patients with type 1 diabetes. N Engl J Med 2005; 353(25):2643–2653.
21. Stratton IM, Adler AI, Neil HAW, et al. Association of glycaemia with macrovascular and microvascular complications of type 2 diabetes (UKPDS 35): prospective observational study. Br Med J 2000; 321:405–412.
22. Huang ES, Meigs JB, Singer DE. The effect of interventions to prevent cardiovascular disease in patients with type 2 diabetes mellitus. Am J Med 2001; 111:633–642.
23. Vijan S, Hayward RA. Treatment of hypertension in type 2 diabetes mellitus: blood pressure goals, choice of agents, and setting priorities in diabetes care. Ann Intern Med 2003; 138:593–602.
24. Tinetti ME. Clinical practice. Preventing falls in elderly persons. N Engl J Med 2003; 348(1): 42–49.
25. Murray MD, Kroenke K. Polypharmacy and medical adherence. J Gen Intern Med 2001; 16:137–139.
26. Anderson RJ, Freedland KE, Clouse RE, Lustman PJ. The prevalence of comorbid depression in adults with diabetes: a meta-analysis. Diabetes Care 2001; 24(6):1069–1078.
27. Stewart R, Liolitsa D. Type 2 diabetes mellitus, cognitive impairment and dementia. Diabet Med 1999; 16:93–112.

28. Brown JS, Seeley DG, Fong J, Black DM, Ensrud KE, Grady D. Urinary incontinence in older women: who is at risk? Study of Osteoporotic Fractures Research Group. Obstet Gynecol 1996; 87(5 Pt 1): 715–721.
29. Greene DA, Stevens MJ, Feldman EL. Diabetic neuropathy: scope of the syndrome. Am J Med 1999; 107(2B):2S–8S.
30. Curb JD, Pressel SL, Cutler JA, et al. Effect of diuretic-based antihypertensive treatment on cardiovascular disease risk in older diabetic patients with isolated systolic hypertension. Systolic Hypertension in the Elderly Program Cooperative Research Group [published erratum appears in J Am Med Assoc 1997; 277(17):1356] [see comments]. JAMA 1996; 276(23):1886–1892.
31. Heart Outcomes Prevention Evaluation Study Investigators. Effects of ramipril on cardiovascular and microvascular outcomes in people with diabetes mellitus: results of the HOPE study and MICRO-HOPE substudy. Lancet 1999; 355:253–259.
32. Vijan S, Hofer TP, Hayward RA. Estimated benefits of glycemic control in microvascular complications in type 2 diabetes. Ann Intern Med 1997; 127(9):788–795.
33. Eastman RC, Javitt JC, Herman WH, et al. Model of complications of NIDDM: II. Analysis of the health benefits and cost-effectiveness of treating NIDDM with the goal of normoglycemia. Diabetes Care 1997; 20(5):735–744.
34. Charlson ME, Pompei P, Ales KL, MacKenzie CR. A new method of classifying prognostic comorbidity in longitudinal studies: development and validation. J Chronic Dis 1987; 40(5):373–383.
35. Covinsky KE, Palmer RM, Fortinsky RH, et al. Loss of independence in activities of daily living in older adults hospitalized with medical illnesses: increased vulnerability with age. J Am Geriatr Soc 2003; 51:451–458.
36. Lee SJ, Lindquist K, Segal MR, Covinsky KE. Development and validation of a prognostic index for 4-year mortality in older adults. JAMA 2006; 295(7):801–808.
37. Shorr RI, Ray WA, Daugherty JR, Griffin MR. Incidence and risk factors for serious hypoglycemia in older persons using insulin or sulfonylureas. Arch Intern Med 1997; 157(15):1681–1686.
38. Turner RC, Cull CA, Frighi V, Holman RR. Glycemic control with diet, sulfonylurea, metformin, or insulin in patients with type 2 diabetes mellitus: progressive requirement for multiple therapies (UKPDS 49). UK Prospective Diabetes Study (UKPDS) Group. JAMA 1999; 281(21):2005–2012.
39. Fried LP, Tangen CM, Walston J, et al. Frailty in older adults: evidence for a phenotype. J Gerontol A Biol Sci Med Sci 2001; 56(3):M146–M156.
40. Saliba D, Elliott M, Rubenstein LV, et al. The vulnerable elders survey: a tool for identifying vulnerable older people in the community. J Am Geriatr Soc 2001; 49:1691–1699.
41. Brauner DJ, Muir JC, Sachs GA. Treating nondementia illnesses in patients with dementia. J Am Med Assoc 2000; 283(24):3230–3235.
42. Harris MI. Epidemiology of diabetes mellitus among the elderly in the United States. Clin Geriatr Med 1990; 6(4):703–719.
43. Eastman RC. Cost-effectiveness of treatment of type 2 diabetes. Diabetes Care 1998; 21(3):464–465.
44. Huang ES, Jin L, Shook M, Chin MH, Meltzer DO. The impact of patient preferences on the cost-effectiveness of intensive glucose control in older patients with new onset diabetes. Diabetes Care 2006; 29(2):259–264.
45. Tsevat J, Dawson NV, Wu AW, et al. Health values of hospitalized patients 80 years or older. J Am Med Assoc 1998; 279(5):371–375.
46. Hardy SE, Gill TM. Recovery from disability among community-dwelling older persons. J Am Med Assoc 2004; 291(13):1596–1602.

21 | Oral Agents and Insulin in Care of Older Adults with Diabetes

Hermes Florez
Divisions of Endocrinology and Geriatric Medicine, University of Miami Miller School of Medicine and Geriatric Research, Education, and Clinical Center, Miami Veterans Affairs Medical Center, Miami, Florida, U.S.A.

Jennifer B. Marks
Divisions of Endocrinology, Diabetes, and Metabolism, University of Miami Miller School of Medicine, and Miami Veterans Affairs Medical Center, Miami, Florida, U.S.A.

CHALLENGES ASSOCIATED WITH GLYCEMIC CONTROL IN THE ELDERLY

Care for elderly patients with diabetes poses a unique clinical challenge (1). The management of older patients with diabetes is complicated by the medical and functional heterogeneity of this group (2,3). The heterogeneity of this population is a key consideration for clinicians developing intervention strategies and establishing clinical targets for elderly patients with diabetes (4–9). The examples of clinical and functional heterogeneity include:

1. Patients who have just shifted from impaired glucose tolerance to diabetes and have a few comorbidities but remain active with excellent functional status
2. Patients who have been recently diagnosed but have had significant hyperglycemia for many years and already have complications at diagnosis
3. Elderly who have developed diabetes in middle age and developed multiple related comorbidities over time
4. Patients who are disabled and frail, with advanced cognitive impairment, multiple comorbidities, and complications. Since many elderly diabetic patients are in between the stages described above, with mild or early functional limitations and multiple risks for worsening morbidity, they require an individualized plan based on their functional status and life expectancy (4,10).

Elderly persons with diabetes have been an undertreated subset of diabetic patients. Data from the Cardiovascular Health Study showed that close to 78% of diabetic patients aged 65 years and older did not meet the American Diabetes Association (ADA) recommendations for glycemic control (11). The goals of physicians and other providers caring for the elderly diabetic patient should be to optimize glycemic control and reduce associated cardiovascular risk factors in an effort to maximize long-term quality of life (4,12). On the other hand, for some frail older patients, particularly those with severe comorbidities and disabilities, aggressive management is not likely to provide benefit and may even result in harm as a consequence of frequent hypoglycemia associated with aggressive glycemic control (13).

MANAGEMENT—GUIDING PRINCIPLES

Several drug therapy options alone and in combination are available for treatment of diabetes in the elderly (4). At first glance, the therapeutic principles for glycemic control in elderly patients with diabetes are not very different from those in younger adults. However, the elderly with diabetes require additional areas of consideration in goal setting and use of treatment modalities. As previously discussed, treatment goals must be individualized, and at times, the enthusiasm for tight glucose control may need to be weighed against safety concerns in the elderly with diabetes. In deciding the best strategy for the intervention, it is important to adjust the regimen and goals periodically as the diabetes progresses and/or complications develop.

The ADA recently published a consensus algorithm for the initiation and adjustment of therapy in patients with type 2 diabetes (14), with emphasis on the achievement and maintenance of normal glycemic goal but not addressing the needs and consideration of elderly patients with diabetes. In these patients, the regimens should be simplified with less frequent dosing, avoiding interaction with other drugs that may affect the treatment effectiveness. The presence of renal, liver, and/or cardiovascular comorbidities may create contraindications and/or increase the risk of hypoglycemia. Other important considerations are cost and effect of these medications on weight and/or lipids. In general, oral agents should be started at the lowest possible effective dose to minimize the risk of adverse events.

ORAL AGENTS FOR GLUCOSE MANAGEMENT

Five classes of oral pharmaceutical agents for the treatment of type 2 diabetes have been approved in the United States by the Food and Drug Administration (FDA) (Table 1) (15–17). In general, there is no clinical evidence of superiority of a particular drug over another in elderly patients. Knowledge of pharmacokinetics, side effects, and potential interactions allow for a safe use of these drugs in older patients with diabetes (18). Two classes of drugs, the sulfonylureas and the meglitinides improve glucose levels by stimulating insulin secretion from

TABLE 1 Noninsulin Agents for Treatment of Type 2 Diabetes

Drug	Dosage	Efficacy (change in HbA1c)
Oral agents		
Sulfonylureas (2nd generation)		−1% to −2%
Glimepiride (Amaryl)	4–8 mg daily (begin 1–2 mg)	
Glipizide (Glucotrol)	2.5–40 mg daily or divided	
(Glucotrol XL)	5–20 mg daily	
Glyburide (Diaβeta, Micronase)	1.25–20 mg daily or divided	
Micronized glyburide (Glynase)	1.5–12 mg daily	
Meglitinides		−1% to −2%
Nateglinide (Starlix)	60–120 mg t.i.d.	
Repaglinide (Prandin)	0.5 mg b.i.d.–q.i.d. if HbA1c < 8% or previously untreated	
	1–2 mg b.i.d.–q.i.d. if HbA1c ≥ 8% or previously treated	
α-Glucosidase Inhibitors		−0.5% to −1%
Acarbose (Precose)	50–100 mg t.i.d., just before meals; start with 25 mg	
Miglitol (Glyset)	25–100 mg t.i.d, with first bite of meal; start with 25 mg	
Biguanides		−1% to −2%
Metformin (Glucophage)	500–2550 mg divided	
(Glucophage XR)	1500–2000 mg daily	
Thiazolidinediones		−1% to −2%
Pioglitazone (Actos)	15 or 30 mg daily; max 45 mg/day as monotherapy, 30 mg/day in combination therapy	
Rosiglitazone (Avandia)	4 mg daily or b.i.d.	
Injectable agents		−0.5% to −1%
Incretin mimetic	5–10 μg s.c. b.i.d.	
Exenatide *(Byetta)*		
Amylin analog	60 μg s.c. before meals	
Pramlintide (Symlin)		

Abbreviations: b.i.d., twice a day; HbA1c, hemoglobin A1c; q.i.d., four times a day; s.c., subcutaneously; t.i.d., three times a day.

TABLE 2 Mechanisms to Lower Blood Glucose by Each Antidiabetic Agent

	Correct insulin deficiency	Stimulate insulin secretion	Increase muscle glucose uptake	Decrease hepatic glucose production	Retard carbohydrate absorption
Sulfonylureas		X			
Meglitinides		X			
Biguanides			(X)	X	
Thiazolidinediones			X	(X)	
Glucosidase inhibitors					X
Incretin mimetics/ amylin analogs		X		X	X
Insulin/insulin analogs	X				

Note: X, main mechanism; (X) less-clear mechanism.

pancreatic β-cells. Other agents target different mechanisms in the underlying pathogenesis of the disease (Table 2), such as the reduction of carbohydrate absorption (α-glucosidase inhibitors) and improvement in insulin sensitivity (biguanides and thiazolidinediones). Any of these agents may be used as first-line monotherapy since most demonstrate equivalent efficacy in improving glycemic control. When monotherapy fails, the addition of a second oral agent from a different drug class is advised to achieve fasting or postprandial glycemic targets. In general, the use of triple therapy is safe but should be used with caution because of the high risk of polypharmacy in the elderly and higher associated costs.

Sulfonylurea

Sulfonylurea preparations have a long record of safety and effectiveness. They work by stimulating insulin secretion by the pancreatic β-cell, binding to an adenosine triphosphate–sensitive potassium channel, which results in its depolarization, a subsequent influx of intracellular calcium, and the release of insulin. Sulfonylureas are effective both as monotherapy and in combination with other agents that have different mechanisms of action. A significant percentage of patients (up to 10% per year) who are initially properly managed with sulfonylurea monotherapy lose glycemic control over time. Their main side effects include hypoglycemia and weight gain (Table 3). Hypoglycemia is a serious adverse effect in the elderly and can trigger serious events such as myocardial infarction and stroke. These drugs must be used cautiously in patients with significant renal and hepatic insufficiency, since the liver is the primary site of metabolism and they are excreted by the kidneys. In these settings, the preferred option may be *glipizide*, whose metabolites are inactive, or *glimepiride*, which is substantially excreted through the bile.

A commonly used sulfonylurea in younger populations, *glyburide*, may have age-related impaired absorption and elimination, and elderly subjects appear to have enhanced insulin responses to the drug as well. This may explain, in part, the age-related exponential increase

TABLE 3 Limiting Factors in the Use of Antidiabetic Agents in the Elderly

	Hypoglycemia	Weight gain	Other
Sulfonylureas	X	X	May impede ischemic preconditioning
Meglitinides	X	X	Frequent dosing may affect compliance; no long-term experience
Biguanides	No	No (wt loss)	Risk of lactic acidosis; diarrhea
Thiazolidinediones	No	XX	Edema; expensive; no long-term experience
Glucosidase inhibitors	No	No	Frequent dosing may affect compliance; intestinal gas; expensive
Incretin mimetics/amylin analogs	No	No (wt loss)	Injection; expensive; no long-term experience

Note: X, main side effect; XX, pronounced side effect.
Abbreviation: wt, weight.

in the frequency of severe or fatal hypoglycemia with this drug. In addition to the type of sulfonylurea, other potential risk factors for hypoglycemia with these drugs in elderly persons include black race, multiple medications, male sex, renal dysfunction, and ethanol consumption. Sulfonylureas should be considered as first-line therapy in lean elderly patients with diabetes. The result in hemoglobin A1c (HbA1c) lowering is approximately 1% to 2% as monotherapy.

Meglitinides

Meglitinides (repaglinide and nateglinide) are nonsulfonylurea drugs that have a distinct β-cell binding profile and stimulate insulin secretion from the β-cell by a mechanism similar to that of sulfonylureas. The potential advantage of this type of drug is that it has a rapid onset and very short duration of action. Meglitinides have been associated with lower frequency of hypoglycemic events when compared with conventional sulfonylureas, presumably because of their shorter duration of action and the fact that the kinetics are not altered with age. *Repaglinide* lowers HbA1c by 1% to 2%, a reduction similar to that of the sulfonylureas, whereas the glucose-lowering effect of *nateglinide* is somewhat less potent. Similar changes in fasting glucose and HbA1c values are seen in middle-aged and elderly subjects, suggesting that there is similar efficacy in each age group. Both repaglinide and nateglinide are extensively metabolized by the liver; therefore, they should be used cautiously in patients with hepatic dysfunction. Meglitinides may be considered as an appropriate strategy for elderly patients who have irregular eating habits or have frequent hypoglycemic events on conventional sulfonylureas. These potential benefits must be balanced against the cost of these newer drugs and the compliance problems that could result from a three-times-a-day dosing schedule, particularly in patients who have impaired memory or take may other drugs.

α-Glucosidase Inhibitors

α-glucosidase inhibitors (miglitol and acarbose) impair the breakdown and limit the absorption of carbohydrates from the gut; therefore their major effect is reduction in postprandial glucose excursions. These drugs are associated with less weight gain and a lower frequency of hypoglycemia than sulfonylureas. The residual carbohydrates in the intestinal lumen cause diarrhea in about 25% of patients taking these drugs. Gradual dose titration is crucial to minimize gastrointestinal side effects and achieve better compliance. Their overall effect on HbA1c concentration is a modest reduction of 0.5% to 1%. In a recent randomized multicenter trial of the α-glucosidase inhibitor *acarbose* in obese elderly patients with diabetes, acarbose reduced HbA1c by about 0.8% when compared with placebo and also resulted in an improvement in insulin sensitivity (19). α-glucosidase inhibitors are useful drugs as primary therapy for elderly patients with modest fasting hyperglycemia, especially if they are obese. They can also be used in patients taking other oral agents to enhance glycemic control. Hypoglycemia may occur if these agents are used in combination with sulfonylureas or insulin; consequently, only glucose should be used for prompt treatment of hypoglycemia because the absorption of other carbohydrates is delayed. Acarbose has minimal systemic absorption, yet some hepatic metabolism occurs and because of rare but possible hepatotoxicity, it is contraindicated in patients with advanced liver disease. In contrast, as much as 50% to 90% of the *miglitol* dose may be absorbed but is not metabolized in the liver but rather eliminated through the kidney. Therefore, miglitol should not be used in patients with renal failure.

Metformin

Metformin is currently the only biguanide available in North America. Its mechanism of action is to improve insulin sensitivity, chiefly by reducing insulin resistance in the liver, thereby decreasing hepatic glucose production. In addition, its glucose-lowering effect is accompanied by a reduction in plasma insulin concentration, and some experts refer to metformin as an insulin sensitizer. Metformin lowers HbA1c by 1% to 2%. Although, the most important side effect associated with biguanides is lactic acidosis, this is rare with metformin; and aging itself does not appear to be a risk factor provided that careful attention is paid to the contraindications for this drug (significant liver, renal, and cardiac disease). Clinical studies suggest that the drug is safe and effective as monotherapy in obese older people. In our view, metformin is an ideal drug for first-line therapy of obese older patients, because it increases insulin sensitivity, assists with weight loss, reduces lipid levels, and does not cause hypoglycemia. The recently published ADA management algorithm suggests the use of metformin, together with lifestyle intervention, as initial monotherapy (14).

In addition, metformin is a useful adjunct for patients who are inadequately controlled on maximum doses of sulfonylureas. Metformin is contraindicated in older subjects with renal insufficiency, in men with a serum creatinine level of 1.5 mg/dL or higher or women with a serum creatinine level of 1.4 mg/dL or higher. Serum creatinine should be measured at least annually and with any increase in dose of metformin. It should be noted, however, that serum creatinine does not adequately reflect the renal function in the elderly. For those aged 80 years or older or those suspected to have reduced muscle mass, a timed urine collection for creatinine clearance should be obtained. Metformin should be avoided if the value is less than 60 mL/ min. Metformin should be temporarily discontinued during radiographic studies that use iodinated contrast agents, during acute illness, and during most hospitalizations. Clinical situations where tissue perfusion is compromised (sepsis, dehydration, pulmonary disease with hypoxemia, and acute or advanced heart failure) also contraindicate the use of metformin.

Thiazolidinediones

Thiazolidinediones (*rosiglitazone* and *pioglitazone*) improve insulin sensitivity primarily in muscles and adipocytes, thereby increasing peripheral uptake and utilization of glucose. They are generally well tolerated and appear to be as effective in older patients as in younger patients, with an approximate 1.5% reduction in HbA1c and with a dose-dependent glucose-lowering effect, which may take four to eight weeks. In addition to benefits of these drugs on cardiovascular and metabolic markers, a recent randomized trial has shown the effect of pioglitazone on the reduction of cardiovascular outcomes in patients with type 2 diabetes (20). Thiazolidinediones do not lead to hypoglycemia unless they are used in conjunction with secretagogues or insulin. Hepatic toxicity has not been reported in elderly subjects, but liver function tests should be monitored regularly. The incidence of edema and anemia is higher in elderly patients than in middle-aged patients treated, and volume status and blood count need to be carefully monitored. Thiazolidinediones-related fluid retention is a major contributor to increased body weight, typically manifests as peripheral edema, and develops predominantly within the first months of treatment. Thiazolidinediones can be a useful first-line therapy in obese elderly patients, particularly for those patients who cannot tolerate metformin or those who have a contraindication to it. In fact, thiazolidinediones can be safely used in patients with renal impairment provided that the cardiac function is preserved. In addition, they may be a beneficial adjunct therapy in elderly patients who have suboptimal glycemic control, despite insulin requirements of 50 or more units per day.

OTHER INJECTABLE AND NEW AGENTS

There are new injectable agents approved by the FDA for use in patients with type 1 or type 2 diabetes that have unique mechanisms of action.

Incretin Mimetic Agents

Incretin mimetic agents activate the glucagon-like peptide-1 (GLP-1) receptor. GLP-1 is normally secreted from the intestine in response to food ingestion. GLP-1 agonists work via several mechanisms: (*i*) enhancement of glucose-mediated pancreatic insulin secretion, (*ii*) inhibition of exaggerated postprandial glucagons secretion, (*iii*) slowing the rate of gastric emptying, and (*iv*) actions on the hypothalamus to decrease appetite. *Exenatide*, the first approved drug in this class, is indicated for the treatment of type 2 diabetes patients who have not achieved glycemic control with metformin and/or a sulfonylurea (21,22). Exenatide is dosed as 5 or 10 μg subcutaneously before meals. It lowers HbA1c levels by about 1%, does not lead to hypoglycemia by itself, and may lead to a modest weight loss. Its major side effects include nausea, vomiting, and diarrhea. Recent data suggest that GLP-1 maintains its ability to enhance glucose-induced insulin release in elderly patients and may also increase insulin sensitivity and non–insulin-mediated glucose uptake (23). Long-term clinical studies are required to determine the role of this peptide in the therapy of diabetes in elderly patients.

Amylin Analogs

Amylin analogs predominantly lower postprandial glucose levels, complementing the effect of insulin. Amylin, a hormone that is made in the pancreatic α-cells, is normally cosecreted with insulin in response to carbohydrates and amino acids, and in the postprandial state produces: (*i*) suppression of glucagon secretion, (*ii*) delay in gastric emptying, and (*iii*) reduction of appetite. *Pramlintide*, a synthetic analog of human amylin, is indicated for use in patients with type 2 or type 1 diabetes treated with insulin (24,25). Its major side effect is hypoglycemia, but in contrast to insulin, it may lead to some weight loss. It has been shown to help patients achieve lower postprandial blood glucose levels resulting in less fluctuation during the day. It is dosed as 15 to 120 μg subcutaneously before each meal. No published data are currently available on the use of pramlintide in elderly patients. In addition, because it requires adding three or more injections per day and more frequent glucose monitoring, compliance may be a problem in the elderly population.

Dipeptidyl Peptidase-IV Inhibitors

Dipeptidyl peptidase-IV (DPP-IV) inhibitors are in various stages of development (26). DPP-IV is the enzyme that degrades native GLP-1. Inhibition of this enzyme can increase GLP-1 levels and potentially improve postprandial glycemic control. In clinical trials, vildagliptin improves glycemic control both as monotherapy and in combination with metformin (27). Analyses of efficacy data for elderly patients in two phase 3 clinical studies (about 500 patients) and safety data from monotherapy studies including 2000 elderly patients revealed significant, consistent and sustained reductions in HbA1c and similar safety and tolerability to that found in younger patients [data presented by Baron MA et al. (28)]. Studies with sitagliptin demonstrated similar benefits in older patients as in younger ones receiving the drug. Further studies are now required to evaluate its long-term durability, effects, safety, and tolerability in comparison with other anti-diabetic agents and in different patient subgroups, including elderly patients with diabetes.

Endocannabinoid Receptor Antagonists

An endocannabinoid receptor antagonist (*Rimonabant*) is currently under review for a new drug application. This is the first in a new class of agents that selectively block the cannibinoid-1 receptor in the endocannabinoid system, an endogenous signaling system involved in lipid and glucose metabolism in adipose tissue (26). It can help regulate food intake and energy balance. Rimonabant has been shown to have significant effect on weight loss and improve lipid profiles and glycemic control (29–31).

INSULIN AND INSULIN ANALOGS

Insulin is frequently initiated when maximum dose of single or combined oral agents fail to control glucose levels (32–34). Diabetes is a progressive disease with continuing loss of β-cell function—patients should be informed that this is the natural history and they have not personally failed. Insulin and insulin analogs are available in a number of long-, intermediate-, and short-acting preparations and in an inhaled form, recently approved by the FDA for use in patients with type 1 or type 2 diabetes.

When initiating the older patient on insulin, the advantages and concerns of treatment need to be reviewed. Aspects such as physical, mental, and visual problems must be carefully assessed; practical and safe glucose targets must be established based on the individual patient's needs and capabilities. Insulin therapy must be individualized based on each patient's glucose levels, prognosis related to coexisting medical conditions, and treatment goals.

   Insulin is often initially used in combination with one or more oral agents. Basal insulin—intermediate- or long-acting—is initially started at bedtime and slowly increased to reach safe morning glucose targets and, if required, a second dose and/or additional fast-acting insulin is added during the day. Complex multiple-dose insulin regimens should be avoided unless essential. A wide variety of insulins is available, from very rapid-acting to very long-acting and premixed combination preparations (Table 4).

   The greatest risk of insulin therapy is hypoglycemia, and evidence suggests that frail older adults are at higher risk of serious hypoglycemia (35) than are healthier, more functional older adults. A practical approach to improve benefit and reduce risk when using insulin therapy includes

- Continuation of use of oral agents. There is evidence that it will enhance effectiveness of residual insulin, reduce glycemic variability, and may help with weight control (36).
- Use of basal insulin early [neutral protamine Hagedorn (NPH) or glargine]. With a starting dose of 10 units bed time (HS) (5 units if frail) or up to 0.25 units/kg weight, then titrating weekly or biweekly to a goal of fasting blood glucose of 120 to 140 mg/dL.
- Use of insulin analogs in patients who require prandial insulin because it may reduce the likelihood of hypoglycemia in those with variable food intake or unpredictable digestion/absorption.

Time for supervised practice for those with motor or visual problems should be provided and can improve the accuracy of insulin administration. The patient's insulin injection technique should be observed on a regular basis to detect a need for adaptive strategies such as additional lighting, magnification, and premixed syringes. Elderly subjects often make errors when trying to mix insulin on their own. The accuracy of insulin injections may be improved in older patients when they are treated with premixed insulin. Family members, home care nurses, and visiting nurses can assist with implementing these techniques at home.

   Physician and educator attitudes are important factors in the acceptance of insulin therapy. Discussing the benefits and potential challenges of insulin therapy may help patients decide about whether to take insulin or not. The need of insulin can be presented as the treatment for the patient's particular stage of diabetes. This approach may help overcome patient resistance to insulin use (i.e., fear of injection, pain, lipohypertrophy, complexity of regimens, etc.). In

TABLE 4   Insulin Preparations

Preparations	Onset	Peak	Duration	Indication
Insulins (Humulin, Novolin)				
Short acting	—	—	—	—
Regular	0.5–1 hr	2–3 hr	6–12 hr	Prandial
Intermediate acting				
NPH	1–1.5 hr	4–12 hr	8–12 hr	Basal
Lente (intermediate acting)	1–2.5 hr	8–12 hr	10–24 hr	Basal
Long acting				
Ultralente	4–8 hr	16–18 hr	36 hr	Basal
Insulin analogs	—	—	—	—
Rapid acting	—	—	—	—
Insulin aspart (NovoLog)	30 min	1–3 hr	3–5 hr	Prandial
Insulin lispro (Humalog)	15 min	0.5–1.5 hr	3–5 hr	Prandial
Insulin glulisine (Apidra)	15 min	0.5–1.5 hr	3–5 hr	Prandial
Long acting	—	—	—	—
Insulin glargine (Lantus)	1–2 hr	—	22–24 hr	Basal
Insulin detemir (Levemir)	1–2 hr	—	14–24 hr	Basal
Premixed combination insulin/analogs	—	—	—	—
NPH and regular insulin mix (70/30 or 50/50)	30 min	2–12 hr	24 hr	Mixed
NPH and insulin analog mix (NPH and lispro 75/25, NPH and aspart 70/30)				

Abbreviation: NPH, neutral protamine Hagedorn (insulin).

addition, it is important to recognize and address the provider's resistance related to lack of time and resources to supervise treatment, skepticism about the effectiveness of insulin, and perceived cardiovascular risk. Finally, understanding medical limitations associated with insulin use (weight gain and risk for hypoglycemia) may help overcome these barriers and target therapy more appropriately.

OTHER MANAGEMENT RECOMMENDATIONS IN THE ELDERLY

Because most elderly patients with diabetes have polypharmacy, including a pharmacist in the diabetes management team can improve detection of redundant therapies and detection of interactions with other diseases, drugs, and food. In addition, a pharmacist can also help identify ways to simplify medication programs for those with comorbidities.

The effectiveness of therapy increases when medications are taken as recommended (37). The following approaches may increase the likelihood of patients taking their medications prescribed:

- Incorporate medication schedule into daily routine.
- Teach patients to understand their prescription labels.
- Devise or procure memory aids such as calendars, pillboxes, or timers.
- Recommend pill-splitting aids or magnifiers, as needed.

It is important to provide brief, easy-to-read written, visual, and verbal information about the specific oral agent that is being used and to inquire about side effects at each visit. When appropriate, family members who are involved in day-to-day care should be included in educational and clinical sessions. These caregivers often are older spouses for whom educational adaptation will also be needed (38). Collaborative goals for management are established by discussing with the patient existing diabetes complications, comorbidities, abilities, and willingness to carry out the treatment plan.

REFERENCES

1. Thearle M, Brillantes AM. Unique characteristics of the geriatric diabetic population and the role for therapeutic strategies that enhance glucagon-like peptide-1 activity. Curr Opin Clin Nutr Metab Care 2005; (1):9–16.
2. Meneilly GS, Tessier D. Diabetes in elderly adults. J Gerontol A Biol Sci Med Sci 2001; 56(1):M5–M13.
3. Piette JD, Kerr EA. The impact of comorbid chronic conditions on diabetes care. Diabetes Care 2006; 29(3):725–731.
4. Brown AF, Mangione CM, Saliba D, et al. California Health Care Foundation/American Geriatrics Society Panel on Improving Care for Elders with Diabetes. Guidelines for improving the care of the older person with diabetes mellitus. J Am Geriatr Soc 2003; 51(suppl 5 Guidelines):S265–S280.
5. Macheledt JE, Vernon SW. Diabetes and disability among Mexican Americans: the effect of different measures of diabetes on its association with disability. J Clin Epidemiol 1992; 45(5):519–528.
6. Gregg EW, Beckles GL, Williamson DF, et al. Diabetes and physical disability among older U.S. adults. Diabetes Care 2000; 23:1272–1277.
7. Maty SC, Fried LP, Volpato S, et al. Patterns of disability related to diabetes mellitus in older women. J Gerontol 2004; 59A:M148–M153.
8. Chou KL, Chi I. Functional disability related to diabetes mellitus in older Hong Kong Chinese adults. Gerontology 2005; 51(5):334–339.
9. Al Snih S, Fisher MN, Raji MA, et al. Diabetes mellitus and incidence of lower body disability among older Mexican Americans. J Gerontol A Biol Sci Med Sci 2005; 60(9):1152–1156.
10. Pogach LM, Brietzke SA, Cowan CL Jr, et al. VA/DoD Diabetes Guideline Development Group. Development of evidence-based clinical practice guidelines for diabetes: the Department of Veterans Affairs/Department of Defense guidelines initiative. Diabetes Care 2004; 27(suppl 2):B82–B89.
11. Smith NL, Heckbert SR, Bittner VA, et al. Antidiabetic treatment trends in a cohort of elderly people with diabetes. The cardiovascular health study, 1989–1997. Diabetes Care 1999; 22(5):736–742.
12. Pitale S, Kernan-Schroeder D, Emanuele N, et al. VACSDM Study Group. Health-related quality of life in the VA Feasibility Study on glycemic control and complications in type 2 diabetes mellitus. J Diabetes Complicat 2005; 19:207–211.
13. Alam T, Weintraub N, Weinreb J. What is the proper use of hemoglobin A1c monitoring in the elderly? J Am Med Dir Assoc 2006; 7(suppl 3):S60–S64.

14. Nathan DM, Buse JB, Davidson MB, et al. Management of Hyperglycemia in Type 2 Diabetes: a Consensus Algorithm for the Initiation and Adjustment of Therapy: a consensus statement from the American Diabetes Association and the European Association for the Study of Diabetes. Diabetes Care 2006; 29(8):1963–1972.
15. DeFronzo RA. Pharmacologic therapy for type 2 diabetes. Ann Intern Med 1999; 131:281–303.
16. Kimmel B, Inzucchi SE. Oral agents for type 2 diabetes: an update. Clin Diabetes 2005; 23:64–76.
17. American Diabetes Association Position Statement. Standards of medical care for diabetes. Diabetes Care 2006; 29(suppl 1):S4–42.
18. Sakharova OV, Inzucchi SE. Treatment of diabetes in the elderly. Addressing its complexities in this high-risk group. Postgrad Med 2005; 118(5):19–26:29.
19. Phillips P, Karrasch J, Scott R, et al. Acarbose improves glycemic control in overweight type 2 diabetic patients insufficiently treated with metformin. Diabetes Care 2003; 26(2):269–273.
20. Dormandy JA, Charbonnel B, Eckland DJ, et al. Secondary prevention of macrovascular events in patients with type 2 diabetes in the PROactive Study (PROspective pioglitAzone Clinical Trial In macroVascular Events): a randomised controlled trial. Lancet 2005; 366(9493):1279–1289.
21. Buse JB, Henry RR, Han J, et al. Exenatide-113 Clinical Study Group. Effects of exenatide (exendin-4) on glycemic control over 30 weeks in sulfonylurea-treated patients with type 2 diabetes. Diabetes Care 2004; 27(11):2628–2635.
22. Kendall DM, Riddle MC, Rosenstock J, et al. Effects of exenatide (exendin-4) on glycemic control over 30 weeks in patients with type 2 diabetes treated with metformin and a sulfonylurea. Diabetes Care 2005; 28(5):1083–1091.
23. Dungan K, Buse JB. Glucagon-like peptide-1based therapies for type 2 diabetes: a focus on exenatide. Clin Diabetes 2005; 23:56–62.
24. Hollander P, Maggs DG, Ruggles JA, et al. Effect of pramlintide on weight in overweight and obese insulin-treated type 2 diabetes patients. Obes Res 2004; 12(4):661–668.
25. Ratner RE, Dickey R, Fineman M, et al. Amylin replacement with pramlintide as an adjunct to insulin therapy improves long-term glycaemic and weight control in Type 1 diabetes mellitus: a 1-year, randomized controlled trial. Diabet Med 2004; 21(11):1204–1212.
26. Lebovitz H. Diabetes: assessing the pipeline. Atheroscler Suppl 2006; 7(1):43–49.
27. Ahren B. Vildagliptin: an inhibitor of dipeptidyl peptidase-4 with antidiabetic properties. Expert Opin Investig Drugs 2006; 15(4):431–442.
28. Baron MA, et al. International Diabetes Federation Congress, December 3–7, 2006; Cape Town, South Affrica.
29. Despres JP, Golay A, Sjostrom L. Rimonabant in Obesity-Lipids Study Group. Effects of rimonabant on metabolic risk factors in overweight patients with dyslipidemia. N Engl J Med 2005; 353(20): 2121–2134.
30. Pi-Sunyer FX, Aronne LJ, Heshmati HM, et al. RIO-North America Study Group. Effect of rimonabant, a cannabinoid-1 receptor blocker, on weight and cardiometabolic risk factors in overweight or obese patients: RIO-North America: a randomized controlled trial. JAMA 2006; 295(7):761–775.
31. Gelfand EV, Cannon CP. Rimonabant: a cannabinoid receptor type 1 blocker for management of multiple cardiometabolic risk factors. J Am Coll Cardiol 2006; 47(10):1919–1926.
32. Saudek CD, Hill GS. Feasibility and outcomes of insulin therapy in elderly patients with diabetes mellitus. Drugs Aging 1999; 14:375–385.
33. Meneilly GS, Tessier D. Diabetes in elderly adults. J Gerontol 2001; 56A:M5–M13.
34. Hirsch IB, Bergenstal RM, Parkin CG, et al. Practical Pointers: a real-world approach to insulin therapy in primary care practice. Clin Diabetes 2005; 23:78–86.
35. Shorr RI, Ray WA, Daugherty JR, et al. Incidence and risk factors for serious hypoglycemia in older persons using insulin or sulfonylureas. Arch Intern Med 1997; 157(15):1681–1686.
36. Yki-Jarvinen H, Ryysy L, Nikkila K, Tulokas T, Vanamo R, Heikkila M. Comparison of bedtime insulin regimens in patients with type 2 diabetes mellitus. A randomized, controlled trial. Ann Intern Med 1999; 130(5):389–396.
37. Wallsten SM, Sullivan RJ Jr, Hanlon JT, et al. Medication taking behaviors in the high- and low-functioning elderly: MacArthur field studies of successful aging. Ann Pharmacother 1995; 29(4):359–364.
38. Silliman RA, Bhatti S, Khan A, et al. The care of older persons with diabetes mellitus: families and primary care physicians. J Am Geriatr Soc 1996; 44(11):1314–1321.

22 | Nutritional Therapy for Diabetes in Older Patients

Ronni Chernoff
Geriatric Research Education and Clinical Center, Central Arkansas Veterans Healthcare System, Department of Geriatrics, Arkansas Geriatric Education Center and Reynolds Institute on Aging, University of Arkansas for Medical Sciences, Little Rock, Arkansas, U.S.A.

INTRODUCTION

Impaired glucose tolerance is associated with advanced age and nearly half of the individuals with type 2 diabetes are over age 60 (1). However, only about 10% of the variability of a response to an oral glucose load can be attributed to age; alterations in glucose tolerance are also affected by activity level and diet (2). Although type 2 diabetes is the prevalent type of diabetes seen in older adults, some elderly individuals do become insulin dependent and must be carefully monitored (3).

Diabetes contributes to a variety of complications that affect nearly all organ systems; vascular compromise is one of the primary etiologies of diabetes-associated conditions. Micro-vascular pathology contributes to cardiovascular disease, blindness, renal disease, peripheral neuropathy, and peripheral vascular disease leading to foot or leg amputation (3). Older adults also have multiple pathologies that contribute to the development of these conditions, thereby making it more difficult to manage them.

One factor closely associated with the onset of later-life diabetes is overweight and obesity (4,5). In large epidemiologic studies, modifiable risk factors of obesity have been identified; they include weight control, dietary alterations, and exercise (6). Older adults with diabetes have been noted to be less overweight and to have a greater degree of insulin insufficiency than do middle-aged adults (1). The link between diabetes and onset of other chronic diseases is so strong that prevention strategies should be implemented in early life, maintained throughout adulthood, and continued into old age. A weight reduction of even 10% has been reported to have benefits such as better glycemic control, a reduction in blood pressure, and an improved lipid profile (7).

DIABETES IN OLDER ADULTS
Age-Related Risk Factors

Aging is associated with changes in body composition that include loss of lean body mass, reduced total body water, decreased bone mass, and increased relative or actual fat mass. Not only is abdominal fat linked to insulin resistance but also visceral fat, which accumulates with advancing age (8).

Metabolism is altered due to the decrease in lean body mass and associated reduction of the total body protein pool. For many years, age was considered a significant factor in glucose intolerance; however, the fasting blood glucose thresholds for diabetes in older adults was lowered (9) and a greater number of older adults were diagnosed as diabetics. Early prevention with continued interventions makes common sense to avoid the onset of diabetes and its consequences in elderly people.

Interventions

Diabetes is a progressive disease and, over time, interventions will need to be adjusted to account for concurrent illnesses and changing lifestyles related to disability, diet, and medications (5). Older adults must be followed up carefully to keep them in good health and to assure a good quality of life.

Many different research reports support the importance of nutrition and exercise in primary prevention of type 2 diabetes; strategies to reduce risk include weight reduction, reduction of dietary fat, and increase in physical activity (6,8). Primary prevention should include beneficial lifestyle habits that begin early in life. Recommendations for primary prevention are also useful. Secondary or tertiary prevention in older adults can contribute to reducing the risk of complications in elderly, type 2 diabetes patients (10).

Treatment of diabetes in elderly adults is actually the same as treatment used for younger adults and includes diet, physical activity, and oral hypoglycemic agents or insulin (1). Treatment goals should be established quickly to control blood glucose levels with a combination of medication, diet, and lifestyle changes. Nationally recommended goals include:

1. Maintain blood glucose within normal limits using HbA1c levels (11).
2. Attain lipid levels within adequate guidelines.
3. Achieve and maintain a healthy body weight.
4. Manage medications as directed by the physician.
5. Incorporate physical activity into lifestyle.

For several years, the trend in diabetic diet recommendations has shifted from low fat and high carbohydrate to lower carbohydrate and higher protein, in combination with an exercise regimen (12). In several studies, greater weight loss has been associated with low-carbohydrate diets despite greater calorie intake (13–16). It has been reported that low-carbohydrate diets contribute to greater glycemic control, which has been associated with a reduced risk of diabetes as well as an improved lipid profile (16,17).

The management of diabetes using a high-protein, low-carbohydrate diet has become more popular recently. However, knowledge of the long-term management of obesity and diabetes using low-carbohydrate diets is somewhat limited due to small sample sizes and poor dietary adherence (12). Additionally, reported studies generally do not include elderly subjects but tend to focus on young and middle-aged adults.

Diets that are very low in carbohydrates do not appear to be as beneficial for adult diabetics as diets that have a more balanced profile of macronutrients. Carbohydrates should come from foods that contain a higher proportion of unrefined starches (whole grains) (18). Studies conducted on the glycemic index (GI) of foods (the rate at which glucose released from the digestion of a food enters the bloodstream) demonstrate that foods with a low GI contribute to a better balance between blood glucose and insulin levels (19–21). Carbohydrate-containing foods should include whole-grain cereals, baked goods, and breads; foods containing more refined carbohydrates (i.e., sugarcoated cereals, baked goods with icing, jellies, and jams) should be only a small proportion of the overall diet.

WEIGHT LOSS AND DIABETES MANAGEMENT

Control of body weight and blood glucose may be associated with a lower risk of late-life dementia (22). Weight loss in older adults is surprisingly controversial; there is no strong indication that obesity in adults over 70 years contributes to increased mortality (23). There is a theory that excess weight may provide available energy or nutritional reserve during periods of stress and illness (24). However, control of blood glucose levels is easier if weight is maintained or a rational weight loss is supported by a plan that the individual can manage without confusion, stress, or major lifestyle changes. Weight loss should be gradual, using a nutritionally complete dietary regimen that includes all essential nutrients and reduces caloric intake to achieve a 1- to 2-pound weight loss per week. Diets that lead to rapid weight loss, by reducing intake from one or more dietary groups, put overall nutritional status and blood glucose control at risk.

In one report, middle-aged and older men who participated in a diet-induced weight-loss program lost 9-kg body weight, reduced their total body fat by 19%, and had an 8% reduction in waist circumference; weight loss led to improved glucose tolerance and insulin action (25). In another prospective study, insulin sensitivity was measured in obese subjects on maintenance, calorie-restriction (800 kcal/day), and severe calorie-restriction (400 kcal/day) diets.

Changes in insulin secretion and insulin sensitivity were substantial after the initial calorie restriction (26).

Evidence indicates that patients are more likely to adhere to dietary changes and weight-loss plans if the recommendation comes from their physician (10,23). One of the most important steps a physician can take when recommending a weight-loss diet to older adults is to assess an individual's readiness to change (27,28). Despite what may seem to be a reasonable solution to overweight, the patient has to be ready and willing to make important lifestyle changes for success. Basically, there are two conditions necessary for weight loss to be achieved: increased activity and decreased caloric intake.

Physical Activity

Increasing activity may seem like an achievable goal; however, each individual must be assessed for conditions that may limit physical activity, whether it is systemic disease, sensory limitations, or physical restrictions. Any plan for exercise must be individualized to accommodate impairments of any type. The most successful weight-loss programs include both calorie restriction and exercise (29). Exercise also has other benefits for older adults including maintenance of bone density, increased strength, and improved function, all of which contribute to a better quality of life (30,31).

Meeting Nutrient Needs

Decreased caloric intake is an essential component of a successful weight-loss program. Commercial weight-loss plans may be expensive; may not accommodate ethnic, religious, or cultural preferences; and may not fit the needs of elderly people. Nutritional requirements in older adults are slightly altered but may also be affected by chronic disease, medications, and ethnic or dietary preferences (32). Calorie-restricted diets may be low in selected nutrients and may contribute to nutritionally inadequate diets. Specific nutrients for which requirements change or for which adequate intakes may be difficult to achieve include protein, vitamin D, vitamin B12, fiber, and fluid.

Protein requirements are higher in elderly persons. The recommended protein requirement is at least 1.0 g protein/kg body weight. This is higher if conditions of healing are present or if the person is restricted to the chair or the bed (32–34). If a reduced diet does not provide enough protein and calories to protect the body's protein content, muscle wasting will occur, immune function may be compromised, healing will be slow, and new tissue will be of poor quality. Even with adequate protein, if there is inadequate energy substrate, protein tissue may be lost.

Older adults also commonly have an inadequate intake of vitamin D. Vitamin D is essential for the maintenance of bone health and immune function (35). The primary dietary source of vitamin D is fortified milk. For those individuals who cannot consume milk and milk products, over-the-counter supplements can be used. It is beneficial to use lower fat (2%, 1%, or skimmed milk) dairy products to lower overall caloric intake while consuming adequate calcium and vitamin D. The recommendation for daily intake of vitamin D is 800 IU. Supplement intake should not exceed daily recommendations and there appears to be no risk of toxicity from high doses (36).

Vitamin B12 is another nutrient that may be deficient in older adults. Inadequate intake may be due to inadequate consumption of red meat and organ meats, (i.e., liver). Older adults may have a decrease in intrinsic factor production, an increased prevalence of atrophic gastritis, and a potential for bacterial overgrowth, all of which impair vitamin B12 absorption (34). For older adults on weight-reduction diets, foods that provide vitamin B12 should be included. The vitamin B12 used in oral supplements is a crystalline form that does not require gastric acid for absorption; generic vitamin supplements that contain the daily recommendation for vitamin B12 are acceptable sources of this vitamin (31).

Fiber intake is important in older adults; it provides bulk in a diet and promotes peristalsis and gastrointestinal function as well as other potential health benefits. In older adults, fiber intake is often inadequate due to a reduction in complex carbohydrate, vegetable, and fruit consumption. Dietary fiber supplements are often used by older adults to provide the peristalsis and bowel regulation that is decreased when dietary fiber is absent. There are many commercial choices available including bran fiber, psyllium, and chemical stimulants that may be used to manage bowel function. The manufacturer-recommended dose for supplemental fiber should be adhered to and adequate dietary fluid should be consumed, particularly if the fiber supplement is a tablet or wafer that is not to be mixed with water. An average dose of supplemental fiber is approximately 20 g (37). Increased dietary fiber is associated with better glycemic control and increased insulin sensitivity (38). This recommended dose of supplemental fiber will not interfere with absorption of any dietary nutrients (39).

Associated with an increase in dietary fiber intake, there is a need for adequate fluid consumption. Although the recommendation of eight glasses of fluid per day (64 ounces) may be an overestimation of the requirements of older adults, many elderly people are taking less than they need. A recommendation of approximately 30 mL/kg/day with a minimum of 1500 mL/day (approximately 6–8-ounce glasses of fluid) seems to be adequate under normal health and climate conditions (40). The challenge of achieving an adequate fluid intake in older persons is that thirst sensitivity diminishes and consuming even this much fluid may be difficult (41).

Weight reduction in overweight or obese elderly adults is not easy, even in individuals who are highly motivated. It is important to make changes in diets that do not compromise nutritional status; that meet nutritional requirements; that contribute to a healthy, sustained decrease in weight; and that contribute to better blood glucose control. Small changes may have positive effects in older subjects.

Strategies

Usually, strategies that include a combination of approaches to control weight and manage glucose levels are most successful. The Dietary Intervention: Evaluation of Technology (DIET) Study was an intensive, two-year longitudinal study of 247 independent, overweight older adults living in two retirement communities, who received a 10-week program of psychological and educational approaches to lifestyle changes. The control group was the retirees who were wait-listed for entry in the program but were asked to complete the same diet diaries, workbooks, and tests as the intervention group. Over a two-year period, all volunteers were exposed to the interventions. The outcomes focused on relapse prevention and maintenance of lifestyle changes. The tools used for the intervention included diet education videotapes, workbooks, food diaries, optional professional counseling, telephone hot lines, and regular weigh-ins (42). Despite a 57% attrition rate during the follow-up period, the program results showed that this intervention was efficacious in maintaining reductions in weight and control of glucose levels of overweight older adults for at least two years (43).

WEIGHT-LOSS OPTIONS FOR OLDER ADULTS

Weight-loss attempts in overweight and obese people are often frustrating, difficult to manage, and unsuccessful. Regardless of sound advice from nutrition professionals, every new diet becomes the faddish thing to try. Weight loss is a big business in the United States with a few, new, quick weight-loss regimens promoted every year. Although some of these fad diets lead to rapid weight loss, they may be based on poor science and may cause health problems over time. The greatest problem is recidivism—weight lost and regained—because a limited diet is unsustainable over long periods. Some of the weight-loss diets may lack essential nutrients and require dietary supplements to provide adequate micronutrients. It is interesting to note that ad-lib fat and protein diets may be hypocaloric due to early satiety associated with a high intake of protein and fat (12).

Quick weight-loss diets may be associated with a very limited dietary regimen that is hypocaloric and will lead to short-term and fast results. If eating patterns are not changed to a more nutritionally balanced diet that can be sustained for a long period without endangering nutritional health, a yo-yo effect occurs, that is, a cycle of rapid weight loss, then weight gain, followed by another rapid weight-loss diet with recurrent weight gain.

Low-carbohydrate weight-loss diets represent a popular trend that has spawned an entire line of food products. The effectiveness and long-term success rate of these diets need to be investigated, particularly in older adults. However, in retrospective data analyses, low-carbohydrate diets do not appear to be as efficacious as first promoted. One study by Kennedy et al. (44) showed that diets high in carbohydrates and low in fat tend to be lower in energy; however, the dietary quality was also higher. Individuals consuming a vegetarian or a high-carbohydrate diet had lower body mass indices than those on a low-carbohydrate diet, belying claims that low-carbohydrate diets are better for weight reduction or health maintenance. In one prospective research report, both young (18–24 years old) and elderly (67–86 years old) subjects receiving a short trial (21–28 days) of a high-carbohydrate, high-fiber diet demonstrated a 143% increase in glucose disposal (45). Longer studies are needed to demonstrate long-term efficacy.

A systematic review of low-carbohydrate diets including the Atkins diet, the South Beach diet, and others revealed that the weight loss that occurs is related to the duration of the diet and the level of energy intake and not the restriction of carbohydrates. When a carbohydrate-restricted diet is compared to a low-fat, calorie-restricted diet, the weight loss is greater for the low-carbohydrate diet after six months but there is no difference after 12 months of either diet (46). For short-term weight reduction, low-carbohydrate diets have been shown to be effective and loss of weight will have a beneficial impact on blood glucose control (47).

Not all of the consequences of low-carbohydrate diets are beneficial. Negative outcomes may include a decrease of total body calcium or a change in lipid profiles; there are reports that both support and discredit these concerns (47). Presently, recommendations by experts are to use low-carbohydrate diets for only short-term interventions (48).

One question as yet unanswered is how well tolerated these types of diets are in older adults. Although risk factors of coronary heart disease become more prevalent with advancing age, a diet high in fat and low in carbohydrates leaves older adults at a risk of deficiency because many important nutrients are left out. High dietary fat intake contributes to increases in body fat in older adults, which may counteract the potential positive effects of weight reduction. Elderly people may experience difficulty chewing meat products that are fibrous and may eliminate whole-grain baked goods, breads and cereals, and fresh vegetables and fruits, thereby limiting dietary fiber, which is important for the maintenance of gastrointestinal tract function.

IMPACT OF PHYSICAL ACTIVITY ON DIABETES MANAGEMENT

Most weight-loss programs should include physical activity as part of the treatment plan; a decrease in caloric intake will be enhanced by an increase in energy expended through exercise, even by simply increasing the number of steps walked in a day. Exercise may contribute to other health benefits such as maintaining bone density, muscle mass, and gastrointestinal function, and lowering fasting blood glucose levels.

Few studies have been conducted in older adults with diabetes but extrapolating the positive results of exercise and diet programs in middle-aged diabetic adults make it seem likely that there are also benefits in older adults (49). Of course, a physical evaluation of the older adult to determine the suitability of different types of exercise is a wise precaution.

ELDERLY PATIENTS WITH SPECIAL DIETARY NEEDS

Older adults commonly have concurrent medical conditions and are more likely to have episodes of acute illnesses, hospitalizations, or sick days. Managing blood glucose levels during these periods is very important and the older patient and caregiver must be provided instructions on how to meet nutritional needs during illness (3). The goal is to maintain tight blood glucose control below 140 mg/dL. This requires careful and close monitoring.

For diabetic patients who require enteral nutrition support, there are unique formulas that have been designed to contribute to the management of blood glucose levels (50,51). The most commonly used formulas have higher protein, slightly lower carbohydrate, and higher fat levels than do standard formulas. The fat tends to be from monounsaturated fatty acids, which have been associated with an improved lipid profile, better glycemic control, and lower insulin levels (3).

Acutely ill elderly diabetics may require parenteral nutritional support. Parenterally infused solutions are based on hypertonic glucose as the primary energy source. To assure control of blood sugar, adequate insulin can be mixed in with the solution or added via a piggy-back line, but the timing of the infusion should be closely managed to avoid either hypo- or hyperglycemia. For individuals requiring simple intravenous fluid support, glucose and insulin should be infused together.

DIETARY COMPLIANCE

Dietary management of diabetes in older adults may require many adjustments for the patient. For older diabetics, changes may need to be made in food choices and meal patterns. They also need to learn how to manage their medications to avoid episodes of hypo- or hyperglycemia. Modifying eating behavior in older adults may be rather difficult; changes in meal patterns and diet may require incorporating new foods, minimizing intake of less healthy choices, or altering familiar meal patterns. Older adults with impaired cognitive function may find that following a complicated diet is quite challenging; it is often difficult to manage meal patterns to coordinate with insulin regimens or count exchanges or carbohydrates. Individuals who have a cognitively intact and competent spouse may have more success managing dietary interventions (3). The older diabetic patient with dementia, unintended weight loss, or failure to thrive may enjoy a better quality of life with a liberalized diet even if blood glucose levels are allowed to be high (52).

A structured meal pattern based on the individual's lifestyle and meal habits, with alternative plans for holidays, travel, or illness, may be easier to manage. Trying to incorporate too many changes may be a recipe for disaster and noncompliance. It is difficult to change eating and meal habits in later life. Restricting intake of lifelong favorite foods or snacks may create resistance to making the necessary changes. It is generally recommended that incorporating change incrementally, allowing time to adjust to new foods or food patterns, will contribute to a higher rate of success in managing diabetic diets. A registered dietitian who has expertise in diabetes care can help by prioritizing the dietary alterations needed. Teaching the modifications with explanations of the reasons and potential benefits from the changes may contribute to successful management of blood glucose levels. Efforts to incorporate ethnic, cultural, or religious preferences are essential to assure dietary compliance.

SUMMARY

Health providers including physicians, nurses, and dietitians have a responsibility to develop a plan for dietary compliance that offers the greatest likelihood of achieving success. Diabetes management is complicated for most patients, but for older adults it may seem daunting. Incorporating medication regimens, dietary changes, and exercise plans may be overwhelming. Plans for treatment should be provided in writing and verbally to patients and primary caregivers as well as members of the extended support system, particularly adult children. Health providers should be readily available, either directly or through a surrogate.

REFERENCES

1. Morley JE. Endocrine aspects of nutrition and aging. In: Chernoff R, ed. Geriatric Nutrition: The Health Professional's Handbook. 3rd ed. Boston: Jones and Bartlett, 2006:345–364.
2. Elahi D, Muller DC. Carbohydrate metabolism in the elderly. Eur J Clin Nutr 2000; 54(suppl 3): S112–S120.
3. Stetson B, Mokshagundam SP. Nutrition and lifestyle change in older adults with diabetes mellitus. In: Bales CW, Ritchie CS, eds. Handbook of Clinical Nutrition and Aging. Totowa, NJ: Humana Press, 2003:487–516.
4. Edelstein SL, Knowler WC, Bain RP, et al. Predictors of progression from impaired glucose tolerance to NIDDM: an analysis of six prospective studies. Diabetes 1997; 46(4):701–710.
5. Ogden CL, Carroll MD, Flegal KM. Epidemiologic trends in overweight and obesity. Endocrinol Metab Clin N Am 2003; 32(4):741–760.
6. Smith GD, Bracha Y, Svendsen KH, et al. Incidence of type 2 diabetes in the randomized multiple risk factor intervention trial. Ann Intern Med 2005; 142:313–322.
7. Wing RR, Goldstein MG, Acton KJ, et al. Behavioral science research in diabetes: lifestyle changes related to obesity, eating behavior, and physical activity. Diabetes Care 2001; 24:1–2.

8. Ryan A. Insulin resistance with aging: effects of diet and exercise. Sports Med 2000; 30(5):327–346.

9. Elahi D, Muller DC, Tzankoff SP, Andres R, Tobin JD. Effect of age and obesity on fasting levels of glucose, insulin, glucagon, and growth hormone in man. J Gerontol 1982; 37(4):385–391.

10. Chernoff R. Nutrition and health promotion in older adults. J Gerontol: Biol Sci Med Sci 2001; 56A(suppl II):47–53.

11. American Diabetes Association. Evidence-based nutrition principles and recommendations for the treatment and prevention of diabetes and related complications. Diabetes Care 2002; 25:202–212.

12. Arora SK, McFarlane SI. The case for low carbohydrate diets in diabetes management. Nutr Metab 2005; 2:16–25.

13. Volek J, Sharman M, Gomez A, et al. Comparison of energy-restricted very low-carbohydrate and low-fat diets on weight loss and body composition in overweight men and women. Nutr Metab (London) 2004; 1:13.

14. Boden G, Sargrad K, Homko C, et al. Effect of low-carbohydrate diet on appetite, blood glucose levels, and insulin resistance in obese patients with type 2 diabetes. Ann Int Med 2005; 142:403–411.

15. Foster GD, Wyatt HR, Hill JO, et al. A randomized trial of a low-carbohydrate diet for obesity. N Engl J Med 2003; 348:2082–2090.

16. Nuttall FQ, Gannon MC. The metabolic response to a high-protein, low-carbohydrate diet in men with type 2 diabetes mellitus. Metabol Clin Experimental 2006; 55:243–251.

17. Franz MJ, Bantle JP, Beebe CA, et al. Evidence-based nutrition principles and recommendations for the treatment and prevention of diabetes and related complications. Diabetes Care 2002; 25:148–198.

18. Ryan-Harshman M, Aldoori W. New dietary reference intakes for macronutrients and fibre. Can Fam Physician 2006; 52(2):177–179.

19. Jenkins DJ, Kendall CW, Augustin LS, et al. Glycemic index: overview of implications in health and disease. Am J Clin Nutr 2002; 76(suppl 1):S266–S273.

20. Salmeron J, Manson JE, Stampfer MJ, et al. Dietary fiber, glycemic load, and risk of non–insulin-dependent diabetes mellitus in women. JAMA 1997; 277:472–477.

21. Salmeron J, Ascherio A, Rimm EB, et al. Dietary fiber, glycemic load, and risk of non-insulin-dependent diabetes mellitus in men. Diabetes Care 1997; 20:545–550.

22. Flicker L, Almeida OP, Acres J, et al. Predictors of impaired cognitive function in men over the age of 80 years: results from the Health in Men Study. Ageing 2005; 34(1):77–80.

23. Kiehn JM, Ghormley CO, Williams EB. Physician-assisted weight loss and maintenance in the elderly. Clin Geriatr Med 2005; 21:713–723.

24. Kennedy RL, Chokkalingham K, Srinivasan R. Obesity in the elderly: who should we be treating, and why, and how? Curr Opin Clin Nutr Metab Care 2004; 7(1):3–9.

25. Colman E, Katzel LI, Rogus E, et al. Weight loss reduces abdominal fat and improves insulin action in middle-aged and older men with impaired glucose tolerance. Metabolism 1995; 44:1502–1508.

26. Kelley DE, Wing R, Buonocore C, et al. Relative effects of calorie restriction and weight loss in noninsulin-dependent diabetes mellitus. J Clin Endocrinol Metabol 1993; 77:1287–1293.

27. Serdula MK, Kahn LK, Dietz WH. Weight loss counseling revisited. J Am Med Assoc 2003; 289(14):1747–1750.

28. Lowe MR, Miller-Kovach K, Frye N, et al. An initial evaluation of a commercial weight loss program: short-term effects on weight, eating behavior, and mood. Obes Res 1999; 7:51–59.

29. Miller W. How effective are traditional dietary and exercise interventions for weight loss? Med Sci Sports Exerc 1999; 31:1129–1134.

30. Kirchengast S, Knogler W, Hauser G. Protective effect of moderate overweight on bone density of the hip joint in elderly and old Austrians. Anthropol Auz 2002; 60(2):187–197.

31. Evans WJ. Exercise training guidelines for the elderly. Med Sci Sports Exerc 1999; 30:992–1008.

32. Chernoff R. Dietary management for older subjects with obesity. Clin Geriatr Med 2005; 21: 725–733.

33. Campbell WW, Carnell NS, Thalacker AE. Protein metabolism and requirements. In: Chernoff R, ed. Geriatric Nutrition: The Health Professional's Handbook. 3rd ed. Boston: Jones & Bartlett, 2006: 15–22.

34. Rosner S. Obesity in the elderly—a future matter of concern? Obes Res 2001; 2(3):183–188.

35. Suter P. Vitamin metabolism and requirements in the elderly: selected aspects. In: Chernoff R, ed. Geriatric Nutrition: The Health Professional's Handbook. 3rd ed. Boston: Jones & Bartlett, 2006: 31–76.

36. Bischoff-Ferrari HA, Willett WC, Giovannucci E, Dietrich T, Dawson-Hughes B. Estimation of optimal 25-hydroxyvitamin D levels for multiple health outcomes. Am J Clin Nutr 2006; 84:18–28.

37. Scarlett Y. Medical management of fecal incontinence. Gastroenterology 2004; 126:S56–S63.

38. Liese AD, Schulz M, Fang F, et al. Dietary glycemic index and glycemic load, carbohydrate and fiber intake, and measures of insulin sensitivity, secretion, and adiposity in the Insulin Resistance Atherosclerosis Study. Diabetes Care 2005; 28(12):2832–2838.

39. Madar Z, Thorene R. Dietary fiber. Prog Food Nutr Sci 1987; 11(2):153–174.

40. Chernoff R. Thirst and fluid requirements in the elderly. Nutr Revs 1994; 52:132–136.

41. Kleiner SM. Water: an essential but overlooked nutrient. Am Dietet Assoc 1999; 99(2):200–206.

42. Wylie-Rosett J, Swencionis C, Peters M, et al. A weight reduction intervention that optimizes use of practitioners' time, lowers glucose level, and raises high-density cholesterol level in older adults. J Am Dietet Assoc 1994; 94(1):37–42.
43. Dornelas EA, Wylie-Rosett J, Swencionis C. The DIET study: long-term outcomes of a cognitive-behavioral weight-control interventions in independent-living elders. Dietary intervention:evaluation technology. J Am Dietet Assoc 1998; 98(11):1276–1281.
44. Kennedy ET, Bowman SA, Spence JT, et al. Popular diets:correlation to health, nutrition, and obesity. J Am Dietet Assoc 2001; 101:411–420.
45. Fukagawa NK, Anderson JW, Hageman G, et al. High-carbohydrate, high-fiber diets increase peripheral insulin sensitivity in healthy young and old adults. Am J Clin Nutr 1990; 52:524–528.
46. Astrup A, Meinert-Larsen T, Harper A. Atkins and other low carbohydrate diets: hoax or an effective tool for weight loss? Lancet 2004; 364(9437):897–899.
47. Kennedy RL, Chokkalingam K, Farshchi HR. Nutrition in patients with type 2 diabetes: are low-carbohydrate diets effective, safe or desirable? Diabetes UK 2005; 22:821–832.
48. Astrup A, Kappagoda CT, Hyson DA, Amsterdam EA. Low-carbohydrate-high protein diets: is there a place for them in clinical cardiology? J Am Coll Cardiol 2004; 43:725–730.
49. Samaras K, Ashwell S, Mackintosh AM, et al. Will older sedentary people with non-insulin-dependent diabetes start exercising? A health promotion model. Diabetes Res Clin Pract 1997; 37: 121–128.
50. Wright J. Total parenteral and enteral nutrition in diabetics. Curr Opin Clin Nutr Metabol Care 2000; 3:5–10.
51. Pohl M, Mertl-Roetzer M, Lauster F, et al. Glycaemic control in type II diabetic tube-fed patients with a new enteral formula low in carbohydrates and high in monounsaturated fatty acids: a randomized controlled trial. Eur J Clin Nutr 2005; 59:1221–1232.
52. Position of the American Dietetic Association: liberalization of the diet prescription improves quality of life for older adults in long-term care. J Am Diet Assoc 2005; 105(12):1955–1965.

23 | Exercise in Older Adults with Diabetes

David W. Dunstan
Department of Epidemiology and Clinical Research, NOT Geriatric Research Education and Clinical Center, Melbourne, Victoria, Australia

Robin M. Daly
School of Exercise and Nutrition Sciences, Deakin University, Melbourne, Victoria, Australia

INTRODUCTION

Exercise is an integral component of diabetes management that also provides a range of additional health and psychosocial benefits that can reduce morbidity and mortality and improve the quality-of-life for adults with this condition. There is now a substantial body of scientific evidence, which indicates that regular physical activity and exercise training has a marked effect on a range of metabolic parameters in adults with type 2 diabetes. These include reducing blood glucose levels and various risk factors for cardiovascular disease (CVD) and improving insulin sensitivity. However, most of the evidence has come from studies in young and middle-aged adults; little is known about the impact of regular exercise for the management (or prevention) of diabetes in older adults and the elderly. This chapter will focus on the role of exercise for the management of diabetes in adults aged over 60 years. Because type 2 diabetes accounts for most of the diabetes cases in older adults, the content of this chapter will exclusively concern this type of diabetes. Current exercise prescription guidelines and recommendations, including the optimal type, frequency, duration, and intensity of exercise, the various contraindications and precautions to exercise, and strategies that may be used to maximize the potential benefits of exercise, will also be discussed. First however, we will briefly review the key physiological changes in body composition that occur with aging and the potential benefits of regular physical activity or exercise for nondiabetic older adults.

BODY COMPOSITION CHANGES ASSOCIATED WITH AGING

Aging is associated with a number of progressive physical and physiological changes that influence the functional status and disease risk of elderly men and women. One of the most striking consequences of aging is the involuntary loss in muscle mass, a condition commonly termed "sarcopenia," which contributes to muscle weakness (decreased muscle strength), loss of muscle power (a reduction in the force-producing capacity of muscle), and reduced muscular endurance (muscle fatigue). The importance of these changes to both health and functional capacity is highlighted by the increasing evidence that they have been linked with a number of metabolic, cardiovascular, and musculoskeletal disorders, in addition to the loss of functional independence and decreased mobility, all which can contribute to increased disability and even mortality in the elderly (1,2).

In both males and females, the age-related loss in muscle mass begins around the fourth decade of life (~30 years of age), with the greatest losses occurring after the age of 50 (3–5). Although there is marked interindividual variability in this loss due to differences in genetic, lifestyle, and disease-related factors, it has been reported that as much as 40% of muscle mass (or size) is lost from around the age of 20 up to 60 to 90 years (4,6–9). It has also been shown that men experience a greater loss than women (10), which may be related to gender differences in hormonal factors, and that there is a preferential loss in muscle mass in the lower extremities (4) due, at least partly, to the age-related reduction in physical activity. Cross-sectional studies also indicate that muscle strength peaks around the age of 30 but is maintained until about the age of 45 to 50 years (11–13). Thereafter, the rate of decline in healthy men and women is approximately 12% to 15% per decade (3,14), with even greater losses (up to 30% over 12 years) reported in some longitudinal studies (15) and the very old (16). The finding that there is a greater reduction in muscle strength compared to mass suggests that other intrinsic factors contribute to the reduction in the force-producing capacity of muscle. For instance, this may be related to reduced neural drive, loss of motor units, or a diminished muscle fiber contractile ability (17–19). Further details regarding the possible mechanisms underlying the age-related changes in muscle can be found in several recent reviews (3,11,18). Importantly however, the reduction in muscle mass or size with aging is due to similar losses in the number of type I (slow twitch) and type II (fast twitch) muscle fibers, but a selective reduction in the size of type II muscle fibers (5). This atrophy of type II muscle may account, at least partly, for the accelerated loss in muscle power with aging. For instance, it has been shown that muscle power declines earlier and more rapidly with age than muscle strength or endurance (20). This is important because most activities of daily living for older adults and the elderly, such as walking, rising from a chair, and climbing stairs, require power and not strength alone.

Accompanying the loss in muscle mass, strength, and power with aging is a decrease in basal metabolic rate and whole body fat oxidation (21), in addition to reduced energy expenditure and physical activity (22,23). These metabolic changes may help to explain the concurrent increase in body weight and fat mass with advancing age; even without a change in body weight, it appears that the amount of fat mass still increases with age (6). In both men and women, weight and fat mass increases progressively from around the age of 20 up until 60 to 65 years, with a gradual decline thereafter (3,24). However, perhaps more important are the changes in body fat distribution. Much of the age-related increase in fat mass is due to abdominal (visceral) fat accumulation, whereas subcutaneous fat in the arms and legs tends to decrease (25). This progressive increase in visceral and truncal fat has been strongly linked to an increased risk of CVD and type 2 diabetes (26,27). Recent data also indicate that there is an age-related increase in intramuscular fat, which is a marker of muscle lipid content (28). This increased fat infiltration within muscle has been shown to be associated with skeletal muscle insulin resistance independent of total or abdominal adiposity (29), and higher values have been observed in adults with type 2 diabetes (30). These findings indicate that the quality of muscle may also be an important determinant of disease risk in older adults.

In summary, aging is associated with a reduction in muscle mass that is accompanied by a decrease in muscle strength, power, and/or endurance, together with an increase in weight and fat mass, including a redistribution of adipose tissue and increased intramuscular fat. Although not reviewed within this chapter, there are also substantial reductions in bone mass; women experience accelerated bone loss during the perimenopausal years, and thereafter there is a gradual decline for both men and women into old age, which has been associated with an increased risk of fragility fractures. These changes in body composition can have serious repercussions on both health and function as they have been strongly linked to the development of chronic diseases such as type 2 diabetes, CVD, hypertension, stroke, dyslipidemia, osteoporosis, and (osteo)arthritis.

HEALTH AND PHYSIOLOGICAL BENEFITS OF EXERCISE FOR OLDER ADULTS AND THE ELDERLY

The importance of physical activity (or inactivity) and regular exercise for health was recognized by Booth et al. (22) who suggested that "... *with the possible exception of diet modification, we know of no single intervention with greater promise than physical exercise to reduce the risk of virtually all chronic diseases simultaneously.*" This statement reflects the large amount of research that has been devoted toward examining the role of physical activity for the management (and prevention) of common chronic diseases. In this section, we will briefly review some of the evidence relating to physical activity and its effects on the primary and secondary prevention of CVD and musculoskeletal disorders. This will also include a brief overview of some of the key physiological changes that occur with physical activity. The importance of exercise for the management of type 2 diabetes will be discussed in detail in subsequent sections.

Cardiovascular Disease

Several recent reviews examining large-scale, long-term prospective observational studies in both men and women have reported that increased levels of physical activity and fitness are associated with reduced mortality from any cause and from CVD (1,2,31). For instance, there is evidence that men who take up light or moderate physical activity (32) or those who maintain or increase physical fitness levels experience significantly reduced mortality (all-cause or CVD-related) (33,34). In middle-aged women followed up for 24 years, physical inactivity (less than one hour per week) was associated with a 52% increase in overall mortality, a doubling of mortality from CVD, and a 29% increase in mortality from cancer (35). There is also substantial evidence from both randomized controlled trial (RCTs) and meta-analyses to support the beneficial effects of exercise in patients with established CVD (36). A recent systematic review and meta-analysis of 48 trials reported that exercise-based cardiac rehabilitation programs reduced all-cause and CVD-related mortality by 20% and 26%, respectively (36).

Regular physical training can also lead to improvements in blood pressure and blood lipid and lipoprotein levels, particularly in those at increased risk due to elevated levels or in patients with coronary heart disease and insulin resistance (37,38). A recent meta-analysis of 72 trials reported that aerobic endurance training for an average of 40 minutes per session, three times per week at an intensity of 65% of maximum performance and lasting 16 weeks, reduced resting systolic and diastolic blood pressure by 3.0 and 2.4 mmHg in the normotensive group, with more pronounced reductions (6.9 and 4.9 mmHg) observed in the hypertensive group (39). Moderate-intensity progressive resistance training has also been reported to have favorable effects on blood pressure, particularly diastolic blood pressure (40). With regard to lipid changes, the available evidence indicates that moderate- to high-intensity aerobic exercise training (30 minutes per session, three to five times per week at 50–80% of maximum for more than 12 weeks) can improve high-density lipoprotein-cholesterol and decrease triglyceride and low-density lipoprotein-cholesterol (37). In those with CVD, other favorable changes associated with exercise training include a reduction in the symptoms of recurrent angina, less breathlessness associated with heart failure and stroke, and a reduction in the severity of claudication pain associated with walking in those with peripheral vascular disease (1,41).

There is also increasing evidence for an inverse, linear dose–response relationship between physical activity and rates of mortality (42,43). It has been reported that an average energy expenditure of about 1000 kcal per week, which is equivalent to engaging in about 30 minutes of moderate-intensity exercise most days of the week, is associated with a 20% to 30% reduction in all-cause mortality rates, with even higher volumes of training (2000 kcal per week) associated with reductions of 50% or more (42). While lower levels of physical activity (about half of what is currently recommended) may also elicit health benefits (42), it appears that the greatest benefits on all-cause mortality are related to moving from sedentary to moderate physical activity or fitness levels (2). Whether there is also a dose–response relationship between physical activity and other health outcomes remains uncertain. There are some data for a dose-related reduction in the risk as total physical activity and brisk walking increase in women (44). However, we must await the outcome of well-designed RCTs to define the minimal (or optimal) dose of exercise required to improve a range of CVD risk factors.

Musculoskeletal Disorders

Musculoskeletal disorders, including sarcopenia, osteoporosis and related fractures, and osteoarthritis, are responsible for significant functional limitations and morbidity in the elderly. For sarcopenia (low muscle mass), there is compelling evidence that physical training, particularly progressive resistance training, results in large improvements in muscle strength (100% or more) and a maintenance or increase (5–10%) in muscle mass or cross-sectional area in both older men and women (45,46) and the very old (47). Furthermore, resistance training can play an important role in weight control by increasing resting metabolic rate and energy requirements and decreasing both total body and visceral fat (48,49).

For the prevention and management of osteoporosis, a recent position statement by the American College of Sports Medicine reported that there is evidence from RCTs that progressive resistance training and regular weight-bearing exercise (e.g., brisk walking, jogging, stair climbing, and/or jumping activities) alone or in combination results in modest increments (1–4%) in bone mineral density (BMD) or an attenuation of bone loss in healthy and at-risk (e.g., those with low BMD) older adults (50). There is also substantial evidence that these modes of exercise are accompanied by large improvements in gait velocity, balance, flexibility, and mobility, which can contribute to improved functional capacity and a reduction in the risk of falls (50,51). However, the evidence for the effectiveness of exercise on fracture risk is less convincing because there have been no large RCT. Despite this, several large longitudinal observational studies have reported that higher levels of physical activity protected against hip and vertebral fractures in both men and women (52,53). There is evidence that older adults with type 2 diabetes mellitus have a higher risk of fracture compared with nondiabetic adults, despite increased BMD (54,55). The paradoxical increase in the risk of fracture may be the result of increased rate of falls among patients with diabetes (56). Whether exercise can prevent fractures in older adults with diabetes is not known, but there is some evidence that resistance training can prevent the loss in BMD and muscle mass associated with weight loss in previously sedentary, overweight adults with type 2 diabetes (57).

EXERCISE FOR THE TREATMENT OF TYPE 2 DIABETES

Extensive epidemiological and experimental evidence supports the importance of regular physical activity and exercise training for the management of type 2 diabetes. In addition to the health benefits described in the previous section, exercise can be an effective tool to achieve and maintain near-normal blood glucose levels and optimal lipid levels, thereby preventing or delaying the development of microvascular, macrovascular, and neural complications (58). In particular, exercise is one of the principal therapies used to acutely lower blood glucose levels, since repeated muscle contractions during exercise can lead to significant improvements in glucose metabolism, which can persist postexercise.

Effects of Acute Exercise on Glucose Metabolism

The metabolic effects of acute exercise on glucose metabolism have recently been reviewed in detail by Sigal et al. (58). Briefly, these changes relate to enhanced insulin-independent and insulin-sensitive muscle glucose uptake through various mechanisms such as increased delivery of glucose from the blood to the muscle, increased transport of glucose across the muscle membrane, and increased phosphorylation of glucose in the muscle. Evidence also exists to suggest that exercise leads to several adaptations within muscle and liver tissue leading to enhanced glucoregulation that persists after the cessation of exercise, primarily through the replenishment of fuel stores, including muscle and liver glycogen (58). However, the benefits of a single bout of exercise on glucose metabolism are short-lived, lasting for approximately 24 to 72 hours, depending on the duration and intensity of the activity (59). Hence, while it is widely accepted that more frequent physical activity (or exercise training) can enhance glucose uptake in muscle through improved insulin sensitivity, this has largely been attributed to a carryover effect of the last exercise session, rather than a long-term training effect (60). Consequently, to achieve sustained glucose-lowering effects and improved insulin sensitivity, it is well accepted that regular exercise should be promoted in adults with type 2 diabetes.

Exercise Training in Adults with Type 2 Diabetes

Numerous trials have been undertaken to evaluate the long-term effects of regular exercise training on metabolic parameters in adults with type 2 diabetes, but the findings have not been consistent. This has been attributed to a number of factors including differences in the mode of training used (e.g., aerobic, resistance, or a combination) or whether dietary intervention (e.g., weight loss) was also part of the intervention (61). Furthermore, many studies involved small sample sizes or utilized poor study designs, including the lack of a control group or non-randomization of participants to treatment groups.

A meta-analysis published in 2001 examined the effect of at least eight weeks of exercise training on glycemic control [hemoglobin A1c (HbA_{1c})] in adults with type 2 diabetes (61). The meta-analysis included 14 (11 randomized, 3 nonrandomized) controlled trials encompassing a total of 504 participants. The mean (SD) of the participants in these studies was 55.0 (7.2) years (range: 39.5–69.4 years), duration of diabetes was 4.3 (4.6) years, and 50% of participants were women. Twelve of the trials examined the effect of aerobic training (typically consisting of walking or cycling at a moderate intensity), while two studies examined the effects of resistance training (consisting of 2–3 sets ranging from 10–20 repetitions). No differences could be identified between the effect of aerobic and resistance training. There was also no dose–response effect on glycemic control in relation to the intensity or duration of training. However, even in the absence of weight loss, when the postintervention results were pooled, HbA_{1c} was significantly lower in the exercise compared to control groups [7.6% vs. 8.3%; weighted mean difference (WMD), –0.66%; $P < 0.001$]. The reduction in HbA_{1c} was similar to that observed following intensive glycemic control with metformin in the United Kingdom Prospective Diabetes Study (UKPDS) (62). In this study, a 0.9% reduction in HbA_{1c} was sufficient to reduce the risk of diabetes-related complications by 32% and diabetes-related mortality by 42% (62).

A separate meta-analysis undertaken by Boule et al. (63) has examined the effects of exercise training on cardiorespiratory fitness from a total of 266 adults with type 2 diabetes (mean age: 55.7 years). Low cardiorespiratory fitness has been shown to be a powerful and independent predictor of mortality in adults with diabetes (64). This meta-analysis included 266 adults with type 2 diabetes from studies that had assessed the effects of at least eight weeks of aerobic training. On average, the training consisted of 3.4 sessions per week at an intensity of 50% to 75% of maximum oxygen uptake (VO_{2max}) for 49 minutes per session for 20 weeks. Overall, they reported a clinically significant 11.8% increase in VO_{2max} in the exercising groups compared with a 1% decrease in control groups. Interestingly, exercise intensity was found to be more important than exercise volume in predicting the postintervention WMD in HbA_{1c}.

There has been no published meta-analysis of the effects of exercise training on lipids or blood pressure in adults with type 2 diabetes. However, as we have described earlier, evidence from meta-analyses undertaken in adults without diabetes indicates that exercise training can have favorable effects on both lipids and blood pressure.

Exercise Training Studies in Older People with Type 2 Diabetes

The majority of studies included in both of the meta-analyses by Boule et al. (61,63) have involved younger and middle-aged adults. Hence, it is uncertain to what extent these findings can be generalized to older adults and the elderly. We have identified 12 published trials in the literature that have assessed the effects of fully or partly supervised exercise training in older adults with type 2 diabetes (as reflected by the mean age in the exercise intervention group being ≥60 years) (65–76). Two of these trials did not use a RCT study design and therefore were not included in our review (66,72). The 10 remaining studies presented in Tables 1 and 2 involved small sample sizes and were restricted to "younger" older adults (i.e., 60–69 years). Furthermore, some studies specifically focused on aerobic training, while others assessed resistance training or the combination of resistance and aerobic training.

Aerobic Training Studies

We identified five studies that have assessed the effects of aerobic exercise training in older adults with type 2 diabetes (Table 1). The intervention duration in all these studies was for six months or less and typically focused on moderate-intensity walking programs undertaken three days per week. Significant improvements in cardiovascular fitness (VO_{2max}) were observed in two of these trials (73,76), and in one study this improvement was sustained through nonsupervised training at home (73). The effects on glycemic control (HbA_{1c}) however were inconsistent; some studies observed an improvement in HbA_{1c} (65,71), while others did not detect any beneficial changes in various glycemic parameters (73,74,76). Improved lipid profiles and blood pressure were also observed in some (73,76), but not all of these trials. In general, the largest reductions in HbA_{1c}, lipids, and blood pressure were observed in those trials which included a specific dietary intervention that led to weight loss (65,71).

Resistance Training Studies

The efficacy of resistance training on glycemic control in older adults with type 2 diabetes has been assessed in three RCTs (Table 2) (67,68,70). In these studies, the duration of the intervention ranged from four months to two years, with training undertaken two to three days per week. Two of these studies reported the effects of high-intensity progressive

TABLE 1 Summary of Randomized Controlled Trials Involving Aerobic Exercise Training in Older Adults with Type 2 Diabetes

Ref.	*n*	Age and gender	Duration	Training program	Glycemic control	Fitness	Lipids	BP
Verity et al. (76)	10	E: 61±4; C: 57±4; Women	4 mo	Walking; moderate intensity (65–80% of predicted cardiac reserve); 60–90 min, 3 times/wk	NC	↑ VO$_{2max}$	↑ HDL-C, Chol/HDL-C ratio	N/A
Ligtenberg et al. (73)	58	E: 63±5; C: 61±5; Men and women	3 phases; 1st: 6 wk	Bicycle ergometer, swimming, treadmill, rowing; moderate (60–80% VO$_{2max}$); 50 min, 3 times/wk	NC	↑ VO$_{2max}$	↓ TG, VLDL-TG, ApoB	N/A
			2nd: 6 wk	Home-based	NC	NC	↓ Chol	N/A
			3rd: 14 wk	Home-based	NC	↑ VO$_{2max}$	NC	N/A
Agurs-Collins et al. (65)	64	E: 62±6; C: 61±6; Men and women	6 mo	Treadmill, stationary cycling, rowing machine; low-impact activity; 20 min, 1 time/wk supervised, 2 times/wk home-based	↓ HbA$_{1c}$	N/A	NC	↓ diastolic BP
Samaras et al. (74)	26	E: 61±8; C: 61±2; Men and women	6 mo (6 mo follow-up)	Low-moderate intensity (up to 50% VO$_{2max}$) activity; duration not reported, 1 time/mo	NC	N/A	NC	N/A
Goldhaber-Fiebert et al. (71)	75	E: 60±10; C: 57±9; Men and women	3 mo	Walking; moderate intensity (brisk); 60 min, 3 times/wk	↓ HbA$_{1c}$, ↓ glucose	N/A	NC	NC

Note: Only significant changes relative to controls (i.e., between group difference) are reported; Age is mean ± SD.
Abbreviations: ↑, increase; ↓, decrease; E, exercise group; C, control group; VO$_{2max}$, maximum oxygen uptake; chol, total cholesterol; HDL-C, high-density lipoprotein-cholesterol; VLDL, very low-density lipoprotein; ApoB, apolipoprotein B; HbA$_{1c}$, glycated hemoglobin; BP, blood pressure; N/A, not assessed or not reported; NC, no changes.

resistance training (three sets of 8–12 repetitions at 70% to 85% of maximum strength) (68,70), whereas the third utilized a low-moderate intensity program (three sets of 8–12 repetitions at 50–70% of maximum strength) (67). Not surprising, all of these studies showed large improvements (30–43%) in muscle strength following training, and some provided evidence that these benefits can be maintained through lower-intensity home-based training (77). Most importantly, supervised progressive resistance training was found to result in marked improvements in HbA$_{1c}$ levels (68,70), but, unlike muscle strength, these changes did not appear to be sustained following a similar period of home-based resistance training (77). These beneficial effects on glycemic control may be related to the associated increases or maintenance of muscle mass (68,70), or possibly intrinsic changes in the muscle (78) resulting from resistance training. Other reported benefits of resistance training in older adults with type 2 diabetes include improvements in physical function and mobility and reduced systolic

TABLE 2 Summary of Randomized, Controlled Trials Involving Resistance or Combined Resistance/Aerobic Training in Older Adults with Type 2 Diabetes

Ref.	n	Age	Duration	Type of intervention	Glycemic control	Fitness	Lipids	BP
Dunstan et al. (70,77)	36	E: 68±5; C: 67±5; Men and women	6 mo (+6 mo home-based)	High-intensity (75–85% of 1RM), 3 times/wk 3 sets of 8–10 repetitions (home-based 3 times/wk)	↓ HbA$_{1c}$ No changes after 12 mo	↑ muscle strength (after 6 and 12 mo)	NC	NC
Castaneda et al. (68)	62	E: 66±2; C: 66±1; Men and women	4 mo	High-intensity (70–80% of 1RM), 3 times/wk; 3 sets of 8 repetitions	↓ HbA$_{1c}$	↑ muscle strength	NC	↓ systolic BP
Brandon et al. (67)	31	E: 66±8; C: 66±7; Men and women	2 yr	Moderate-intensity (50–70% of 1RM), 0–6 mo: 3 days/wk; 6–24 mo 2–3 times/wk); 3 sets of 8–12 repetitions	N/A	↑ muscle strength, downstairs mobility	N/A	N/A
Tessier et al. (75)	39	E: 69±4; C: 70±4; Men and women	4 mo	Moderate-intensity (brisk) walking (20 min)+resistance exercise (20 min—2 sets of 20 repetitions); 3 times/wk	NC	↑ time on treadmill	N/A	N/A
Cuff et al. (69)	28	AE+RT: 63±2; AE: 59±2; C: 60±3; Women	4 mo	AE+RT—Total time 75 min: moderate (60–75% of heart-rate reserve) treadmill, bicycle, stepper, rowing exercise+moderate resistance training (2 sets of 12 repetitions); AE: 75 min (as above); 3 times/wk	AE+RT vs. C: ↑ glucose disposal; no changes in HbA$_{1c}$	NC	NC	N/A

Note: Only significant changes relative to controls (i.e., between group difference) are reported; Age is mean ± SD. ↑, increase; ↓, decrease.

Abbreviations: AUC, area under the curve; AE, aerobic exercise; BP, blood pressure; C, control group; E, exercise group; HbA$_{1c}$, glycated hemoglobin; NC, no changes; N/A, not assessed or not reported; RM, repetition maximum; RT, resistance exercise; VO$_{2max}$, maximum oxygen uptake.

blood pressure (68). No changes in lipid profiles have been observed following resistance training in older adults with type 2 diabetes.

Combination Training

Two studies utilized training protocols involving a combination of aerobic and resistance training in older adults with type 2 diabetes (Table 2) (69,75). In both of these trials, participants completed three sessions per week for four months, with the total time split between moderate-intensity aerobic exercise (walking/stationary cycling/stepper/rowing machine) and moderate-intensity resistance training (two sets of between 12–20 repetitions). The study by Cuff et al. (69) made direct comparisons between combined training, aerobic training alone, and a usual care control group. In that study, cardiorespiratory fitness improved similarly in the combined and aerobic training groups, and muscle strength improved in the combination group only (69). However, HbA$_{1c}$ levels did not change in any of the groups, which may be attributable to the short follow-up periods. Nevertheless, in the study by Cuff et al. (69), improved insulin sensitivity (increased glucose disposal) was observed in the combination group (but not the aerobic-only group) relative to the control group (69). Neither of these studies reported the effects of combined training on lipids or blood pressure. To determine whether aerobic, resistance, or the combination of both is more effective for improving metabolic and body composition parameters, additional intervention studies with four groups (aerobic, resistance, combination, and control group), longer durations, and larger sample sizes are needed.

In conclusion, exercise training for the treatment of type 2 diabetes in the older adult is difficult to assess because the published data are from studies that utilized small sample sizes and short-term training periods (less than six months). Furthermore, there is no published data that pertain directly and specifically to elderly or very old people with type 2 diabetes. Despite these limitations, the available evidence suggests that in older adults with type 2 diabetes, regular aerobic and/or progressive supervised resistance training can lead to clinically important improvements in glycemic control and insulin sensitivity that could reduce the risk of microvascular and macrovascular diabetes complications.

EXERCISE RECOMMENDATIONS

In the past decade, there has been increased interest in defining the optimal mode, frequency, volume, and intensity of exercise for improving glycemic control and other related risk factors in adults with type 2 diabetes (58,79,80). In 2006, the American Diabetes Association (ADA) published a consensus statement containing revised exercise recommendations for people with type 2 diabetes (81) based on an earlier technical review of the evidence available in the literature (58). These recommendations are consistent with earlier recommendations published by the American College of Sports Medicine (ACSM) (79). A summary of the current exercise recommendations is provided below.

Frequency

The current physical activity guidelines for the general population recommend that adults accumulate 30 minutes or more of moderate-intensity activity (defined as that which will cause a slight, but noticeable, increase in breathing and heart rate) on most, ideally all, days of the week (82). While most adults with type 2 diabetes should be encouraged to follow these guidelines, the ADA recommend that exercise should be distributed over at least three days per week, with no more than two consecutive days without exercise (81). The rationale for this recommendation is based on data derived from several successful RCTs, which have typically included a training frequency of three sessions per week. Most of the benefits of a single bout of exercise are lost within 24 to 72 hours (59). Furthermore, the recommendation that adults with type 2 diabetes exercise at least three days per week is based on the assumption that many people may find it easier to schedule fewer longer sessions rather than five or more weekly shorter sessions (81).

Type and Amount of Exercise

Both the ADA (81) and the ACSM (79) recommend that a well-rounded exercise program for people with type 2 diabetes should incorporate both aerobic and resistance exercise. This reflects the increasing evidence from rigorous RCTs that a range of specific health benefits can be derived from both types of exercise.

Aerobic Exercise

For aerobic exercise (e.g., walking, jogging, cycling) to elicit improvements in glycemic control and body composition and reduce the risk of CVD-related complications, it is recommended that adults with type 2 diabetes engage in at least 150 minutes per week of moderate-intensity aerobic exercise (40–60% of VO_{2max} or 50–70% of maximum heart rate) and/or at least 90 minutes per week of vigorous aerobic exercise (>60% of VO_{2max} or >70% of maximum heart rate) if accustomed to this level of activity (81). Furthermore, for CVD risk reduction, performing moderate to vigorous aerobic and/or resistance exercise for four hours or more per week is more effective than lower exercise volumes (81). If long-term maintenance of major weight loss is desired, at least seven hours per week of moderate or vigorous aerobic exercise is recommended, if it can be tolerated (81).

Resistance Exercise

As already highlighted, there is compelling scientific evidence that moderate- to high-intensity progressive resistance training is a safe and effective training modality for adults (including older adults) with type 2 diabetes. The ADA recommends that in the absence of any contraindications, adults with type 2 diabetes should be encouraged to perform resistance exercise three times a week, targeting all major muscle groups, and progressing to three sets of 8 to 10 repetitions at a weight that cannot be lifted more than 8 to 10 times (81). Previously, concerns have been raised about the safety of high-intensity progressive resistance exercise in older adults with or at risk of diabetes, hypertension, and CVD because of issues related to the acute rises in blood pressure associated with lifting heavy weights. The risks include provoking a stroke, myocardial ischemia, or retinal hemorrhage (58). However, in the recent technical review by Sigal et al. (58), there was no evidence that resistance training actually increased these risks. Furthermore, there are currently no data for any serious adverse events associated with high-intensity progressive resistance training in older adults with type 2 diabetes (68,70).

In both of the studies involving high-intensity resistance training in older adults with type 2 diabetes, the training was progressive in nature [i.e., the resistance (or workload) was gradually increased over time] (68,70). Each session was supervised by an exercise specialist and included a five-minute warm-up and cool-down period consisting of light aerobic activity (e.g., cycling) with and without flexibility exercises, and 35 to 45 minutes of resistance training (five to nine exercises involving all the major muscle groups) using a combination of free and machine weights. Furthermore, the training initially (first two to eight weeks) commenced at a low- to moderate-intensity (40–60% of maximum strength) and focused largely on correct lifting technique, after which the training was progressively increased to higher intensities (70–80% of maximum). If warranted (e.g., for the obese, previously sedentary individuals, or the elderly), a more conservative approach could be to begin with one set of 10 to 15 repetitions two to three times per week at moderate intensity (50–75% of maximum) for several weeks, progressing to two sets of 10 to 15 repetitions two to three times per week, and then three sets of 8 to 10 repetitions at a weight that cannot be lifted more than 8 to 10 times with correct technique (58). In all situations, continual education on appropriate training techniques should be provided, with particular emphasis on avoiding sustained isometric contractions, and breath-holding and Valsalva maneuvers (58).

EXERCISE CONSIDERATIONS
Contraindications

When prescribing exercise for older adults with type 2 diabetes, consideration must also be given to certain risks associated with exercise. Before increasing usual patterns of physical activity or embarking on a new exercise program, individuals with diabetes should undergo a medical examination to carefully assess the potential risks versus benefits (58,81,83). It is generally recommended that before beginning a program of physical activity more vigorous than brisk walking, adults with diabetes should be assessed for conditions that are associated with CVD or might contraindicate certain types of exercise or predispose to injury (81). These conditions include severe autonomic neuropathy, severe peripheral neuropathy, and preproliferative or proliferative retinopathy. A detailed description of what should be included in the pre-exercise medical evaluation is well documented (83). This includes review of medical history, physical examination, assessment of orthopedic problems and the presence of diabetes complications, exercise history, medication use, and glycemic control.

Additionally, to assist practitioners in determining suitability to exercise, guidelines have been developed to identify health conditions, which may be contraindications to exercise participation (Table 3) (83,84). For certain individuals, the risks of exercise participation can outweigh the potential benefits. In general, individuals with absolute contraindications should not commence a new exercise program until such conditions are stabilized or adequately

TABLE 3 Contraindications to Exercise Participation

Absolute	Relative
A recent change in the resting ECG suggesting significant ischemia, recent myocardial infarction (within 2 days), or other acute cardiac event	Fasting blood glucose > 16.7 mmol/L (300 mg/dL) or >13.9 mmol/L (>250 mg/dL) with urinary ketone bodies present
Unstable angina	Uncontrolled severe arterial hypertension (i.e., systolic BP of >200 mmHg and/or a diastolic BP of >110 mmHg) at rest
Uncontrolled cardiac dysrhythmias causing symptoms or hemodynamic compromise	Severe autonomic neuropathy with exertional hypotension
Symptomatic severe aortic stenosis	Left main coronary stenosis
Uncontrolled symptomatic heart failure	Moderate stenotic valvular heart disease
Suspected or known dissecting aneurysm	Hypertrophic cardiomyopathy and other forms of outflow tract obstruction
Acute myocarditis or pericarditis	Tachyarrhythmia or bradydysrhythmia
Acute thrombophlebitis or intracardiac thrombi	High-degree atrioventricular block
Acute pulmonary embolus or pulmonary function	Ventricular aneurysm
Untreated high-risk proliferative retinopathy	Electrolyte abnormalities (hypokalemia, hypomagnesemia)
Recent significant retinal hemorrhage	Uncontrolled metabolic disease (e.g., thyrotoxicosis and myxedema)
Acute or inadequately controlled renal failure	Chronic infectious diseases (e.g., mononucleosis, hepatitis, and AIDS)
Acute systemic infection, accompanied by fever, body aches, or swollen lymph glands	Neuromuscular, musculoskeletal, or rheumatoid disorders that are exacerbated by exercise
	Mental or physical impairment leading to inability to exercise adequately
	Complicated pregnancy

Abbreviations: BP, blood pressure; ECG, electrocardiogram.
Source: From Ref. 83.

treated (83). For individuals with relative contraindications, careful evaluation of the risk-to-benefit ratio is necessary to ascertain suitability to participate (83,84). Following such an evaluation, adaptations to the exercise prescription (e.g., commencing at a lower exercise intensity) may be required to allow individuals to exercise, but with caution.

Whether stress testing should be performed prior to beginning an exercise program in adults with diabetes has been debated extensively (58,80,83,84). The current view is that there is no evidence that such testing is routinely necessary for those planning moderate-intensity aerobic activity such as walking, but it should be considered for previously sedentary individuals at moderate- to high-risk of CVD who want to undertake vigorous aerobic exercise exceeding the demands of everyday living (81). For those planning to undertake resistance training, there is little or no evidence as to whether stress testing is necessary and given that typical stress testing protocols are based on aerobic exercise, the relevance of such tests for resistance exercise is questionable (81).

Precautions

In general, for most people with type 2 diabetes, the risks associated with not exercising are greater than those associated with exercising. However, additional precautions are warranted when dealing with older adults with type 2 diabetes. Detailed description of these are available in the literature (58,79,80), but we provide a brief summary of the key considerations and subsequent exercise recommendations below.

Hyperglycemia

The current ADA guidelines recommend that vigorous exercise be avoided in the presence of ketosis; however, in the absence of very severe insulin deficiency, light- or moderate-intensity exercise may have beneficial effects on glucose levels. Assuming that the individual is well-hydrated and the urine and/or blood ketones are negative, exercise can be recommended even in the presence of hyperglycemia (81).

Hypoglycemia

While the likelihood of hypoglycemia is rare in those who are not treated with insulin or insulin secretagogues, caution is warranted in those who are taking these medications since exercise may lead to hypoglycemia if medication dose or carbohydrate consumption is not altered (58,85). It is recommended that for individuals on insulin and/or insulin secretagogues, additional carbohydrate should be ingested if pre-exercise glucose levels are less than 5.6 mmol/L (100 mg/dL) (81). Additionally, capillary blood glucose should be checked before, after, and several hours after exercise, at least initially, to develop an understanding of the usual glycemic response to specific exercise regimens. The most recent guidelines conclude that supplementary carbohydrate is generally not necessary for individuals treated only with diet, metformin, α-glucosidase inhibitors, and/or thiazolidinediones without insulin or insulin secretagogues (81).

Medications

It is not uncommon for individuals with type 2 diabetes to take multiple medications in addition to oral hypoglycemic agents or insulin. Those taking concomitant medications who engage in exercise training, particularly those with chronic complications, should be aware that many commonly used medications may cause significant alterations in the metabolic, cardiovascular, and hemodynamic responses to exercise, sometimes affecting exercise performance (85). The more commonly used medications that need to be considered for adults with type 2 diabetes include diuretics, β-adrenergic blockers, calcium-channel blockers, angiotensin-converting enzyme inhibitors, glucocorticoids, lipid-lowering agents, salicylates, and nonsteroidal analgesics (85). High doses of diuretic agents may induce hyperglycemia through multiple mechanisms, including decreased insulin secretion and impaired insulin sensitivity (85). Diuretics can also interfere with fluid and electrolyte balance. β-adrenergic blockers may decrease exercise capacity, lower peak heart rate and blood pressure, and can blunt the adrenergic symptoms of hypoglycemia, possibly increasing risk of hypoglycemia unawareness (58,85). Some people with angina or coronary artery disease may experience better exercise capacity because of the relief of symptoms. ACE inhibitors have been shown to improve insulin sensitivity, and both ACE inhibitors and high doses of aspirin (4–6 g/day) may increase risk of hypoglycemia through unclear mechanisms (58,85). Glucocorticoids, in supraphysiological and pharmacological doses, cause insulin resistance and compensatory hyperinsulinemia in non-diabetic individuals or in subjects with impaired glucose tolerance (85). Progressive worsening of pre-existing hyperglycemia via multiple effects on liver, adipose tissue, and muscle can occur with progressive increases in the dosage of glucocorticoids. In rare cases, myositis may arise with use of statins, especially in combination with fibrates (58). Nonsteroidal anti-inflammatory drugs have the potential of causing renal injury and inducing hyperkalemia in older patients with type 2 diabetes or those with underlying renal disease (85).

Retinopathy

Participation in vigorous aerobic or resistance exercise (e.g., heavy lifting and straining or high-impact aerobics), which may lead to increases in systolic blood pressure or intraocular pressure, may be contraindicated in those with proliferative or severe nonproliferative diabetic retinopathy because of the risk of triggering vitreous hemorrhage or retinal detachment (81). For these individuals, it is recommended that they participate in moderate, low-impact aerobic (e.g., walking, cycling, or water activities) or resistance activities or moderate leisure activities that do not require excessive lifting or placing the head below waist level.

Peripheral Neuropathy

The most common activities, which are contraindicated for adults with peripheral neuropathy due to risk of foot/limb injury, are weight-bearing, high-impact activities, including jogging or running, step exercise, and jumping (58). Thus, non–weight-bearing activities such as resistance training (seated), swimming, bicycling, and arm or chair exercises may be more appropriate in the presence of severe peripheral neuropathy. It is also important that these individuals regularly check their feet after each exercise bout to reduce the risk of foot injury.

Autonomic Neuropathy

Autonomic neuropathy can lead to a number of important physiological changes that must be considered before prescribing exercise, including decreasing cardiac responsiveness to exercise, postural hypotension, altered thermoregulation due to impaired skin blood flow and sweating, and impaired thirst leading to an increased risk of dehydration (81). Currently it is recommended that individuals with diabetic autonomic neuropathy who plan to increase their exercise levels or undertake intensive exercise should first undergo cardiac investigation (81).

Microalbuminuria and Nephropathy

In general, there may be no need for any specific exercise restrictions for adults with diabetic kidney disease (81). In fact, there is some evidence that aerobic and progressive resistance training may have beneficial effects on those with renal disease (86). However, due to the risk of silent cardiac ischemia, an exercise stress test is recommended in previously sedentary individuals with microalbuminuria and proteinuria who are planning to begin a more intensive exercise program that is greater than the demands of everyday living (81).

THE CHALLENGES OF PROMOTING AND MAINTAINING EXERCISE

Despite the reported benefits of physical activity and exercise training for the management of type 2 diabetes, motivating individuals to commence and then maintain regular physical activity remains an important and challenging issue for many health-care professionals. The poor long-term adherence and marked attrition in many studies, including structured exercise programs (67,73,74,77), may be due in part to the failure of many of these studies to utilize known theories of behavior modification, which have proven to be effective in the adoption and maintenance of physical activity (87). Although there is no universal consensus about the most effective way to promote and maintain physical activity, a large body of research supports the use of the transtheoretical model of behavioral change (88). This model postulates that each individual is at a different cognitive stage in their readiness to adopt and maintain a particular behavior (i.e., exercise), which ranges from precontemplation and contemplation to preparation, action, and maintenance (88). The model includes three mediators of behavior change: (*i*) self-efficacy: confidence in the ability to change; (*ii*) decisional balance: understanding the pros and cons of change; and (*iii*) processes of change: strategies and techniques used to change, such as social support. Recent studies in older adults without diabetes have consistently demonstrated that matching an intervention to an individual's level of motivational readiness (transtheoretical model) is a more effective approach for increasing and maintaining physical activity levels than a one-treatment-fits-all approach in which all individuals receive the same intervention regardless of their motivation to change their activity levels (89,90).

Recently, physical activity counselling interventions based on the transtheoretical model using stage-tailored strategies and techniques have been shown to be effective for promoting and maintaining physical activity levels in adults with type 2 diabetes (91,92). In addition to improved physical activity levels, these studies have also observed long-term (one to two years) improvements in HbA$_{1c}$ and systolic blood pressure in those who received counselling compared to a usual care control group. Another study used pedometers as a self-monitoring and feedback tool and reported improvements in physical activity participation (as reflected by the number of steps taken per day), but did not observe any changes in glycemic control, lipids, or blood pressure after the four-month intervention (93).

Notwithstanding the promising findings from trials using physical activity counseling, most of the success from clinical trials in older adults with type 2 diabetes has been observed in structured group or center-based settings. Adherence rates typically decrease once the structured, supervised context is removed (77). Therefore, when prescribing exercise, consideration must be given to the potential interaction between each individual's characteristics and the exercise setting. For instance, some individuals may prefer to exercise in a structured setting (e.g., fitness center), which could include social interaction (e.g., exercising with a partner), while others may prefer a less formal and less-exposed setting (e.g., a park). Other potential approaches that may be considered include telephone-supervised home-based programs or programs that combine both a group-based program and a home-based program; or gradually sequenced programs designed to encourage independence with periodical refresher sessions (90).

SUMMARY

For decades, exercise has been considered a cornerstone of diabetes management, because it can lower blood glucose concentrations and make the contracting muscles more sensitive to insulin. It can also impart favorable effects on many of the physiological and body compositional changes that accompany advancing age and has a positive influence on reducing the risk of many other chronic diseases.

The limited evidence available from studies conducted in older persons with type 2 diabetes indicates that exercise training interventions involving aerobic and/or progressive resistance exercise, at least in the short-term (≤6 months), can lead to a number of favorable health benefits such as improved glycemic control, increased cardiorespiratory fitness, increased muscle strength, maintenance of muscle mass, decreased fat mass (including visceral fat), and improved lipid profiles and blood pressure, even in the absence of weight loss.

In the absence of contraindications, older adults with type 2 diabetes should be encouraged to undertake both aerobic and resistance exercise. Specifically, the frequency should be at least three times per week, encompassing at least 150 min/wk of moderate-intensity aerobic exercise (40–60% of VO_2max or 50–70% of maximum heart rate) and/or resistance exercise three times a week, including all major muscle groups, progressing to three sets of 8 to 10 repetitions at a weight that cannot be lifted more than 8 to 10 times.

Before increasing usual patterns of physical activity or embarking on a new exercise program more vigorous than brisk walking, older adults with type 2 diabetes should undergo a medical examination to identify conditions that might contraindicate certain types of exercise or where the risks of exercise may outweigh the benefits.

Approaches based on known theories of behavior modification strategies such as the transtheoretical model may be helpful in enhancing the adoption and maintenance of regular physical activity.

REFERENCES

1. Pedersen BK, Saltin B. Evidence for prescribing exercise as therapy in chronic disease. Scand J Med Sci Sports 2006; 16 (suppl 1):3–63.
2. Warburton DE, Nicol CW, Bredin SS. Health benefits of physical activity: the evidence. CMAJ 2006; 174(6):801–809.
3. Doherty TJ. Invited review: aging and sarcopenia. J Appl Physiol 2003; 95(4):1717–1727.
4. Janssen I, Heymsfield SB, Wang ZM, et al. Skeletal muscle mass and distribution in 468 men and women aged 18–88 yr. J Appl Physiol 2000; 89(1):81–88.
5. Lexell J, Taylor CC, Sjostrom M. What is the cause of the aging atrophy? Total number, size and proportion of different fiber types studied in whole vastus lateralis muscle from 15- to 83-year-old men. J Neurol Sci 1988; 84(2–3):275–294.
6. Gallagher D, Ruts E, Visser M, et al. Weight stability masks sarcopenia in elderly men and women. Am J Physiol Endocrinol Metab 2000; 279(2):E366–E375.
7. Porter MM, Vandervoort AA, Lexell J. Aging of human muscle: structure, function and adaptability. Scand J Med Sci Sports 1995; 5(3):129–142.
8. Young A, Stokes M, Crowe M. Size and strength of the quadriceps muscles of old and young women. Eur J Clin Invest 1984; 14(4):282–287.
9. Young A, Stokes M, Crowe M. The size and strength of the quadriceps muscles of old and young men. Clin Physiol 1985; 5(2):145–154.
10. Gallagher D, Visser M, De Meersman RE, et al. Appendicular skeletal muscle mass: effects of age, gender, and ethnicity. J Appl Physiol 1997; 83(1):229–239.
11. Deschenes MR. Effects of aging on muscle fibre type and size. Sports Med 2004; 34(12):809–824.
12. Larsson L, Grimby G, Karlsson J. Muscle strength and speed of movement in relation to age and muscle morphology. J Appl Physiol 1979; 46(3):451–456.
13. Lindle RS, Metter EJ, Lynch NA, et al. Age and gender comparisons of muscle strength in 654 women and men aged 20–93 yr. J Appl Physiol 1997; 83(5):1581–1587.
14. Hughes VA, Frontera WR, Wood M, et al. Longitudinal muscle strength changes in older adults: influence of muscle mass, physical activity, and health. J Gerontol A Biol Sci Med Sci 2001; 56(5): B209–B217.

15. Frontera WR, Hughes VA, Fielding RA, et al. Aging of skeletal muscle: a 12-yr longitudinal study. J Appl Physiol 2000; 88(4):1321–1326.
16. Murray MP, Duthie EH Jr, Gambert SR, et al. Age-related differences in knee muscle strength in normal women. J Gerontol 1985; 40(3):275–280.
17. Doherty TJ, Brown WF. The estimated numbers and relative sizes of thenar motor units as selected by multiple point stimulation in young and older adults. Muscle Nerve 1993; 16(4):355–366.
18. Kamel HK. Sarcopenia and aging. Nutr Rev 2003; 61(5 Pt 1):157–167.
19. Larsson L, Li X, Frontera WR. Effects of aging on shortening velocity and myosin isoform composition in single human skeletal muscle cells. Am J Physiol 1997; 272(2 Pt 1):C638–C649.
20. Metter EJ, Conwit R, Tobin J, et al. Age-associated loss of power and strength in the upper extremities in women and men. J Gerontol A Biol Sci Med Sci 1997; 52(5):B267–B276.
21. Poehlman ET, Toth MJ, Fonong T. Exercise, substrate utilization and energy requirements in the elderly. Int J Obes Relat Metab Disord 1995; 19(suppl 4):S93–S96.
22. Booth FW, Gordon SE, Carlson CJ, et al. Waging war on modern chronic diseases: primary prevention through exercise biology. J Appl Physiol 2000; 88(2):774–787.
23. Klausen B, Toubro S, Astrup A. Age and sex effects on energy expenditure. Am J Clin Nutr 1997; 65(4):895–907.
24. Hughes VA, Frontera WR, Roubenoff R, et al. Longitudinal changes in body composition in older men and women: role of body weight change and physical activity. Am J Clin Nutr 2002; 76(2):473–481.
25. Kotani K, Tokunaga K, Fujioka S, et al. Sexual dimorphism of age-related changes in whole-body fat distribution in the obese. Int J Obes Relat Metab Disord 1994; 18(4):207–202.
26. Hernandez-Ono A, Monter-Carreola G, Zamora-Gonzalez J, et al. Association of visceral fat with coronary risk factors in a population-based sample of postmenopausal women. Int J Obes Relat Metab Disord 2002; 26(1):33–39.
27. Pi-Sunyer FX. The epidemiology of central fat distribution in relation to disease. Nutr Rev 2004; 62(7 Pt 2):S120–S126.
28. Goodpaster BH, Carlson CL, Visser M, et al. Attenuation of skeletal muscle and strength in the elderly: the Health ABC Study. J Appl Physiol 2001; 90(6):2157–2165.
29. Goodpaster BH, Thaete FL, Simoneau JA, et al. Subcutaneous abdominal fat and thigh muscle composition predict insulin sensitivity independently of visceral fat. Diabetes 1997; 46(10):1579–1585.
30. Goodpaster BH, Thaete FL, Kelley DE. Thigh adipose tissue distribution is associated with insulin resistance in obesity and in type 2 diabetes mellitus. Am J Clin Nutr 2000; 71(4):885–892.
31. Kesaniemi YK, Danforth E Jr, Jensen MD, et al. Dose-response issues concerning physical activity and health: an evidence-based symposium. Med Sci Sports Exerc 2001; 33(suppl 6):S351–S358.
32. Wannamethee SG, Shaper AG, Walker M. Changes in physical activity, mortality, and incidence of coronary heart disease in older men. Lancet 1998; 351(9116):1603–1608.
33. Blair SN, Kohl HW III, Barlow CE, et al. Changes in physical fitness and all-cause mortality. A prospective study of healthy and unhealthy men. JAMA 1995; 273(14):1093–1098.
34. Myers J, Kaykha A, George S, et al. Fitness versus physical activity patterns in predicting mortality in men. Am J Med 2004; 117(12):912–918.
35. Hu FB, Willett WC, Li T, et al. Adiposity as compared with physical activity in predicting mortality among women. N Engl J Med 2004; 351(26):2694–2703.
36. Taylor RS, Brown A, Ebrahim S, et al. Exercise–based rehabilitation for patients with coronary heart disease: systematic review and meta-analysis of randomized controlled trials. Am J Med 2004; 116(10):682–692.
37. Leon AS, Sanchez OA. Response of blood lipids to exercise training alone or combined with dietary intervention. Med Sci Sports Exerc 2001; 33:S502–S520.
38. Pescatello LS, Franklin BA, Fagard R, et al. American College of Sports Medicine position stand. Exercise and hypertension. Med Sci Sports Exerc 2004; 36(3):533–553.
39. Cornelissen VA, Fagard RH. Effects of endurance training on blood pressure, blood pressure-regulating mechanisms, and cardiovascular risk factors. Hypertension 2005; 46(4):667–675.
40. Cornelissen VA, Fagard RH. Effect of resistance training on resting blood pressure: a meta-analysis of randomized controlled trials. J Hypertens 2005; 23(2):251–259.
41. Briffa TG, Maiorana A, Sheerin NJ, et al. Physical activity for people with cardiovascular disease: recommendations of the National Heart Foundation of Australia. Med J Aust 2006; 184(2):71–75.
42. Lee IM, Skerrett PJ. Physical activity and all-cause mortality: what is the dose-response relation? Med Sci Sports Exerc 2001; 33(suppl 6):S459–S471; discussion S493–S454.
43. Oguma Y, Shinoda-Tagawa T. Physical activity decreases cardiovascular disease risk in women: review and meta-analysis. Am J Prev Med 2004; 26(5):407–418.
44. Hu FB, Stampfer MJ, Colditz GA, et al. Physical activity and risk of stroke in women. JAMA 2000; 283(22):2961–2967.
45. Charette SL, McEvoy L, Pyka G, et al. Muscle hypertrophy response to resistance training in older women. J Appl Physiol 1991; 70(5):1912–1916.
46. Frontera WR, Meredith CN, O'Reilly KP, et al. Strength conditioning in older men: skeletal muscle hypertrophy and improved function. J Appl Physiol 1988; 64(3):1038–1044.

47. Fiatarone MA, O'Neill EF, Ryan ND, et al. Exercise training and nutritional supplementation for physical frailty in very elderly people. N Engl J Med 1994; 330(25):1769–1775.

48. Campbell WW, Crim MC, Young VR, et al. Increased energy requirements and changes in body composition with resistance training in older adults. Am Soc Clin Nutr 1994; 60:167–175.

49. Treuth MS, Hunter GR, Kekes-Szabo T, et al. Reduction in intra-abdominal adipose tissue after strength training in older women. J Appl Physiol 1995; 78(4):1425–1431.

50. Kohrt WM, Bloomfield SA, Little KD, et al. American College of Sports Medicine Position Stand: physical activity and bone health. Med Sci Sports Exerc 2004; 36(11):1985–1996.

51. Gregg EW, Pereira MA, Caspersen CJ. Physical activity, falls, and fractures among older adults: a review of the epidemiologic evidence. J Am Geriatr Soc 2000; 48(8):883–893.

52. Gregg EW, Cauley JA, Seeley DG, et al. Physical activity and osteoporotic fracture risk in older women. Study of Osteoporotic Fractures Research Group. Ann Intern Med 1998; 129(2):81–88.

53. Paganini-Hill A, Chao A, Ross RK, et al. Exercise and other factors in the prevention of hip fracture: the Leisure World study. Epidemiology 1991; 2(1):16–25.

54. Schwartz AV, Sellmeyer DE, Ensrud KE, et al. Older women with diabetes have an increased risk of fracture: a prospective study. J Clin Endocrinol Metab 2001; 86(1):32–38.

55. Strotmeyer ES, Cauley JA, Schwartz AV, et al. Nontraumatic fracture risk with diabetes mellitus and impaired fasting glucose in older white and black adults: the health, aging, and body composition study. Arch Intern Med 2005; 165(14):1612–1617.

56. Schwartz AV, Hillier TA, Sellmeyer DE, et al. Older women with diabetes have a higher risk of falls: a prospective study. Diabetes Care 2002; 25(10):1749–1754.

57. Daly RM, Dunstan DW, Owen N, et al. Does high-intensity resistance training maintain bone mass during moderate weight loss in older overweight adults with type 2 diabetes? Osteoporos Int 2005; 16(12):1703–1712.

58. Sigal RJ, Kenny GP, Wasserman DH, et al. Physical activity/exercise and type 2 diabetes. Diabetes Care 2004; 27(10):2518–2539.

59. Schneider SH, Amorosa LF, Khachadurian AK, et al. Studies on the mechanism of improved glucose control during regular exercise in Type 2 (Non-Insulin-Dependent) Diabetes. Diabetologia 1984; 26:355–360.

60. Ivy J. Role of exercise training in the prevention and treatment of insulin resistance and non-insulin-dependent diabetes mellitus. Sports Med 1997; 24:321–336.

61. Boule NG, Haddad E, Kenny GP, et al. Effects of exercise on glycemic control and body mass in type 2 diabetes mellitus. A meta–analysis of controlled clinical trials. JAMA 2001; 286:1218–1227.

62. Stratton IM, Adler AI, Neil HA, et al. Association of glycaemia with macrovascular and microvascular complications of type 2 diabetes (UKPDS 35): prospective observational study. Br Med J 2000; 321(7258):405–412.

63. Boule NG, Kenny GP, Haddad E, et al. Meta-analysis of the effect of structured exercise training on cardiorespiratory fitness in Type 2 diabetes mellitus. Diabetologia 2003; 46(8):1071–1081.

64. Wei M, Gibbons LW, Kampert JB, et al. Low cardiorespiratory fitness and physical inactivity as predictors of mortality in men with type 2 diabetes. Ann Intern Med 2000; 132(8):605–611.

65. Agurs-Collins TD, Humanyika SK, Ten Have TR, et al. A randomized controlled trial of weight reduction and exercise for diabetes management in older African-American subjects. Diabetes Care 1997; 20:1503–1511.

66. Balducci S, Leonetti F, Di Mario U, et al. Is a long-term aerobic plus resistance training program feasible for and effective on metabolic profiles in type 2 diabetic patients? Diabetes Care 2004; 27(3):841–842.

67. Brandon LJ, Gaasch DA, Boyette LW, et al. Effects of long-term resistive training on mobility and strength in older adults with diabetes. J Gerontol A Biol Sci Med Sci 2003; 58(8):740–745.

68. Castaneda C, Layne JE, Munoz-Orians L, et al. A randomized controlled trial of resistance exercise training to improve glycemic control in older adults with type 2 diabetes. Diabetes Care 2002; 25(12):2335–2341.

69. Cuff DJ, Meneilly GS, Martin A, et al. Effective exercise modality to reduce insulin resistance in women with type 2 diabetes. Diabetes Care 2003; 26(11):2977–2982.

70. Dunstan DW, Daly RM, Owen N, et al. High-intensity resistance training improves glycemic control in older patients with type 2 diabetes. Diabetes Care 2002; 25(10):1729–1736.

71. Goldhaber-Fiebert JD, Goldhaber-Fiebert SN, Tristan ML, et al. Randomized controlled community-based nutrition and exercise intervention improves glycemia and cardiovascular risk factors in type 2 diabetic patients in rural Costa Rica. Diabetes Care 2003; 26(1):24–29.

72. Honkola A, Forsen T, Eriksson J. Resistance training improves the metabolic profile in individuals with type 2 diabetes. Acta Diabetol 1997; 34:245–248.

73. Ligtenberg PC, Hoekstra JB, Bol E, et al. Effects of physical training on metabolic control in elderly type 2 diabetes mellitus patients. Clin Sci Lond 1997; 93(2):127–135.

74. Samaras K, Ashwell S, Mackintosh AM, et al. Will older sedentary people with non-insulin-dependent diabetes mellitus start exercising? A health promotion model. Diabetes Res Clin Pract 1997; 37:121–128.

75. Tessier D, Menard J, Fulop T, et al. Effects of aerobic physical exercise in the elderly with type 2 diabetes mellitus. Arch Gerontol Geriatr 2000; 31:121–132.

76. Verity LS, Ismail AH. Effects of exercise on cardiovascular disease risk in women with NIDDM. Diabetes Res Clin Pract 1989; 6:27–35.
77. Dunstan DW, Daly RM, Owen N, et al. Home-based resistance training is not sufficient to maintain improved glycemic control following supervised training in older individuals with type 2 diabetes. Diabetes Care 2005; 28(1):3–9.
78. Holten MK, Zacho M, Gaster M, et al. Strength training increases insulin-mediated glucose uptake, GLUT4 content, and insulin signaling in skeletal muscle in patients with type 2 diabetes. Diabetes 2004; 53(2):294–305.
79. Albright A, Franz M, Hornsby G, et al. American College of Sports Medicine position stand. Exercise and type 2 diabetes. Med Sci Sports Exerc 2000; 32(7):1345–1360.
80. Zinman B, Ruderman N, Campaigne BN, et al. Physical activity/exercise and diabetes. Diabetes Care 2004; 27(suppl 1):S58–S62.
81. Sigal RJ, Kenny GP, Wasserman DH, et al. Physical activity/exercise and type 2 diabetes: a consensus statement from the American Diabetes Association. Diabetes Care 2006; 29(6):1433–1438.
82. U.S. Department of Health and Human Services. Physical activity and health: A report of the Surgeon General. Atlanta, GA: U.S. Department of Health and Human Services, Centers for Disease Control and Prevention, National Center for Chronic Disease Prevention and Health Promotion, 1996.
83. Gordon NF. The exercise prescription. In: Ruderman N, Devlin JT, Schneider SH, Kriska A, eds. Handbook of Exercise in Diabetes. 2nd ed. Alexandria, Virginia: American Diabetes Association, 2002:269–288.
84. Whaley MH, Brubaker PH, Otto RM. ACSM's Guidelines for Exercise Testing and Prescription. 7th ed. Baltimore, Maryland: Lippincott, Williams & Wilkins, 2006.
85. Ganda O. Patients on various drug therapies. In: Ruderman N, Devlin JT, Schneider SH, Kriska A, eds. Handbook of Exercise in Diabetes. 2nd ed. Alexandria, Virginia: American Diabetes Association, 2002:587–599.
86. Castaneda C, Gordon PL, Uhlin KL, et al. Resistance training to counteract the catabolism of a low-protein diet in patients with chronic renal insufficiency. A randomized, controlled trial. Ann Intern Med 2001; 135(11):965–976.
87. Clark DO. Physical activity efficacy and effectiveness among older adults and minorities. Diabetes Care 1997; 20(7):1176–1182.
88. Prochaska JO, Marcus BH. The transtheoretical model: Applications to exercise. In: Dishman RK, ed. Advances in Exercise Adherence. Illinois: Human Kinetics, 1994:161–180.
89. King AC. Interventions to promote physical activity by older adults. J Gerontol A Biol Sci Med Sci 2001; 56(spec no. 2):36–46.
90. King AC, Rejeski WJ, Buchner DM. Physical activity interventions targeting older adults. A critical review and recommendations. Am J Prev Med 1998; 15(4):316–333.
91. Di Loreto C, Fanelli C, Lucidi P, et al. Validation of a counseling strategy to promote the adoption and the maintenance of physical activity by type 2 diabetic subjects. Diabetes Care 2003; 26(2):404–408.
92. Kirk A, Mutrie N, MacIntyre P, et al. Effects of a 12-month physical activity counselling intervention on glycaemic control and on the status of cardiovascular risk factors in people with Type 2 diabetes. Diabetologia 2004; 47(5):821–832.
93. Tudor-Locke C, Bell RC, Myers AM, et al. Controlled outcome evaluation of the First Step Program: a daily physical activity intervention for individuals with type II diabetes. Int J Obes Relat Metab Disord 2004; 28(1):113–119.

24 | Diabetes Education in Older Adults

Lilya Sitnikov
Section of Behavioral and Mental Health Research, Joslin Diabetes Center, Boston, Massachusetts, U.S.A.

Katie Weinger
Section of Behavioral and Mental Health Research, Joslin Diabetes Center and Department of Psychiatry, Harvard Medical School, Boston, Massachusetts, U.S.A.

INTRODUCTION

Diabetes presents many serious challenges to older adults; challenges that affect the persons with diabetes, their family, and the course of the disease. The science of diabetes education for the elderly is underdeveloped as little research has investigated social, emotional, physical, cognitive, and other factors associated with aging and their impact on the delivery of education and on the benefits that the elderly receive from diabetes education. In this chapter, we first discuss components of the diabetes education plan for older adults. We then review various factors that impact how older individuals and families learn to manage diabetes. Finally we describe how diabetes interventions may be individualized for older people.

DIABETES EDUCATION FOR OLDER PERSONS WITH DIABETES

In general, the diabetes education plan includes (*i*) a comprehensive assessment of the individual's knowledge, skills, attitudes, beliefs, and psychosocial and physical status; (*ii*) assisting persons with diabetes and their family to develop and prioritize self-care goals; (*iii*) formulating a plan based on the assessment that is individualized, proactive, and designed to maximize the person's and family's ability to manage diabetes; and (*iv*) a complete evaluation that includes reassessment and revision of the plan based on the reassessment.

Assessment

Older adults with diabetes are heterogeneous with respect to their social, psychological, clinical, and functional status and the type and duration of diabetes. For older adults with diabetes, the risk for developing complications secondary to diabetes increases with age (1,2); however, many of these patients remain highly functional, leading active and productive lives.

A comprehensive assessment necessary for the development of a diabetes education plan for older patients includes assessment of functional and cognitive status as well as physical and psychosocial factors such as health beliefs, attitudes, and family support (Table 1). The developmental phase of aging differs from that of other age groups in that physical and cognitive abilities decrease over time rather than improve, and the development of comorbidities and complications is common. Thus, frequent thorough assessment is very important for older people. Further, the American Geriatric Society and the California Healthcare Foundation panel (6) on improving care for elders with diabetes recommends that assessment of older adults incorporate screening and management of six areas that are typically more common in older adults with diabetes than in those without diabetes: polypharmacy, cognitive impairment, depression, falls, urinary incontinence, and pain.

The process of educational assessment of older adults with diabetes is not substantially different from that of middle-aged patients with diabetes, except that greater emphasize is placed on understanding the effects of the aging process in general as well as in the context of diabetes. Moreover, because the health status of older patients can deteriorate rapidly, assessment is an ongoing process that, when appropriate, includes family members, caregivers, and other health-care providers. To help older adults assimilate diabetes care into their lifestyle and,

TABLE 1 Important Assessment Areas for Older Adults with Diabetes

Area	Comments
Cognitive status	Assess for cognitive impairment
	Standardized screening instruments such as the Mini Mental state examination and/or the clock drawing test are useful
	Reassess cognitive status if increased difficulty with self-care tasks is noted
Learning	Assess understanding of key points using open-ended questions: "How will you use your glucose monitoring results to adjust your insulin?" "What will you do differently with your meal plan?"
	Ask the patient to demonstrate previously reviewed skills
Family and social support	Assess the relationship with family. Is it antagonistic or supportive?
	Assess who the person lives with, how much support the person wants, and how much support the person receives
	Assess social networks and community groups
	Assess utilization of community resources: meals on wheels, visiting nurses, etc.
Depression	Note if the older adult is tearful, sad, or angry
	Ask two validated questions, "During the past month, have you been bothered by feeling down, depressed or hopeless?" and "During the past month, have you been bothered by little interest or pleasure in doing things?"
	Administer the geriatric depression scale
	Refer to a mental health professional who understands diabetes
Stress	Diabetes-related distress and other common psychosocial issues in diabetes can be assessed with items from the problem areas in diabetes[a]
	Identify any life events that are perceived by the individual as stressors: deaths, loss of job, divorce, etc.
Attitudes toward diabetes and self-care tasks	How important are self-care tasks to older patients? What level of importance does the person apply to diabetes self-care?
	Assess, which domains of diabetes self-care are most important to the older adult with diabetes (e.g., diet, exercise, and medications)
	Prioritize and individualize educational goals and identify perceived barriers to diabetes self-care
Literacy	Assesses whether the person can read and in what language(s)
	Some may try to conceal their low reading ability and difficulty with comprehension by becoming defensive, claiming the light is not good, or that they forgot their reading glasses
	The short test of functional health literacy[b] is useful for assessing health literacy
	Literacy is not necessarily equated with the level of intelligence
Current knowledge/ behavior	Does the patient understand diabetes and self-care recommendations and prescriptions?
	Assess what the patient currently does: the rationale for and frequency of doing self-care behaviors is important
	Assess patients mastery of diabetes management skills (e.g., checking blood glucose levels, preparing and administering insulin dose, and taking medications)
Physical status	Assess for any hearing or vision impairments
	Multiple diabetes-related comorbidities and other chronic conditions may limit patient's capability for self-care, including activities of daily living, exercise, and ability to attend medical appointments
	Assess patient's exercise preferences and any relevant physical limitations
	Consider cardiac clearance before recommending an intensive exercise program

[a]From Refs. 3, 4.
[b]From Ref. 5.

when necessary, adapt their lifestyle to follow therapeutic recommendations, assessment focuses on identifying current psychosocial and physical status, support systems, and barriers to self-care. The ultimate purpose of assessment is to understand patients' needs, preferences, and beliefs in order to tailor the educational intervention and maximize its impact.

Assessment is also a critical first step in the process of empowerment. Patient empowerment posits that patients have the knowledge, personal control, and experience to set and implement their own goals and priorities (7–9). Older adults often experience physiological and psychosocial changes, related and unrelated to diabetes, that may restrict their independence and threaten their sense of self-efficacy and personal control (10). Encouraging older patients with diabetes to express their preferences during initial assessment and formulate treatment goals may help increase older patients' feelings of independence and competency, which are associated with increased adherence to healthcare behavior recommendations and improved metabolic control (11,12).

Self-Management Goal Setting

Goal setting goes beyond identifying patient preferences. Goal setting allows the person with diabetes to have a voice in the management of diabetes. Diabetes self-management by its nature must be integrated into one's life. Once the person with diabetes has a basic understanding of what is required to manage diabetes, setting diabetes self-management goals helps that person to cope with diabetes self-care to the best of his or her ability at that particular time and to maintain control over self-care. However, some older adults may have cognitive impairment associated with diabetes (13–16), have unrelated degenerative dementia such as Alzheimer's disease, or show the minimal cognitive decline associated with the normal aging process (17,18). Consequently, setting mutual educational goals and individualizing the educational plan must take into account the multifaceted assessment aimed at identifying patients' abilities, needs, preferences, and potential barriers to learning and to self-care. The role of the educator is to help guide the person with diabetes in setting goals that are specific, realistic, and measurable; these goals serve to provide structure to the process of learning about and maximizing diabetes self-care.

Intervention

The ideal education program for elderly persons with diabetes includes a multidisciplinary team that works together to coordinate care. Team members include the physician, nurse, nutritionist, and psychosocial counselor, and if possible an exercise physiologist. Communication among the team, support services, and other health-care providers such as podiatrist, cardiologist, or neurologist is extremely important to provide consistent educational and medical approaches for the patient and family (19).

Interventions for older adults use the same principles of adult learning that apply to younger adults. Content areas that should be included in an educational plan for any person with diabetes are summarized in Table 2. Two important components of following therapeutic recommendations are actually knowing what the advice or therapeutic recommendations are and understanding how to implement that advice. Many patients do not recall therapeutic recommendations given during an appointment (20–22). Kravitz et al. (23) found that 96% of patients with diabetes recalled being prescribed medications, although only 91% of those reported taking medications; 80% recalled nutrition recommendations and 69% of those followed the recommendations; 74%, 77%, and 56% recalled receiving advice on exercise, avoidance of tobacco, and regularly checking feet while only 19%, 8%, and 64% of those recalling the advice, respectively, adhered to it. However, utilizing strategies that maximize patients' ability to remember advice received during a medical/educational visit (20) can help facilitate patients' knowledge and diabetes self-care management (Table 3). Moreover, many older adults believe that their symptoms can be managed outside of the medical care system by utilizing over-the-counter medications, dietary home remedies, and lay consultations from family and friends (24). Thus, educating older patients about the potential danger of medicine misuse as well as correcting any misconceptions about the efficacy of lay treatment strategies for diabetes is

TABLE 2   Summary of Key Content Areas for Educational Plan for the Elderly

Glucose monitoring and pattern management
Medications
Physical activity
Meal planning/nutrition
Preventing and detecting acute and chronic complications
Coping with diabetes
Problem-solving skills
Maximizing quality of life and social support
How to prepare for a medical education appointment

TABLE 3 Reinforcing Diabetes Educational and Medical Advice

Primacy—things presented first are remembered better
Perceived importance—more important advice is remembered better
Simplicity—simple advice is remembered better than complex advice
Repetition—repeated advice is remembered better
Specific—specific advice is remembered better than general advice
Those with more medical knowledge remember advice better

important. Similarly, patients' education should include a discussion of safety issues (e.g., preventing lows and minimizing the risk for injuries).

Educational strategies and interventions aimed at older adults with diabetes must take into account the often deteriorating physical, social, and cognitive status of this population. Successful strategies include providing structured learning, reinforcement, and assessment of understanding. Materials should use large print, be clearly written, and directly relevant to person. Orienting older adults to the health-care system, helping them understand when to call, and how to prepare for a medical appointment are important issues that diabetes education can address. Education sessions may need to be shorter with smaller amounts of information given at each visit so that patients do not feel overwhelmed. For some elderly patients, important information such as that regarding recognition and treatment of hypoglycemia may need to be repeated frequently, often at every clinic visit.

Family support for the person with diabetes is important. Older adults achieve better glycemic control, greater increase in diabetes-related knowledge, and greater adherence to treatment recommendations when family members and peers participate in diabetes education (25,26). Making diabetes education directly relevant to the learner is even more important for the elderly than for younger age groups. Older adults typically want to learn about the impact of diabetes on them and their families rather than general information that is not directly related to them.

An important issue is whether elderly persons can benefit from group diabetes education. Group education serves two main functions: (*i*) to provide an efficient and successful forum for the provision of and reinforcement of diabetes self-management, and (*ii*) to provide a social outlet that serves to normalize living with diabetes (27). Group education must be engaging and interactive. In a systematic review, Sarkisian et al. found that successful self-care interventions for older individuals with diabetes included group counseling or support, although the mean age was 70 years or younger in all of the studies (28). Whether these findings apply to individuals over 80 years is not clear. A nonrandomized observation study found that individuals over 80 years of age who participated in group education did only as well as those who were not eligible for group education because of cognitive dysfunction of problems following treatment recommendations in terms of improvement in glycemic control and the frequency of glucose monitoring (29). However, the authors did not discuss if family or other caregivers were providing care to either group. More research is needed to identify characteristics of older individuals who are most likely to succeed in group education. Status of cognitive function especially executive function (the ability to plan, organize, and integrate new information into behavior) is likely to impact how much the elderly benefit from group education.

Evaluation

Assessment of learning and of self-care skills is important whether the person attends group or individual education. Having the person with diabetes (or the caregiver) summarize the key points particularly stating, which specific behaviors or activities will be done at home is an effective way to assess understanding. Having the person demonstrate specific skills such as drawing-up insulin is important to assess the ability to deliver the correct dose. Providing written information about specific self-care tasks that need to be done at home is also helpful.

Follow-up assessment allows the educator to determine if the person and/or the caregiver is/are able to carry out self-care at home and to assess barriers to self-care. For example, if the individual lives in an assisted living or nursing home facility, they may not have control over meals. The educator may need to contact the facility to clarify the person's self-care and nutritional requirements. The education plan, and, in some cases, the treatment plan may need to be adjusted based on the follow-up assessment.

FACTORS ASSOCIATED WITH DIABETES EDUCATION IN THE OLDER ADULTS

Several aspects of daily life influence how individuals with diabetes learn about and manage their diabetes. Within each area are factors that serve as barriers to learning or to self-management and other factors that support the older person's ability to perform diabetes self-care behaviors.

Cognitive Status

As individuals with diabetes age, they are at an increased risk of decline in memory, learning, psychomotor speed, and executive functioning (15,30). The prevalence of cognitive impairment is greater in older adults with diabetes than in healthy older adults without diabetes (13,30–34). Recent studies suggest that longer duration of diabetes and biomedical complications such as retinopathy are associated with cognitive dysfunction (14,15,35).

Although the capacity to learn new information remains throughout life, cognitive deficits often seen in older adults with diabetes may affect the ability to process and retain information and to integrate self-care behaviors into their lifestyles. One study found that older adults with diabetes with a low score on Minimental State Examination (MMSE), which assesses, among other things, attention and calculation, recall, language, and visual construction were significantly less likely to engage in diabetes self-care or attend a specialist diabetes clinic. They were also significantly more likely to have been hospitalized in the previous year and to require help with self-care (36). Moreover, changes in learning and memory skills associated with normal aging as well as degenerative dementia may interact with diabetes-related cognitive changes to manifest a greater level of cognitive impairment.

Older adults with diabetes can be assessed for cognitive impairments with standardized screening instruments such as the MMSE (37,38) and the Clock Drawing Test (36,39). These relatively short and easy to administer cognitive assessments can detect overt cognitive dysfunction in older adults with diabetes. Frequent reassessment of cognitive status is important, especially if increased difficulty with self-care tasks or significant decline in health status occurs.

As individuals age, memory and executive functioning may diminish. Executive function is the ability to engage in independent, purposive behavior (40). Executive function includes skills that are necessary to establish and implement diabetes self-care behaviors such as the ability to identify a need and have a future vision: plan, organize, and implement. Subtle changes in executive function, particularly in planning capabilities, may be enough to interfere with one's ability to institute and maintain the complex problem-solving skills required for diabetes self-care (41).

Preliminary studies have demonstrated that gross disruption in cognitive and executive function in the elderly interferes with diabetes self-care (36) and emerging evidence suggests that more subtle effects may also impair glycemic control (42). In addition to including caregivers and family members in education sessions, using structured education approaches with clear, simple instructions and recommendations can help older adults understand their self-care better. Moreover, providing simple written instructions that repeat the verbal information is important. More work needs to be done in examining the impact of subtle changes in executive function on the ability to learn and implement diabetes self-care behaviors and in developing sensitive and easily interpreted assessment tools for cognitive and executive function in the elderly with diabetes.

Literacy and Health Literacy

Literacy and health literacy impacts how people learn and how people manage their diabetes. Clinicians must assess if the person and/or family members can read and in what languages. Health literacy is the degree to which individuals have the capacity to read, comprehend, and implement basic health-related information such as instructions on prescription bottles and educational brochures (6). The prevalence of inadequate health literacy is high among older adults; many older adults struggle to read and comprehend even the simplest health-related materials (43,44). Recent studies suggest that older adults with low health literacy and chronic illnesses have less knowledge of their disease and its treatment, fewer correct self-management skills, and higher medical costs (45–48). To further patients' knowledge and understanding of their self-care recommendations, health-care providers and educators often rely on written instructions and educational materials, placing patients with low health literacy at considerable disadvantage. Tailoring educational materials to the literacy level of the person and family is important. Those with low literacy may need pictorials, video or audiotapes, or materials written in elementary language (second- to fourth-grade level) (49). Some individuals who are otherwise literate struggle with numeracy, a key component for understanding medication prescriptions (47). Further, some patients with low literacy may not admit they have difficulty reading because of shame (50). Asking the individual and/or family members to state in their own words their understanding of medications, the dosing, and timing is very important.

Psychosocial Status

Psychosocial factors such as depression (51–54), anxiety (55–57), diabetes-related emotional distress and pessimistic attitudes (3,58), lack of readiness to change behavior (59), introversion and social isolation (60,61) are associated with poor glycemic control and may interfere with the performance of recommended self-care behaviors. Consequently, to individualize care and incorporate patients' goals and preferences into the treatment plan, assessing patients' knowledge and understanding of their treatment recommendations as well as psychological barriers (e.g., depression and stress) and supportive factors for carrying out self-care behaviors is important. Because older adults often depend on family, friends, and caregivers to help them with self-care tasks as well as provide emotional and at times financial support, diabetes education should include family and other caregivers.

Depression
Older adults with diabetes are at an increased risk for major depression than those without diabetes (2,62–65). The presence of depression is associated with poor glycemic control, increased number of complications, and an increase in functional impairments and mortality (65–67). Depression is often undiagnosed and undertreated (52,68). Depression adversely affects self-care behaviors (e.g., adherence to diet and exercise) (69). Moreover, untreated depression may add to the financial burden associated with having a chronic illness by increasing medical costs (70,71). Thus a comprehensive assessment of older adults should include standardized screening tools such as the Geriatric Depression Scale (72). When a more thorough assessment is not available, simply asking two validated questions as a depression screen is useful in clinical settings, "During the past month, have you been bothered by feeling down, depressed, or hopeless?" and "during the past month, have you been bothered by little interest or pleasure in doing things?" (73). If depression is suspected, referral to a mental health professional is important and helpful.

Symptoms of depression should not be used to exclude older adults from educational interventions. A recent study examining the impact of depression on older patients' ability to benefit from diabetes education in a large sample of ethnically diverse older adults with diabetes found that depression did not effect patients' ability to benefit from the intervention (74).

Stress
The relationship between stress and diabetes is multifaceted and reciprocal (58,75–80). If major life events and daily hassles are appraised by individuals as stressful, they may negatively affect glycemic control. Feelings of anxiety and depression associated with events that are perceived as stressful and threatening can lead to emotion-focused and avoidant coping strategies (81,82). The use of avoidant coping strategies such as eating too much when feeling stressed negatively affects adherence to self-care behaviors and glycemic control (79,83). Similarly, the way in which a person appraises his or her ability to cope with diabetes is likely to influence the level of diabetes-related emotional distress; consequently the level of diabetes-related

distress will influence how well individuals adjust to the impact of diabetes on their life and is strongly predictive of glycemic outcome (3,4,58). Moreover, experiences of stress may lead to other negative health behaviors such as increase in alcohol and tobacco consumption (84,85), this, in turn, further disrupts regimen adherence and increases the risk of developing diabetes complications.

Stressful life events may put older adults already predisposed to developing diabetes at even greater risk for developing the disease (86,87). Among older adults living with diabetes, stressful life events and diabetes-related emotional distress are associated with feelings of frustration and inability to maintain self-care behaviors (60). Older individuals under stress report feeling overwhelmed by the complexity of their disease management requirements, often altering dietary and exercise behaviors and engaging in other behaviors that are detrimental to glycemic control (75,88,89). Further, the onset of diabetes-related complications in older adults, coexisting medical conditions, and the associated decline in physical health can often become a significant source of sustained stress and further deplete coping resources (90–92).

Stress, diabetes-related distress, and coping are important predictors of diabetes self-care behaviors (3,58,79). Studies suggest that patients experiencing high levels of diabetes-related distress report feeling unmotivated to carry out self-care behaviors such as healthy eating and exercise (93). Because stress is known to interfere with everyday self-care tasks and diabetes self-management itself may become a source of assessment of stress levels is particularly important as part of self-management education for older adults. Educators should help older individuals identify life events and self-management tasks that they perceive as stressors. Moreover, the educator can help older adults with diabetes develop an understanding of the relationship among stress, coping mechanisms, and blood glucose levels (94).

Social and Family Support

Support from family and friends has been positively linked to greater individual adherence to self-care recommendations and treatment prescriptions (86,95–97). Several studies suggest that for older individuals, social support improves psychosocial adaptation to the illness by serving as a buffer against the negative effect of stress and depression related to diabetes (75,98–102). Perceived availability of social support may help individuals with chronic illness to interpret stressful situations associated with self-management regimens as less threatening and provide additional resources for coping with stressors (97,103). Assessment should focus on evaluating the older patients' support network and financial resources as they relate to their ability to follow therapeutic recommendations, and if the older adult with diabetes feels he or she receives the amount of help needed (75,94). Further, culture-specific issues may impact diabetes self-care including the attitude toward diabetes, readiness, and ability to make changes (104), thus culture must be taken into account during assessment.

Older adults with diabetes, especially those with cognitive and functional impairments, often depend on family members to help them with self-care tasks. Among older adults with diabetes, social support is positively linked to diabetes-related knowledge and perceived quality of life (25,105,106). Moreover, diabetes-specific social support is a strong predictor of self-care behaviors (103). Family involvement and peer support maximize the positive effects of educational interventions. For example, older patients with spouses who participated in diabetes education showed greater improvement in knowledge, family involvement, and stress levels than those without participating spouses (25).

Incorporating peer support into an educational intervention may be beneficial to patients with chronic diseases. Mutual exchange of knowledge, experiences, feelings, and challenges among individuals with diabetes has been shown to improve adherence to therapeutic recommendations (27,107–109). In older patients attending diabetes education classes, peer support was associated with weight reduction and improved glycemic control (12,27). Social support may be particularly important in domains for which perceived barriers to implementing self-care behaviors exist, specifically diet and exercise (23,25,110,111). Wen et al. reported that older Hispanic adults with diabetes who had higher levels of family support for dietary self-care reported fewer barriers to following dietary recommendations (26).

Not all older adults with diabetes require or desire a great deal of social support. At times, too much social support from family and friends will be perceived as nagging and may become a burden (94). Furthermore, when help that is not wanted is provided, older adults may feel overwhelmed and that they are perceived as incompetent, thereby limiting their sense of autonomy and perceived control, which may negatively impact diabetes self-care (103,112–114). Similarly, feelings of helplessness and incompetence may be detrimental to the educational process, which focuses on empowering the patient to take charge of their own care (7,115).

Financial Considerations

For older adults with diabetes, the burden of out-of-pocket expenditures associated with diabetes care can be high (116). Moreover, in older adults, financial strain has been associated with symptoms of depression and stress (117). Older patients', many of whom are retired and are Medicare recipients with no supplemental income, often cite financial limitations as barriers to adherence with therapeutic recommendations including dietary (118–120). Older adults with low income frequently must choose between expensive prescription drugs and a healthy diet (121,122). Consequently, some older adults are forced to eat more canned foods, frozen foods, and fast foods. Similarly, for lower-income older Medicare recipients, payments and other out-of-pocket costs for prescription medications were associated with lower rates of use of these medications than for higher-income adults (123). When creating an individualized self-care plan for older patients, educators must take into account the financial burden associated with loss of income and its impact on the ability of older patients to follow treatment recommendations. Referral to support services or a social worker can be helpful when older people and their families need assistance in applying for free care, free or discounted medications, and other available services.

Physical Limitations

In older adults, diabetes is associated with a high prevalence of physical disability (124). Older adults are more prone to chronic complications secondary to diabetes, even when the onset of diabetes occurs after the age of 65 (2,125). A high proportion of older adults with diabetes have hypertension, hyperlipidemia, atherosclerotic arterial disease, diabetic renal disease, peripheral neuropathy, and other diabetes-related complications (126,127). Many older patients with diabetes report functional disability and limited mobility related to these complications of diabetes and coexisting chronic conditions (128). One study also reported a positive link between diabetes and the risk of falls in older adults (129). In the context of educational intervention, functional status should be assessed with respect to older patients' capabilities for self-care and physical limitations that may affect the efficacy of education. Moreover, recognizing and addressing physical limitations that are perceived by patients as barriers to diabetes education is important. In a recent study, older adults with diabetes identified poor vision and hearing loss as the most common barriers to diabetes education (130). Accordingly, incorporating vision and hearing screening as part of initial assessment of patients' educational needs may be necessary. For example, older adults with diminished vision will often report experiencing difficulty with driving to their appointments, reading food labels for nutrition information, and checking their feet (131). If vision impairment is found to be a barrier, strategies using "talking meter" or large print reading material can achieve better results.

When setting educational goals, educators' should take into consideration the presence of multiple comorbidities and their effect on patients' functional level. The goal of diabetes education is to provide the individual with the knowledge, skills, and the tools to self-manage their disease. However, the presence of significant comorbid problems among older adults with diabetes may cause functional difficulties and impede successful diabetes self-management. Functional assessment should include assessment of activities of daily living (ADL) (e.g., bathing, grooming, dressing, feeding, and toileting) and assessment of instrumental ADL (e.g., shopping, finances, and housework) (132).

Exercise and physical activity are directly linked to improvements in age-associated physiologic changes and impairments as well as mortality and disability (133–135). Exercise is also a key component of most intervention programs for diabetes and has been shown to improve glycemic control, especially among adults with type 2 diabetes (136). Although the objective and subjective benefits of exercise, especially weight lifting and resistance training (137), as part of a lifestyle intervention for older patients with diabetes have been shown (138,139), an exercise program should be developed only after assessing patients' preferences, physical limitations, and setting realistic goals that the exercise program will help to achieve. Many older adults tolerate gradual increase in physical activity and do not require cardiac work-up before starting low impact exercise. Before initiation of an intensive exercise program, older adults should undergo a comprehensive medical screening that includes assessment of risk for cardiac events.

SUMMARY

The goal of diabetes education is to improve self-care behaviors and the quality of life of individuals with diabetes. This goal is met by assisting older adults with diabetes to integrate into their life styles a well-planned, individualized intervention that addresses their specific needs and barriers. The diabetes education plan begins with a comprehensive assessment of patients' life activities and priorities, including physiological and psychosocial changes associated with aging, and then determining whether these support or interfere with diabetes self-care. The health-care provider and the older patient mutually set and prioritize individualized behavioral goals to reflect treatment requirements and patient preferences. Although the educational plan for older adults incorporates unique methods for teaching older adults with different comorbidities and functional impairments, the focus of diabetes education still remains on providing the patient and family the tools and the skills to successfully self-manage their disease.

ACKNOWLEDGMENT

Work on this chapter by grant number NIH R01DK60115 from the National Institutes of Health National Institute of Diabetes and Digestion and Kidney Disease.

REFERENCES

1. Quinn L. Type 2 diabetes: epidemiology, pathophysiology, and diagnosis. Nurs Clin North Am 2001; 36(2):175–192.
2. Meneilly GS, Tessier D. Diabetes in elderly adults. J Gerontol A Biol Sci Med Sci 2001; 56(1): M5–M13.
3. Polonsky WH, Anderson BJ, Lohrer PA, et al. Assessment of diabetes-related distress. Diabetes Care 1995; 18(6):754–760.
4. Welch GW, Jacobson AM, Polonsky WH. The Problem Areas in Diabetes Scale. An evaluation of its clinical utility. Diabetes Care 1997; 20(5):760–766.
5. Parker RM, Baker DW, Williams MV, et al. The test of functional health literacy in adults: a new instrument for measuring patients' literacy skills. J Gen Intern Med 1995; 10(10):537–541.
6. Health literacy: report of the Council on Scientific Affairs. Ad Hoc Committee on Health Literacy for the Council on Scientific Affairs, American Medical Association. JAMA 1999; 281(6):552–557.
7. Anderson RM, Funnell MM, Butler PM, et al. Patient empowerment. Results of a randomized controlled trial. Diabetes Care 1995; 18(7):943–949.
8. Funnell MM, Anderson RM. Patient empowerment: a look back, a look ahead. Diabetes Educ 2003; 29(3):454–458, 460, 462 passim.
9. Funnell MM, Anderson RM, Arnold MS, et al. Empowerment: an idea whose time has come in diabetes education. Diabetes Educ 1991; 17(1):37–41.
10. Mirowsky J, Ross CE. Control or defense? Depression and the sense of control over good and bad outcomes. J Health Soc Behav 1990; 31(1):71–86.
11. Grembowski D, Patrick D, Diehr P, et al. Self-efficacy and health behavior among older adults. J Health Soc Behav 1993; 34(2):89–104.
12. Garcia R, Suarez R. Diabetes education in the elderly: a 5-year follow-up of an interactive approach. Patient Educ Couns 1996; 29(1):87–97.
13. Crooks VC, Buckwalter JG, Petitti DB. Diabetes mellitus and cognitive performance in older women. Ann Epidemiol 2003; 13(9):613–619.
14. Ryan CM, Geckle M. Why is learning and memory dysfunction in Type 2 diabetes limited to older adults? Diabetes Metab Res Rev 2000; 16(5):308–315.

15. Ryan CM. Diabetes, aging, and cognitive decline. Neurobiol Aging 2005; 26(suppl 1):21–25.
16. Ryan CM, Freed MI, Rood JA, et al. Improving metabolic control leads to better working memory in adults with type 2 diabetes. Diabetes Care 2006; 29(2):345–351.
17. Verhaeghen P, Salthouse TA. Meta-analyses of age-cognition relations in adulthood: estimates of linear and nonlinear age effects and structural models. Psychol Bull 1997; 122(3):231–249.
18. Salthouse TA. Age-related differences in basic cognitive processes: implications for work. Exp Aging Res 1994; 20(4):249–255.
19. Mensing C, Boucher J, Cypress M, et al. National standards for diabetes self-management education. Diabetes Care 2006; 29(suppl 1):S78–S85.
20. Ley P. Satisfaction, compliance and communication. Br J Clin Psychol 1982; 21(Pt 4):241–254.
21. Page P, Verstraete DG, Robb JR, et al. Patient recall of self-care recommendations in diabetes. Diabetes Care 1981; 4(1):96–98.
22. Ruggiero L, Glasgow R, Dryfoos JM, et al. Diabetes self-management. Self-reported recommendations and patterns in a large population. Diabetes Care 1997; 20(4):568–576.
23. Kravitz RL, Hays RD, Sherbourne CD, et al. Recall of recommendations and adherence to advice among patients with chronic medical conditions. Arch Intern Med 1993; 153(16):1869–1878.
24. Stoller EP, Pollow R, Forster LE. Older people's recommendations for treating symptoms: repertoires of lay knowledge about disease. Med Care 1994; 32(8):847–862.
25. Gilden JL, Hendryx M, Casia C, et al. The effectiveness of diabetes education programs for older patients and their spouses. J Am Geriatr Soc 1989; 37(11):1023–1030.
26. Wen LK, Parchman ML, Shepherd MD. Family support and diet barriers among older Hispanic adults with type 2 diabetes. Fam Med 2004; 36(6):423–430.
27. Wilson W, Pratt C. The impact of diabetes education and peer support upon weight and glycemic control of elderly persons with noninsulin dependent diabetes mellitus (NIDDM). Am J Public Health 1987; 77(5):634–635.
28. Sarkisian CA, Brown AF, Norris KC, et al. A systematic review of diabetes self-care interventions for older, African American, or Latino adults. Diabetes Educ 2003; 29(3):467–479.
29. Sedlak M, Raml A, Schmekal B, et al. Metabolic control in insulin-treated type 2-diabetic patients aged over 80 years and without participation in a structured diabetic teaching program. Wien Med Wochenschr 2005; 155(1–2):26–29.
30. Helkala EL, Niskanen L, Viinamaki H, et al. Short-term and long-term memory in elderly patients with NIDDM. Diabetes Care 1995; 18(5):681–685.
31. Perlmuter LC, Hakami MK, Hodgson-Harrington C, et al. Decreased cognitive function in aging non-insulin-dependent diabetic patients. Am J Med 1984; 77(6):1043–1048.
32. U'Ren RC, Riddle MC, Lezak MD, et al. The mental efficiency of the elderly person with type II diabetes mellitus. J Am Geriatr Soc 1990; 38(5):505–510.
33. Leibson CL, Rocca WA, Hanson VA, et al. The risk of dementia among persons with diabetes mellitus: a population-based cohort study. Ann NY Acad Sci 1997; 826:422–427.
34. Ott A, Stolk RP, Hofman A, et al. Association of diabetes mellitus and dementia: The Rotterdam Study. Diabetologia 1996; 39(11):1392–1397.
35. Grodstein F, Chen J, Wilson RS, et al. Type 2 diabetes and cognitive function in community-dwelling elderly women. Diabetes Care 2001; 24(6):1060–1065.
36. Sinclair AJ, Girling AJ, Bayer AJ. Cognitive dysfunction in older subjects with diabetes mellitus: impact on diabetes self-management and use of care services. All Wales Research into Elderly (AWARE) Study. Diabetes Res Clin Pract 2000; 50(3):203–212.
37. Folstein MF, Folstein SE, McHugh PR. "Mini-mental state." A practical method for grading the cognitive state of patients for the clinician. J Psychiatr Res 1975; 12(3):189–198.
38. Tombaugh TN, McIntyre NJ. The mini-mental state examination: a comprehensive review. J Am Geriatr Soc 1992; 40(9):922–935.
39. Shulman KI. Clock-drawing: is it the ideal cognitive screening test? Int J Geriatr Psychiatry 2000; 15(6):548–561.
40. Lezak MD. Neuropsychological Assessment. 3rd ed. New York: Oxford University Press, Inc., 1995.
41. Munshi M, Grande L, Ayres D, et al. Depression and undiagnosed executive dysfunction are important barriers to optimal diabetes care in older adults. Diabetes 2005; 54(suppl 1):A40.
42. Munshi M, Grande L, Hayes M, et al. Cognitive Dysfunction is associated with poor diabetes control in older adults. Diabetes Care 2006; 29:1794–1799.
43. Gazmararian JA, Baker DW, Williams MV, et al. Health literacy among Medicare enrollees in a managed care organization. JAMA 1999; 281(6):545–551.
44. Williams MV, Parker RM, Baker DW, et al. Inadequate functional health literacy among patients at two public hospitals. JAMA 1995; 274(21):1677–1682.
45. Howard DH, Gazmararian J, Parker RM. The impact of low health literacy on the medical costs of medicare managed care enrollees. Am J Med 2005; 118(4):371–377.
46. Gazmararian JA, Williams MV, Peel J, et al. Health literacy and knowledge of chronic disease. Patient Educ Couns 2003; 51(3):267–275.

47. Williams MV, Baker DW, Parker RM, et al. Relationship of functional health literacy to patients' knowledge of their chronic disease. A study of patients with hypertension and diabetes. Arch Intern Med 1998; 158(2):166–172.
48. Williams MV, Baker DW, Honig EG, et al. Inadequate literacy is a barrier to asthma knowledge and self-care. Chest 1998; 114(4):1008–1015.
49. Hosey GM, Freeman WL, Stracqualursi F, et al. Designing and evaluating diabetes education material for American Indians. Diabetes Educ 1990; 16(5):407–414.
50. Parikh NS, Parker RM, Nurss JR, et al. Shame and health literacy: the unspoken connection. Patient Educ Couns 1996; 27(1):33–39.
51. Lustman PJ, Freedland KE, Griffith LS, et al. Predicting response to cognitive behavior therapy of depression in type 2 diabetes. Gen Hosp Psychiatry 1998; 20(5):302–306.
52. Jacobson AM, Weinger K. Treating depression in diabetic patients: is there an alternative to medications? Ann Intern Med 1998; 129(8):656–657.
53. Cohen SJ. Potential barriers to diabetes care. Diabetes Care 1983; 6(5):499–500.
54. Cohen ST, Welch G, Jacobson AM, et al. The association of lifetime psychiatric illness and increased retinopathy in patients with type I diabetes mellitus. Psychosomatics 1997; 38(2):98–108.
55. Mazze RS, Lucido D, Shamoon H. Psychological and social correlates of glycemic control. Diabetes Care 1984; 7(4):360–366.
56. Niemcryk SJ, Speers MA, Travis LB, et al. Psychosocial correlates of hemoglobin Alc in young adults with type I diabetes. J Psychosom Res 1990; 34(6):617–627.
57. Hamburg BA, Inoff GE. Coping with predictable crises of diabetes. Diabetes Care 1983; 6(4):409–416.
58. Weinger K, Jacobson AM. Psychosocial and quality of life correlates of glycemic control during intensive treatment of type 1 diabetes. Patient Educ Couns 2001; 42(2):123–131.
59. Ruggiero L. Helping people with diabetes change behavior: from theory to practice. Diabetes Spectrum 2000; 13:125–132.
60. Orr DP, Golden MP, Myers G, et al. Characteristics of adolescents with poorly controlled diabetes referred to a tertiary care center. Diabetes Care 1983; 6(2):170–175.
61. Lane JD, Stabler B, Ross SL, et al. Psychological predictors of glucose control in patients with IDDM. Diabetes Care 1988; 11(10):798–800.
62. Anderson RJ, Freedland KE, Clouse RE, et al. The prevalence of comorbid depression in adults with diabetes: a meta-analysis. Diabetes Care 2001; 24(6):1069–1078.
63. Amato L, Paolisso G, Cacciatore F, et al. Non-insulin-dependent diabetes mellitus is associated with a greater prevalence of depression in the elderly. The Osservatorio Geriatrico of Campania region group. Diabetes Metab 1996; 22(5):314–318.
64. Lloyd CE, Dyer PH, Barnett AH. Prevalence of symptoms of depression and anxiety in a diabetes clinic population. Diabet Med 2000; 17(3):198–202.
65. Rosenthal MJ, Fajardo M, Gilmore S, et al. Hospitalization and mortality of diabetes in older adults. A 3-year prospective study. Diabetes Care 1998; 21(2):231–235.
66. de Groot M, Anderson R, Freedland KE, et al. Association of depression and diabetes complications: a meta-analysis. Psychosom Med 2001; 63(4):619–630.
67. Lustman PJ, Anderson RJ, Freedland KE, et al. Depression and poor glycemic control: a meta-analytic review of the literature. Diabetes Care 2000; 23(7):934–942.
68. Lustman PJ, Harper GW. Nonpsychiatric physicians' identification and treatment of depression in patients with diabetes. Compr Psychiatry 1987; 28(1):22–27.
69. Lin EH, Katon W, Von Korff M, et al. Relationship of depression and diabetes self-care, medication adherence, and preventive care. Diabetes Care 2004; 27(9):2154–2160.
70. Katon W, Unutzer J, Fan MY, et al. Cost-effectiveness and net benefit of enhanced treatment of depression for older adults with diabetes and depression. Diabetes Care 2006; 29(2):265–270.
71. Simon GE, Katon WJ, Lin EH, et al. Diabetes complications and depression as predictors of health service costs. Gen Hosp Psychiatry 2005; 27(5):344–351.
72. Brown AF, Mangione CM, Saliba D, et al. Guidelines for improving the care of the older person with diabetes mellitus. J Am Geriatr Soc 2003; 51(5 suppl Guidelines):S265–S280.
73. Whooley MA, Avins AL, Miranda J, et al. Case-finding instruments for depression. Two questions are as good as many. J Gen Intern Med 1997; 12(7):439–445.
74. Trief PM, Morin PC, Izquierdo R, et al. Depression and glycemic control in elderly ethnically diverse patients with diabetes: The Ideatel Project. Diabetes Care 2006; 29(4):830–835.
75. Lo R. Correlates of expected success at adherence to health regimen of people with IDDM. J Adv Nurs 1999; 30(2):418–424.
76. Surwit RS, van Tilburg MA, Zucker N, et al. Stress management improves long-term glycemic control in type 2 diabetes. Diabetes Care 2002; 25(1):30–34.
77. Delamater AM, Cox D. Psychological stress, coping, and diabetes. Diabetes Spectrum 1994; 7:18–49.
78. Lloyd CE, Dyer PH, Lancashire RJ, et al. Association between stress and glycemic control in adults with type 1 (insulin-dependent) diabetes. Diabetes Care 1999; 22(8):1278–1283.

79. Peyrot M, McMurry JF Jr, Kruger DF. A biopsychosocial model of glycemic control in diabetes: stress, coping and regimen adherence. J Health Soc Behav 1999; 40(2):141–158.

80. Lloyd CE, Smith J, Weinger K. Stress and diabetes: a review of the links. Diabetes Spectrum 2005; 18(2):121–127.

81. Lazarus RS, Folkman S. Stress, Appraisal and Coping. New York: Springer Publishing Company, 1984:464.

82. Aspinwall LG, Taylor SE. Modeling cognitive adaptation: a longitudinal investigation of the impact of individual differences and coping on college adjustment and performance. J Pers Soc Psychol 1992; 63(6):989–1003.

83. Peyrot MF, McMurry JF Jr. Stress buffering and glycemic control. The role of coping styles. Diabetes Care 1992; 15(7):842–846.

84. Spangler JG, Summerso JH, Bell RA, et al. Smoking status and psychosocial variables in type 1 diabetes mellitus. Addict Behav 2001; 26(1):21–29.

85. Smith J. The enemy within: stress in the lives of women with diabetes. Diabet Med 2002; 19(suppl 2): 98–99.

86. Wang CY, Fenske MM. Self-care of adults with non-insulin-dependent diabetes mellitus: influence of family and friends. Diabetes Educ 1996; 22(5):465–470.

87. Mooy JM, de Vries H, Grootenhuis PA, et al. Major stressful life events in relation to prevalence of undetected type 2 diabetes: The Hoorn Study. Diabetes Care 2000; 23(2):197–201.

88. Jacobson AM. The psychological care of patients with insulin-dependent diabetes mellitus. N Engl J Med 1996; 334(19):1249–1253.

89. Travis T. Patient perceptions of factors that affect adherence to dietary regimens for diabetes mellitus. Diabetes Educ 1997; 23(2):152–156.

90. Jacobson AM, Rand LI, Hauser ST. Psychologic stress and glycemic control: a comparison of patients with and without proliferative diabetic retinopathy. Psychosom Med 1985; 47(4):372–381.

91. Aikens JE, Wallander JL, Bell DS, et al. Daily stress variability, learned resourcefulness, regimen adherence, and metabolic control in type I diabetes mellitus: evaluation of a path model. J Consult Clin Psychol 1992; 60(1):113–118.

92. Wulsin LR, Jacobson AM, Rand LI. Psychosocial aspects of diabetic retinopathy. Diabetes Care 1987; 10(3):367–373.

93. Albright TL, Parchman M, Burge SK. Predictors of self-care behavior in adults with type 2 diabetes: An Rrnest Study. Fam Med 2001; 33(5):354–360.

94. Polonsky WH. Diabetes Burnout: What To Do When You Can't Take It Anymore. Alexandria, VA: American Diabetes Association, 1999.

95. Tillotson LM, Smith MS. Locus of control, social support, and adherence to the diabetes regimen. Diabetes Educ 1996; 22(2):133–139.

96. Glasgow RE, Toobert DJ. Social environment and regimen adherence among type II diabetic patients. Diabetes Care 1988; 11(5):377–386.

97. Willoughby DF, Kee C, Demi A. Women's psychosocial adjustment to diabetes. J Adv Nurs 2000; 32(6):1422–1430.

98. Griffith LS, Field BJ, Lustman PJ. Life stress and social support in diabetes: association with glycemic control. Int J Psychiatry Med 1990; 20(4):365–372.

99. Ruggiero L, Spirito A, Bond A, et al. Impact of social support and stress on compliance in women with gestational diabetes. Diabetes Care 1990; 13(4):441–443.

100. Garay-Sevilla ME, Nava LE, Malacara JM, et al. Adherence to treatment and social support in patients with non-insulin dependent diabetes mellitus. J Diabetes Complicat 1995; 9(2):81–86.

101. Littlefield CH, Rodin GM, Murray MA, et al. Influence of functional impairment and social support on depressive symptoms in persons with diabetes. Health Psychol 1990; 9(6):737–749.

102. Bailey TS, Yu HM, Rayfield EJ. Patterns of foot examination in a diabetes clinic. Am J Med 1985; 78(3):371–374.

103. Connell CM, Davis WK, Gallant MP, et al. Impact of social support, social cognitive variables, and perceived threat on depression among adults with diabetes. Health Psychol 1994; 13(3):263–273.

104. Brown SA, Garcia AA, Kouzekanani K, et al. Culturally competent diabetes self-management education for Mexican Americans: The Starr County Border Health Initiative. Diabetes Care 2002; 25(2):259–268.

105. Gilden JL, Hendryx MS, Clar S, et al. Diabetes support groups improve health care of older diabetic patients. J Am Geriatr Soc 1992; 40(2):147–150.

106. Trief PM, Himes CL, Orendorff R, et al. The marital relationship and psychosocial adaptation and glycemic control of individuals with diabetes. Diabetes Care 2001; 24(8):1384–1389.

107. Joseph DH, Griffin M, Hall RF, et al. Peer coaching: an intervention for individuals struggling with diabetes. Diabetes Educ 2001; 27(5):703–710.

108. Keyserling TC, Ammerman AS, Samuel-Hodge CD, et al. A diabetes management program for African American women with type 2 diabetes. Diabetes Educ 2000; 26(5):796–805.

109. Heisler M, Piette JD. "I help you, and you help me": facilitated telephone peer support among patients with diabetes. Diabetes Educ 2005; 31(6):869–879.

110. Glasgow RE, Ruggiero L, Eakin EG, et al. Quality of life and associated characteristics in a large national sample of adults with diabetes. Diabetes Care 1997; 20(4):562–567.
111. Dalewitz J, Khan N, Hershey CO. Barriers to control of blood glucose in diabetes mellitus. Am J Med Qual 2000; 15(1):16–25.
112. Smith GC, Kohn SJ, Savage-Stevens SE, et al. The effects of interpersonal and personal agency on perceived control and psychological well-being in adulthood. Gerontologist 2000; 40(4):458–468.
113. Connell CM. Psychosocial contexts of diabetes and older adulthood: reciprocal effects. Diabetes Educ 1991; 17(5):364–371.
114. Boehm S, Schlenk EA, Funnell MM, et al. Predictors of adherence to nutrition recommendations in people with non-insulin-dependent diabetes mellitus. Diabetes Educ 1997; 23(2):157–165.
115. Anderson RM, Funnell MM. Patient empowerment: reflections on the challenge of fostering the adoption of a new paradigm. Patient Educ Couns 2005; 57(2):153–157.
116. Bernard DM, Banthin JS, Encinosa WE. Health care expenditure burdens among adults with diabetes in 2001. Med Care 2006; 44(3):210–215.
117. Krause N. Chronic financial strain, social support, and depressive symptoms among older adults. Psychol Aging 1987; 2(2):185–192.
118. Moss SE, Klein R, Klein BE. Factors associated with having eye examinations in persons with diabetes. Arch Fam Med 1995; 4(6):529–534.
119. Musey VC, Lee JK, Crawford R, et al. Diabetes in urban African-Americans. I. Cessation of insulin therapy is the major precipitating cause of diabetic ketoacidosis. Diabetes Care 1995; 18(4):483–489.
120. Lynch T. Medication costs as a primary cause of nonadherence in the elderly. Consult Pharm 2006; 21(2):143–146.
121. Fuchs VR. Provide, provide: the economics of aging. Cambridge, MA: National Bureau of Economic Research, 1998.
122. Stitt S, O'Connell C, Grant D. Old, poor and malnourished. Nutr Health 1995; 10(2):135–154.
123. Brown AF, Gross AG, Gutierrez PR, et al. Income-related differences in the use of evidence-based therapies in older persons with diabetes mellitus in for-profit managed care. J Am Geriatr Soc 2003; 51(5):665–670.
124. Gregg EW, Beckles GL, Williamson DF, et al. Diabetes and physical disability among older US adults. Diabetes Care 2000; 23(9):1272–1277.
125. Gu K, Cowie CC, Harris MI. Mortality in adults with and without diabetes in a national cohort of the US population, 1971–1993. Diabetes Care 1998; 21(7):1138–1145.
126. Moritz DJ, Ostfeld AM, Blazer D II, et al. The health burden of diabetes for the elderly in four communities. Public Health Rep 1994; 109(6):782–790.
127. Fillenbaum GG, Pieper CF, Cohen HJ, et al. Comorbidity of five chronic health conditions in elderly community residents: determinants and impact on mortality. J Gerontol A Biol Sci Med Sci 2000; 55(2):M84–M89.
128. Wray LA, Ofstedal MB, Langa KM, et al. The effect of diabetes on disability in middle-aged and older adults. J Gerontol A Biol Sci Med Sci 2005; 60(9):1206–1211.
129. Maurer MS, Burcham J, Cheng H. Diabetes mellitus is associated with an increased risk of falls in elderly residents of a long-term care facility. J Gerontol A Biol Sci Med Sci 2005; 60(9):1157–1162.
130. Rhee MK, Cook CB, El-Kebbi I, et al. Barriers to diabetes education in urban patients: perceptions, patterns, and associated factors. Diabetes Educ 2005; 31(3):410–417.
131. Schoenberg NE, Drungle SC. Barriers to non-insulin dependent diabetes mellitus (NIDDM) self-care practices among older women. J Aging Health 2001; 13(4):443–466.
132. Stuck AE, Siu AL, Wieland GD, et al. Comprehensive geriatric assessment: a meta-analysis of controlled trials. Lancet 1993; 342(8878):1032–1036.
133. Paffenbarger RS Jr, Hyde RT, Wing AL, et al. The association of changes in physical-activity level and other lifestyle characteristics with mortality among men. N Engl J Med 1993; 328(8):538–545.
134. Frontera WR, Meredith CN, O'Reilly KP, et al. Strength conditioning in older men: skeletal muscle hypertrophy and improved function. J Appl Physiol 1988; 64(3):1038–1044.
135. Leveille SG, Guralnik JM, Ferrucci L, et al. Aging successfully until death in old age: opportunities for increasing active life expectancy. Am J Epidemiol 1999; 149(7):654–664.
136. Boule NG, Haddad E, Kenny GP, et al. Effects of exercise on glycemic control and body mass in type 2 diabetes mellitus: a meta-analysis of controlled clinical trials. JAMA 2001; 286(10):1218–1227.
137. Willey KA, Singh MA. Battling insulin resistance in elderly obese people with type 2 diabetes: bring on the heavy weights. Diabetes Care 2003; 26(5):1580–1588.
138. Agurs-Collins TD, Kumanyika SK, Ten Have TR, et al. A randomized controlled trial of weight reduction and exercise for diabetes management in older African-American subjects. Diabetes Care 1997; 20(10):1503–1511.
139. Ivy JL, Zderic TW, Fogt DL. Prevention and treatment of non-insulin-dependent diabetes mellitus. Exerc Sport Sci Rev 1999; 27:1–35.

25 | Hypoglycemia and Self-Care in Elderly Patients with Diabetes Mellitus

Mark R. Burge, Leslie Gamache, and Hemanth Pai
Department of Medicine, Endocrinology Division, University of New Mexico Health Sciences Center, Albuquerque, New Mexico, U.S.A.

Alissa Segal
College of Pharmacy, University of New Mexico Health Sciences Center, Albuquerque, New Mexico, U.S.A.

INTRODUCTION

Diabetes mellitus is one of the major health problems in older adults, as evidenced by its high prevalence and an increasing incidence in the geriatric population. Estimates from the Centers for Disease Control and Prevention indicate that in 1998, 12.7% of patients older than 70 years had a diagnosis of diabetes mellitus (1). In the National Health and Nutrition Examination Survey of 1999 to 2002, 35% of all patients with diabetes were between the ages of 60 and 74, and 17% were over the age of 75 (2). By the year 2050, the prevalence of diabetes is expected to rise from 11 million to 29 million, with the largest percentage increase in patients over the age of 75 (3). Mortality in this population of older patients with diabetes is higher than its counterpart without diabetes. A population-based study using Medicare data from 1994 to 1996 showed that patients older than 65 years of age with diabetes suffered excess mortality at every age group (4). As the prevalence of diabetes increases and as treatment guidelines call for more and more rigorous glycemic control, rates of hypoglycemia and concern over how to appropriately prevent and treat hypoglycemia will continue to grow.

A morbidity and mortality survey conducted amongst the elderly U.S. Medicare population between 1994 and 1996 reported that the overall mortality rate in diabetic patients above 65 years of age was 62.3 per 1000 person-years in women and 81.8 per 1000 person-years in men. Additionally, hypoglycemia was the most frequent metabolic complication noted in the elderly diabetic individuals, occurring at a rate of 28.3 events per 1000 person-years (4). A cross-sectional study of Medicare beneficiaries aged 65 years and above in the United States demonstrated that health-care costs for individuals with diabetes were 1.5 times greater than for nondiabetic persons, with acute-care hospitalization costs accounting for 60% of the total expenditure and outpatient and physician services accounting for 7% and 33% of the costs, respectively (5).

Evidence is mounting that hypoglycemia among elderly subjects is a very real and costly concern. A recent study details all Emergency Room visits for severe hypoglycemia in a German Community of 200,000 between 1997 and 2000 (6). Severe hypoglycemia was defined as a symptomatic event requiring intravenous glucose or glucagon for treatment. Among patients receiving insulin, the incidence of severe hypoglycemia was 14.1 per 100,000 patient-years, and the incidence among sulfonylurea users was 5.6 per 100,000 patient-years. Because of the preponderance of type 2 diabetes in the population, however, 56% of the cases of severe hypoglycemia occurred in patients with type 2 diabetes and only 35% occurred in patients with type 1 diabetes. Among hospitalized patients, the investigators found that patients with type 2 diabetes had longer hospital stays than patients with type 1 diabetes (9.5 ± 10.6 days vs. 2.3 ± 5.3 days) and that direct medical costs for severe hypoglycemia were greater in patients with type 2 diabetes than in patients with type 1 diabetes. The average cost for each hospitalization was approximately \$1500. The authors conclude that "elderly, multimorbid patients with a long history of type 2 diabetes are at a high risk of developing hypoglycemia." If applied to the approximately 15 million Americans with type 2 diabetes, these data suggest that at least

$1,260,000 in direct medical costs accrue each year as a result of severe hypoglycemia among patients with type 2 diabetes. Although patient education and aggressive management of diabetes mellitus may ultimately result in improved glycemic control and decreased rates of diabetes complications, severe hypoglycemia will become an increasing occurrence and concern as a result of these same interventions (7,8). In fact, hypoglycemia is the major complication of intensive management of diabetes and remains the major barrier to achieving normoglycemic goals in elderly patients with diabetes.

This article will review the problem of hypoglycemia among elderly individuals. The general physiology of glucose homeostasis and the pathophysiology of hypoglycemia in diabetes will be first reviewed, followed by a discussion of the known risks and causes of hypoglycemia in patients with type 2 diabetes. Finally, diabetes self-care and hypoglycemia prevention and management strategies will be considered.

DEFINITION AND CLASSIFICATION OF HYPOGLYCEMIA

Hypoglycemia is defined by Whipple's triad of (*i*) symptoms of hypoglycemia in conjunction with (*ii*) an abnormally low plasma glucose concentration (generally <50 mg/dL or 2.8 mmol/L), and (*iii*) relief of those symptoms after glucose levels normalize. Clinically, hypoglycemia is classified as (*i*) asymptomatic or biochemical hypoglycemia, (*ii*) mild-to-moderate symptomatic hypoglycemia, and (*iii*) serious or severe hypoglycemia. Diabetic subjects with asymptomatic or "biochemical" hypoglycemia have abnormally low plasma glucose in the absence of warning symptoms. Patients with mild-to-moderate hypoglycemia experience the typical neurogenic (autonomic) warning symptoms of hypoglycemia and are able to take appropriate action to correct their plasma glucose concentration. Conversely, patients who experience severe or serious hypoglycemia require external assistance to correct their plasma glucose concentration.

CLINICAL MANIFESTATIONS OF HYPOGLYCEMIA

Clinical manifestations of hypoglycemia can be categorized as neurogenic or neuroglycopenic. Neurogenic symptoms are further classified as those secondary to adrenergic or cholinergic responses. Adrenergic symptoms include tremulousness, palpitations, and anxiety. Cholinergic symptoms include sweating, tingling, and hunger. Patients develop neuroglycopenic symptoms when the blood glucose supply to the brain falls below a critical level. Patients are typically weak, tired, and drowsy and may experience difficulty thinking or speaking as well as confusion, incoordination, and odd behavior. If the necessary steps to correct hypoglycemia are not taken in a timely fashion, patients with neuroglycopenia may experience seizures, coma, or death (9). The common symptoms of hypoglycemia are listed in Table 1.

UTILIZATION OF GLUCOSE BY THE BRAIN

The brain transports roughly three times more glucose from the circulation across the blood–brain barrier than is needed to satisfy the normal metabolism (10). This is largely an insulin-independent process that is facilitated by glucose transport protein 1 (GLUT 1), which is only minimally insulin responsive (11,12). When a critical glucose threshold is reached, centers in the hypothalamus sense the fall in systemic glucose concentrations and stimulate the release of glucagon and epinephrine. As the arterial plasma glucose concentration falls below a critical value of approximately 3.7 mmol/L (67 mg/dL) in nondiabetic humans, glucose transport across the blood–brain barrier becomes rate limiting to brain metabolism (13–15). Maintaining the plasma glucose concentration above this critical value is crucial for survival.

NORMAL PHYSIOLOGY OF GLUCOSE HOMEOSTASIS

The ambient plasma glucose concentration is an aggregate result of the rate of glucose appearance into the circulation (i.e., the sum of endogenous hepatic glucose production and exogenous glucose delivery from the gut) and the rate of glucose utilization via tissue extraction and urinary loss (16). The interplay of a variety of hormones and other mechanisms establishes and maintains normal glucose homeostasis, including insulin, glucagon, epinephrine, growth

TABLE 1 Classification of Hypoglycemic Symptoms

Neurogenic	Neuroglycopenic
Adrenergic	Difficulty thinking
Tremulousness	Confusion
Palpitations	Drowsiness
Anxiety	Weakness
	Warmth
Cholinergic	Difficulty speaking
Sweating	Clumsiness
Tingling	Odd behavior
Hunger	Seizure
	Coma
	Death

hormone (GH), and cortisol. The so-called counterregulatory hormones are complemented by glucose autoregulation to effectively prevent or correct the occurrence of hypoglycemia (16). The role of each of these will be discussed in detail below.

The Role of Endogenous Insulin

Insulin is the major glucose-regulating hormone in the fed state, and it acts to stimulate glucose utilization in insulin-sensitive tissues such as skeletal muscle and adipose tissue. Insulin also inhibits glycogenolysis and gluconeogenesis, thereby suppressing endogenous glucose production (17). When glucose production rates exceed the ambient rates of glucose utilization, plasma glucose concentrations tend to rise, and when glucose utilization rates exceed those of production, plasma glucose concentrations tend to fall (16). Suppression of insulin secretion is the earliest response to declining glucose concentrations (18). Heller and Cryer have demonstrated that the rate of recovery from hypoglycemia is inversely related to plasma insulin concentrations. Thus, inhibition of insulin is the first important step in the defense against hypoglycemia (19).

The Role of Glucagon

Glucagon plays a primary role in the recovery from acute hypoglycemia. It induces hepatic glycogenolysis and gluconeogenesis, thus promoting endogenous glucose production. Although it is important for normal recovery from hypoglycemia, it has been demonstrated that a deficient glucagon response does not completely prevent such a recovery (20,21).

The Role of Epinephrine

Epinephrine plays the most significant role during short-term hypoglycemia and also contributes to recovery from prolonged hypoglycemia. Its role is also crucial in preventing severe hypoglycemia in diabetic patients with acquired glucagon deficiency. Epinephrine acts directly through α- and β-adrenergic receptors to cause hepatic gluconeogenesis and glycogenolysis. Further, it inhibits insulin secretion and stimulates glucagon secretion, thereby restoring euglycemia (22,23). Finally, epinephrine reduces glucose utilization by reducing blood flow to insulin-sensitive tissues such as skeletal muscle (24). In experimental models of short-term hypoglycemia, recovery was reduced when glucagon secretion was absent and epinephrine responses were blocked pharmacologically (20,21). As further evidence of the importance of these two hormones, patients with type 1 diabetes have a 25-fold increase in the frequency of severe iatrogenic hypoglycemia when both glucagon and epinephrine secretion is deficient (24,25).

During the late phase of hypoglycemia, epinephrine also induces lipolysis, mobilizing substrates such as lactate, glycerol, alanine, and free fatty acids from peripheral tissues to sustain hepatic glucogenesis. The increase in free fatty-acid concentrations results in decreased glucose utilization in peripheral tissues via substrate competition and also serves as an alternate fuel source for the brain (26,27).

The Roles of GH and Cortisol

Both GH and cortisol are counterregulatory hormones that are operative as late responses to hypoglycemia. These hormones are not essential for the correction or prevention of acute hypoglycemia in adults when other counterregulatory hormones are intact, but they play an important role in the restoration of euglycemia during prolonged episodes of hypoglycemia such as may occur during starvation or after sulfonylurea overdose (28).

PHYSIOLOGY OF THE COUNTERREGULATORY HORMONES

Counterregulatory hormones play essential roles in the restoration of glucose homeostasis following a hypoglycemic stress, and there is a well-established hierarchical hormonal response to hypoglycemia. It should be noted that most of the current knowledge about the physiology of glucose homeostasis and hypoglycemia counterregulation has been gleaned from studies of young adults, with relatively few studies having been performed on the elderly population. These studies demonstrate that the most important of all the counterregulatory hormones in the defense of acute hypoglycemia is glucagon. Other hormones that play a role in the restoration of euglycemia during hypoglycemia, in order of importance, are epinephrine, GH, and cortisol. A schematic representation of normal physiology of glucose counterregulation is shown in Figure 1.

The exact relationship between a fall in the plasma glucose concentration and the activation of counterregulatory hormones, the initiation of warning symptoms, or the onset of deterioration in cerebral function is complex. Cryer and coworkers have characterized the kinetics of glucose counterregulation. Mitrakou et al. demonstrated, for example, that activation of glucagon, epinephrine, norepinephrine, and GH began at an average plasma glucose concentration of 68 ± 2 mg/dL in normal, nondiabetic volunteers (29). Figure 2 depicts the relationship between plasma glucose and counterregulatory hormones in these subjects. Neurogenic symptoms (anxiety, palpitations, sweating, irritability, and tremors) began at glucose concentrations of 58 ± 2 mg/dL, and neuroglycopenic symptoms (hunger, dizziness, tingling, blurred vision, difficulty in thinking, and fainting) began at glucose concentrations of 51 ± 3 mg/dL. Deterioration of cognitive function began at glucose concentrations of 49 ± 2 mg/dL. Figure 3 shows the onset of neurogenic and neuroglycopenic symptoms at different glucose concentrations in nondiabetic subjects. Such a hierarchy would effectively counteract and maximize the defense against hypoglycemia (18,29).

GLUCOSE AUTOREGULATION

Glucose autoregulation is defined as the process of hypoglycemia itself directly increasing endogenous glucose production. Glucose autoregulation is independent of counterregulatory hormones and is observed only during conditions of severe hypoglycemia. During glucose autoregulation, hepatic gluconeogenesis is inversely related to plasma glucose concentrations (30,31).

DAWN AND SOMOGYI PHENOMENA

Counterregulatory hormones can also cause hyperglycemia by additional mechanisms, namely the Dawn and Somogyi phenomena. The dawn phenomenon, defined as an increased insulin

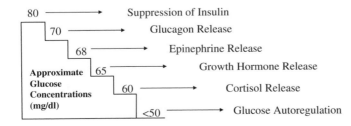

FIGURE 1 Schematic representation of the hierarchical response to hypoglycemia in nondiabetic individuals. *Source*: From Ref. 9.

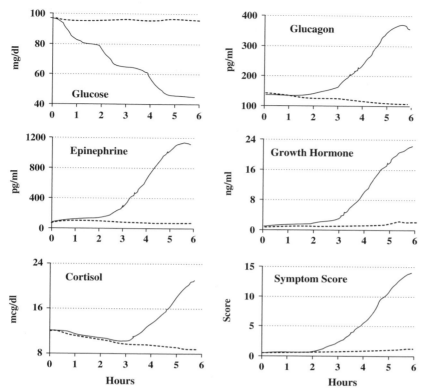

FIGURE 2 Schematic depiction of counterregulatory hormone and symptom responses during euglycemia (*dashed line*) and stepped hypoglycemia (*solid line*) in normal, nondiabetic subjects. *Source*: From Ref. 29.

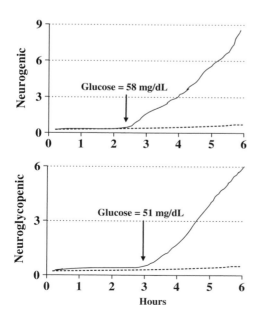

FIGURE 3 Schematic depiction of neurogenic and neuroglyc-openic symptom scores during euglycemia (*dashed line*) and stepped hypoglycemia (*solid line*) in normal, nondiabetic subjects. *Source*: From Ref. 29.

requirement between 0400 and 0800 hours, results from the early morning release of GH, which induces insulin resistance in hepatic and extrahepatic tissues (32).

In 1930, Somogyi observed that insulin-dependent diabetic subjects developed posthypoglycemic hyperglycemia. He postulated that antecedent hypoglycemia caused release of counterregulatory hormones that antagonized insulin action, causing insulin resistance. Subsequent studies have confirmed that counterregulatory hormones cause insulin resistance, leading to posthypoglycemic hyperglycemia (21,32,33). Although glucagon is the most important anti-insulin hormone during acute hypoglycemia, studies have also shown that the insulin-antagonist effect of glucagon is transient, lasting less than two hours. Insulin resistance induced by epinephrine, however, typically persists for four to six hours and is subsequently sustained by cortisol and GH for up to 12 hours.

RISK FACTORS FOR HYPOGLYCEMIA IN ELDERLY DIABETES PATIENTS

The strongest predictors of severe hypoglycemia are advanced age, recent hospitalization, and polypharmacy (34). As shown in Table 2, Shorr et al. have developed a list of the relevant risk factors for severe hypoglycemia associated with the treatment of diabetes among elderly Tennessee Medicare enrollees. In this cohort, the crude rate of hypoglycemia was almost 7 per 100 person-years during the first 30 days after discharge from the hospital. Among persons aged 80 years and more, the risk of severe hypoglycemia was 8.7 per 100 person-years within the first 30 days following hospital discharge. Similarly, persons using five or more therapeutic

TABLE 2 Risks Associated with Hypoglycemia in Elderly Type 2 Diabetes Patients

Variable	Relative risk (95% confidence interval)
Drug	
Sulfonylurea	1.0 (reference value)
Insulin	2.1 (1.8–2.5)
Insulin plus sulfonylurea	2.9 (1.6–9.2)
Age (years)	
65–69	1.0
70–74	1.1 (0.9–1.4)
75–79	1.5 (1.2–1.9)
>79	1.8 (1.4–2.3)
Gender	
Male	1.0
Female	0.8 (0.7–1.0)
Race	
White	1.0
Black	2.0 (1.7–2.4)
County of residence	
Rural	1.0
Urban	0.9 (0.7–1.1)
Days since hospital discharge	
>365	1.0
31–365	1.7 (1.4–2.0)
1–30	4.5 (3.5–5.7)
Nursing home resident	
No	1.0
Yes	1.0 (0.8–2.3)
Number of concomitant medications	
0–4	1.0
>4	1.3 (1.1–1.5)
New hypoglycemic drug therapy	
No	1.0
Yes	1.4 (1.0–1.9)

Source: From Ref. 35.

TABLE 3 Risk Factors for Hypoglycemia in Elderly Type 2 Diabetes Patients

Advanced age
Polypharmacy
Recent hospitalization
Use of sulfonylurea and/or insulin
Poor nutrition or fasting
Intercurrent illness
Chronic liver, renal, or cardiovascular disease
Prolonged physical exercise
Alcohol
Endocrine deficiency (thyroid, adrenal, and pituitary)
Loss of normal counterregulation
Hypoglycemic unawareness

classes of medications were at an increased risk of developing severe hypoglycemia (relative risk 1.3). The risk of drug-associated hypoglycemia is accentuated by intercurrent illness and polypharmacy. Potential mechanisms for the findings of the Shorr study include age-associated decreases in hepatic oxidative enzyme activity interfering with metabolism of sulfonylurea agents. Similarly, an age-related decline in renal function may impair excretion of insulin or sulfonylureas. The finding of a twofold increase in risk among black subjects also suggests the possibility of racial differences in drug metabolism or in the recognition of hypoglycemia. The risk factors for hypoglycemia are listed in Table 3.

The pharmacologic agents most often associated with hypoglycemia include sulfonylureas and insulin or combination therapy with one of these agents. Theoretically, monotherapy of type 2 diabetes with a biguanide, a thiazolidinedione, or an α-glucosidase inhibitor should not cause hypoglycemia. However, rare hypoglycemia has been reported with metformin (35,36). The novel incretin mimetic, exenatide, has also been associated with a low frequency of hypoglycemia. Specifically, when exenatide was added to metformin, the incidence of mild-to-moderate hypoglycemia was similar to that with placebo therapy and there were no severe hypoglycemic events (37). When exenatide was added to both sulfonylurea and metformin, however, the incidence of mild/moderate hypoglycemia was 28% with the 10 μg dose, 19% with the 5 μg dose, and 13% in the placebo group. Rates of hypoglycemia were apparently lower in the group of subjects who were assigned to a minimally effective sulfonylurea dose versus the group that received a maximally effective dose of sulfonylurea (38).

Unfortunately, the antidiabetic agents that do not cause hypoglycemia have numerous limitations including high cost, limited efficacy when used as monotherapy (α-glucosidase inhibitors), high prevalence of gastrointestinal side effects (α-glucosidase inhibitors, biguanides), risk of exacerbating congestive heart failure (thiazolidinediones), and risk of lactic acidosis (biguanides). Therefore, these agents are often either avoided in elderly patients or combined with agents that are associated with a higher risk of hypoglycemia, such as sulfonylureas or insulin. The most common drugs that cause hypoglycemia are listed in Table 4.

INTENSIVE DIABETES MANAGEMENT AND HYPOGLYCEMIA

Casparie and Elving studied a mixed population of type 1 and 2 diabetes subjects to determine the causes of severe hypoglycemia (39). They identified several such causes, of which the most

TABLE 4 Common Pharmacological Agents Associated with Hypoglycemia

Insulin
Sulfonylureas
Combination therapy with insulin and/or sulfonylureas
Drugs that potentiate sulfonylureas
Incretin mimetics (exenatide)
Certain antibiotics (sulfonamides, gatifloxacin, and pentamidine)

important was the overzealous use of insulin or the use of improper combinations of insulin. This was a factor in about 20% of the patients who experienced severe hypoglycemia, and a total of 28% of the severe hypoglycemia reactions were attributable to patient errors in insulin dosing. Missed meals or excessive exercise with improper adjustment of insulin dosing were common scenarios.

The Diabetes Control and Complications Trial (DCCT) reported an incidence of severe hypoglycemia that was three times higher in the patients receiving intensified diabetes management compared with conventional therapy in type 1 diabetes patients. There were 16.3 episodes of coma or seizures per 100 patient-years in the intensive-therapy group versus 5.4 such episodes per 100 patient-years in the conventional-therapy group (7). Similarly, the United Kingdom Prospective Diabetes Study (UKPDS) reported that rates of severe hypoglycemia episodes were increased in type 2 diabetes patients receiving intensive therapy with sulfonylureas (2.4%) or insulin (1.8%) compared to patients receiving conventional therapy (0.7%) (8). Moreover, the type 2 diabetes patients in this study often did not achieve target glycemic goals because of a high incidence of insulin-induced hypoglycemia. Risk factors for insulin-induced hypoglycemia in elderly diabetic patients are enumerated in Table 5.

Sulfonylurea-Induced Hypoglycemia

An estimated 50% to 66% of patients with type 2 diabetes use sulfonylureas alone or in combination with some other therapy, and hence, the study of hypoglycemia in patients with type 2 diabetes has been closely associated with the study of sulfonylureas (40). Although sulfonylureas are well tolerated by patients, are dosed once or twice daily, and remain relatively inexpensive, the mechanisms of occurrence of sulfonylurea-associated hypoglycemia remain poorly understood.

Retrospective studies have identified advanced age and caloric restriction as the main factors that predispose sulfonylurea-treated patients with type 2 diabetes to severe hypoglycemia, but the factors that predispose such patients to unanticipated, mild hypoglycemia on any given day are not known (36). Such unanticipated hypoglycemia is different from the prolonged, severe, and life-threatening hypoglycemia that results from intentional sulfonylurea overdose.

Data from Sweden and Switzerland indicate that the incidence of severe hypoglycemia due to sulfonylureas is about 0.22 per 1000 patient-years as compared with an incidence of about 100 per 1000 patient-years in case of insulin (41,42). Risk factors for sulfonylurea-induced hypoglycemia include an age greater than 60 years, disability, poor nutrition, and polypharmacy (43). Seltzer reviewed 1418 cases of drug-induced hypoglycemia and found that 15% of sulfonylurea users were taking multiple drugs predisposing one to severe hypoglycemia. He

---

TABLE 5   Risk Factors for Insulin-Induced Hypoglycemia in Elderly Patients with Diabetes

Insulin dosing errors
  Excessive insulin dose
  Improper timing of insulin relative to timing of food intake
  Injection of wrong insulin type (e.g., rapid-acting in place of long-acting insulin)
Decreased glucose influx
  Missed meals
  Fasting
  Gastroparesis with delayed carbohydrate absorption
Increased insulin sensitivity
  Weight loss
  Intensive insulin therapy
  Increased exercise
Delayed insulin clearance and erratic insulin absorption
  Renal failure
  Insulin injection in hypertrophic sites
Decreased endogenous glucose production
  Severe liver disease
  Defective glucagon or epinephrine counterregulation
  Alcohol ingestion

also reported a mortality rate of 7.5% among patients experiencing sulfonylurea-induced severe hypoglycemia (36). The overall mortality rate in cases of severe sulfonylurea-induced hypoglycemia is approximately 10% (44).

Van Staa et al. found that 605 of 34,052 sulfonylurea users experienced hypoglycemia during therapy, which converts to an annual risk of 1.8% (45). People aged 65 years or older experienced a rate of 427 cases of hypoglycemia per 21,706 persons-years of sulfonylurea therapy, which is equivalent to an annual risk of 2.0% compared to an annual risk of 1.4% for people aged less than 65 years.

When individual sulfonylurea agents are considered, drugs with longer time-action characteristics have an increased potential for causing hypoglycemia. Glyburide (glibenclamide) exhibited an incidence of severe hypoglycemia of 16.6%, a rate that was twice that of glipizide and fivefold greater than the rate for tolbutamide (46). Stahl and Berger report that the odds ratio for severe hypoglycemia requiring hospital admission per 1000 years was three times higher in those treated with long-acting sulfonylureas among Swedish patients in their analysis (47).

Jennings et al. reported that the rate of hypoglycemic symptoms experienced by sulfonylurea-treated type 2 diabetes patients during any given month was 5.9% (48). Additionally, mean glycosylated hemoglobin and postprandial plasma glucose were reduced in patients reporting hypoglycemic symptoms compared to those without symptoms. On the other hand, Burge et al. performed a prospective, randomized, placebo-controlled study of three of the major risk factors for sulfonylurea-induced hypoglycemia, including maximal-dose sulfonylurea ingestion, advanced age, and missed meals (i.e., breakfast and lunch) among 52 type 2 diabetic subjects during a 23-hour fast. The study found that this combination of risk factors does not result in hypoglycemia in otherwise healthy elderly diabetic subjects receiving maximal doses of once-daily oral sulfonylureas (49).

Potentiators of Sulfonylureas

Many drugs potentiate the action of sulfonylureas through a variety of mechanisms. Known mechanisms of prolonged sulfonylurea action include displacement of sulfonylureas from their protein-binding sites, decreased sulfonylurea clearance rates, and decreased sulfonylurea metabolism rates (50). All sulfonylureas are extensively bound to albumin. The first-generation sulfonylureas (such as chlorpropamide and tolbutamide) exhibit ionic binding with the plasma proteins. Therefore, charged drugs such as warfarin and salicylates are able to readily displace the first generation sulfonylureas, thus predisposing subjects to hypoglycemia. On the other hand, the second-generation sulfonylureas (such as glipizide and glyburide) exhibit nonionic binding to plasma proteins and so are not easily displaced. This property of the second-generation sulfonylureas effectively minimizes drug interactions. Table 6 lists known drug–drug interactions that potentiate the hypoglycemic action of sulfonylureas.

Except for acetohexamide, the liver metabolizes all sulfonylureas. Chronic liver disease causes decreased sulfonylurea clearance, prolonged sulfonylurea half-life, and increased free drug concentrations due to hypoalbuminemia, resulting in increased risk of hypoglycemia (41). The half-life of sulfonylureas is also prolonged in renal disease. Glyburide and tolazamide have active metabolites that accumulate when the glomerular filtration rate falls below 30 mL per minute, but glipizide and tolbutamide are excreted only in small amounts by the kidneys, and because their metabolites are less active, these drugs may be preferable in the setting of moderate-to-severe renal insufficiency (41). Regardless, sulfonylureas should be used with extreme caution in the setting of renal insufficiency.

Unanticipated Hypoglycemia with Sulfonylurea Therapy

Unanticipated hypoglycemia may be disabling to patients, is widely recognized as the primary adverse effect of sulfonylurea therapy, and is frequently cited by physicians and patients alike as a reason for not achieving better glycemic control (41). Brodows has noted that nearly 10% of ambulatory home blood glucose readings were 4.5 mmol/L or less among his elderly patients using sulfonylureas, suggesting that elderly patients are at a significant risk of unanticipated hypoglycemia on a daily basis (51). Furthermore, elderly people may develop hypoglycemia

TABLE 6 Drugs that Potentiate the Hypoglycemic Action of Sulfonylureas

Drugs	Interaction
Clofibrate Phenylbutazone Salicylates Sulfonamides	Displacement of sulfonylurea from plasma proteins
Dicumarol Chloramphenicol MAO Inhibitors Sulfaphenazole Phenylbutazone	Reduces hepatic sulfonylurea metabolism
Allopurinol Probenecid Phenylbutazone Salicylates Sulfonamides	Decreases urinary excretion of sulfonylureas or their metabolites
Insulin Alcohol β-Adrenergic antagonists Salicylates MAO Inhibitors Guanethidine	Have intrinsic hypoglycemic activity

Abbreviation: MAO, monoamine oxidase.
Source: From Ref. 51.

during periods of light activity such as golfing or grocery shopping. This phenomenon may be the result of an age-related decline in β-adrenergic receptor function (52).

ANTIHYPERTENSIVES AND HYPOGLYCEMIA

About 73% of adults with diabetes have hypertension, and people with diabetes have heart-disease death rates two to four times higher than adults without diabetes. Blood-pressure control is central to diabetic-patient care in that it can reduce the risk of cardiovascular disease (heart disease or stroke) by 33% to 50% (53). Therefore, the concern that antihypertensives, specifically β-blockers and ACE inhibitors, might increase the risk of hypoglycemia has been an important one in the treatment of elderly diabetics. Anxiety over β-blocker therapy has centered on its potential to blunt the autonomic warning symptoms of hypoglycemia. Alternatively, an increase in insulin sensitivity has been the mechanism thought to cause potential hypoglycemia with ACE inhibitor therapy.

Two large studies have addressed the risk of antihypertensive therapy and hypoglycemia in the elderly population. In a retrospective cohort study with 13,559 elderly diabetic patients, Shorr et al. found no significant increase in risk of serious hypoglycemia with the use of any class of antihypertensive drugs including β-blockers and ACE inhibitors (54). Additionally, a case-control study of 3477 elderly (mean age 71.4 years), hospitalized patients showed no significant association between antihypertensive therapy and occurrence of hypoglycemia (55). With the known cardiovascular and renal protection by β-blockers and ACE inhibitors, these studies support the current opinion that their use should not be restricted in patients with diabetes based on concern of their becoming affected with hypoglycemia.

ALCOHOL-ASSOCIATED HYPOGLYCEMIA

Alcohol intake impairs glucose counterregulation during insulin-induced hypoglycemia in type 1 diabetes and so may be considered to be a risk factor for hypoglycemia. Rasmussen et al., however, did not find oral alcohol ingestion to impair recovery from insulin-induced hypoglycemia in early type 2 diabetes patients (56). Conversely, Burge et al. demonstrated that minimum plasma glucose concentrations were reduced in 10 elderly type 2 diabetes patients when low-dose ethanol was infused intravenously during hours 14 and 15 of a 24-hour fast compared to

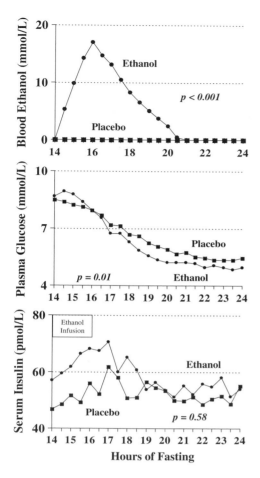

FIGURE 4 Concentrations of blood ethanol, plasma glucose, and serum insulin during the final 10 hours of a 24-hour fast among 10 elderly subjects with type 2 diabetes receiving low-dose intravenous ethanol or placebo in addition to sulfonylurea therapy. Squares represent the placebo study and circles represent the ethanol study. *Source*: From Ref. 57.

placebo infusion (4.4 ± 1.2 mmol/L vs. 5.0 ± 1.4 mmol/L; $p = 0.01$) (57). As shown in Figure 4, these results suggest that low doses of ethanol predispose fasted, elderly type 2 diabetic patients to low blood glucose during a short-term fast. Further studies have demonstrated that glucose production is suppressed by low-dose intravenous ethanol infusion in subjects with type 2 diabetes, but not in nondiabetic subjects, during recovery from insulin-induced hypoglycemia (58). Moreover, peak epinephrine responses to hypoglycemia were delayed following the glycemic nadir in subjects with type 2 diabetes during the ethanol study compared to the placebo study, but no such delay was observed in nondiabetic subjects (59). These results suggest that contrary to the situation in nondiabetic subjects, low-dose ethanol delays recovery from hypoglycemia in subjects with type 2 diabetes. These observations are at least partially attributable to impaired glucose counterregulation, secondary to ethanol.

ANTIBIOTICS AND HYPOGLYCEMIA

Several case reports of sulfonamide-induced hypoglycemia have been published in the literature. Similar to sulfonylureas, these antibiotics are thought to cause hypoglycemia by increasing pancreatic secretion of insulin (60). Its occurrence usually happens in the setting of decreased renal function, although other risk factors include prolonged fasting, malnutrition, and concomitant sulfonylurea use (61). More recently, attention has focused on the association of gatifloxacin, a fluoroquinolone, with both hypoglycemia and hyperglycemia. In a nested case control study, gatifloxacin use was associated with a fourfold increase in hypoglycemia when compared to the use of macrolide antibiotics (62). Animal studies suggest that the mechanism for this hypoglycemia is the stimulation of insulin secretion by inhibition of pancreatic β-cell adenosine triphosphate–sensitive potassium channels (63). More studies will be needed to ascertain if other medications in the fluoroquinolone class confer the same risk of dysglycemia. For now, gatifloxacin use should be avoided in the elderly diabetic patient since there are several other broad spectrum antibiotics available that have not been associated with hypoglycemia. Finally, intravenous pentamidine has well-documented toxic effects on pancreatic β cells and can cause hypoglycemia as insulin is released from damaged cells (64).

EXERCISE AND HYPOGLYCEMIA

One prospective study found no increase in the tendency to hypoglycemia among 25 obese, sulfonylurea-receiving type 2 diabetes subjects who performed 90 minutes of aerobic exercise on a treadmill after an overnight fast (65). Nevertheless, Katz postulates that elderly diabetic patients who exercise may have (*i*) inappropriately high insulin concentrations despite increased insulin sensitivity after exercise, (*ii*) increased insulin absorption from injection sites over exercising muscle, and/or (*iii*) increased insulin secretion and more avid glucose utilization (66). All of these factors may predispose patients to delayed hypoglycemia after exercise. In a study of 37 type 2 diabetes patients treated with insulin, Herz et al. found that patients utilizing a prepared 25/75 mixture of insulin lispro and neutral protamine hagedorn (NPH) were less inclined to experience hypoglycemia when insulin was injected three hours prior to moderate exercise than were patients receiving a 70/30 mixture of NPH and regular insulin (0.7 ± 0.2 episodes/month vs. 1.2 ± 0.3 episodes/month; $p = 0.04$) (67).

DEFECTIVE COUNTERREGULATORY MECHANISMS

Type 1 diabetes patients are at a high risk of developing severe hypoglycemia when counterregulatory mechanisms fail to respond appropriately. More than 50% of patients with longstanding type 1 diabetes exhibit some degree of deficient counterregulatory mechanisms. Specifically, they are unable to secrete glucagon due to (*i*) defective glucose sensing by the pancreatic α cells, and (*ii*), minimal or absent β-cell function to complement and facilitate normal glucagon secretion (68–70). The absence of a glucagon response to declining plasma glucose concentrations, in conjunction with the presence of (exogenous) hyperinsulinemia, is a critical pathophysiologic feature of defective counterregulation in type 1 diabetes. Attenuation of the epinephrine response also eventually occurs after repeated exposure to hypoglycemia. A vast majority of patients with type 1 diabetes for more than five years exhibit an abnormality in epinephrine secretion in response to hypoglycemia. Type 1 diabetes patients with a combination of acquired glucagon and epinephrine deficiencies are at a 25-fold or greater risk of developing severe hypoglycemia compared to patients with intact counterregulatory mechanisms (24,25).

Two separate studies have demonstrated an age-related impairment in epinephrine and glucagon secretion in healthy, nondiabetic elderly individuals (71,72). The magnitude of this deficit is depicted in Figure 5. Meneilly et al. studied the counterregulatory hormone responses of elderly diabetic patients and found that there was reduced incremental secretion of glucagon

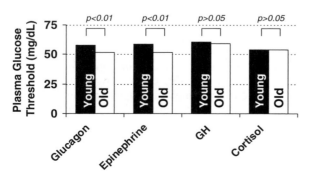

FIGURE 5 Plasma glucose thresholds for the release of glucagon and epinephrine are reduced in healthy older patients. *Abbreviation*: GH, growth hormone. *Source*: From Ref. 71.

and GH at a glucose concentration of 2.0 mmol/L, but that epinephrine and cortisol responses were increased (73). More recently, Segel et al. demonstrated that, as is the case in type 1 diabetes, the glucagon response to hypoglycemia was virtually absent in type 2 diabetes patients approaching the insulin-deficient end of the disease spectrum (74). In the same study, there was also a shift to higher glycemic thresholds (i.e., lower glucose concentrations, or greater degrees of hypoglycemia, are required to elicit a response) for autonomic and symptomatic responses to hypoglycemia precipitated by recent antecedent hypoglycemia, thus predisposing patients to a vicious cycle of iatrogenic hypoglycemia. A different study attempted to determine the effects of glycemic control on counterregulatory responses to hypoglycemia in patients with type 2 diabetes. The study showed that poorly controlled type 2 diabetes patients have exaggerated counterregulatory responses to declining blood glucose concentrations even during normoglycemia (75). After glycemic control is improved in these patients, their counterregulatory responses are diminished, thereby narrowing the gap between the onset of symptoms and the onset of cognitive impairment. The authors postulate that this phenomenon predisposes insulin dependent type 2 patients to asymptomatic and potentially severe hypoglycemia.

Similarly, another study evaluated the effect of a short-term improvement in glycemic control on plasma glucose thresholds for symptomatic and hormonal responses to hypoglycemia in patients with type 2 diabetes (76). Of the elderly patients, 10 with type 2 diabetes were admitted for an eight-day inpatient protocol. All subjects underwent insulin-induced hypoglycemia before and after the short-term implementation of intensified diabetes management. As shown in Figure 6, plasma glucose thresholds for epinephrine release during insulin-induced hypoglycemia is higher compared to baseline following the week of intensive management (3.7 ± 0.5 mmol/L vs. 3.1 ± 0.3 mmol/L, $p < 0.05$). The plasma glucose threshold for hypoglycemic symptoms was also increased by intensive therapy from a glucose concentration (5.3 ± 1.2 mmol/L vs. 3.3 ± 0.6 mmol/L, $p = 0.003$). Thus, rapid changes in prevailing glycemia appear to increase the risk of developing severe hypoglycemia in patients with type 2 diabetes.

HYPOGLYCEMIC UNAWARENESS

Hypoglycemic unawareness is defined as a lack of appropriate autonomic warning signals before the development of neuroglycopenia. According to Gerich, the predisposing factors to

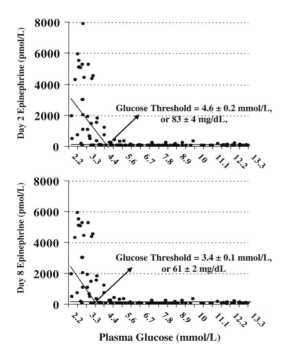

FIGURE 6 Pooled results for plasma epinephrine as a function of plasma glucose during insulin-induced hypoglycemia following one week of baseline diabetes therapy (*Top*) and one week of intensive diabetes therapy (*Bottom*) in 10 elderly subjects with type 2 diabetes. $P < 0.001$ for glucose threshold for epinephrine release on baseline therapy versus intensive therapy by unpaired Student's t-test. *Source*: From Ref. 76.

hypoglycemic unawareness are an increased prevalence of antecedent, severe hypoglycemia; a longer duration of diabetes; a lower hemoglobin A_{1C} (HbA$_{1C}$) level; and the utilization of intensified diabetes management (77). In his stepped hypoglycemic clamp study of 43 type 1 diabetes patients, he demonstrated that counterregulatory hormone responses, neuroglycopenic symptoms, and cognitive dysfunction began at lowered plasma glucose concentrations in the unaware patients. Moreover, the magnitude of plasma catecholamine responses and autonomic symptoms were reduced in patients who lacked awareness of hypoglycemia.

Gold et al. prospectively studied type 1 diabetes patients with hypoglycemic unawareness to determine their frequency of severe hypoglycemia (78). They reported an overall annual incidence of 2.8 episodes per patient per year. This study also reported that type 1 diabetes patients with hypoglycemia unawareness possessed a sixfold increase in the risk of developing severe hypoglycemia. Such patients are more prone to severe hypoglycemia at any time of the day, but these events occur most often after supper (i.e., between 6 P.M. and midnight). Veneman et al. also found that frequent episodes of asymptomatic nocturnal hypoglycemia caused higher plasma glucose thresholds for counterregulatory hormone release, reduced the magnitude of autonomic and neuroglycopenic symptoms, and delayed cognitive dysfunction, thus predisposing the patients to hypoglycemic unawareness (79).

All of the above studies involved young, type 1 diabetes subjects. Unfortunately, there have been no definitive studies of the extent or magnitude of hypoglycemia unawareness in type 2 diabetic subjects on insulin, although recent data suggest that an analogous situation exists in insulin-requiring type 2 diabetes patients (74).

GUIDELINES FOR GLUCOSE MONITORING AMONG ELDERLY PATIENTS WITH DIABETES

Self-monitoring of blood glucose (SMBG) is an integral part of diabetes self-management programs. SMBG is utilized to determine patterns and maintain glucose levels for short- and long-term–assessment glycemic control (80). SMBG also gives patients a sense of autonomy and control over their disease as well as a feedback on the impact of their lifestyle on control of their diabetes. Studies have demonstrated that routine SMBG results in improved problem-solving ability among patients, and the immediate feedback of SMBG gives patients and providers the ability to detect and prevent severe hypoglycemia and hyperglycemia (81–86). SMBG also has utility in the adjustment of care based on individual responses to lifestyle or pharmacologic intervention (80).

Successful evaluations of intensive insulin therapy have utilized SMBG as a component of their management programs (7,8,87). As shown in Figure 7, Burge demonstrated that self-reported adherence to recommended self-monitoring frequency is inversely related to physician visits and hospitalizations (88). Numerous consensus guidelines and recommendations have evaluated SMBG efficacy in the care of patients with diabetes. SMBG is widely recommended for insulin-treated patients (80,89–92). The American Diabetes Association

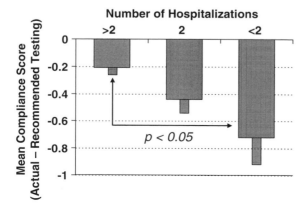

FIGURE 7 Hospitalization rates increase as compliance with self-monitoring of blood glucose recommendations declines. *Source*: From Ref. 88.

(ADA) recommends that SMBG be performed three or more times each day for patients on multiple insulin injections. Increased testing is also recommended when adjustments are made to the regimen, during illness, and when glycemic control is not at target levels (80). The frequency of SMBG ultimately depends on the type of therapy being employed, the risk of hypoglycemia, and the presence or absence of hypoglycemia unawareness. A recent report from a global consensus conference provides more specific guidelines for SMBG (93). This report's recommendation for SMBG in patients managed with insulin pumps or multiple insulin injections is more than three to four times daily. Specifically, blood glucose testing should include preprandial and postprandial assessments in addition to occasional assessments at 2 to 3 A.M.

The need for routine SMBG in patients with type 2 diabetes on oral and/or nonpharmacological therapy is controversial. Although a number of studies now support the practice of SMBG in non–insulin-treated patients with type 2 diabetes, several other studies have not supported its use in this patient population (80,82,85,94–100). The lack of appropriate education on proper SMBG technique and interpretation may account for some of the discrepancy between these studies. Two recent meta-analyses and a large retrospective cohort study have demonstrated that patients utilizing SMBG as part of their diabetes management had greater reductions in their HbA_{1C} levels, and SMBG was further associated with a decrease in diabetes-related morbidity and all-cause mortality (101–103). Murata has also demonstrated that episodes of hypoglycemia might be predicted by increased variability in glycemic excursions among patients with type 2 diabetes (104). Hence, the ADA recommends routine SMBG in patients receiving oral and nonpharmacological treatment for diabetes but remains unclear as to the optimal frequency of such testing (80). Conversely, the global consensus conference report provides guidelines on SMBG for patients receiving less-intensive insulin and oral treatment regimens. Recommendations for patients receiving only one injection of insulin daily, either in conjunction with oral agents or alone, are stratified by glycemic control. If a patient is above target glycemic goals, SMBG should be performed two or more times daily (93). Once target glycemic goals are achieved, SMBG should be completed one or more times daily, including preprandial and postprandial levels on more than one day per week (82,85). In cases where patients are treated with only nonpharmacological management, assessments of blood glucose levels in response to diet and exercise are recommended on a weekly basis (93). All of the consensus statements and guidelines encourage more frequent monitoring during acute or concurrent illness, when glycemic control fails to achieve targets, and during adjustment of therapeutic regimens.

The ADA and recent consensus statement both mention the option of reducing the frequency of monitoring in older adults (80,93). In 2003, a panel from the California Healthcare Foundation and the American Geriatrics Society provided guidelines for improving diabetes care in older adults (105). These guidelines recommend stratification of older patients based on life expectancy and functional status, in addition to consideration of the patient's goals and preferences for treatment. A less stringent HbA_{1C} target level of less than 8% was recommended for patients with life expectancy of less than five years, but a target of less than 7% was retained for individuals with a life expectancy greater than five years (105). Huang et al. evaluated the stratification of older adults by physician-estimated life expectancy, age in years, number of activities of daily living that required assistance, and the Modified Charleston Co-morbidity Index Score. Of the patients, 61% to 83% achieved the target goal of HbA_{1C} less than 8% in this study (106). Recommendations for SMBG frequency in elderly patients with diabetes are shown in Table 7. Development of a standardized stratification plan for older adults and the impact that these less-stringent recommendations will have on patients' quality of life are still under investigation. Currently, such determinations should be made on a case-specific basis, depending on the presence of hypoglycemia unawareness, the frequency of hypoglycemic episodes, the risk of hypoglycemia associated with the selected treatment regimen, and the patient barriers to SMBG.

BARRIERS TO SMBG FACED BY ELDERLY PATIENTS

As discussed earlier, SMBG is essential for the glycemic control of patients with diabetes, particularly those patients utilizing insulin therapy (7,80). Nevertheless, the practice of

TABLE 7   Summary of Guidelines for Self-Monitoring Blood Glucose in Elderly Diabetes Patients

American Diabetes Association	
Target HbA$_{1c}$ level	<7%
Daily self-monitoring blood glucose frequency	
Intensive insulin treatment (type 1 or type 2 diabetes)	≥3 times[a]
Less-intensive insulin treatment/oral treatment	Enough to maintain control[a]
Report of global consensus conference on glucose-monitoring panel	
Self-monitoring blood glucose frequency	
Type 1 diabetes mellitus	
Type 2 diabetes mellitus	3–4 times[a,b]
At target glycemic control	
Treatment with single insulin injection and/or oral therapy	
Not at target glycemic control	≥1 time[a,c]
Single insulin injection and/or oral therapy	≥2 times[a,c]
California Healthcare Foundation/American Geriatrics Society modification of target A1c levels for older adults by life expectancy	
Life expectancy:	Target *A1c* level
>5 yr	<7%
<5 yr	<8%

[a]Increased frequency is recommended during adjustments in treatment, acute illness, and when glycemic control is not at target levels.
[b]Include in monitoring pre-/postprandial and occasional 2–3 A.M. levels. Increased frequency of monitoring with multiple episodes of hypoglycemia.
[c]A weekly profile of pre-/postprandial levels on ≥1 day/wk should be included in frequency.
Abbreviation: HbA$_1$c, hemoglobin A$_1$c.

self-monitoring among elderly patients with diabetes has not changed despite increasing evidence of its efficacy (86,107). In general, those patients who are at highest risk of poor glycemic control and diabetes complications are not monitoring their blood sugars regularly (7,86,108–110). Karter et al. found that an age greater than 65 years was an independent risk factor of not adhering to SMBG practices (110). To improve SMBG in such patients, education and diabetes self-care should be adopted for older adults (90).

There are numerous barriers to self-care behaviors in diabetes, including SMBG, identified in the literature. The barriers can be classified into health beliefs and self-efficacy, cost, and physical barriers (108,111,112).

Health Beliefs and Self-Efficacy

SMBG requires self-motivated action by patients as well as an ability to gain knowledge of the appropriate technique and interpretation of the results. Perception that the efficacy of SMBG is limited is a common health-belief barrier. In the time permitted during provider visits, it can be difficult to identify this barrier. Comments that "my sugar never changes, so why do I need to check it?," or "I can tell when my blood sugar is high or low without checking it," may indicate to a provider that the patient does not adhere to SMBG recommendations due to this health belief (113,114). But older adults are at a high risk of hypoglycemic unawareness. In one survey, older patients reported that adherence to SMBG was more important than diet and exercise. These patients identified independence in activities of daily living and a goal to be healthy as primary health-care goals, potentially influencing the high level of self-monitoring in this study (83%) (115). The importance of recognizing episodes of hypoglycemia, frequent education about patient-specific hypoglycemia symptoms, and the importance of the information provided by SMBG might ultimately decrease this barrier.

The ability to accurately interpret and react to SMBG data is imperative for using it to effectively prevent and treat hypoglycemia. Skelly et al. found that less than 30% of older adults in a rural community were shown how to interpret their SMBG data (111). Hence, diabetes education should be adopted for older adults by providing increased episodes of knowledge transfer and opportunities for the patients to demonstrate the self-monitoring technique and the interpretation of blood glucose results. Providers should also provide positive feedback to reinforce patients' belief in their capability to complete the tasks involved in self-monitoring. Assistance with SMBG by family members or caregivers may be necessary for individuals who are unable to effectively complete the tasks involved in SMBG (81). In addition, family members can provide reinforcement of self-monitoring education in between provider visits.

Physical Barriers to Diabetes Self-Care
Vision
Diabetes is a leading cause of visual impairment in the United States. In 2003, three million adults with diabetes reported visual impairment. Approximately 28% of adults older than 75 years reported visual impairment even with their corrective lenses (116). Visual impairment further complicates self-care practices. Adequate vision is essential in the process of SMBG. Patients must be able to read and code their glucose meter, lance their finger, locate the lanced site, and properly apply the blood droplet to a test strip.

Patients should have visits for dilated eye exams and visual acuity tests at least yearly to continually assess the presence and/or extent of visual impairment, in addition to the provision of interventions that may stabilize or improve vision, such as laser photocoagulation and cataract removal. During SMBG education and followup, patients should learn to handle the glucose meter and describe the aspects of the meter, use frames of reference for placement of the test strip and other supplies, directly observe the process, and provide feedback (117,118). Selection of glucose meters is important for patients with visual impairment. As elucidated in Table 8, several glucose meters are now available with features that decrease the impact of visual impairment on the accuracy and frequency of self-monitoring (119).

Adaptive devices can also assist patients with visual impairment in other aspects of their diabetes control. Caps are available for insulin vials with a guided hole for assistance in placement of the syringe. Devices are also available to fill syringes to a set amount. Magnifiers are available for both syringes and insulin pens to enlarge print or font. The Innolet device and various insulin pens with auditory indicators help ensure injection of the correct dosage of insulin. Some insulin pumps are also equipped with the ability to increase font size, provide auditory alerts, and assist with catheter placement (120).

Fine Motor Agility and Coordination
Although most of the barriers to self-monitoring focus on visual impairment, there are other physical changes that require adjustment of self-monitoring techniques or tools. Older adults may experience a decrease in their dexterity due to musculoskeletal or neurological conditions such as arthritis, stroke, and Parkinson's disease. These impairments result in decreased ability to handle the smaller glucose meters, difficulty calibrating the glucose meters, and difficulty handling test strips. Technological advances in glucose meters may decrease these barriers by providing automatic calibration, preloaded test strips (Accuchek Compact or Ascensia meters), and/or larger test strips with physical guides for placement of the blood droplet (Comfort Curve test strips) (117,121).

Some glucose meters are capable of testing at alternative sites such as the forearm or thigh. Testing at these sites should be limited to SMBG during a fasting state because of decreased sensitivity to detect rapid changes in glucose levels following meals or during episodes of hypoglycemia (122–124). Alternative testing sites may prove useful for patients who have not been self-monitoring regularly because of the physical discomfort associated with testing procedures. Continuous glucose monitoring (CGM) devices assess shifts in blood

TABLE 8   Desirable Features of Glucose Meters for Visually Impaired Patients

---

Adjustable or larger font size and thickness
Touchable test strip
No requirement for coding
Ability to apply additional blood to sample
Auditory alert for adequate blood sample and/or completion of test
Voice output

---

glucose levels throughout the day, but they do not provide immediate feedback to alert the patient of a hypoglycemic or hyperglycemic event. The accuracy of CGM is not equivalent to that obtained with finger-stick glucose monitoring, particularly at lower blood glucose levels, and these devices are not approved for use in adjusting insulin doses (125–127).

Language
The inability to communicate in English has been identified as a barrier to SMBG. Participants in a survey of patients with diabetes receiving pharmacological treatment from Kaiser Permanente Northern California Region found that limited English fluency resulted in less-frequent SMBG (110). Historically, educational materials and instruction manuals have been available in only a few languages, but this is no longer the case. Some glucose meters have the capability to switch languages, and numerous translations of educational documents and instruction manuals are available (128).

Cognitive Function
Hypoglycemia has been associated with cognitive dysfunction, which may contribute to reduced self-care and ability to monitor and interpret self-monitoring data. Pramming et al. have reported that cognitive dysfunction occurs acutely even during asymptomatic bouts of hypoglycemia (129). A prospective study of cognitive function in elderly diabetes patients reported that diabetic subjects have diminished global cognitive performance as compared to their nondiabetic counterparts (130). Although mild hypoglycemia is well tolerated, patients who undergo repeated episodes of hypoglycemia are likely to be emotionally distressed, and this distress may ultimately manifest as increased caloric intake and poorly controlled diabetes (77). Careful attention to cognitive ability during the assessment of elderly patients allows for extra educational support to be provided or for family members to become involved in the patient's self-care when necessary.

Cost

Cost barriers relate to both monetary and time impact on the performance of self-care behaviors. Inconvenience is frequently reported as a barrier to patients testing their blood glucose (131,132). Older patients are less likely to experience difficulty integrating blood testing into a work schedule or between group activities, and peer pressure is also lower among older adults than among younger patients with diabetes (132,133). The addition of testing to an older patient's daily activities, however, may make the patient uncomfortable, resulting in a lack of testing.

Patients of lower socioeconomic status are less likely to participate in SMBG, a fact that may be partially attributable to a limited access to health care (134). The expense of test strips or a lack of insurance coverage for the appropriate number of test strips often limits the practice of SMBG (110,135). Manufacturers of glucose meters and test strips have decreased this barrier by providing rebates and meter exchanges, but test strips remain too costly for many patients. Fortunately, most elderly patients are specifically protected against this barrier because Medicare now covers the cost of test strips.

In summary, frequent reassessment and reinforcement of teaching as well as the use of family members or chronic caregivers as intermediaries may increase the likelihood of effective self-care activities as patients age.

STRATEGIES TO PREVENT HYPOGLYCEMIA IN ELDERLY DIABETIC SUBJECTS
Patient Education

Education is the key to preventing recurrent and severe hypoglycemia. Thomson et al., in their study of elderly diabetics, have shown that 88% of patients receiving oral hypoglycemic agents and 32% of patients receiving insulin therapy did not possess any significant knowledge regarding hypoglycemia (136). This study highlights the need for intensive education programs specifically targeting elderly patients with diabetes. Elderly patients should be taught to recognize the symptoms of hypoglycemia and its appropriate treatment. Emphasis should be placed on the importance of periodic home blood glucose monitoring, especially when symptoms that may be attributable to hypoglycemia occur. Family, friends, and colleagues should also be aware of appropriate hypoglycemia management. Safe driving should be emphasized, and elderly patients who are prone to hypoglycemia should routinely check their blood glucose before driving.

Schillinger and colleagues found that 30% of type 2 diabetic patients with poor glycemic control had inadequate health literacy (134). Patients with inadequate health literacy were less likely to achieve acceptable glycemic control (adjusted odds ratio = 0.57). Similarly, Colleran et al. performed the Michigan Diabetes Knowledge Test on 77 subjects with type 2 diabetes and found an inverse correlation between number of correct responses and HbA_{1c} values. For each additional question answered correctly, HbA_{1c} decreased by 0.239% (r = −0.337, $P < 0.003$) (137). These results suggest that improved diabetes knowledge improves glycemic control.

The same study reports a high incidence of diabetic complications among patients with poor health literacy. This study stresses the urgent need to critically evaluate and remodel current patient education methods. All health-care workers must be encouraged to actively participate in patient education.

Role of Physicians and Health-Care Providers

At each follow-up visit, physicians should inquire about the occurrence of hypoglycemia. They should evaluate possible causes of hypoglycemia, including inappropriate insulin dosing, inappropriate combination therapy, or the use of long-acting sulfonylureas. Providers should also make an effort to assess for possible drug interactions and should query the patient about his/her eating habits and caution about the danger of erratic eating behavior. Finally, the existence of comorbid diseases such as renal or hepatic disease that increase the risk of hypoglycemia, should be sought.

Because elderly people may be prone to forgetfulness, physicians should take the time to review and reinforce recognition and treatment of hypoglycemic symptoms. Specific instructions such as how to avoid exercise-induced hypoglycemia and caution about the use of ethanol should be routinely provided. Patients on insulin should be instructed to assess their blood glucose before, during, and after exercise. Additionally, insulin-requiring patients should be advised to administer their insulin into the abdomen or another nonexercising area in order to avoid rapid absorption by the exercising muscles. Reducing insulin doses by 50% or ingesting supplemental carbohydrate will usually provide adequate safeguards against hypoglycemia (66).

The incidence of serious hypoglycemia by long-acting sulfonylureas is higher when compared to short-acting sulfonylureas. In order to prevent serious hypoglycemic episodes, it is prudent to switch the patients on long-acting sulfonylureas, who experience repeated hypoglycemic episodes, to short-acting sulfonylureas (34,35,45–47,138,139).

One recent randomized, controlled trial of insulin glargine versus NPH in combination with glimepiride has demonstrated a decrease in the frequency of nocturnal hypoglycemia among patients using glargine. Specifically, the frequency of nocturnal hypoglycemia was reduced from 23% with bedtime NPH to 17% with insulin glargine (140). Another study reported that only 30% of the patients on bedtime insulin glargine experienced hypoglycemic episodes compared to 50% of patients receiving NPH insulin (141).

Because of the reduced risk of hypoglycemia associated with insulin glargine, it may be the long-acting insulin of choice in elderly patients with type 2 diabetes. Insulin detemir is a new long-acting insulin that has also been shown to be associated with reduced risk of hypoglycemia compared to NPH insulin, but head-to-head comparisons with insulin glargine or among elderly patients have not been performed.

Because metformin has recently been demonstrated to have several potential metabolic benefits including reductions in relevant glycemic and macrovascular endpoints and possibility of weight loss, many diabetes care providers now preferentially use metformin as first-line therapy for obese patients with type 2 diabetes (8,141). Although metformin can be used as first-line therapy in elderly subjects, physicians should keep the potential side effects of metformin in mind, especially in view of the fact that creatinine clearance decreases with age. Careful periodic monitoring of renal function should occur when elderly patients are receiving this drug.

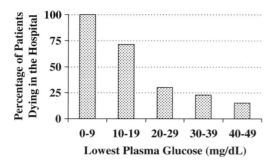

FIGURE 8 Mortality rates according to severity of hypoglycemia for 94 hospitalized patients experiencing at least one episode of documented hypoglycemia (glucose < 50 mg/dL) during their hospitalization. *Source*: From Ref. 142.

Fischer's study of hypoglycemia in hospitalized patients found that 90% of the hypoglycemic episodes that occur in the hospital setting were attributable to the excessive administration of insulin (142). The study also states that renal insufficiency unrelated to diabetes was the second commonest cause for hypoglycemia in hospitalized patients. There are currently no established guidelines for the treatment of diabetes in hospitalized patients, but some studies strongly suggest improved outcomes if glycemia is tightly controlled in the hospital setting. When diabetic patients are hospitalized, it is a common practice to continue them on the same regimen they receive at home. During a hospital stay, however, normal lifestyle is disrupted. Specifically, patients tend to eat less. Caloric intake may be markedly reduced secondary to the illness itself or the comorbid conditions, not to mention the common need for fasting status as a prerequisite for diagnostic tests. Thus, a better approach to the treatment of diabetes in the hospital is to tailor therapy according to the individual patient needs. In some patients, dosing fast-acting insulin analogs after meal ingestion may be appropriate if caloric intake is variable and unpredictable. Provision of long-acting background insulin along with a variable dose of rapid-acting insulin is often the most expedient way to address all these concerns. Figure 8 depicts the mortality risk associated with hypoglycemia in hospitalized patients.

Elderly patients who are prone to repeated hypoglycemic episodes or nocturnal hypoglycemia should receive a thorough evaluation to ascertain and treat the underlying causes of hypoglycemia. Many recent studies have convincingly shown that strict avoidance of repetitive hypoglycemia and meticulous followup can successfully restore hypoglycemic awareness, at least in part (143–145). These same studies also demonstrate that target glycemic goals can often be achieved even while working to scrupulously avoid hypoglycemia.

One particular topic that is unique to elderly diabetes patients is the issue of diabetes care in the nursing home. Benbow et al. reported that at least 10% of the diabetic residents in a British nursing home study were at an increased risk of hospitalization (146). Moreover, protocols for treating hypoglycemia were often not available and nursing staffs were often unable to contact the proper physician in the event of a hypoglycemic event, and many nursing homes lacked appropriate supervision by diabetes-trained personnel. Hospital discharge summaries were inadequate and rarely included a future plan of care, and records often reached the wrong destination (146). The few existing protocols that addressed various aspects of diabetes management were generally very extensive, rigid, and cumbersome. In his accompanying editorial, Tattersall recommended that hospital discharge plans should include a problem list and a management plan that is communicated appropriately to the nursing home staff (147). Additionally, a protocol for diabetes management and treatment of hypoglycemia should be established, and nursing home staff should be associated with a local diabetes team for managing the complex problems of elderly diabetes patients.

SUMMARY

Numerous studies have now demonstrated the feasibility and the desirability of achieving near-normal glycemia in patients with types 1 and 2 diabetes. Among these, the Kumamoto study documented a significant reduction in microvascular complications among type 2 diabetes patients receiving intensified management with multidose insulin compared to conventionally treated, insulin-receiving type 2 patients, although the odds ratio for severe hypoglycemia was increased to 1.6 in the intensively treated group (148). Similarly, the UKPDS reported a significant reduction in microvascular endpoints in intensively managed type 2 diabetes patients as compared to conventionally treated patients (8). Finally, the DCCT documented that a mean 1% decrease in the HbA_{1C} was associated with a 45% decrease in microvascular complications (7). Whether or not these findings apply to elderly patients with diabetes remains to be determined. As always, glycemic goals should be individualized for each patient. At a minimum, diabetes therapy should be targeted to reduce symptoms of hyperglycemia (such as polyuria and polydipsia) in the elderly, and as a practical rule, glucose concentrations should be maintained as close to normal as possible without undue disruption of the patient's lifestyle or safety.

Although, taken together, these studies have revolutionized diabetes management and have improved the prospects for a healthy life with diabetes, the application of these results to older patients with diabetes is far from universal. Because of the generally younger age groups in all of these studies and because the studies often excluded older patients with chronic disease (e.g., angina, heart failure, severe concurrent illnesses, and renal disease), extrapolation of the perceived risks and benefits of intensified diabetes management to elderly patients with diabetes is limited, at best.

In general, otherwise healthy elderly diabetes patients should aim for near-normal fasting plasma glucose concentrations of less than 110 mg/dL and a HbA_{1C} of less than 7%, but treatment goals must be individualized for all patients with diabetes, and reduced cognitive or physical ability, reduced life expectancy, and/or a heavy burden of comorbid disease may necessitate increasing target glycemic goals in elderly diabetes patients. Because of its great capacity to disrupt health and quality of life, however, every step to avoid hypoglycemia should be taken for elderly diabetes patients as a matter of course. In this patient population, the prevention of hypoglycemia has great potential to enhance the quality of remaining life and to optimize compliance with the treatment program than in perhaps any other age group (149).

REFERENCES

1. Mookad AH, Ford ES, Bowman BA, et al. Diabetes trends in the U.S. 1990–98. Diabetes Care 2000; 23:1278–1283.
2. Resnick HE, Foster GL, Bardsley J, Ratner RE. Achievement of the American Diabetes Association clinical practice recommendations among U.S. adults with diabetes, 1999–2002: the national health and nutrition examination survey. Diabetes Care 2006; 29:531–537.
3. Boyle JP, Honeycutt AA, Narayan KM, et al. Projection of diabetes burden through 2050: impact of changing demography and disease prevalence in the U.S. Diabetes Care 2001; 24:1936–1940.
4. Bertoni AG, Krop JS, Anderson GF, Brancati FL. Diabetes-related morbidity and mortality in a national sample of US elders. Diabetes Care 2002; 25:471–475.
5. Krop JS, Powe NR, Weller WE, Shaffer TJ, Saudek CD, Anderson GF. Patterns of expenditures and use of services among older adults with diabetes: implications for to transition to capitated managed care. Diabetes Care 1998; 21:747–752.
6. Holstein A, Plaschke A, Egberts EH. Incidence and costs of severe hypoglycemia. Diabetes Care 2002; 25:2109–2110.
7. The Diabetes Control and Complications Trial Research Group. The effect of intensive treatment of diabetes on the development and progression of long-term complications in insulin-dependent diabetes mellitus. N Engl J Med 1993; 329:977–986.
8. The UKPDS Study Group. Intensive blood glucose control with sulfonylureas or insulin compared with conventional treatment and risk of complications in patients with type 2 diabetes (UKPDS 33). Lancet 1998; 352:837–853.
9. Cryer PE, Gerich JE. Hypoglycemic in insulin-dependent diabetes mellitus: Interplay of insulin excess and compromised glucose counterregulation. In: Porte D, Sherwin RS, eds. Ellenburg and Rifkin's Diabetes Mellitus: Theory and Practice. 5th ed. Appleton and Lange 1997:745–760.
10. Herbel G, Boyle PJ. Hypoglycemia: pathophysiology and treatment. Endocrinol Metab Clin N Am 2000; 29:725–743.
11. Pardridge WM. Brain metabolism: a perspective from the blood-brain barrier. Physiology Rev 1983; 63:1481–1535.
12. Pardridge WM, Boado RJ, Farrell CR. Brain-type glucose transporter (GLUT-1) is selectively localized to the blood brain barrier: studies with quantitative western blotting and in situ hybridization. J Biol Chem 1990; 265:18035–18040.

13. Borg MA, Sherwin RS, Borg WP, Tamborlane WV, Shulman GI. Local ventromedial hypothalamus glucose perfusion blocks counterregulation during systemic hypoglycemia in awake rats. J Clin Invest 1997; 99:361–365.

14. Borg WP, During MJ, Sherwin RS, Borg MA, Brines ML, Shulman GI. Ventromedial hypothalamus lesions in rats suppress counterregulatory hormone responses to hypoglycemia. J Clin Invest 1994; 93:1677–1682.

15. Borg WP, Sherwin RS, During MJ, Borg MA, Shulman GI. Local ventromedial hypothalamus glycopenia triggers counterregulatory hormone release. Diabetes 1995; 44:180–184.

16. Cryer PE. Glucose counterregulation: prevention and correction of hypoglycemia in humans. Am J Physiol 1993; 264(2 Pt 1):E149–E155.

17. Rizza RA, Mandarino LJ, Gerich JE. Dose-response characteristics for the effects of insulin on production and utilization of glucose in man. Am J Physiol 1981; 240:E630–E639.

18. Schwartz NS, Clutter WE, Shah SD, Cryer PE. Glycemic thresholds for activation of glucose counterregulatory systems are higher than the threshold for symptoms. J Clin Invest 1987; 79:777–781.

19. Heller SR, Cryer PE. Hypoinsulinemia is not critical to glucose recovery from hypoglycemia in humans. Am J Physiol 1991; 261:E41–E48.

20. Gerich J, Davis J, Lorenzi M, et al. Hormonal mechanisms of recovery from insulin induced hypoglycemia in man. Am J Physiol 1979; 236:E380–E385.

21. Rizza R, Cryer PE, Gerich JE. Role of Glucagon, epinephrine and growth hormone in human glucose counterregulation: effects of somatostatin and adrenergic blockade on plasma glucose recovery and glucose flux rates following insulin induced hypoglycemia. J Clin Invest 1979; 64:62–71.

22. Rizza RA, Cryer PE, Haymond MW, Gerich JE. Adrenergic mechanisms for the effect of epinephrine on glucose production and clearance in man. J Clin Invest 1980; 65:682–689.

23. Rizza RA, Cryer PE, Haymond MW, Gerich JE. Differential effects of physiological concentration of epinephrine on glucose production and disposal in man. Am J Physiol 1979; 237:E356–E362.

24. White NH, Skor DA, Cryer PE, et al. Identification of type 1 diabetic patients at increased risk for hypoglycemia during intensive therapy. N Engl J Med 1983; 308:485–491.

25. Bolli GB, DeFeo P, DeCosmo S, et al. A reliable and reproducible test for adequate glucose counterregulation in type 1 diabetes mellitus. J Clin Invest 1985; 75:1623–1631.

26. Caprio S, Gelfand RA, Tamborlane WV, Sherwin RS. Oxidative fuel metabolism during mild hypoglycemia: critical role of free fatty acids. Am J Physiol Endocrinol Metab 1989; 256:E413–E419.

27. Fanelli CG, De Feo P, Porcellati F, et al. Adrenergic mechanisms contribute to the late phase of hypoglycemic glucose counterregulation in humans by stimulating lipolysis. Clin Invest 1992; 89:2005–2013.

28. Boyle PJ, Cryer PE. Growth hormone, cortisol, or both are involved in defense against, but are not critical to recovery from, hypoglycemia. Am J Physiol 1991; 260:E395–E402.

29. Mitrakou A, Ryan C, Veneman T, et al. Hierarchy of glycemic thresholds for counterregulatory hormone secretion, symptoms, and cerebral dysfunction. Am J Physiol 1991; 260:E67–E74.

30. Bolli GB, DeFeo P, Perriello G, et al. Role of hepatic autoregulation in defense against hypoglycemia in humans. J Clin Invest 1985; 75:1623–1631.

31. Hansen I, Firth R, Haymond M, Cryer PE, Rizza R. The role of autoregulation of hepatic glucose production in man: response to a physiologic decrements in plasma glucose. Diabetes 1986; 35:186–191.

32. Campbell PJ, Bolli GB, Cryer PE, Gerich JE. Pathogenesis of the dawn phenomenon in patients with insulin-dependent diabetes mellitus: accelerated glucose production and impaired glucose utilization due to nocturnal surges in growth hormone secretion. N Engl J Med 1985; 312:1473–1479.

33. Bolli GB, Gottesman IS, Campbell PJ, Haymond MW, Cryer PE, Gerich JE. Glucose counterregulation and waning of insulin in the Somogyi phenomenon (posthypoglycemic hyperglycemia). N Engl J Med 1984; 311(19):1214–1219.

34. Shorr RI, Ray WA, Daugherty JR, Griffin MR. Incidence and risk factors for serious hypoglycemia in older persons using insulin or sulfonylureas. Arch Intern Med 1997; 157:1681–1686.

35. Zimmerman BR. Sulfonylureas. Endocrinol Metab Clin N Am 1997; 26:511–522.

36. Seltzer HS. Drug-induced hypoglycemia. A review of 1418 cases. Endocrinol Metab Clin N Am 1989; 18:163–183.

37. DeFronzo RA, Ratner RE, Kim HJ, et al. Effects of exenatide (exendin 4) on glycemic control and weight over 30 weeks in metformin-treated patients with type 2 diabetes. Diabetes Care 2005; 28:1092–1100.

38. Kendall DM, Riddle MC, Rosenstock J, et al. Effects of exenatide (exendin 4) on glycemic control over 30 weeks in patients with type 2 diabetes treated with metformin and a sulfonylurea. Diabetes Care 2005; 28:1083–1091.

39. Casparie AF, Elving LD. Severe hypoglycemic in diabetic patients: frequency, causes, prevention. Diabetes Care 1985; 8:141–145.

40. Fertig BJ, Simmons DA, Martin DB. Therapy for diabetes. In: Diabetes in America. Chapter 25. 2nd ed. Bethesda, MD: DHHS (NIH) Publication No. 95-1468, 1995:519–540.

41. Gerich JE. Oral hypoglycemic agents. N Engl J Med 1989; 321:1231–1241.

42. Wiholm BE, Westerholm B. Drug utilization and morbidity statistics for the evaluation of drug safety in Sweden. Acta Scand 1984; 683(suppl):107–117.
43. Berger W. Incidence of severe side effects during therapy with sulfonylureas and biguanides. Hormone Metab Res 1985; 17(suppl 15):111–115.
44. Campbell IW. Metformin and the sulfonylureas: the comparative risk. Hormone Meta Res 1985; 17(suppl 15):105–111.
45. Van Staa T, Abenhaim L, Monette J. Rates of hypoglycemia in users of sulfonylureas. J Clin Epidemiol 1997; 50:735–741.
46. Shorr RI, Ray WA, Daugherty JR, Griffin MR. Individual sulfonylureas and serious hypoglycemia in older people. J Am Geriatr Soc 1996; 44:751–755.
47. Stahl M, Berger W. Higher incidence of severe hypoglycemia leading to hospital admission in type 2 diabetic patients treated with long-acting versus short-acting sulfonylureas. Diabet Med 1999; 16:586–590.
48. Jennings AM, Wilson RM, Ward JD. Symptomatic hypoglycaemia in NIDDM patients treated with oral hypoglycaemic agents. Diabetes Care 1989; 12:203–208.
49. Burge MR, Schmitz-Fiorentino K, Fischette C, et al. A prospective trial of risk factors for sulfonylurea-induced hypoglycemia in type 2 diabetes mellitus. JAMA 1998; 279:137–143.
50. Walter MW. Hypoglycemia: still a risk in the elderly. Geriatrics 1990; 45:69–75.
51. Brodows RG. Benefits and risks with glyburide and glipizide in elderly NIDDM patients. Diabetes Care 1992; 15:75–80.
52. Heinsmer JA, Lefowitz RJ. The impact of aging and adrenergic receptor function: clinical and biochemical aspects. J Am Geriatr Soc 1985; 33:184–188.
53. Centers for Disease Control and Prevention. National diabetes fact sheet: general information and national estimates on diabetes in the United States, 2005. Atlanta, GA: U.S. Department of Health and Human Services, Centers for Disease Control and Prevention, 2005.
54. Shorr RI, Wayne AR, Daugherty JR, Griffin MR. Antihypertensives and the risk of serious hypoglycemia in older persons using insulin or sulfonylureas. JAMA 1997; 278:40–43.
55. Corsonello A, Pedone C, Corica F, et al. Antihypertensive drug therapy and hypoglycemia in elderly diabetic patients treated with insulin and/or sulfonylureas. Eur J Epidemiol 1999; 15:893–901.
56. Rasmussen BM, Orskov L, Schmitz O, Hermansen. Alcohol and glucose counterregulation during acute insulin induced hypoglycemia in type 2 diabetes subjects. Metabolism 2001; 50:451–457.
57. Burge MR, Zeise TM, Sobhy TA, Rassam AG, Schade DS. Low dose ethanol predisposes elderly fasted patients with type 2 diabetes to sulfonylurea-induced low blood glucose. Diabetes Care 1999; 22:2037–2043.
58. Sood V, Sobhy TA, Schade DS, Burge MR. Low dose ethanol delays recovery from hypoglycemia in type 2 diabetes. Diabetes 2000; 49(suppl 1):A66.
59. Sood V, Sobhy T, Schade DS, Burge MR. Low dose ethanol alters epinephrine responses and decreases glucose production during hypoglycemia in patients with type 2 diabetes. Diabetes 2001; 50(suppl 1):A139.
60. Mathews WA, Manint JE, Kleiss J. Trimethoprim-sulfamethoxazole-induced hypoglycemia as a cause of altered mental status in an elderly patient. J Am Board Fam Pract 2000; 13:211–212.
61. Lee AJ, Maddix DS. Trimethoprim/sulfamethoxazole-induced hypoglycemia in a patient with acute renal failure. Ann Pharmacother 1997; 31:727–732.
62. Park-Wylie LY, Juurlink DN, Kopp A, et al. Outpatient gatifloxacin therapy and dysglycemia in older adults. N Engl J Med 2006; 354:1352–1361.
63. Saraya A, Yokokura M, Gonoi T, Seino S. Effects of fluoroquinolones on insulin secretion and β-cell ATP-sensitive K+ channels. Eur J Pharmacol 2004; 497:111–117.
64. O'Brien JG, Dong BJ, Coleman RL, Gee L, Balano KB. A 5-year retrospective review of adverse drug reactions and their risk factors in human immunodeficiency virus-infected patients who were receiving intravenous pentamidine therapy for Pneumocystis carinii pneumonia. Clin Infect Dis 1997; 24:854–859.
65. Riddle MC, McDaniel PA, Tive LA. Glipizide GITS does not increase the hypoglycemic effect of mild exercise during fasting in NIDDM. Diabetes Care 1997; 20:992–994.
66. Katz MS, Lowenthal DT. Influences of Age and exercise on glucose metabolism: implications for management of older diabetics. Southern Med J 1994; 87:S70–S73.
67. Herz M, Profozic V, Arora V, et al. Effects of a fixed mixture of 25% insulin lispro and 75% NPL on plasma glucose during and after moderate physical exercise in patients with type 2 diabetes. Curr Med Res Opin 2002; 18:188–193.
68. Gerich JE, Langlois M, Noacco C, et al. Lack of glucagon response to hypoglycemia in diabetes: evidence for an intrinsic pancreatic β cell defect. Science 1973; 182:171–173.
69. Fukuda M, Tanaka A, Tahara Y, et al. Correlation between minimal secretory capacity of pancreatic β-cells and stability of diabetic control. Diabetes 1988; 37:81–88.
70. Robertson RP, Porte D Jr. The Glucose receptor: a defective mechanism in diabetes mellitus distinct from the β-adrenergic receptor. J Clin Invest 1973; 52:870–876.

71. Meneilly GS, Cheung E, Tuokko H. Altered response to hypoglycemia of healthy elderly people. J Clin Endocrinol Metab 1994; 78:1341–1348.

72. Marker JC, Cryer PE, Clutter WE. Attenuated glucose recovery from hypoglycemia in the elderly. Diabetes 1992; 41:671–678.

73. Meneilly GS, Cheung E, Tuokko H. Counterregulatory hormone responses to hypoglycemia in the elderly patient with diabetes. Diabetes 1994; 43:403–410.

74. Segel SA, Deanna SP, Paramore S, Cryer PE. Hypoglycemia-associated autonomic failure in advanced type 2 diabetes. Diabetes 2002; 51:724–733.

75. Korzon-Burakowska A, Hopkins D, Matyka K, et al. Effects of glycemic control on protective responses against hypoglycemia in type 2 diabetes. Diabetes Care 1998; 21:283–290.

76. Burge MR, Sobhy TA, Qualls CR, Schade DS. Effect of short-term glucose control on glycemic thresholds for epinephrine and hypoglycemic symptoms. J Clin Endocrinol Metab 2001; 86:5471–5478.

77. Mokan M, Mitrakou A, Veneman T, et al. Hypoglycemia unawareness in IDDM. Diabetes Care 1994; 17:1397–1403.

78. Gold AE, MacLeod KM, Frier BM. Frequency of severe hypoglycemia in patients with type I diabetes with impaired awareness of hypoglycemia. Diabetes Care 1994; 17:697–703.

79. Veneman T, Mitrakou A, Mokan M, Cryer PE, Gerich J. Induction of hypoglycemia unawareness by symptomatic nocturnal hypoglycemia. Diabetes 1993; 42:1233–1237.

80. American Diabetes Association. Standards of medical care in diabetes. Diabetes Care 2006; 29: S4–S42.

81. Mayfield J, Havas, for the AAFP Panel of Self-Monitoring of Blood Glucose. Self-control: A Physicians's Guide to Blood Glucose Monitoring in the Management of Diabetes. American Family Physician Monograph. Available at: http://www.aafp.org/x25813.xml. Accessed June 19, 2006.

82. Guerci B, Drouin P, Grange V, et al., for the ASIA group. Self-monitoring of blood glucose significantly improves metabolic control in patients with type 2 diabetes mellitus: the auto-surveillance intervention active (asia) study. Diabetes Metab 2003; 29:587–594.

83. Owens D, Barnett AH, Pickup J, et al. Blood glucose self-monitoring in type 1 and type 2 diabetes: reaching a multidisciplinary consensus. Diabetes Prim Care 2004; 6:8–16.

84. Poulsen MK, Henriksen JE, Hother-Nielsen O, Beck-Nielsen H. The combined effect of triple therapy with rosiglitazone, metformin, and insulin aspart in type 2 diabetic patients. Diabetes Care 2003; 26:3274–3279.

85. Schwedes U, Siebolds M, Mertes G, for the SMBG Study Group. Meal-related structured self-monitoring of blood glucose: effect on diabetes control in non-insulin treated type 2 diabetic patients. Diabetes Care 2002; 25:1928–1932.

86. Adams AS, Mah C, Soumerai SB, Zhang F, Barton MB, Ross-Degnan D. Barriers to self-monitoring of blood glucose among adults with diabetes in an HMO: a cross sectional study. BMC Health Serv Res 2003; 3:6.

87. Riddle MC, Rosenstock J, Gerich J. The treat-to-target trial: randomized addition of glargine or human NPH insulin to oral therapy of type 2 diabetic patients. Diabetes Care 2003; 26:3080–3086.

88. Burge MR. Lack of compliance with home blood glucose monitoring predicts hospitalization in diabetes mellitus. Diabetes Care 2001; 24:1502–1503.

89. American Association of Clinical Endocrinologists and the American College of Endocrinology. Medical guidelines for the management of diabetes mellitus: the AACE system of intensive diabetes self-management-2002 update. Endocr Pract 2002; 8:40–82.

90. American Association of Diabetes Educators. Position statement: special considerations for the education and management of older adults with diabetes. Diabetes Educ 2000; 26:37–39.

91. Burgers JS, Bailey JV, Klazinga NS, Van Der Bij AK, Grol R, Feder G, for the AGREE Collaboration. Inside guidelines: comparative analysis of recommendations and evidence in diabetes guidelines from 13 countries. Diabetes Care 2002; 25:1933–1939.

92. Canadian Diabetes Association. Canadian diabetes association 2003 clinical practice guidelines for the prevention and management of diabetes in Canada. Can J Diabet 2003; 27:S1–S152.

93. Bergenstal RM, Gavin JR, for the Global Consensus Conference on Glucose Monitoring Panel. The role of self-monitoring of blood glucose in the care of people with diabetes: report of a global consensus conference. Am J Med 2005; 118:1S–6S.

94. Coster S, Gulliford MC, Seed PT, Powrie JK, Swaminathan R. Self-monitoring in type 2 diabetes mellitus: a meta-analysis. Diabet Med 2000; 17:755–761.

95. Faas A, Schellevis FG, Van Eijk JT. The efficacy of self-monitoring of blood glucose in NIDDM: a criteria-based literature review. Diabetes Care 1997; 20:1482–1486.

96. Karter AJ, Ackerson LM, Darbinian JA, et al. Self-monitoring of blood glucose levels and glycemic control: the Northern California kaiser permanente diabetes registry. Am J Med 2001; 111:1–9.

97. Murata GH, Shah JH, Hoffman RM, et al. Intensified blood glucose monitoring improves glycemic control in stable insulin-treated veterans with type 2 diabetes: the diabetes outcomes in veterans study (DOVES). Diabetes Care 2003; 26:1759–1763.

98. Fontbonne A, Billault B, Acosta M, et al. Is glucose self-monitoring beneficial in non-insulin-treated diabetic patients? Results of a randomized comparative trial. Diabet Metab 1989; 15:255–260.

99. Miles P, Everett J, Murphy J, Kerr D. Comparison of blood or urine testing by patients with newly diagnosed non-insulin dependent diabetes: patient survey after randomized crossover trial. Br Med J 1997; 315:348–349.

100. Wing RR, Epstein LH, Nowalk MP, Scott N, Koeske R, Hagg S. Does self-monitoring of blood glucose levels improve dietary compliance for obese patients with type II diabetes? Am J Med 1986; 81:830–836.

101. Sarol JN Jr, Nicodemus NA Jr, Tan KM, Grava MB. Self-monitoring of blood glucose as part of a multi-component therapy among non-insulin requiring type 2 diabetes patients: a meta-analysis (1966-2004). Curr Med Res Opin 2005; 21:173–184.

102. Welschen LM, Bloemendal E, Nijpels G, et al. Self-monitoring of blood glucose in patients with type 2 diabetes who are not using insulin: a systematic review. Diabetes Care 2005; 28:1510–1517.

103. Martin S, Schneider B, Heinemann L, et al. for the ROSSO Study Group. Self-monitoring of blood glucose in type 2 diabetes and long-term outcome: an epidemiological cohort study. Diabetologia 2006; 49:271–278.

104. Murata GH, Hoffman RM, Shah JH, Wendel CS, Duckworth WC. A probilistic model for predicting hypoglycemia in type 2 diabetes mellitus: the diabetes outcomes in veterans study (DOVES). Arch Intern Med 2004; 164:1445–1450.

105. Brown AF, Mangione CM Sa Brown AF, Mangione CM, Saliba D, Sarkisian C. California Healthcare Foundation/American Geriatrics Society Panel on Improving Care for Elders with Diabetes. Guidelines for improving the care of the older person with diabetes mellitus. J Am Geriatr Soc 2003; 51(suppl 5):S265–S280.

106. Huang ES, Sachs GA, Chin MH. Implications of new geriatric diabetes care guidelines for the assessment of quality of care in older patients. Med Care 2006; 44:373–377.

107. United States Department of Health. Center for Disease Control and Prevention. National Center for Chronic Disease Prevention and Health Promotion. National Diabetes Surveillance System. Preventative care practices: age-adjusted rates of annual dilated eye exam, daily self-monitoring of blood glucose, foot exam in the last year, and doctor visit for diabetes in the last year per 100 adults with diabetes, United States, 1994–2004. Available at: http://www.cdc.gov/diabetes/statistics/preventive/fX.htm. Accessed on June 2, 2006.

108. Goldstein DE, Little RR, Lorenz RA, Malone JI, Nation D, Peterson CM. Tests of glycemia in diabetes. Diabetes Care 1995; 18:896–909.

109. Harris MI, Cowie CC, Howie LJ. Self-monitoring of blood glucose by adults with diabetes in the United States population. Diabetes Care 1993; 16:1116–1123.

110. Karter AJ, Ferrara A, Darbinian JA, Ackerson LM, Selby JV. Self-monitoring of blood glucose: language and financial barriers in a managed care population with diabetes. Diabetes Care 2000; 23:477–483.

111. Skelly AH, Arcury TA, Snively BM, et al. Self-monitoring of blood glucose in a multiethnic population of rural older adults with diabetes. Diabetes Educ 2005; 31:84–90.

112. Vincze G, Barner JC, Lopez D. Factors associated with adherence to self-monitoring of blood glucose among persons with diabetes. Diabetes Educ 2004; 30:112–125.

113. Aljasem LI, Peyrot M, Wissow L, Rubin RR. The impact of barriers and self-efficacy on self-care behaviors in type 2 diabetes. Diabetes Educ 2001; 27:393–404.

114. O'Connell KA, Hamera EK, Schorfheide A, Guthrie D. Symptom beliefs and actual blood glucose in type II diabetes. Res Nurs Health 1990; 13:145–151.

115. Huang ES, Gorawara-Bhat R, Chin MH. Self-reported goals of older patients with type 2 diabetes mellitus. J Am Geriatr Soc 2005; 53:306–311.

116. United States Department of Health. Center for Disease Control and Prevention. National Center for Chronic Disease Prevention and Health Promotion. National Diabetes Surveillance System. Visual impairment: prevalence of visual impairment per 100 adults with diabetes, by age, United States, 1997–2003. Available at: http://www.cdc.gov/diabetes/statistics/visual/fig3.htm. Accessed on June 2, 2006.

117. Sokol-McKay D, Buskirk K, Whittaker P. Adaptive low-vision and blindness techniques for blood glucose monitoring. Diabetes Educ 2003; 29:614–630.

118. Uslan M, Eghtesadi C, Spiker A, Schnell K, Burton D. Product evaluation: managing diabetes with a visual impairment. Access World; 2002:3. Available at: http://www.afb.org/afbpress/pub.asp?DocID=AW030503&select=1. Accessed on June 2, 2006.

119. American Diabetes Association Resource Guide 2006. Blood glucose meters and data management systems. Diabetes Forecast 2006; 59:RG40–RG59.

120. American Diabetes Association Resource Guide 2006. Insulin delivery. Diabetes Forecast 2006; 59: RG23–RG39.

121. American Diabetes Association. Tests of glycemia in diabetes. Diabetes Care 2004; 27:S91–S93.

122. Bina DM, Anderson RL, Johnson ML, Bergenstal R, Kendall DM. Clinical impact of prandial state, exercise, and site preparation on the equivalence of alternative-site blood glucose testing. Diabetes Care 2003; 26:981–985.

123. Ellison JM, Stegmann JM, Colner SL, et al. Rapid changes in postprandial blood glucose produce concentration differences at finger, forearm, and thigh sampling sites. Diabetes Care 2002; 25:951–964.

124. Jungheim K, Koschinsky T. Glucose monitoring at the arm: risk delays of hypoglycemia and hyperglycemia detection. Diabetes Care 2002; 25:956–960.

125. Wilson DM, Block J. Real-time continuous glucose monitor use and patient selection: what have we learned and where are we going? Diabetes Technol Therap 2005; 7:788–791.

126. Klonoff DC. A review of continuous glucose monitoring technology. Diabetes Technol Therap 2005; 7:770–775.

127. Potts Ro, Tamada JA, Tierney MJ. Glucose monitoring by reverse iontophoresis. Diabetes Metab Res Rev 2002; 18:S49–S53.

128. Foster SA, Goode J-VR, Small RE. Home blood glucose monitoring. Ann Pharmacother 1999; 33:355–363.

129. Pramming S, Thorsteinsson B, Theilgaard A, Pinner EM, Binder C. Cognitive function during hypoglycaemia in type I diabetes mellitus. Br Med J 1986; 292:647–650.

130. Fontbonne A, Berr C, Ducimetiere P. Poorer cognitive performance evolution over four years in elderly diabetics compared to controls with normal or impaired fasting blood glucose. Diabetes 2000; 49(suppl 1):A191–A192.

131. Nyomba BLG, Berard L, Murphy LJ. The cost of self-monitoring of blood glucose is an important factor limiting glycermic control in diabetic patients. Diabetes Care 2002; 25:1244–1245.

132. Tu K-S, Barchard K. An assessment of diabetes self-care barriers in older adults. J Comm Health Nurs 1993; 10:113–118.

133. Whetstone WR, Reid JC. Health promotion of older adults: perceived barriers. J Adv Nurs 1991; 16:1343–1349.

134. Coonrod BA, Betschart J, Harris MI. Frequency and determinants of diabetes patient education among adults in the U.S. population. Diabetes Care 1994; 17:822–858.

135. Simmons D, Peng A, Ara C, Garland B. The personal costs of diabetes; a significant barrier to care in South Auckland. N Z Med J 1999; 112:383–385.

136. Thomson FJ, Masson EA, Leeming JT, Boulton AJM. Lack of knowledge of symptoms of hypoglycemia by elderly diabetic patients. Age Ageing 1991; 20:404–406.

137. Colleran KM, Starr B, Burge MR. Putting diabetes to the test: analyzing glycemic control based on patients' diabetes knowledge. Diabetes Care 2003; 26:2220–2221.

138. Rosenstock J, Shen GS, Gatlin MR, Foley JE. Combination therapy with nateglinide and a thiazolidinedione improves glycemic control in type 2 diabetes. Diabetes Care 2002; 25:1529–1533.

139. Saloranta C, Kenneth H, Ball M, Dickinson S, Holmes D. Efficacy and safety of nateglinide in type 2 diabetic patients with modest fasting hyperglycemia. J Clin Endocrinol Metab 2002; 87:4171–4176.

140. Frische A, Schweitzer MA, Häring HU, and the 4001 study group. Glimepiride combined with morning insulin glargine, bedtime neutral protamine hagedorn insulin, or bedtime insulin glargine in patients with type 2 diabetes. Ann Intern Med 2003; 138:952–959.

141. Yki-Jarvinen H, Dressler A, Ziemen M, and the HOE 901/3002 study group. Less nocturnal hypoglycemia and better post-dinner glucose control with bedtime insulin glargine compared with bedtime NPH insulin during insulin combination therapy in type 2 diabetes. Diabetes Care 2000; 23:1130–1136.

142. Fischer KF, Lees JA, Newman JH. Hypoglycemia in hospitalized patients. N Engl J Med 1986; 315:1245–1250.

143. Davis SN, Shavers C, Davis B, Costa F. Prevention of an increase in plasma cortisol during hypoglycemia preserves subsequent counterregulatory responses. J Clin Invest 1997; 100:429–438.

144. Dagogo-Jack S, Rattarasarn C, Cryer PE. Reversal of hypoglycemia unawareness, but not defective glucose counterregulation, in IDDM. Diabetes 1994; 43:1426–1434.

145. Cranston I, Lomas J, Maran A, et al. Restoration of hypoglycaemia awareness in patients with long-duration insulin-dependent diabetes. Lancet 1994; 344:283–287.

146. Benbow SJ, Walsh A, Gill GV. Diabetes in the institutionalised elderly: a forgotten population? Br Med J 1997; 315:1868–1870.

147. Tattersall R, Simon P. Managing diabetes in residential and nursing homes: presents a complex set of problems with no one solution. Br Med J 1998; 316:89.

148. Shichiri M, Kishikawa H, Ohkubo Y, Wake N. Long-term results of the Kumamoto Study on optimal diabetes control in type 2 diabetic patients. Diabetes Care 2000; 23(suppl 2):B21–B29.

149. Cryer PE, Davis SN, Shamoon H. Hypoglycemia in diabetes: technical review. Diabetes Care 2003; 26:1902–1912.

150. Schillinger D, Grumbach K, Piette J, et al. Association of health literacy with diabetes outcomes. JAMA 2002; 288:475–482.

26 | Care of Community-Living Racial/Ethnic Minority Elders

Monica E. Peek and Marshall H. Chin
Section of General Internal Medicine, The University of Chicago, Chicago, Illinois, U.S.A.

INTRODUCTION

The number of minority elders is projected to increase by 300% over the next three decades, with older African Americans comprising 9% of the U.S. population (1). Many of these elders will have type 2 diabetes. Current estimates show that between 40% and 45% of persons over 65 years have either type 2 diabetes or impaired glucose tolerance (2,3). The increasing diversity of our nation's elderly population creates tremendous challenges and opportunities for clinicians and our systems of health care. Cultural differences in health beliefs and practices as well as disparities in the health status and health care of our racial/ethnic minority elders are prevalent and must be understood and addressed in order to care for this population in a compassionate, cost-effective manner.

Multidisciplinary health-care teams are increasingly being utilized to manage patients with diabetes and can help ensure that culturally competent, high-quality care is delivered to elderly minority patients with this disease. Each member of the team—including primary care physicians (PCPs), endocrinologists, geriatricians, nurses, social workers, and health educators—who masters the skill set unique to cultural competency will be a more effective provider and make significant contributions to reducing the disproportionate diabetes morbidity and mortality burden among this vulnerable population. This chapter provides a framework for health-care providers to understand issues relevant to the care of racial/ethnic minority elders with diabetes. Specifically, we seek to

- provide an overview of racial disparities in diabetes health outcomes among the elderly;
- illustrate sociocultural issues from both the patient and the provider perspective, which are relevant to the clinical management of minority elders;
- describe barriers and potential interventions in the areas of diabetes self-management, exercise, and nutrition among racial/ethnic minority elders; and
- address geriatric syndrome–management issues relevant to minority elders.

This chapter offers providers the core competencies necessary for understanding and treating racial/ethnic minority elders within a sociocultural context. It does not address the issue of potential racial variation in health outcomes due to biological or genetic differences. Although providers often use race as a proxy to estimate an individual's genetic risk for disease and treatment response, recent studies of genetic variation indicate that genetic composition is only modestly correlated with race but is highly correlated with geographic ancestry (4). Consequently, geographic ancestry and explicit genetic information are more appropriate alternatives to race for clinicians in making health-care decisions that involve the estimating of genetic risk. Current evidence supports the concept that disease prevalence and racial/ethnic health disparities are largely due to sociological and environmental influences (5–7), and it is within this paradigm that we address the specific needs of community-dwelling elderly minority persons living with diabetes. Although we attempt to describe the issues relevant to treating minority elders, it is beyond the scope of this chapter to cover any single racial/ethnic group in its entirety. Moreover, we recognize the inherent heterogeneity that exists "within" all racial/ethnic groups, including non-Hispanic whites, and caution must be used to not overgeneralize our findings to all members of any ethnic group.

EPIDEMIOLOGY OF TYPE 2 DIABETES

Racial/ethnic minority elders with diabetes have a greater burden of disease than whites due to higher incidence and prevalence rates as well as worse diabetes health outcomes, including glycemic control, comorbid conditions, and complications. Hence, providing high-quality care to this population should be a public health priority. Unfortunately, there is evidence of poor quality of care for this population, although recent trends indicate that such disparities may be decreasing (8,9).

Diabetes Incidence and Prevalence

Within the United States, persons aged 65 years and older have the highest diabetes prevalence and expected increase in prevalence when compared to other age groups. By 2050, diabetes will have increased by 252% among women aged 65 to 74 years and by 537% among men 75 years of age and older (10). Among the elderly, the highest incidence and prevalence rates are observed within racial and ethnic minorities (11). There is, however, significant intragroup variation within the racial/ethnic minority groups based on nationality. For example, among Hispanics, the diabetes prevalence rates have ranged from reports of 16% among Cuban Americans to 25% among Mexican Americans and Puerto Ricans aged 45 to 74 years (12). Unfortunately, there is little national, representative data about Native Americans (NA)/Alaskan natives and other racial/ethnic groups (i.e., Asian Indians), but preliminary data indicates that higher rates exist in comparison to whites. For example, the prevalence rates among the Navajo have been estimated at 41% among those aged 65 years and above, and among Northern Plains NA, diabetes prevalence is 33% for men and 40% for women aged 45 to 74 years (13). One study of Asian Indians in Atlanta found an 18.3% prevalence of diabetes for all ages (14).

Diabetes Complications and Comorbid Conditions

Little data exists about diabetes complications among the elderly, and we are unaware of literature about racial/ethnic differences in complications within this age group. We can, however, extrapolate from data about diabetes complications among all adults where racial/ethnic minorities have poorer glycemic control (15) and higher rates of diabetes complications including retinopathy, nephropathy, neuropathy and limb amputation, and higher disease-specific mortality rates (16–18). Renal disease and blindness are two to four times higher among African Americans and Latinos with diabetes than among non-Hispanic whites and African Americans have twice the amputation and amputation-associated mortality rates than non-Hispanic whites (16).

As with diabetes complications, there is little information about comorbid conditions among the elderly, but evidence shows that disparities do exist. For example, among persons aged 65 to 84 years, black men are 83% more likely to have hypertension and black women are 71% more likely to have this disease (19). Extrapolating information about adults in general, racial/ethnic minorities have higher rates of dyslipidemia and hypertension, both of which are more poorly controlled (19,20), as well as cerebrovascular disease (21) and premature coronary-artery-disease mortality (22). Higher burdens of comorbid illness may translate into more complicated disease management for these elderly subpopulations.

Differences in Quality of Diabetes Care

Although the reason for the observed disparities in diabetes health outcomes among racial/ethnic minorities is multifactorial, it has been partly attributed to differences in the quality of care delivered to these groups. The Institute of Medicine recently reviewed the health disparities' literature and, in its report "Unequal Treatment: Confronting Racial and Ethnic Disparities in Health Care," found that although health-care access and demographic variables account for some of the disparity, there is a persistent, residual gap in outcomes attributed to differences in the quality of care received (23).

There is specific evidence documenting that African Americans, Latinos, Asian Americans, and NA receive poorer diabetes-related quality of care. For example, African Americans with diabetes have fewer visits to PCPs and ophthalmologists, fewer measurements of glycosylated hemoglobin and low-density lipoprotein cholesterol, and lower rates of influenza vaccination (24–27). Puerto Rican adults in New York state are less likely to receive annual HgbA1c testing (72.7% vs. 84.9%), cholesterol testing (67.5% vs. 87.2%), antihypertensive medications (82.4% vs. 91.9%), and pneumococcal vaccinations (19.3% vs. 28.5%) despite having equal access to health care (insurance, medical home, and frequency of physician visits) (28). Among Medicare beneficiaries, African Americans were 30% less likely than whites to have an eye-care visit (29). There has been little research into whether racial differences in other processes of care such as referrals for nutritional counseling, exercise programs, and weight reduction also exist and account for some of the observed disparities in diabetes health outcomes.

The Agency for Healthcare Research and Quality report, "Strategies for Improving Minority Healthcare Quality," calls for more quality improvement interventions with a focus on diseases with significant health disparities, such as diabetes (30). Early research indicates that generic diabetes quality improvement initiatives have the potential to improve health outcomes among racial/ethnic minorities and reduce health disparities (31–34). More research is needed to understand the full impact of such programs, and culturally tailoring interventions may increase their effectiveness among vulnerable elderly populations with diabetes (35,36).

SOCIOCULTURAL ISSUES: THE PATIENT PERSPECTIVE

The reasons for racial disparities in quality of diabetes care and health outcomes are likely multifactorial and sociocultural in nature. The cultural and economic context in which the United States exists impacts the quality and the quantity of opportunities afforded to social groups that are defined by race, gender, and ethnicity, and shapes the cultural norms, health beliefs, and behaviors of both patients and providers alike. Significant variation in cultural beliefs and expectations, family and gender-based role behaviors, and relationship structures and behaviors can have a major impact on how diabetes is understood and managed by patients and their families (37). Incongruent expectations between patients and providers have been shown to foster misunderstandings, mistrust, and lack of treatment adherence (38–40). Patient-centered health care can address such patient/provider incongruences and includes understanding patients' expectations, feelings, and the way they understand the illness (41,42). Patient-centered care redefines the role of patients as collaborators (41,42) and has been shown to have positive health outcomes in diabetes and other chronic diseases (43,44).

This next section reviews sociocultural issues that may affect minority elders' understanding, experience, and management of their diabetes. These issues are important for clinicians to be familiar with and comfortable addressing within the clinical encounter. Although the entire spectrum of sociocultural issues is too broad to cover in this chapter, we provide meaningful insight for clinicians by addressing issues of explanatory models (EMs) of disease, aging/cohort effects, family/social support, religion/spirituality, and complementary/alternative medicine use (Table 1) and refer the reader to additional sources for a more in-depth discussion of these issues (45,46).

Explanatory Models

A valuable step for clinicians in approaching diabetes care for racial/ethnic minority elders is to understand the various EMs of disease that exist among different cultures. Kleinman conceptualizes EMs as ideas and beliefs about a disease that help persons understand and make sense of an illness within a cultural context (39). Although it is important to appreciate such EMs, it is often difficult to apply such knowledge to heterogeneous ethnic groups and to individualize care without oversimplifying cultural norms and unconsciously utilizing stereotypes (47). Such inadvertent actions may actually hinder, rather than enhance, the medical encounter (48). Thus, care must be taken by clinicians to balance efforts to incorporate and address cultural beliefs with attempts to individualize patient experiences and tailor plans of medical care.

We describe here two case studies of EMs that have been explored among Mexican Americans and Chinese Americans. These models are not generalizable to all members of these groups and may vary, in particular, by level of acculturation, but serve as examples of how cultural beliefs may impact clinical care.

TABLE 1   Several Key Domains for Exploration during the Clinical Encounter

Domain	Example questions
Sociocultural background	"Where did you grow up? (→ How long have you been in the United States?) What was that experience like?" "Is there a language other than English that you prefer to use?" "Do you want to tell me anything about yourself or your previous experiences that would help me take better care of you?"
Explanatory models of diabetes	"Tell me about your diabetes." "What do you think causes your diabetes?" "What do you think is the best way to treat your diabetes? Why?" "Are there things about your life with diabetes that are important for me to know?"
Aging/cohort effects	"You grew up in a different time period than me. Do you think that people in your generation have different ideas about how to keep yourself healthy? Give me some examples."
Family/social support	"Are there family members or friends that you want to have with us during our visits? Who?" "Who helps you manage your diabetes at home?" "How has your family adjusted to you having diabetes?"
Religion/spirituality	"Do you use spirituality or religion to help you deal with your diabetes in any way? How?" "Is there a spiritual advisor or religious person that helps you understand, cope with, or treat your diabetes? Who? How do they help?"
Complementary/alternative medicine use	"Many people use natural remedies or other treatments to help manage their diabetes. Other than what a doctor may prescribe, do you use anything else to treat your diabetes? Which ones?"

Qualitative research among subgroups of Mexican Americans has identified an EM of diabetes where disease causality is attributed to emotional distress such as "susto," defined as a sudden deep fright triggered by an extremely traumatizing event or near-death experience (49–51). Traditionally Western concepts of nutrition, exercise, and obesity have been described within the context of changing cultural norms and lifestyles where the peaceful, healthy "old ways" of Mexico have been replaced by contemporary lifestyles marked by socioeconomic stressors such as unemployment, poverty, urban living conditions, and reduced availability of fresh, natural foods (49,52).

Ethnographic studies of Chinese Americans have also provided insight into some EMs that exist within this population. Based on ancient Chinese philosophy, a holistic approach toward health exists that combines herbs, acupuncture, diet change, massotherapy, and therapeutic exercise to modulate energy flow ("qi") through the body's multiple meridians to cure disorders and promote health (53,54). Within this framework, health is defined as a state of spiritual and physical harmony with nature, and the role of the physician is to look for yin/yang imbalances within each meridian (53,54). It is within this context that different EMs of diabetes often arose. For example, in one study, participants described diabetes medications as nephrotoxic agents that should be avoided if possible (55). Increased elimination of these toxins was believed to occur by drinking more water and by exercising to sweat and "pass water." Focusing on the therapeutic benefits of exercise can be a culturally appropriate way to encourage physical activity, particularly because exercise may be viewed as a traditional form of medical therapy. Another EM that emerged focused on "sugar control," partly because diabetes translates in Chinese as the "sugar-in-urine" disorder (55). The alternative use of the term "metabolic syndrome" (which is identified as a kind of "ti-zhi" or constitution) may be more culturally acceptable terminology that reduces the misconception that diabetes management is focused on reduced intake of sugar.

Aging Perceptions/Cohort Effects

There is evidence that different cultures perceive the process of aging, and its associated diseases, differently. For example, African Americans are three times more likely to attribute heart disease to overwork and stress and more likely to attribute arthritis to environmental exposures and harsh working conditions than non-Hispanic whites, who are more likely to attribute these conditions to a normal part of aging (56). Studies also show that ethnic minority families are more likely to understand dementia in terms other than biomedical models, such as folk and mixed biomedical/folk models, and more likely to "normalize" dementia as an aging process rather than a distinct disease entity (57).

However, some of the differences in attitudes about aging are due to cohort effects. It is important to recognize that today's elderly population is aging differently than future generations, having lived through two world wars, the Great Depression, and significant changes in family relationships and norms. Shorter life expectancies, an industrial-based economy, and institutional discrimination impacted options regarding education, occupation, and lifestyles that continue to affect the health and health behaviors of the elderly today. Additionally, many racial/ethnic minority elders in the United States are immigrants who may have experienced torture, genocide, or other traumatizing events that led to their emigration. Consequently, it is important to recognize that society has changed for the current cohort of elders, many of whom may have established behavioral norms and attitudes that are discordant with today's standards. Attitudes about leisure time activity, exercise, nutrition and other health behaviors may be more challenging to address among the elderly because of such cohort effects. For example, cigarette smoking was initially marketed as a healthy activity, promoted by physicians, and distributed by the federal government to young men in the military. The cohort that matured during this era may have different attitudes about smoking than young adults today.

The Role of the Family and Social Support

The importance of familial support in chronic disease management crosses cultures. Among those with diabetes, the role of family has been shown to be important in African Americans, Chinese immigrants, Mexican Americans, NA, and European Americans (58–61). However, the importance of family may be more pronounced among racial/ethnic minorities (62). One study of racial/ethnic differences in the role of family members in health-care decision making among the elderly reported that 91% of whites preferred to express their own health-care wishes (without input from the family) in comparison to 85% of Hispanics, 83% of Asians, and 67% of blacks (63). An alternative decision maker was identified for 8% of whites and 15% of Hispanics and Asians, and approximately one-third of African Americans (63).

There is additional work that supports the primacy of the family among racial/ethnic minority groups. For example, one study found that African American middle-class women reported receiving much higher levels of family support than any other racial/ethnic group (64), and a systematic review found that African Americans tend to rely more heavily than whites do on their informal social networks for preventive care and to meet their disease-management needs (65).

Cultural differences in the role of the family and in understanding of health and illness also account for some of these differences (62). Research has shown that many non-Western cultures perceive life through a holistic worldview where their world is interconnected within a larger context (66). For example, work among urban Canadian aboriginal people, NA in Oklahoma, and the Haida people in British Columbia show that diabetes is seen as existing not only within oneself but also within the family and the larger community; it pervades the community and affects everyone, even those not diagnosed with the disease (67–69).

Enhanced social support networks have been shown to have positive health outcomes (65,70). Social support is thought to facilitate self-care and adaptation to illness (71–73); research among African Americans found significant associations between social support and improved diabetes management (65). Among the Navajo, cooking for an individual often signifies a caregiving role and reflects Navajo values of interconnectedness (74). Researchers found that among these NA, when family members cooked the majority of the meals for those with diabetes, the respondents had better control of their diabetes and dyslipidemia than those who prepared their own meals (75).

There can, however, be negative health consequences of social networks when the importance of family well-being takes precedence over a patient's commitment to diabetes self-management. Qualitative studies of Puerto Ricans and Chinese Americans showed a tendency to prioritize family matters and other life needs over diabetes management (76,77).

For example, patients often reported protecting the quality and taste of the family's food as a significant concern, and described accommodating the family by "eating around" meals, taking their portions out of the cooked family meal before adding oils and spices and discreetly selecting their needed foods to avoid having others accommodate them (77). Krause found a curvilinear relationship among African American women where initial support may alleviate stress, but after a threshold, such support systems exacerbate symptoms and have negative health effects (78,79). Among women, there may be a higher personal cost for using social support because of expected reciprocity, given the traditional role of women as caretakers (79).

The Role of Religion and Spirituality

Like familial and social support networks, spirituality and religion have been shown to have prominent roles cross-culturally. Spirituality has been utilized as a coping strategy that ameliorates the stress and the uncertainty of the illness trajectory, moving one from despair and fear to hope and possibility (80). In a study of multiethnic elderly persons, approximately half reported using cultural religious traditions as a method of healing: NA used sweat lodges, traditional healing ceremonies, and dance rituals; rural whites appealed to God for intervention; and Hispanics prayed during mass (62,81).

However, there is evidence that the role of spirituality may be particularly important to some racial/ethnic minority groups and impact how chronic diseases such as diabetes are managed.

This may be especially true for African Americans, where several studies have documented higher levels of religious practices and beliefs in comparison to whites, including more frequent prayer and higher importance placed on the role of prayer (82,83). The majority of African Americans have been found to read religious materials and watch or listen to religious programs at least once a week (84).

Spirituality can have both positive and negative impacts on diabetes self-management behavior (46). For many African Americans, God is the ultimate controller of illness and health (85,86). Those who "turn it over to God" may do so entirely and have fewer self-management practices; these persons are more likely to be elderly and members of lower socioeconomic groups (87–90). However, religion can also enhance diabetes self-management, as persons strive to protect their bodies (seen as "God's temples") and interpret the role of the physician as a healer being used as God's instrument (87,88,90,91). Some patients may have a need for religious counseling arising from diabetes-related issues, such as feeling that their diabetes is a sign of being abandoned by God (46). Because most clinicians have no training in this area, addressing patients' need for religious/spiritual counseling is usually most appropriate through referrals to clergy, other pastoral-care professionals, or nonreligious support systems such as family counselors (46).

Complementary and Alternative Medicine Use

Complementary and alternative medicine (CAM) use is a fairly common practice in the United States, where approximately 42% of the population uses some form of CAM (92). Higher CAM use has been reported among women, the elderly, those with higher education, and persons with more comorbidities (93,94). People with diabetes are 1.6 times as likely to use CAM as those without the disease (95). However, despite the high prevalence of CAM utilization, physicians typically have limited knowledge and acceptance of traditional/CAM medicine (96). There are mixed reports about racial/ethnic variations in CAM use within the United States. Although cultural traditions, historic exclusion from traditional medical care, and lower CAM cost may facilitate increased usage among minority groups, some researches document less use among these groups, especially in the management of chronic diseases (97,98). However, one survey of primary-care patients reported the following rates of CAM use: 50% of Hispanics, 50% of Asians, 41% of whites, and 22% of African Americans (99). Within this study, whites were more likely to report their CAM use than non-whites, with disclosure rates of 67% in comparison to 45% of African Americans and 31% of Hispanics and Asians (99). Thus, although Hispanics were the most likely to use traditional herbal medications, they were the least likely to tell their physicians about such practices. Studies report that 66% to 69% of Hispanics using traditional therapies choose not to tell their PCP primarily due to fear of physician disapproval (100,101).

One survey reported that 33% to 56% of Mexican Americans surveyed report CAM use for the treatment of diabetes, with nopales (prickly pear cactus) as the most commonly used hypoglycemic agent (50). Interestingly, research has demonstrated efficacy of nopales in lowering blood glucose levels in patients with diabetes (102). Chaya (green leafy shrub), aloe vera, oregano teach, and lime juice with textohiztle bark have also been reported as herbal remedies among Mexican Americans for the treatment of diabetes (103). Cultural competence should also include incorporating evidence-based CAM while dispelling myths and misconceptions about both alternative and Western medicine.

SOCIOCULTURAL ISSUES: THE PROVIDER PERSPECTIVE

The preceding section highlighted some of the cultural issues that may impact elderly minority patients with diabetes. Having an understanding and appreciation for these issues and cultural differences is important to effectively treat these populations and is an essential component of cultural competency. It is also important for clinicians to be able to look introspectively and understand how their own cultural views and biases impact the patient/provider relationship and effective diabetes management.

Cultural Competency

Campinha-Bacote describes cultural competence as having five components: (*i*) "cultural awareness": learning to value and understand other cultures, in part through awareness of personal biases hindering this process, (*ii*) "cultural knowledge": acquiring a basic educational foundation about other cultures, (*iii*) "cultural skills": the ability to apply cultural information in patient health-care assessments, (*iv*) "cultural encounters": gaining experience through cross-cultural interactions, and (*v*) "cultural desire": having the motivation to pursue the above (104).

There are a variety of provider and health-system characteristics and actions that facilitate cultural competence, including linguistic skills, educational materials that are linguistically and culturally appropriate, coordination of services with traditional healers, inclusion of appropriate family members in health-care decisions, and optimizing of racial/ethnic concordance (Table 2) (105–107). Limited English proficiency (LEP) is a significant barrier to quality of care, patient satisfaction, and health outcomes; addressing the linguistic needs of patients is an important component of cultural competency (45,108,109). The use of untrained ad hoc interpreters (i.e., family members or untrained support staff) is an insufficient remedy that can result in increased medical errors (109). Trained professional interpreters can positively affect LEP patients' satisfaction, quality of care, and health outcomes (109), although they can compromise certain aspects of communication when compared to bilingual health-care providers. Bilingual physicians are more likely to elicit patient problems and concerns than those without linguistic skills, even those utilizing professional interpreter services (108,110). This underscores the importance of having a diverse physician workforce who can provide language and cultural concordance within the health-care encounter.

Limited cultural competence can hamper clinical care of patients through a variety of mechanisms including diagnostic errors arising from language/communication barriers, lack of knowledge of culture-specific symptom presentation and epidemiology, failure to account

TABLE 2   Core Skills in Cultural Competency

Ability to elicit, understand, and work with culturally specific health beliefs and practices
Self-awareness of cultural perspectives and potential biases
Familiarity with culturally specific communication styles and methods of showing respect
Utilization of bilingual, bicultural staff or persons
Incorporation of family members and/or significant others into the health-care encounter
Working effectively with interpreter services (i.e., onsite and toll-free telephone programs)
Utilization of culturally tailored education materials and, when available, community health workers

for differing responses to medications, and lack of knowledge about traditional remedies that can interact with prescription medications (111–113). One study found that Mexican American patients using CAM feared telling their primary-care doctors because of concerns of being scolded (50). Even patients using only Western medications wished their physicians knew more about herbal medications and were willing to use both systems (50).

Provider Bias/Discrimination

In addition to being knowledgeable about the sociocultural background of patients, it is important that providers are aware of how their own cultural background and potential biases may impact the patient–provider relationship. For example, Waitzkin showed that persons from middle-class backgrounds tend to be more verbally explicit, whereas those from working-class backgrounds communicate more implicitly through nonverbal signals (114). There is a growing body of research that documents the use of negative stereotypes about African-American patients by physicians (115–120). One study asked nearly 200 physicians to rate over 800 patients on a variety of characteristics. After controlling for confounding variables, the researchers found that African Americans were more likely to be rated as less educated, less intelligent, more likely to abuse drugs and alcohol, and less likely to adhere to treatment regimens (115). Such stereotyping has not gone unnoticed by patients. Racial/ethnic minorities frequently report racial discrimination within the health-care system; 13% to 69% of African Americans report discrimination in comparison to 1% to 2% of whites (121–123).

Although reports of racial discrimination and mistrust within the health-care system are not new, provider bias is only recently being explored as a potentially important contributor to health-care disparities. A landmark study of PCP from around the United States utilized trained patient actors in a computer-simulation model to investigate potential racial differences in recommendation for cardiac catheterization (124). Researchers found that African Americans were 40% less likely to be recommended for cardiac catheterization than whites, despite identical clinical scenarios (risk factors, symptoms, and stress-test results) (124). African American women were 60% less likely than white men to receive an angiogram recommendation, indicating a race–gender interaction (124). Perceived discrimination has been positively correlated with poor mental and physical health measures such as psychological distress, depression, decreased life satisfaction, self-rated health, days spent unwell in bed, high blood pressure/hypertension, cigarette use, risk of preterm delivery, and severity of AIDS-related symptoms (121,125–128). Self-reports of discrimination within the health-care system have been associated with delays in prescription medication utilization and medical testing/treatment and lower levels of patient satisfaction, indicating that discrimination may represent an additional barrier to accessing appropriate health care (128–130). To date, no research has investigated the relationship of provider bias/discrimination and diabetes outcomes. However, as noted earlier in this chapter, there is documented evidence of disparities in the quality of diabetes care delivered to racial/ethnic minorities in comparison to whites (124–127).

CLINICAL APPROACHES TO DIABETES MANAGEMENT AMONG RACIAL/ETHNIC MINORITY ELDERS

Thus far, we have provided a framework for understanding the sociocultural context in which the patient–provider relationship occurs and diabetes management takes place. We now move on to the clinical application of such principles. This section reviews the epidemiology, barriers, and interventions for diabetes self-management (i.e., self glucose monitoring, foot care, symptom management, etc.), physical activity, and nutrition that pertain to the care of racial/ethnic minority elders. It also addresses aspects of diabetes geriatric syndromes that are relevant to minority elders. We begin, however, with a brief overview of providing an individualized approach to diabetes care among this population.

Individualizing Diabetes Management Among Racial/Ethnic Minority Elders

We have discussed the importance of cultural competence in providing optimal care to minority elders. Shared decision making (SDM) takes this concept one step further by ensuring that patients' individual needs and cultural preferences are incorporated into the treatment plan through a collaborative effort between patients and their providers.

Patients differ in how they value and assess different treatment options, side effects, and health outcomes (131,132). There is also significant diversity in patients' medical histories and comorbid disease burdens, their levels of readiness to change, and cultural backgrounds (133). These factors make individualizing treatment plans an important component of chronic disease management, especially for complicated management regimens that address diabetes care. Such tailored plans should incorporate an SDM process where the patient collaborates with the health-care team to create a plan of care that includes patient preferences (133). This is particularly relevant for the elderly, where tight glycemic control may be associated with short-term morbidity due to the increased risk of hypoglycemic episodes and may not result in long-term benefits since the reduction in microvascular complications requires six to eight years of consistent glycemic control (134,135). Elderly patients may choose goals that enhance quality of life (i.e., reducing polypharmacy), treat symptoms, and reduce diabetes-related syndromes rather than goals that focus exclusively on lowering blood sugar levels (136). Although SDM has been linked to enhanced patient satisfaction, adherence, and health outcomes, research has shown that racial/ethnic minorities and the elderly have less SDM than their white, younger counterparts (137,138). Thus, increasing the SDM process of minority elders is an important, and often missing, part of the clinical encounter and patient–provider relationship that can facilitate the development of a tailored plan of care.

Diabetes Self-Management
Epidemiology
There are mixed reports about racial disparities in diabetes self-management and little data about such activities among the elderly. Some research indicates that African Americans are 20% "more" likely to take a self-management class and 30% more likely to check their feet regularly than whites, whereas Hispanics are 60% "less" likely to take a diabetes self-management course, perform daily glucose monitoring, and check their feet for sores or irritation (139). There is fairly consistent evidence, however, that diabetes education may not effectively translate into enhanced knowledge or health behaviors among older, low-income, and/or minority populations (76). One study of Latinos and African Americans who monitored their blood glucose found that few modified their diet, physical activity, or medications in response to their glucose readings (140,141). This may reflect a need for culturally tailored, literacy-appropriate diabetes education that can improve knowledge and practices among these populations.

Barriers
A myriad of barriers to diabetes self-management have been identified among racial/ethnic minorities, many of which also apply to diet and physical activity adherence. Quantitative data specific to racial/ethnic minorities with type 2 diabetes suggest that culture, ethnicity, socioeconomic status, and psychosocial factors (i.e., social support, self-efficacy, and coping skills) play a large role in explaining diabetes self-care and health outcomes.

"Economic barriers" are more common in poor/minority communities and pose a challenge to those managing diabetes (142,143). This is particularly pronounced among the elderly, who are more likely to live on reduced, fixed incomes. Higher out-of-pocket costs can reduce patients' ability to obtain appropriate diabetes medications and monitoring supplies (144,145). One study found that 16% to 40% of low-income African American and Latino patients limited their diabetes care because of concerns about money (141).

"Literacy" is another barrier more common to the racial/ethnic minorities (particularly immigrants with LEP), the poor, and the elderly (146,147). Low-literate patients have problems reading prescription labels and educational materials and following physician instructions for care. They have lower quality and less satisfaction with health care and are at an increased risk of hospitalization (146–148). Low-literacy is particularly common among persons with diabetes and is associated with poor diabetes knowledge and worse health outcomes such as poor glycemic control and retinopathy (147,149). For example, in a study of two urban public hospitals, 55% of patients with diabetes had inadequate functional health literacy; of these, 50% were unaware of the symptoms of hypoglycemia, 62% did not know how to treat hypoglycemia, and

42% could not recall the normal glucose range despite the fact that 73% had attended diabetes education classes (150).

"Health status" is a barrier to diabetes self-management that is particularly relevant to older persons. Among elderly patients attending an urban diabetes clinic comprised primarily of low-income African Americans, 74% reported poor vision and 19% reported hearing problems as major obstacles to diabetes education (151). Among the elderly, these barriers may be more common among racial/ethnic minorities because relevant conditions such as diabetic retinopathy are more common among these subpopulations (151).

As noted earlier in the chapter, "psychosocial barriers" to diabetes self-management can arise from the demands of prioritizing familial demands over personal needs and from stressors arising from the caretaker role. This is particularly prevalent among racial/ethnic minority elders who are more likely to be the primary caretakers of their grandchildren and extended family members. Studies of older African American and Puerto Rican women multicaregivers found that stress due to care provided to family and friends in and outside the home acted as a barrier to appropriate diabetes self-management (76). Having diabetes did not translate into reduced expectations from such care-giving roles.

Interventions/Approaches to Management

In response to the multitude of barriers to self-management among the elderly, Medicare recently began funding diabetes self-management education. Such training may be particularly relevant for minorities and limited-English/immigrant communities and should incorporate participation from caregivers and family members, particularly of the frail elderly.

It is important, however, to underscore that although many racial/ethnic minorities attend diabetes education classes, most have low diabetes knowledge and self-efficacy (148). Consequently, receiving generic diabetes education may not be sufficient; diabetes programs should be tailored to the specific educational needs of racial/ethnic minority elders. There are many strategies to help clinicians develop such tailored education (Table 3). For example, physicians can incorporate the use of stories in the education process (152). Many non-Western cultures utilize storytelling as a means to communicate cultural norms, pass on cultural wisdom, and assist the community in achieving wellness and harmony (153). Storytelling has been a successful method of health education for non-English diabetes patients (154). Clinicians can also address limited literacy issues with the use of pictographs, videos, and slides rather than print materials (155). This is also more appropriate for many older persons who are more likely to have limited eyesight to get their health information from television rather than print media (152).

Physical Activity
Epidemiology

Less than 40% of adults aged 65 years and older routinely exercise, and there has been little success over the past 20 years at increasing these numbers (156). Among older people who do

TABLE 3   Culturally Relevant Clinician Interventions to Enhance Diabetes Management

---

Adapt dietary recommendations to incorporate cultural foods and flavors so that patients are modifying, rather than replacing, traditional recipes

Utilize culturally tailored, literacy-appropriate, bilingual education materials

Utilize racially/ethnically concordant health educators

Incorporate the use of stories in the education process

Address limited literacy with pictographs, videos and slides, rather than print materials

Focus on a single concept message at each visit (i.e., "eat less fat" or "walk at least 10 min each day")

Use "teach back" methods to ensure comprehension and reinforce educational goals

Emphasize the health benefits of exercise (instead of weight loss)

Involve family members and peers, and encourage social contact among learners

Train self and staff to be culturally competent

Where appropriate, incorporate a role for the religious community

Where available, utilize patient navigators to help with logistical barriers (i.e., transportation and scheduling difficulties)

Work with social workers to facilitate use of community services for low-cost meal planning/preparation and exercise/recreation

Advocate health systems and health policy changes that can positively impact care delivery for racial/ethnic minorities (i.e., Medicaid reimbursement for diabetes education)

---

start to exercise, adherence rates are 15% among women and 30% among men (157). Despite the demonstrated benefits of exercise in glucose control, patients with diabetes are more likely to be inactive than those without the disease (158). Little data exist about racial differences in exercise among the elderly, but studies show older Asians have lower rates of physical activity in comparison to whites (159), and older Mexican Americans and African Americans are half as likely as whites to engage in vigorous leisure-time physical activity (160,161).

Barriers

As with diabetes self-management, several barriers to physical activity have been identified that are particularly salient to racial/ethnic minority elders. "Poor health and pain" are the primary reasons for physical inactivity among surveys of older community-dwelling adults (162). The poorer health status of minority elders, including such disorders as diabetic retinopathy, peripheral neuropathy, and cardiovascular disease, indicates that poor health status may be a particularly important barrier to exercise within these communities (163).

"Psychosocial and cultural barriers" to physical activity also exist. Many elderly have negative attitudes about exercise and sweating that reflect their cohort experience (163,164). For example, older African Americans may view being overweight as a sign of robustness and health; such cultural beliefs can hinder exercise interventions, which may be better marketed as strategies to improve health rather than lose weight (152). In addition, low aging expectations, low self-esteem, and low self-efficacy have been shown to predict low levels of physical activity among the elderly and racial/ethnic minorities (133,160).

"Economic barriers" to engaging in physical activity exist among many minority elders with diabetes. For example, racial/ethnic minorities are more likely to live in low-income neighborhoods that may be physically unsafe for exercise (due to crime, busy streets, etc.) and have limited recreational facilities (i.e., parks, golf courses, and recreation centers) (162,165). Proximity of recreational facilities is especially relevant to the elderly, whose daily activities tend to exist within a short radius of their home.

Interventions/Approaches to Management

Physician advice has been shown to be especially effective among the elderly, who typically hold doctors in high esteem and have more visits with their PCP than the nonelderly (166). Although only 62% of surveyed Medicare beneficiaries report receiving physician recommendations to exercise (136), 40% of those who began exercising did so exclusively because of doctor advice (167). Correlates of exercise among elderly racial/ethnic minorities include seeing others in their neighborhood exercising, free/low-cost programs, culturally tailored and age-appropriate interventions, facilitated transportation, and participation in church/religious services (Table 3) (165,168).

Nutrition
Epidemiology

There is evidence that racial/ethnic minorities, such as African Americans and Latinos, are more likely to have diets inconsistent with guidelines of the American Diabetes Association (169). For example, African Americans are less likely to eat five or more fruits and vegetables each day, and are more likely to obtain above 30% of their daily calories from fat and above 10% from saturated fat in comparison to whites (169). Although there has been some controversy about the optimal diet for adults with type 2 diabetes (i.e., high fiber, glycemic index approaches, and low vs. moderate fat), there has been a general consensus about increasing the consumption of fruits and vegetables and decreasing the daily consumption of saturated fats (170,171).

Barriers

As with self-management and physical activity, several barriers to diet adherence have been identified. "Economic barriers" are again cited as a prominent barrier among minority elders.

One study reported that nearly one-third of study participants living in East Harlem reported skipping meals due to finances; this practice was associated with poorer health-related quality of life and a 15% increased likelihood of poorer health status (141).

"Food availability" is a related but separate issue for minority elders seeking adherence to a diabetic diet. For example, within African American neighborhoods, there is a positive association between the intake of fruits and vegetables and the number of supermarkets in the neighborhood (172); yet African American neighborhoods have fewer supermarkets than white neighborhoods (173). Moreover, the available grocery stores within these communities are less likely to have foods appropriate to maintaining a diabetic diet. Only 18% of grocery stores in East Harlem carry five recommended diabetes food items as compared to 58% of stores on the Upper East Side of New York (173).

"Cultural barriers" to nutrition adherence also exist. Older Puerto Ricans surveyed had misconceptions that traditional foods could not be incorporated into a diabetic diet and reported that taste preferences were a significant barrier to dietary adherence (76). Within the African American community, many traditional food practices originate from slavery when discarded animal parts (i.e., pigs' feet and intestines, turkey necks, and ox tails) and lard were staple items in the diet provided by the slave owners (174). These food items and their preparation have been passed down through generations as cultural/traditional cooking methods (174). Among Chinese Americans, cultural traditions prioritize protecting the quality and the taste of the food for the larger family because of the communal eating arrangements. Accommodating the family often takes precedence over individual diabetic dietary needs (175).

Interventions/Approaches to Management

Nutrition interventions among racial/ethnic minorities have met with limited success in comparison to similar interventions targeting non-Hispanic whites (176). Researchers have proposed that successful nutrition and weight-loss programs depend, in part, on addressing educational and health literacy needs as well as a range of attitudes, beliefs, and sociocultural factors such as focusing on health benefits instead of weight loss, inclusion of ethnic foods, and incorporating sociocultural lifestyle situations (Table 3) (177–179).

Management of Diabetes-Related Geriatric Syndromes Among Minority Elders

Racial/ethnic minority elders living in a community may experience higher rates of diabetic geriatric syndromes than whites because of the lower rates of nursing home placement among many racial/ethnic groups, even among patients with comparable need. For example, among community-dwelling older people, racial/ethnic minorities have lower functional levels than whites, a disparity that has been attributed to differential patterns of chronic illness (180,181). One study found that African Americans and Asians have a lower risk of institutionalization (in comparison to whites) despite the fact that all patients in the study were nursing-home certifiable and low-income persons (182). African Americans are more likely than whites to use formal and informal home health services rather than skilled nursing facilities when assistance is needed (183), although home service use does not fully compensate for the differences in nursing home use (184). These findings are unrelated to social class. Differences in preference or access are likely the causes, but this has not been fully investigated (183–185).

This section will briefly review the following diabetic geriatric syndromes: depression, polypharmacy, cognitive impairment, urinary incontinence, and falls.

Rates of depression among the elderly do not vary by race/ethnicity (186), although one study reported that the African American race was associated with diabetes/depression comorbidity (187). There is evidence, however, that disparities in depression "treatment" exist. African Americans, Hispanics, Medicaid patients, and the elderly are especially vulnerable to undertreatment of depression and are more likely to be treated with older tricyclic antidepressants (TCAs) than the newer class of selective serotonin reuptake inhibitors that are associated with fewer side effects (188–192). Increased TCA use may put racial/ethnic minority elders at increased risk of sedation, decreased cognition, and falls. Some of the disparity in treatment rates may be due to patient factors. Researchers found that African Americans were less likely to fill a prescription for depression medication despite equivalent physician delivery of prescriptions to patients of all racial/ethnic groups (193). This same study, however, found that Hispanics were less likely to receive any treatment or an adequate course of psychotherapy (193).

Polypharmacy is common in the elderly, especially those with diabetes. Racial/ethnic minority elders with diabetes generally have more associated comorbidities, which may put them at an even increased risk of polypharmacy. Clinically important side effects often result from polypharmacy among the elderly. In addition to African-American race and advanced age, polypharmacy is a significant risk factor for severe hypoglycemia (194).

Little data exist on racial/ethnic differences in cognition among the elderly. It has become clear, however, that it is important to have culturally appropriate norms in evaluating cognition among the elderly. One study of community-dwelling, nondemented African Americans and white elders found that African Americans had significantly lower scores on cognitive testing that were not due to medical history, occupation, socioeconomic status, or other sociodemographic factors (195).

Studies show that whites are "more" likely to report the geriatric syndrome of urinary incontinence than non-whites, up to twice as much as African Americans (196). It is unclear whether these lower rates are due to differences in prevalence or underdetection among racial/ethnic minorities. Consequently, we recommend screening for urinary incontinence as part of standard diabetes geriatric care for racial/ethnic minority elders.

Older patients with diabetes are at an increased risk of falls due to functional disability, decreased vision, peripheral neuropathy, hypoglycemia, and polypharmacy (136). A higher prevalence of these complications among racial/ethnic minorities may lead to an increased risk of falls. In addition, the sedative effects of TCAs, which are more commonly prescribed for depression among racial/ethnic minorities, may put minority elders at an increased risk of falls.

Community Resources

Community services, especially those involving meal planning or preparation, education, and exercise/recreation activities, are important for diabetic elders' well-being, and they may be particularly relevant to community-dwelling minority elders with diabetes who have higher functional needs (197,198). Yet, minority elders have lower use of community services than whites, particularly in the areas of meal and recreation services, two areas that can impact diabetes management through nutrition and exercise adherence (199). Clinicians and case managers can facilitate the utilization of such services among minority elders with diabetes.

Patient navigators are members of the health-care team that help patients navigate complex medical systems by addressing patient barriers in real time from the initiation to the termination of treatment. They were pioneered, for example, to enhance screening mammography utilization among medically underserved populations and have been successful in assisting patients throughout cancer screening, prevention, and treatment process; the model has recently been applied to chronic-disease management as well (200,201).

Patient navigators can be effective additions to the clinical-care team in maximizing diabetes care delivered to minority elders. Potential barriers that can be addressed include providing medical homes for the uninsured and underinsured, assisting patients with lower health literacy, facilitating to overcome communication difficulties in the patient–provider relationship arising from language barriers or mistrust/cultural issues, and overcoming logistical barriers such as transportation and scheduling difficulties.

CONCLUSIONS

Racial/ethnic disparities in diabetes prevalence, quality of care, and health outcomes exist among our nation's elderly. Understanding sociocultural barriers and incorporating tailored interventions to enhance nutrition, physical activity, and other aspects of diabetes management will help health-care providers deliver better care to minority elders and reduce the health disparities that currently exist among these populations.

ACKNOWLEDGMENTS

Support was provided by the National Institute of Diabetes and Digestive and Kidney Diseases, grants K23 DK075006-01, K24 DK071933-01, and P60 DK20595, and the Robert Wood Johnson Foundation Harold Amos Medical Faculty Development Program, grant 53056.

REFERENCES

1. U.S. Bureau of Census. Statistical Abstracts of the United States: 1995. 115th ed. Washington, DC: U.S. Government Printing Office, 1995.
2. Harris MI, Flegal KM, Cowie CC, et al. Prevalence of diabetes, impaired fasting glucose, and impaired glucose tolerance in U.S. adults. Diabetes Care 1998; 21:518–524.
3. Fain J. National trends in diabetes: an epidemiologic perspective. Nurs Clin North Am 1993; 28:1–7.
4. Bamshad M. Genetic influences on health: does race matter? JAMA 2005; 294:937–946.
5. Bradley EH, Herrin J, Wang Y, et al. Racial and Ethnic differences in time to acute reperfusion therapy for patients hospitalized with myocardial infarction. JAMA 2004; 292(13):1563–1572.
6. Cooper RS. Social inequality, ethnicity, and cardiovascular disease. Int J Epidemiol 2001; 30:S48–S52.
7. Sankar P, Cho MK, Condit CM, et al. Genetic research and health disparities. JAMA 2004; 291:2985–2989.
8. Trivedi AN, Zaslavsky AM, Schneider EC, Ayanian JZ. Trends in the quality of care and racial in Medicare Managed Care. N Engl J Med 2005; 353:692–700.
9. Heisler M, Smith DM, Hayward RA, Krein SL, Kerr EA. Racial disparities in diabetes care processes, outcomes, and treatment intensity. Med Care 2003; 41:1221–1232.
10. Boyle JP, Honeycutt AA, Venkat Narayan KM, et al. Projections of diabetes burden through 2050. Diabetes Care 2001; 24:1936–1940.
11. McBean AM, Li S, Gilbertson DT, Collins AJ. Differences in diabetes prevalence, incidence, and mortality among the elderly of four racial/ethnic groups: whites, blacks, Hispanics, and Asians. Diabetes Care 2004; 27:2317–2324.
12. American Diabetes Association. National diabetes facts and figures among Latinos. www.diabetes.org/main/info/facts/facts_latinos.jsp, 2003.
13. Lee ET, Oopik AJ, Howard BV, et al. Diabetes and impaired glucose intolerance in three American Indian populations aged 45–74 years. Diabetes Care 1995; 18(5):599–610.
14. Venkataraman R, Nanda NC, Baweja G, Parikh N, Bhatia V. Prevalence of diabetes mellitus and related conditions in Asian Indians living in the United States. Am J Cardiol 2004; 94:977–980.
15. Weatherspoon LJ, Kumanyika SK, Ludlow R, Schatz D. Glycemic control in a sample of black and white clinic patients in NIDDM. Diabetes Care 1994; 17:1148–1153.
16. Carter JS, Pugh JA, Monterrosa A. Non-insulin dependent diabetes mellitus in minorities in the United States. Ann Intern Med 1996; 125:221–232.
17. Lanting LC, Joung IMA, Mackenbach JP, Lamberts SWJ, Bootsma AH. Ethnic differences in mortality, end-stage complications, and quality of care among diabetic patients. Diabetes Care 2005; 28:2280–2288.
18. Lavery LA, Ashry HR, Van Houtum W, et al. Variation in the incidence and proportion of diabetes-related amputations in minorities. Diabetes Care 1996; 19:48–52.
19. Sundquist J, Winkleby MA, Pudaric S. Cardiovascular disease risk factors among older black, Mexican-American, and white women and men: an analysis of NHANES III, 1988–1994. Third National Health and Nutrition Examination Survey. J Am Geriatr Soc 2001; 49:109–116.
20. Centers for Disease Control and Prevention. Racial/ethnic and socioeconomic disparities in multiple risk factors for heart disease and stroke—United States, 2003. MMWR Morb Mortal Wkly Rep 2005; 54:113–117.
21. Centers for Disease Control and Prevention. Disparities in premature deaths from heart disease—50 states and the District of Columbia, 2001. MMWR Morb Mortal Wkly Rep 2004; 53:121–125.
22. Harris C, Ayala C, Dai S, Croft JB. Disparities in deaths from stroke among persons aged < 75 years—United States, 2002. MMWR Morb Mortal Wkly Rep 2005; 54:477–481.
23. Smedley BD, Stith SY, Nelson AR, eds. Committee on Understanding and Eliminating Racial and Ethnic Disparities in Health Care. Institute of Medicine. Unequal Treatment: Confronting Racial and Ethnic Disparities in Health Care. Washington, DC: National Academy Press, 2002.
24. Gary TL, McGuire M, McCauley J, Brancati FL. Racial comparisons of health care and glycemic control for African American and white diabetic adults in an urban managed care organization. Dis Manag 2004; 7:25–34.
25. Chin MH, Zhang JX, Merrell K. Diabetes in the African-American Medicare population: morbidity, quality of care, and resource utilization. Diabetes Care 1998; 21:1090–1095.
26. Baumann LC, Chang MW, Hoebeke R. Clinical outcomes for low-income adults with hypertension and diabetes. Nurs Res 2002; 51:191–198.
27. Gavin JR III. Diabetes in minorities: reflections on the medical dilemma and the healthcare crisis. Transac Am Clin Climatol Assoc 1995; 107:213–225.
28. Hosler AS, Melnik TA. Population-based assessment of diabetes care and self-management among Puerto Rican adults in New York City. Diabetes Educ 2005; 31:418–426.
29. Wang F, Javitt JC. Eye care for elderly Americans with diabetes mellitus: failure to meet current guidelines. Ophthalmology 1996; 103:1744–1750.
30. Beach MC, Cooper LA, Robinson KA, et al. Strategies for improving minority healthcare quality. Summary, Evidence Report/Technology Assessment No. 90. AHRQ Publication No. 04-E009-01. Rockville, MD: Agency for Healthcare Research and Quality, 2004.

31. Peek ME, Cargill A, Huang ES. Diabetes health disparities: a systematic review of health care interventions. Med Care Res Rev 2007.

32. Rith-Najarian S, Branchaud C, Beaulieu O, et al. Reducing lower-extremity amputations due to diabetes: application of the staged diabetes management approach in a primary care setting. J Fam Practice 1998; 47:127–132.

33. Piette JD, Weinberger M, McPhee SJ, et al. Do automated calls with nurse follow-up improve self-care and glycemic control among vulnerable patients with diabetes? Am J Med 2000; 108:20–27.

34. Pettitt DJ, Wollitzer AO, Jovanovic L, et al. Decreasing the risk of diabetic retinopathy in a study of case management: the California medical type 2 diabetes study. Diabetes Care 2005; 28:2819–2822.

35. Jenkins C, McNary S, Carlson BA, et al. Reducing disparities for African Americans with diabetes: progress made by the REACH 2010 Charleston and Georgetown diabetes coalition. Public Health Rep 2004; 119:322–330.

36. McNabb WL, Quinn MT, Rosing L. Weight loss program for inner-city black women with non-insulin-dependent diabetes mellitus: PATHWAYS. J Am Diet Assoc 1993; 93:75–77.

37. Kleinman A, Eisenberg L, Good B. Culture, illness and care: clinical lessons from anthropologic and cross-cultural research. Ann Intern Med 1978; 88:251–258.

38. Reimann JO, Talavera GA, Salmon M, Nunez JA, Velasquez RJ. Cultural competence among physicians treating Mexican Americans who have diabetes: a structural model. Soc Sci Med 2004; 59:2195–2205.

39. Kleinman A. Patients and Healers in the Context of Culture. Berkeley: University of California Press, 1980.

40. Freeman J, Loewe R. Barriers to communication about diabetes mellitus: patients' and physicians' different view of disease. J Fam Pract 200; 49:507–512.

41. McWhinney IR, ed. Clincal method. In: A Textbook of Family Medicine. New York: Oxford University Press, 1997:129–178.

42. Susman JL, Helseth LD. Reducing the complications of type II diabetes: a patient centered approach. Am Fam Physician 1997; 56:471–480.

43. Stewart MA. Effective physician-patient communication and health outcomes: a review. Can Med Assoc J 1995; 152:1423–1433.

44. Greenfield S, Kaplan SH, Ware JE, et al. Patients' participation in medical care: effects on blood sugar control and quality of life in diabetes. J Gen Intern Med 1988; 3:448–457.

45. Xakellis G, Brangman SA, Hinton WL, et al. Curricular framework: core competencies in multicultural geriatric care. J Am Geriatr Soc 2004; 52:137–142.

46. Quinn MT, Cook S, Nash K, Chin MH. Addressing religion and spirituality in African Americans with diabetes. Diabetes Educ 2001; 27:643–644,647–648, 655.

47. Chin MH, Humikowski CA. When is risk stratification by race or ethnicity justified in medical care? Acad Med 2002; 77:202–208.

48. Shapiro J, Lenahan P. Family medicine in a culturally diverse world: a solution-oriented approach to common cross-cultural problems in medical encounters. Fam Med 1996; 28:249–255.

49. Daniulaityte R. Making sense of diabetes: cultural models, gender and individual adjustment to type 2 diabetes in a Mexican community. Soc Sci Med 2004; 59:1899–1912.

50. Poss JE, Jezewski MA, Stuart AG. Home remedies for type 2 diabetes used by Mexican Americans in El Paso, Texas. Clin Nurs Res 2003; 12:304–323.

51. Arcury TA, Skelly AH, Gesler WM, Dougherty MC. Diabetes meanings among those without diabetes: explanatory models of immigrant Latinos in rural North Carolina. Soc Sci Med 2004; 59:2183–2193.

52. Brown SA, Harrist RB, Villagomez ET, Segura M, Barton SA, Hanis CL. Gender and treatment differences in knowledge, health beliefs, and metabolic control in Mexican Americans with type 2 diabetes. Diabetes Educ 2000; 26:425–438.

53. Koo LC. The use of food to treat and prevent disease in Chinese culture. Soc Sci Med 1984; 18:757–766.

54. Zhang J, Verhoef MJ. Illness management strategies among Chinese immigrants living with arthritis. Soc Sci Med 2002; 55:1795–1802.

55. Lai WA, Lew-Ting CY, Chie WC. How diabetic patients think about and manage their illness in Taiwan. Diabet Med 2005; 22:286–292.

56. Goodwin JS, Black SA, Satish S. Aging versus disease: the opinions of older black, Hispanic, and non-Hispanic white Americans about the causes and treatment of common medical conditions. JAGS 1999; 47:973–979.

57. Hinton L, Franz CE, Yeo G, Levkoff SE. Conceptions of dementia in a multiethnic sample of family caregivers. J Am Geriatr Soc 2005; 53:1405–1410.

58. Ford ME, Tilley BC, McDonald PE. Social support among African American adults with diabetes. Part 2: a review. J Natl Med Assoc 1998; 90:425–432.

59. Teufel NI, Ritenbaugh CK. Development of a primary prevention program: insight gained in the Zuni Diabetes Prevention Program. Clin Pediatr (Phila) 1998; 37:131–141.

60. Rankin SH, Galbraith ME, Huang P. Quality of life and social environment as reported by Chinese immigrants with non-insulin-dependent diabetes mellitus. Diabetes Educ 1997; 23:171–177.

61. Fitzgerald JT, Anderson RM, Funnell MM, et al. Differences in the impact of dietary restrictions on African Americans and Caucasians with NIDDM. Diabetes Educ 1997; 23:41–47.

62. Struthers R, Hodge FS, Geishirt-Cantrell B, De Cora L. Participant experiences of talking circles on type 2 diabetes in two Northern Plains American Indian Tribes. Qual Health Res 2003; 13: 1094–1115.

63. Hornung CA, Eleazer GP, Strothers HS III, et al. Ethnicity and decision-makers in a group of frail older people. J Am Geriatr Soc 1998; 46:280–286.

64. Snapp MB. Occupational stress, social support, and depression among black and white professional-managerial women. Womens Health 1992; 18:41–79.

65. Ford ME, Tilley BC, McDonald PE. Social support among African-American adults with diabetes. Part 1: theoretical framework. J Natl Med Assoc 1998; 90:361–365.

66. Lowe J. Balance and harmony through connectedness: the intentionality of Native American nurses. Holist Nurs Pract 2002; 16:4–11.

67. Gregory D, Whalley W, Olson J, et al. Exploring the experience of type II diabetes in urban aboriginal people. Can J Nurs Res 1999; 31:101–115.

68. Parker J. The lived experience of Native Americans with diabetes within a transcultural nursing perspective. J Transcult Nurs 1994; 6:5–11.

69. Grams GD, Herbert C, Heffernan C, et al. Haida perspective on living with non-insulin–dependent diabetes. Can Med Assoc J 1996; 55:1563–1568.

70. Kang SH, Bloom JR, Romano PS. Cancer screening among African-American women: their use of tests and social support. Am J Public Health 1994; 84:101–103.

71. McDonald PE, Wykle ML, Mistra R, Suwonroop N, Burant CJ. Predictors of social support, acceptance, health promoting behaviors, and glycemic control in African Americans with type 2 diabetes. J Natl Black Nurses Assoc 2002; 13:23–30.

72. Hornquist JO, Wikby A, Stenstrom U, Andersson PO, Akerlind I. Type II diabetes and quality of life: a review of literature. Pharmacoeconomics 1995; 8:12S–16S.

73. Trief PM, Grant W, Elbert K, Weinstock RS. Family environment, glycemic control, and the psychosocial adaptation of adults with diabetes. Diabetes Care 1998; 19:241–245.

74. Connell CM. Psychosocial contexts of diabetes and older adulthood: reciprocal effects. Diabetes Educ 1991; 17:364–371.

75. Epple C, Wright AL, Joish VN, Bauer M. The role of active family nutritional support in Navajos' type 2 diabetes metabolic control. Diabetes Care 2003; 26:2829–2834.

76. von Goeler DS, Rosal MC, Ockene JK, Scavron J, De Torrijos F. Self-management of type 2 diabetes: a survey of low-income urban Puerto Ricans. Diabetes Educ 2003; 29:663–672.

77. Kagitcibasi C. Individualism and collectivism. In: Berry JW, Poortinga YH, Pandey J, eds. Handbook of Cross-Cultural Psychology. 2nd ed. Boston: Allen and Bacon, 1997.

78. Krause N. Assessing stress-buffering effects: a cautionary note. Psychol Aging 1995; 10:518–526.

79. Fugate N, Lentz M, Mitchell E, Oakely LD. Depressed mood and self-esteem in young Asian, black and white women in America. Health Care Women Int 1994; 15:243–262.

80. Lackey NR, Gates MF, Brown G. African American women's experiences with the initial discovery diagnosis, and treatment of breast cancer. Oncol Nurs Forum 2001; 28:519–527.

81. Schoenberg NE, Stoller EP, Kart CS, Perzynski A, Chapleski EE. Complementary and alternative medicine use among a multi-ethnic sample of older adults with diabetes. J Altern Complement Med 2004; 10:1061–1066.

82. Levin JS, Taylor RJ, Chatters LM. A multi-dimensional measure of religious involvement for African Americans. Sociol Q 1995; 36:157–173.

83. Mansfield CJ, Mitchell J, King DE. The doctor as God's mechanic? Beliefs in the southeastern United States. Soc Sci Med 2002; 54:399–409.

84. Taylor RJ, Chatters LM. Non-organizational religious participation among elderly black adults. J Gerontol Soc Sci 1991; 46:S103–S111.

85. Davis RE. Coming to a place of understanding: the meaning of health and illness for African American women. J Mutlicult Nurs Health 1998; 4:32–41.

86. Woodward EK, Sowell R. God is in control: women's perspectives on managing HIV infection. Clin Nurs Res 2001; 10:233–250.

87. Potts RG. Spirituality and the experiences of cancer in an African American community: implications for psychosocial oncology. J Psychosoc Oncol 1996; 14:1–17.

88. Samuel-Hodge CG, Headen SW, Skelly AH, et al. Influences on day-to-day management of type 2 diabetes among African-American women. Diabetes Care 2000; 23:928–933.

89. Bekhius T, Cook H, Holt K, et al. Ethnicity, church affiliation, and beliefs about the causal agents of health: a comparative study employing a multivariate analysis of covariance. Health Educ Res 1995; 10:73–82.

90. McAuley W, Pecchoni J, Grant L. Personal account of the role of God in health and illness among older African American and white residents. J Cross Cult Gerontol 2000; 15:13–35.

91. Ashing-Giwa K, Ganz PA. Understanding the breast cancer experience of African American women. J Psychosoc Oncol 1997; 15:19–35.

92. Eisenberg DM, Davis RB, Ettner SL, et al. Trends in alternative medicine used in the United States, 1996–1997. JAMA 1998; 280:1569–1575.

93. Barnes PM, Powell-Griner E, McFann K, Nahin RL. [no. 343] Advance data from vital and health statistics. Complementary and Alternative Medicine Use Among Adults: United States, 2002. Hyattsville, MD: National Center for Health Statistics, 2004:343.

94. McMahan S, Lutz R. Alternative therapy use among the young old (65 to 74): an evaluation of the MIDUS database. J Appl Gerontol 2004; 23:91–103.

95. Egede LE, Ye X, Zheng D, Silverstein MD. The prevalence and pattern of complementary and alternative medicine use in individuals with diabetes. Diabetes Care 2002; 25:324–329.

96. Berman BM, Singh BB, Hartnoll SM, Singh BK, Reilly D. Primary care physicians and complementary-alternative medicine: training, attitudes, and practice patterns. J Am Board Fam Pract 1998; 11:272–281.

97. Cherniack EP, Senzel RS, Pan CX. Correlates of use of alternative medicine by the elderly in an urban population. J Altern Complement Med 2001; 7:277–280.

98. Hunt LM, Arar NH, Akan LL. Herbs, prayer, and insulin. J Family Pract 2000; 49:216–223.

99. Kuo GM, Hawley ST, Weiss LT, Balkrishnan R, Volk RJ. Factors associated with herbal use among urban multiethnic primary care patients: a cross-sectional survey. BMC Complement Altern Med 2004; 4:18.

100. Marsh WW, Hentges K. Mexican folk remedies and conventional and conventional medical care. Am Fam Physician 1988; 37:257–262.

101. Rivera JO, Ortiz M, Lawson ME, Verma KM. Evaluation of the use of complementary and alternative medicine in the largest United States-Mexican border city. Pharmacotherapy 2002; 22:256–264.

102. Shapiro K, Gong WC. Natural products used for diabetes. J Am Pharm Assoc 2002; 42:217–226.

103. Benavides-Vaello S, Garcia AA, Brown SA, Winchell M. Using focus groups to plan and evaluate diabetes self-management interventions for Mexican Americans. Diabetes Educ 2004; 30:238, 242–234, 247–250 passim.

104. Campinha-Bacote J. A model and instrument for addressing cultural competence in health care. J Nurs Educ 1999; 38:203–207.

105. Brach C, Fraser I. Can cultural competency reduce racial and ethnic health disparities? A review and conceptual model. Med Care Res Rev 2000; 57(S1):181–217.

106. Cooper-Patrick L, Gallo JJ, Gonzales JJ, et al. Race, gender, and partnership in the patient-physician relationship. JAMA 1999; 282:583–589.

107. Saha S, Komaromy M, Koepsell TD, Bindman AB. Patient-physician racial concordance and the perceived quality and use of health care. Arch Intern Med 1999; 159:997–1004.

108. Green AR, Ngo-Metzger Q, Legedza AT, et al. Interpreter services, language concordance, and health care quality. Experiences of Asian Americans with limited English proficiency. J Gen Intern Med 2005; 20:1050–1056.

109. Flores G. The impact of medical interpreter services on the quality of health care: a systematic review. Med Care Res Rev 2005; 62:255–299.

110. Fernandez A, Schillinger D, Grumbach K, et al. Physician language ability and cultural competence. An exploratory study of communication with Spanish-speaking patients. J Gen Intern Med 2004; 19:167–174.

111. Brondino MJ, Henggeler SW, Rowland MD, et al. Multisystemic therapy and the ethnic minority client: culturally responsive and clinically effective. In: Wilson DK, Rodrigue JR, Taylor WC, eds. Health-Promoting and Health-Compromising Behavior Among Minority Adolescents. Application and Practice in Health Psychology. Washington DC: American Psychological Association, 1997.

112. Holland L, Courtney R. Increasing cultural competence with the Latino community. J Community Health Nurs 1998; 15:45–53.

113. Lavizzo-Mourey R, Mackenzie ER. Cultural competence: essential measurements of quality for managed care organizations. Ann Intern Med 1996; 124:919–921.

114. Waitzkin H. Information giving in medical care. J Health Soc Behav 1985; 26:81–101.

115. van Ryn M, Burke J. The effect of patient race and socio-economic status on physicians' perceptions of patients. Soc Sci Med 2000; 50:813–828.

116. Finucane TE, Carrese JA. Racial bias in presentation of cases. J Gen Intern Med 1990; 5:120–121.

117. Rathore SS, Lenert LA, Weinfurt KP, et al. The effects of patient sex and race on medical students' ratings of quality of life. Am J Med 2000; 108:561–566.

118. van Ryn M, Hanan E, Burke J, Besculides M. An examination of factors associated with physician recommendation for revascularization. Washington, DC: American Public Health Association, 1999.

119. Bogart LM, Kelly JA, Catz SL, Sosman JM. Impact of medical and non-medical factors on physician decision for HIV/AIDS antiretroviral treatment. J Acquir Immune Defic Syndr 2000; 23:396–404.

120. van Ryn M. Research on the provider contribution to race/ethnicity disparities in medical care. Med Care 2002; 40:I140–1151.

121. Greenfield S, Kaplan SH, Ware JE. Expanding patient involvement in care: effects on patient outcomes. Ann Intern Med 1985; 102:520–528.

122. Taira DA, Safran DG, Seto TB, et al. The relationship between patient income and physician discussion of health risk behaviors. JAMA 1997; 87:782–786.

123. O'Malley MS, Earp JA, Hawley ST, Schell MJ, Mathews HF, Mitchell J. The association of race/ ethnicity, socioeconomic status, and physician recommendation for mammography: who gets the message about breast cancer screening? Am J Public Health 2001; 91:49–54.

124. Schulman KA, Berlin JA, Harless W, et al. The effect of race and sex on physicians' recommendations for cardiac catheterization. N Engl J Med 1999; 340:618–626.

125. Adams RJ, Smith BJ, Ruffin RE. Impact of the physician's participatory style in asthma outcomes and patient satisfaction. Ann Allergy Asthma Immunol 2001; 86:263–271.

126. Committee on Quality of Health Care in America. Institute of Medicine. Crossing the Quality Chasm: A New Health System for the 21st Century. Washington, DC: National Academy Press, 2001.

127. Stewart M, Brown JB, Donner A, et al. The impact of patient-centered care on outcomes. J Fam Pract 2000; 49:796–804.

128. Safran DG, Taira DA, Rogers WH, et al. Linking primary care performance to outcomes of care. J Fam Pract 1998; 47:213–220.

129. Levinson W, Roter DL, Mullooly JP, et al. Physician-patient communication: the relationship with malpractice claims among primary care physicians and surgeons. JAMA 1997; 277:553–559.

130. Kaplan SH, Greenfield S, Gandek B, et al. Characteristics of physicians with participatory decision-making styles. Ann Intern Med 1996; 124:497–504.

131. Hayward RA, Manning WG, Kaplan SH, Wagner EH, Greenfield S. Starting insulin therapy in patients with type 2 diabetes: effectiveness, complications, and resource utilization. JAMA 1997; 278:1663–1669.

132. Eddy DM. Clinical decision making: from theory to practice. Designing a practice policy. Standards, guidelines, and options. JAMA 1990; 263:3081–3084.

133. Huang ES, Gorawara-Bhat R, Chin MH. Practical challenges of individualizing diabetes care in older patients. Diabetes Educ 2004; 30:558,560,562 passim.

134. Huang ES. Goal setting in older adults with diabetes. In: Geriatric Diabetes Book, Chapter 20.

135. UK Prospective Diabetes Study (UKPDS) Group. Intensive blood-glucose control with sulfonylureas or insulin compared with conventional treatment and risk of complications in patients with type 2 diabetes (UKPDS 33). Lancet 1998; 352:837–853.

136. California Healthcare Foundation/American Geriatrics Society Panel on Improving Care for Elders with Diabetes. Guidelines for improving the care of the older person with diabetes mellitus. JAGS 2003; 51:S265–S280.

137. Kraetschmer N, Sharpe N, Urowitz S, Deber RB. How does trust affect patient preferences for participation in decision-making? Health Expect 2004; 7:317–326.

138. Johnson RL, Roter D, Powe NR, Cooper LA. Patient race/ethnicity and quality of physician communication during medical visits. Am J Public Health 2004; 94:2084–2090.

139. Thackery R, Merrill RM, Neiger BL. Disparities in diabetes management practice between racial and ethnic groups in the United States. Diabetes Educ 2004; 30:665–675.

140. Bernal H, Woolley S, Schensul JJ, Dickinson JK. Correlates of self-efficacy in diabetes self-care among Hispanic adults with diabetes. Diabetes Educ 2000; 26:673–680.

141. Horowitz CR, Williams L, Bickell NA. A community-centered approach to diabetes in Harlem. J Gen Intern Med 2003; 18:542–548.

142. Brown SA, Garcia AA, Kouzekanani K, Hanis CL. Culturally competent diabetes self-management education for Mexican Americans. Diabetes Care 2002; 25:259–268.

143. Hiss RG, Anderson RM, Hess GE, Stepien CJ, Davis WK. Community diabetes care: a 10 year-old perspective. Diabetes Care 1994; 17:1124–1134.

144. Saadine JB, Engelgau MM, Beckles GL, Gregg EW, Thomspon TJ. A diabetes report card for the United States: quality of care in the 1990's. Ann Inn Med 2002; 136:565–574.

145. Karter AJ, Ferrara A, Darbinian JA, Acerson LM, Selfy JV. Self-monitoring of blood glucose. Language and financial barriers in a managed care population with diabetes. Diabetes Care 2000; 23:477–483.

146. Kirsch IS, Jungeblut A, Jenkins L, Kolstad A. Adult literacy in America. Washington, DC: National Center for Education Statistics, US Department of Education, 2002. NCES publication 1993–275.

147. Schillinger D, Grumback K, Piette J, et al. Association of health literacy with diabetes outcomes. JAMA 2002; 288:475–482.

148. Rothman R, Malone R, Bryant B, Horlen C, DeWalt D, Pignone M. The relationship between literacy and glycemic control in a diabetes disease-management program. Diabetes Educ 2004; 30:263–273.

149. Hawthorne K, Tomlinson S. Pakistani Moslems with type 2 diabetes mellitus: effect of sex, literacy skills, known diabetic complications and place of care on diabetic knowledge, reported self-monitoring management and glycaemic control. Diabetic Med 1999; 16:591–597.

150. Williams MV, Baker DW, Parker RM, Nurss JR. Relationship of functional health literacy to patients' knowledge of their chronic disease. A study of patients with hypertension and diabetes. Arch Intern Med 1998; 158:166–172.

151. Rhee MK, Cook CB, El-Kebbi I, et al. Barriers to diabetes education in urban patients: perceptions, patterns, and associated factors. Diabetes Educ 2005; 31:410–417.

152. Hughes HE, Love A, Peabody K, Kardong-Edgren S. Diabetes education programs for African American women: what works? Diabetes Educ 2001; 27:46,48–50,52–54.
153. Carter J, Perez G, Gilland S. Communicate through stories: experience of the native american diabetes project. Diabetes Educ 1999; 25:179–187.
154. Greenhalgh T, Collard A, Begum N. Sharing stories: complex intervention for diabetes education in minority ethnic groups who do not speak English. BMJ 2005; 330:628–633.
155. Houts P, Bachrach R, Witmer J, et al. Using pictographs to enhance recall of spoken medical instructions. Patient Educ Counsel 1998; 35:83–88.
156. Sheppard L, Senior J, Park CH, Mockenhaupt R, Chodzko-Zajko W, Bazzare T. The National Blueprint Consensus Conference summary report: strategic priorities for increasing physical activity among adults aged > or = 50. Am J Prev Med 2003; 25:209–213.
157. U.S. Department of Health and Human Services. Physical activity and health; A Report of the Surgeon General. Atlanta GA: U.S. Department of Health and Human Resources, Centers for Disease Control and Prevention National Center for Chronic Disease Prevention and Health Promotion; 1996.
158. Brawley LR, Rejeski WJ, King AC. Promoting physical activity for older adults: the challenges for changing behavior. Am J Prev Med 2003; 25:172–183.
159. Hui SS, Morrow JR. Levels of participation and knowledge of physical activity in Hong Kong adults and their associations with age. JAPA 2001; 9:372–385.
160. Dergance JM, Mouton CP, Lichtenstein MJ, Hazuda HP. Potential mediators of ethnic differences in physical activity in older Mexican Americans and European Americans: results from the San Antonio longitudinal study of aging. J Am Geriatr Soc 2005; 53:1240–1247.
161. Crespo CJ, Keteyian SJ, Heath GW, Sempos CT. Leisure-time physical activity among U.S. adults: results from the third national health and nutrition examination survey. Arch Intern Med 1996; 156:93–98.
162. Schutzer KA, Graves BS. Barriers and motivations to exercise in older adults. Prev Med 2004; 39:1056–1061.
163. Booth ML, Bauman A, Owen N, Gore CJ. Physical activity preferences, preferred sources assistance, and perceived barriers to increased activity among physically inactive Australians. Prev Med 1997; 26:131–137.
164. Cohen-Mansfield J, Marx MS, Guralnik JM. Motivators and barriers to exercise in an older community-dwelling population. JAPA 2003; 11:242–253.
165. Wilbur J, Chandler PJ, Dancy B, Lee H. Correlates of physical activity in urban Midwestern Latinas. Am J Prev Med 2003; 25:69–76.
166. Pinto BM, Goldstein MG, Ashba J, Sciamanna CN, Jette A. Randomized controlled trial of physical activity counseling for older primary care patients. Am J Prev Med 2005; 29:247–255.
167. Burton LC, Shapiro S, German PS. Determinants of physical activity initiation and maintenance among community-dwelling older persons. Prev Med 1999; 29:422–430.
168. Wilcox S, Oberrecht L, Bopp M, Kammermann SK, McElmurray CT. A qualitative study of exercise in older African American and white women in rural South Carolina: perceptions, barriers, and motivations. J Women Aging 2005; 17:37–53.
169. Nelson KM, Reiber G, Boyko EJ. Diet and exercise among adults with type 2 diabetes. Diabetes Care 2002; 25:1722–1728.
170. American Diabetes Association. Evidence-based nutrition principles and recommendations for the treatment and prevention of diabetes and related complications (position statement). J Am Diet Assoc 2002; 102:109–118.
171. Nutrition and your health: dietary guidelines for Americans. Washington, DC, U.S. Department of Agriculture, U.S. Department of Health and Human Services, 1995 (Home and Garden Bulletin no. 232).
172. Morland K, Wing S, Diez Rouz A, Poole C. Neighborhood characteristics associated with the location of food stores and food service places. Am J Prev Med 2002; 22:23–29.
173. Horowitz CR, Colson KA, Hebert PL, Lancaster K. Barriers to buying healthy foods for people with diabetes: evidence of environmental disparities. Am J Public Health 2004; 94:1549–1554.
174. Veal YS. African Americans and diabetes: reasons, rationale and research. J Natl Med Assoc 1996; 88:203–204.
175. Chesla CA, Chun KM. Accommodating type 2 diabetes in the Chinese American family. Qual Health Res 2005; 15:240–255.
176. McNabb W, Quinn M, Tobian J. Diabetes in African American women: the silent epidemic. Womens Health 1997; 3:275–300.
177. Gylys JA, Gylys BA. Cultural influences and the medical behavior of low-income groups. J Natl Med Assoc 1974; 66:308–312.
178. McNabb WL. Delivering more effective office weight-loss program for black American women. Diabetes Spectr 1994; 7:332–333.
179. Kumanyika S, Charleston JB. Lose weight and win: a church-based weight loss program for blood pressure control among black women. Patient Educ Couns 1992; 19:19–32.

180. Bryant LL, Shetterly SM, Baxter J, Hamman RF. Changing functional status in a biethnic rural population. The San Luis Valley health and aging study. Am J Epidemiol 2002; 155:361–367.

181. Keil JE, Gazes SE, Sutherland PF, et al. Predictors of physical disability in elderly black and white of the Charleston Heart Study. J Clin Epidemiol 1989; 42:521–529.

182. Friedman SM, Steinwachs DM, Rathouz PJ, Burton LC, Mukamel DB. Characteristics predicting nursing home admission in the program of all-inclusive care for elderly people. Gerontologist 2005; 45:157–166.

183. Cagney KA, Agree EM. Racial differences in skilled nursing care and home health use: the mediating effects of family structure and social class. J Gerontol B Psychol Sci Soc Sci 1999; 54:S223–S236.

184. Wallace SP, Levy-Storms L, Kington RS, Andersen RM. The persistence of race and ethnicity in the use of long-term care. J Gerontol 1998; 53B:S104–S112.

185. Fox K, Hinton WL, Levkoff S. Take up the caregiver's burden: stories of care for urban African American elders with dementia. Cult Med Psychiatry 1999; 23:501–529.

186. Zhang X, Norris SL, Gregg EW, Cheng YJ, Beckles G, Kahn HS. Depressive symptoms and mortality among persons with and without diabetes. Am J Epidemiol 2005; 161:652–660.

187. Blazer DG, Moody-Ayers S, Craft-Morgan J, Burchett B. Depression in diabetes and obesity: racial/ethnic/gender issues in older adults. J Psychosom Res 2002; 53:913–916.

188. Young AS, Klap R, Sherbourne CD, Wels KB. The quality of care for depressive and anxiety disorders in the United States. Arch Gen Psychiatry 2001; 58:55–61.

189. Melfi C, Croghan T, Hanna MP, Robinson RL. Racial Variation in antidepressant treatment in a Medicaid population. J Clin Psychiatry 2000; 61:16–21.

190. Wells K, Klap R, Koike A, Sherbourne C. Ethnicity and the prescribing of antidepressant pharmacology: 1992–1995. Am J Psychiatry 2001; 158:2027–2032.

191. Weilburg JB, O'Leary KM, Meigs JB, Hennen J, Stafford R. Evaluation of the adequacy of out patient antidepressant treatment. Psychiatr Serv 2003; 54:1233–1239.

192. Fortney JC, Rost K, Zhang M. The impact of geographic accessibility on the intensity and quality of depression treatment. Med Care 1999; 37:884–893.

193. Harman JS, Edlund MJ, Fortney JC. Disparities in the adequacy of depression treatment in the United States. Psychiatr Serv 2004; 55:1379–1385.

194. Saudek CD, Hill Golden S. Feasibility and outcomes of insulin therapy in elderly patients with diabetes mellitus. Drugs Aging 1999; 14:375–385.

195. Manly JJ, Jacobs DM, Sano M, et al. Cognitive test performance among nondemented elderly African Americans and whites. Neurology 1998; 50:1238–1245.

196. Melville JL, Katon W, Delaney K, Newton K. Urinary incontinence in US women: a population-based study. Arch Intern Med 2005; 165:537–542.

197. Funnell MM, Merritt JH. The challenges of diabetes in older adults. Nurs Clin North Am 1993; 28:45–60.

198. Laramee SH. Position of the American Diabetic Association: nutrition services in managed care. J Am Diet Assoc 1996; 96:391–395.

199. Nickens HW. The role of race/ethnicity and social class in minority health status. Health Serv Res 1995; 30:151–162.

200. Ell K, Vourlekis B, Muderspach L, et al. Abnormal cervical screen follow-up among low-income Latinas: project SAFE. J Womens Health Gend Based Med 2002; 11:639–651.

201. Frelix GD, Rosenblatt R, Solomon M, Vikram B. Breast cancer screening in underserved women in the Bronx. J Natl Med Assoc 1999; 10:195–200.

27 Management of Diabetes in Chronic Care Settings

Virginia K. Cummings
Division of Gerontology, Beth Israel Deaconess Medical Center, Boston, Massachusetts, U.S.A.

INTRODUCTION

Of the elderly population, 4.5% resides in nursing facilities at any one time, and a further 5% of elders live in supported senior housing communities of some sort, including independent living senior communities, continuing care retirement communities, assisted living, and dementia-specialty assisted-living facilities (1). Studies have estimated the prevalence of diabetes in this population anywhere from 14.5% to 26.7% (2–4) and all studies were in agreement that diabetes and impaired glucose tolerance are underrecognized in chronic care settings. Institutionalized diabetics are much sicker than their nondiabetic counterparts, averaging 6.4 medical diagnoses, as opposed to 2.4 in nondiabetics, and 90% of institutionalized diabetics have coronary artery disease, cerebrovascular disease, or peripheral vascular disease (5). Diabetes is an independent risk factor for hospitalization (6), nursing home placement (6,7) and for a host of comorbidities including cognitive decline, falls, low vision, and renal failure. The Centers for Disease Control and Prevention estimate the cost of diabetic treatment in nursing facilities to be $6 billion annually (8). Despite this expenditure, there is strong evidence that diabetes is undertreated (9–11) as well as underrecognized in nursing homes and assisted-living communities. There is convincing evidence that treatment of diabetes slows or prevents disease progression (12). In theory, the standards and practices for diagnosis and management of diabetes in institutionalized elderly do not differ from those used in ambulatory elderly. However, a number of factors specific to each chronic care setting may modify the goals of diabetes therapy. Additionally, unique barriers to care exist for patients in chronic care facilities, and greater physician awareness of these potential roadblocks may improve implementation of diabetes treatment. Theoretically, the availability of monitoring and medication administration by trained staff in chronic care settings should facilitate the management of diabetes in this population, despite its frailty and medical complexity. This chapter will address recognition and treatment of diabetes in assisted-living facilities, transitional-care, and post-acute-care facilities, and long-term care facilities, with particular emphasis on barriers to optimal care and suggestions for quality improvement systems implementation.

ASSISTED-LIVING FACILITIES

There are approximately 33,000 assisted-living facilities operating in the United States in 2006 (13), serving just under one million seniors. The assisted-living industry is growing rapidly and is soon predicted to house more seniors than nursing homes (14). There are many different names for these facilities (Table 1), but all provide meal service, housekeeping, custodial services, and recreational activities. The vast majority provide assistance with activities of daily living, and some basic types of health monitoring as well. However, licensure and regulations vary from state to state, as do the services that can be provided and the staffing levels required. About 70% employ an registered nurse or licensed practical nurse, and 22 states allow unlicensed staff to administer medication. Only 15 states have minimum staffing requirements (13,15), and skilled nursing is available in only 60%, usually via a medicare-regulated contract agency, such as a visiting nurse association and not via facility-employed staff (13). As these facilities have become more numerous and more competitive, the demographics of the population have changed significantly. In the 1980s, when these facilities first became prevalent, they served the needs of the deinstitutionalized mentally ill under state Medicaid programs or

TABLE 1 Alternate Names for Assisted-Living Facilities

Residential care
Continuing care retirement communities
Adult congregate living care
Board and care homes
Domiciliary care
Adult living facilities
Supported care homes
Enhanced care homes
Community-based retirement facilities
Adult foster care
Group homes
Retirement residences
Senior housing facilities

elderly patients who were independent with activities of daily living (16). Now, however, the average resident of an assisted-living facility is white, female, in her early 80s, and is paying, privately, an average of $4000 per month for the facility and its services (13). Approximately 60% of residents need assistance with one to three activities of daily living, and 75% need assistance with medications (13). Residents average 5 to 6.1 medications daily, a rate similar to that seen in skilled nursing facilities (SNF) (14). Cognitive impairment is extremely prevalent, averaging 50% to 60% (15), and 25% of assisted-living facilities have a dedicated unit for cognitively impaired residents. Average length of stay is approximately three years. Annually, 11% of residents will need hospitalization, 26% will die in the facility, and 26% to 40% will require transfer to a SNF (13), either because of medical decline or because of depletion of financial resources. Forty percent of the residents have hypertension and 20% to 40% have either a recent fracture or a psychiatric diagnosis (15).

Unfortunately, assisted-living facility policies, regulations, and staffing patterns have not kept pace with the increasing frailty and complexity of this population. Since more than 50% of these facilities are for-profit institutions, there is pressure on the staff to maintain declining residents in the facility and allow for "aging in place" despite increasing, and possibly unmet, medical needs. As in SNF, staff turnover is high, approximately 45% yearly (13), and education is not a priority—only 11 states mandate staff education on topics related to aging (13). Additionally, facility-wide supervision of care by a physician is not mandated in any state, as it is for SNF, nor is monitoring or review of facility medication practices by a pharmacist. Although 45 states have regulations in place for food and nutrition services, a recent review by the Nutritional Services at the Massachusetts Executive Office of Elder Affairs did not find adequate oversight policies in place for any state (14).

Goals of Treatment

The goals of treatment in assisted-living settings do not differ substantially from those of ambulatory elderly patients and include

1. Establishing a stable regimen for maintaining glycemic control and preventing microvascular complications
2. Monitoring and adjusting the regimen to optimize glycemic control while avoiding hypoglycemic episodes
3. Coordinating diabetes health maintenance compliance including eye and foot care
4. Controlling associated comorbidities such as hypertension and hyperlipidemia
5. Screening for high-risk complications including vascular-related cognitive impairment, renal disease, malnutrition, and infection

See Chapters 20 and 21 for more detailed information on goal setting and maintenance of glycemic control.

Barriers to Optimal Treatment of Diabetes Mellitus in Assisted-Living Facilities

No studies have been published that specifically address treatment of diabetes in the assisted-living setting, but studies of the treatments of other prevalent chronic diseases including congestive heart failure, coronary artery disease, osteoporosis, stroke, and dementia (15,16) suggest that undertreatment is substantial, and that 37% to 76% of residents were not being treated for these diagnosed conditions. The rates of undertreatment were similar to those found in community-dwelling elderly despite access to licensed nursing staff for medication assistance (15). There is data to show that patients in assisted-living facilities may be at a risk of a more rapid decline in health status than those with similar comorbidities living in SNF (17), in part due to the discrepancy between the availability of health services and the perception that such services are being provided. Although there is no data available on the treatment of diabetes in assisted-living facilities, it is likely that undertreatment rates equal or exceed those found in the community. This is in contrast to SNF, where blood glucose control as measured by hemoglobin A1c (HgA1c) has been shown to be substantially better than that of an ambulatory diabetic population (5). The barriers to optimal treatment of diabetes mellitus in assisted-living facilities are outlined and discussed below.

Underdiagnosis

Although there are no specific data on the prevalence of diabetes in assisted-living facilities, studies of community-dwelling elders and elders admitted to nursing homes find the prevalence of undiagnosed diabetes in this population to be around 12% to 22% (18,19) and the total prevalence to be 14% to 26.7% (2–4,18,19). It can be assumed that rates in the assisted-living facilities are in line with these findings. Diabetes in the elderly remains underrecognized by health-care providers at all levels, and the lack of coordinated nursing and physician oversight of patient care in assisted-living facilities prevents implementation of policies to address this concern. Diagnosis of diabetes in residents of assisted-living facilities remains the responsibility of the primary physician, and the barriers to diagnosis that apply in the community are equally applicable to this population. (See Chapter 4 for more information on diagnosis of diabetes.)

Cognitive Impairment

The prevalence of cognitive impairment is 50% to 60% in assisted-living facilities as compared to 15% in the community (16). Of more concern, a recent study of seven assisted-living facilities in Nebraska noted that 63% of residents with cognitive impairment on mini-mental states exam had no diagnosis of dementia, and 75% with cognitive impairment were on no treatment. This affects management of diabetes in multiple ways. Patients with diabetes and cognitive impairment due to microvascular disease would clearly benefit from tight glucose control as well as aggressive blood pressure and lipid-lowering therapy (12). However, ignorance of cognitive impairment may lead caregivers away from attempts at aggressive medical management despite its particular importance in this setting, for fear of inducing side effects. Additionally, cognitively impaired patients are at a risk of serious medication noncompliance. In the Nebraska study, 22% of patients with known cognitive impairment were nonetheless responsible for self-administration of, on an average, more than five medications. With no state-mandated oversight of medication, the responsibility for diabetes management in the cognitively impaired falls on caregivers and physicians, just as it does in the community. However, since the symptoms of progressive diabetes may be subtle, patients with cognitive impairment, particularly if unrecognized by staff and caregivers, may be untreated or undertreated for longer periods of time than in case of community-dwelling patients.

Physician Misperception of Facility Capabilities

Assisted-living facilities are a relatively new and unresearched entity, and the regulations regarding care provision vary greatly from state to state. Additionally, since there is no federal oversight and very little state oversight, care capabilities may vary significantly from facility to facility. Many physicians have little or no idea what services the facilities provide. Current medical training, even geriatric training, does not mandate any familiarity with this level of care. Physicians may assume that assisted-living facilities have capabilities similar to skilled nursing facilities and mistakenly delegate such care issues as capillary blood glucose monitoring, sliding scale insulin administration, glucagon administration, and dietary education to facility staff who have no training or resources with which to deliver this care. This population is similar in frailty and impairment to the skilled nursing population (15). However, the principles of physician management need to be those used for elders in the ambulatory setting. Patients in assisted-living facilities "may" have access to on-site services such as podiatry, optometry, nutrition, physical therapy, and skilled nursing. However, no facility is mandated to provide the services, and it is the primary physician's responsibility to oversee this care and monitor patient compliance and utilization. Table 2 outlines some important differences between SNF and assisted-living facilities.

Caregiver Misperception of Facility Capabilities

Family members and community caregivers often misperceive the capabilities of assisted-living facilities. Placement in a facility of any kind is often a response to a medical event or significant psychosocial stressor (7), and it frequently reflects the inability of the caregivers to sustain the patient's care in the community due to "burnout" or medical illness. Unfortunately, placement in an assisted-living facility does not alleviate the need for caregiving to the degree that placement in a SNF may. Data suggests that caregivers of patients in assisted living spend more time monitoring the health, well-being, and finances of their loved one, and rate their caregiver burden higher than caregivers of nursing home patients (20). It is still the responsibility of the patient and/or caregiver to coordinate medications, physician visits, and compliance with care plans. Assisted-living facilities may be able to provide or assist with health-care services, but usually at extra cost (21) and only at the request of the patient or caregiver. Many caregivers assume that patient medical needs can be met by the facility without the need for their ongoing involvement. They may also assume that because the facility staff is managing personal care needs and activities of daily living, they are also managing and monitoring chronic medical issues. Again, some facilities may be capable of this, but there is no consistent oversight or regulation of care delivery (13). Furthermore, the majority of patients in assisted living pay privately for services and will move to skilled nursing facilities when finances are depleted (7,21). Patients and families may be reluctant to spend scarce resources for care that they perceive the facility should be providing, such as nutrition counseling or foot care. Physicians need to be aware that caregivers may be unwilling or unable to continue to provide the support and oversight to assisted-living patients that they provided in the community setting. This inability to provide care may have resulted in the facility placement. Without it,

TABLE 2 Assisted-Living Facilities Vs. Skilled Nursing Facilities

Requirement	Skilled nursing facility	Assisted-living facility
Physician oversight	Federal requirement	No requirement, few provide the service
Registered nurse presence	Federal requirement at least 8 of 24 hr	No federal requirement
Licensed staff (LPN or RN) presence	Federal requirement	Only 22 states require
Food services overseen by licensed dietician	Federal requirement	No requirement
Medical or special diets available	Federal requirement	No requirement, few facilities provide the service
Medicare-defined skilled services provided	Federal requirement credentialed and overseen by medical director	No requirement, no facility-specific oversight mandated
Allied health services onsite (i.e., podiatry, dental, etc.)	Federal requirement credentialed and overseen by medical director	No requirement, individual facilities vary, no mandated credentialing
Medical visits mandated	Federal requirement every 60 days, some states require it more frequently	No requirement, individual facilities may require patients to designate a primary physician
Pharmacy onsite, or emergency medication available onsite	Federal requirement, state oversight	No requirement, some states expressly prohibit facility-dispensed medication
Medical records maintained	Federal requirement, state oversight	No requirement

Abbreviations: LPN, licensed practical nurse; RN, registered nurse.

however, diabetics in assisted living may not receive the level of care they received in the community, where both physicians and caregivers were aware of their responsibilities.

Lack of Flexible Nutrition Services

One of the most common patient complaints about any type of facility is the food service. Institutional food is, of course, unable to please everyone all the time. Assisted-living facilities, especially those that are for profit, take a purely consumer-oriented approach to food services. Nutrition oversight is underregulated in the industry (14); the driving force for change is more often patient preference than concern for patient well-being. Large portion sizes, high-sugar, and high-fat offerings are common, and their constant availability and visibility may lead to poor food choices. Special diets such as low-salt food, ground food, low-protein food, and "no concentrated sweets" are not widely available in the vast majority of facilities. Facility staff have no consistent ability to regulate anyone's food intake or prevent patients from making inappropriate food choices. Additionally, many facilities are set up such that patients may prepare their own food in their apartment or room if desired, free of any monitoring whatsoever. The opposite problem exists as well—patients may be faced with food choices that they dislike and may eat inconsistently from day to day, leading to fluctuations in blood glucose and the need to reduce dosing to avoid episodic hypoglycemia. Inconsistent intake is especially common among patients with cognitive impairment, patients with dental or swallowing problems, patients with chronic pain, and patients with gastrointestinal issues such as gastroparesis (22,23). Physicians need to be aware that their patients in assisted-living facilities need the same level of nutrition intervention and counseling, if not more, than their peers in the community.

Strategies for Quality Improvement
Implementation of Federal Standards for Assisted-Living Facilities

Variability in care provision will continue to be an issue until the federal government mandates standards of care for assisted-living facilities. Physicians should join with patients, caregivers, families, and staff to lobby for improved oversight of these facilities.

Integration of Community Programs into Assisted-Living Facilities

Many programs for diabetes management exist in the community for ambulatory patients. Unfortunately, frail, impaired seniors in assisted-living facilities may be unable to take advantage of these programs due to a lack of mobility or knowledge of resource availability. Many community programs could meet at assisted-living facilities rather than physician offices, public libraries, senior centers, etc., thereby benefiting both ambulatory and facility-bound patients.

Staff and Caregiver Education

The signs and symptoms of diabetes may be subtle and unrecognized by staff and caregivers. Education on what to monitor and information on goals of treatment, side effects, and risks and benefits of different glucose control strategies will help staff to develop individual care strategies that take into account patient, family, and facility preferences and limitations.

SUMMARY

Diabetic patients residing in assisted-living facilities offer a unique challenge to physicians. They represent a population as frail and complex as that in SNF but which must be managed as if they were still living in the community. Assisted-living facilities vary widely in their ability to provide services for the management of diabetes. At their best, they provide licensed nursing staff able to offer significant aid to diabetics, including medication administration and on-site ancillary health services. Too often, however, physicians and caregivers have an overly optimistic view of the services provided and neglect to oversee these patients as diligently as those in the community.

POST-ACUTE CARE AND TRANSITIONAL-CARE FACILITIES

Discharge from acute hospitalization to post-acute care in a chronic care hospital or SNF has become increasingly common. Currently, 33% of Medicare beneficiaries are discharged to a post-acute-care setting following hospitalization, and post-acute care accounts for approximately 11% of Medicare spending annually (24). The average length of stay for these patients is 24.6 days, and 50% utilize home care services after discharge. Diabetes is common in this setting; 18% of patients over age 35 with an in-hospital diagnosis-related group of diabetes will be discharged to a post-acute-care facility (25), and a diagnosis of diabetes is a significant risk factor for rehospitalization or progression to long-term care (6,7). It is well known that hyperglycemia from uncontrolled diabetes delays wound healing, increases risk of infection, and can lead to dehydration and impaired cognition (26). Appropriate management of diabetes in the post-acute setting is crucial for improvement in patient functional status and achievement of rehabilitation goals.

Treatment Goals

The treatment goals for diabetics in post-acute care settings are straightforward, since these encounters are, by nature, time-limited. They include

1. Reestablishing a stable regimen for maintaining glycemic control. This may differ from the prehospitalization regimen due to changes in patient health status. Occasionally, diabetes is a new diagnosis. (See Chapter 21 for information about establishing a maintenance regimen for the first time.)
2. Reviewing new diagnoses and medications resulting from the hospitalization to determine their impact on glycemic control and diabetic health maintenance.
3. Monitoring and adjusting the regimen as indicated by patient status. This is of particular importance in the post-acute care setting, where patient status may change significantly in a short time.
4. Educating the patient and caregivers regarding their diabetes regimen, especially emphasizing changes due to new diagnoses and medications.
5. Screening for comorbidities such as hypertension, cognitive impairment, and hyperlipidemia, which may have been missed in the hospital or the ambulatory setting.
6. Monitoring and adjusting treatment of comorbidities as indicated by patient status. Again, status may change significantly over the course of the encounter, and multiple medication adjustments may be necessary.
7. Communicating with the community interdisciplinary team, including the primary physician, endocrinologist, and home care providers to ensure that all members are aware of changes in regimen and status.

A step-by-step strategy for reestablishment of a stable regimen is outlined in Table 3.

Barriers to Optimal Care of Diabetes Mellitus in Post-Acute Care Settings

Post-acute care provides a level of support between that of the acute hospital and that of the ambulatory or long-term care setting. Increased staffing levels and availability of enhanced laboratory, pharmacy, and therapy services should allow clinicians to closely monitor and adjust the diabetes regimen in ways not possible in the community. Unfortunately, many barriers exist that prevent optimal care of diabetes in this setting. Some of the more important of these are outlined below.

Fragmented Care Transitioning

As lengths of stays in hospitals have decreased and discharge to post-acute care has become more prevalent, the use of hospitalists and post-acute care specialists has increased. The traditional model of the primary physician following his/her patients through the continuum of care is becoming less feasible, especially since reimbursement for post-acute care has not kept pace with the acuity level of the patient population (24,25). This has led to fragmentation of care and gaps in the flow of information from one setting to the next (27). Diabetes management is particularly prone to this type of fragmented care, since it is extremely common practice during an acute hospitalization to suspend the outpatient regimen and treat with short-acting insulin via a sliding scale (see Chapter 12 for more information on management of diabetes in the acute

TABLE 3   Reestablishing a Stable Regimen for Glycemic Control

1. Appraise the hospital discharge regimen	
No regimen, but diagnosis of diabetes	Institute q.i.d. fingerstick glucose monitoring and sliding scale regular insulin coverage
Sliding scale regular insulin only	Institute q.i.d. fingerstick glucose monitoring, continue sliding scale regular insulin coverage
Oral agent or long-acting insulin with sliding scale regular insulin	Institute q.i.d. fingerstick glucose monitoring, continue regimen as ordered
Oral agent or long-acting insulin without sliding scale regular insulin	Institute q.i.d. fingerstick glucose monitoring and sliding scale regular insulin coverage
2. Obtain patient's pre-hospital regimen and review changes in medication and status that may necessitate changes	
3. Re-evaluate patient and admission regimen after a minimum of 72 hr and a maximum of 1 wk	
Patient stable, eating reliably	Re-start previous regimen (or institute initial regimen as per Chapter 21). Continue q.i.d. fingerstick monitoring and sliding scale regular insulin
Patient unstable, unable to maintain nutrition	Continue q.i.d. fingersticks, sliding scale regular insulin. Discontinue oral agent or long-acting insulin. Reevaluate patient as per step 3 until able to restart previous regimen
4. Re-evaluate patient and new regimen after a minimum of 72 hr and maximum of 1 wk	
Patient stable, no sliding scale insulin administered	Decrease fingerstick glucose monitoring to b.i.d. Continue sliding scale regular insulin
Patient receiving sliding scale insulin	Increase oral agent(s) or long-acting insulin (see Chapter 21). Continue q.i.d. fingerstick glucose and sliding scale regular insulin
5. Reevaluate patient and new regimen as per step 4 until desired glycemic control is achieved. Discontinue sliding scale regular insulin when patient has been free of administration >72 hr	

hospital). With hospital stays averaging 5.4 days nationally (24), patients seldom have their outpatient regimens reinstated prior to admission to post-acute care. The facility physician may or may not have access to the outpatient medication information and may not have any documentation of glucose control during the hospitalization. Additionally, changes in patient status, such as weight loss or addition of medications, may mandate changes in the previous regimen. If this information is not communicated first to the post-acute physician, and then to the primary physician upon discharge, medication mismanagement and inappropriate treatment may occur.

Delirium

Delirium in the elderly is extremely common during acute hospital stays. It is estimated to be present at admission or develop in the hospital in up to 25% of patients over age 65 and up to 40% of patients over age 85 (28). There is less data on the prevalence of delirium in post-acute care, but estimates place it between 20% and 38% of all admissions. Delirium doubles the chance of discharge to post-acute care (29), and increases the risk of nursing home placement within one year by almost three times (30). Additionally, delirium may persist long after the inciting event has been diagnosed and treated; less than 50% of patients with in-hospital delirium have complete resolution of all symptoms within six months (31). Delirium has been clearly shown to increase length of stay at the acute hospital and the post-acute care (29–31) and to lead to decreased functional recovery and increased comorbidity as compared to the nondelirious elderly. Delirium adds an average of three medications to the patient's regimen and increases the risk of infection, falls, and skin breakdown (28–31).

Presence of delirium has particular significance for the management of diabetes in post-acute care. The fluctuations in the level of consciousness that are the hallmark of delirium may lead to inconsistent oral intake and delay institution of a stable diabetic regimen. Poor oral intake also leads to poor nutrition and dehydration, which further impair glucose control.

Also, patients with delirium are frequently agitated and psychotic, leading to utilization of the atypical antipsychotic medications such as risperidone, olanzepine, and quetiapine, which have been linked with hyperglycemia, increased risk of stroke (a particular risk for diabetics). and increased mortality. Olanzepine, in particular, has been associated with hyperglycemia and should be avoided in diabetics, especially when attempting to stabilize the glycemic regimen. Lastly, the persistence of delirium may impede attempt at patient education and lead to discharge of patients who are unable to appropriately comply with glycemic control in the community. Physicians caring for patients in post-acute care need to be vigilant for delirium symptoms in their diabetic patients and change management strategies accordingly.

Malnutrition/Increased Nutritional Needs

Multiple studies have documented the extremely high prevalence of malnutrition in post-acute care. Two recent large studies, involving over 1500 patients, documented outright malnutrition or high-risk nutritional status in approximately 90% of the patients (32,33). Poor nutrition increases the risks of infection, skin breakdown, poor functional recovery, and in-facility mortality (34). Diabetics are at a particular risk of poor nutrition because of the common practice of dietary limitation in institutional settings. Although the majority are admitted to the facility with concurrent malnutrition and increased nutritional demand (for wound healing, infection, etc.), they are frequently placed on low-calorie, fat-restricted diets, which do not meet their increased metabolic needs. The decreased palatability of these diets may lead to further nutritional losses, and their utilization is not recommended in the post-acute setting. Associated hypoalbuminemia may lead to increased side effects from oral hypoglycemic agents, delaying institution of a stable regimen. Additionally, diabetics are at a risk of infections and gastrointestinal issues such as gastroparesis, which prevent optimal oral intake. Physicians need to be aware of the high risks of malnutrition faced by diabetic patients and encourage individualized diets overseen by nutritionists that provide adequate calories, fat, and protein to facilitate healing and functional recovery.

Lack of Trained/Educated Staff

Post-acute care is becoming more common, and the number of post-acute care beds has increased substantially. The majority of the growth has occurred in SNF, with utilization of SNF-level post-acute care doubling since 1990 (25). Although minimum staffing requirements for post-acute care are mandated under federal and state regulations, staff education and training is not mandated. The vast majority of staff in SNF are licensed nurses, with 12 to 18 months of education, rather than registered nurses, with an associate or bachelor degree. SNF is only required to have one registered nurse in the building per 24-hour period, with 8 hours required onsite and 16 hours of off-site availability. Additionally, the majority of direct patient care in post-acute units is provided by certified nursing assistants, with training varying from 6 to 12 weeks. Licensed nursing staff provides supervision, patient education, and medication administration (35). Staff varies widely in knowledge and experience, particularly with regard to diabetes management. Symptoms of hyper-/hypoglycemia may go unrecognized, and appropriate glucose monitoring may not be done. Additionally, the acuity level and care burden in this setting is high, and the number of medications utilized in post-acute care, an average of 9.1 per patient, increases the likelihood of medication errors. A common error in this setting is the mistiming of insulin administration with regard to glucose monitoring and oral intake, especially when insulin is administered several times per day via a sliding scale. One study found that between 22% and 41% of residents had inappropriate timing of insulin administration (36). Furthermore, staffing patterns vary across shifts and on weekends, so that consistency in management is often unavailable, and patients may receive conflicting education and care (37).

Lack of Physician Presence

Regulation of physician presence in post-acute care facilities has not kept up with the realities of the acuity and complexity of this population. Poor reimbursement, as compared to acute hospital care and ambulatory care, has further limited physician willingness to spend time in these facilities (25). Current Medicare regulations require new patients to be seen within 48 hours of admission, every 30 days for the first 90 days, then every 60 days subsequently.

However, post-acute patients frequently require much more intensive physician management to achieve optimal outcomes. Many physicians and facilities have sought to address this shortage with physician extenders such as nurse practitioners and physician assistants. Studies of physician extenders in long-term care have documented their efficacy and cost effectiveness (38). However, this is not as well documented for post-acute care. Diabetic patients, with their need for frequent monitoring and regimen adjustment and multiple comorbidities, may be at a particular risk of undertreatment in post-acute facilities where physicians are not regularly present and involved.

Strategies for Quality Improvement
Increased Communication Across Continuum
Optimal management of diabetes in the post-acute care setting depends on receipt of appropriate information from the acute hospital on admission and communication of appropriate information to community physicians at discharge. Development of systems that improve ease and accuracy of this communication, such as electronic medical records and standardized transfer forms, will allow providers to have immediate access to this important information and ensure continuity of the glycemic regimen and diabetes-health maintenance care.

Increased Physician Presence
Utilization of post-acute care is increasing, and financial issues are driving down lengths of stay (25,26). Increasing physician presence and involvement in care will lead to better outcomes. This can be achieved by the physician lobbying (along with organizations such as the American Medical Directors Association) for reimbursement that is more consistent with time and complexity of the physician visits. Additionally, many physicians are choosing to delegate post-acute care to a physician specialist, similar to hospitalists in acute care. Physician extenders may also serve to increase care delivery, but further research is needed to verify that this level of care is appropriate in the post-acute setting.

Staff Education and Policy Development
Physicians should take an active role in staff education and policy development in post-acute care facilities. All facilities are mandated to provide staff education, but there is no specific "curriculum" for post-acute care. Physician communication with nursing directors and staff educators regarding perceived educational deficits among staff can guide development of in-services. Furthermore, case-based educational sessions may be especially helpful to staff, and physicians should take a lead role in identifying cases for staff review and analysis. Case identification is important for quality improvement initiatives as well, and physicians need to be involved in the quality improvement process. Lastly, implementation of current evidence-based guidelines can improve diabetes care. Physicians need to be familiar with the post-acute care literature and work with facility educators to incorporate evidence-based medicine into practice.

Patient and Family Education and Involvement
Although a significant percentage of diabetic patients admitted to post-acute care remain institutionalized after rehabilitation, the majority do return to the community. Successful discharge to the ambulatory setting is dependent on patient and caregiver education, and physicians should be familiar with staff education policies and assist in the development of patient education materials. Also, physicians should stress the need for ongoing patient and caregiver education in the ambulatory setting and help the facilities to form linkages with community programs that help maintain frail elderly diabetics in the community.

SUMMARY

Post-acute care is an increasingly common discharge setting for elderly diabetic patients. In theory, a level of care between acute hospitalization and return to the community should allow for reestablishment and adjustment of an optimal diabetes maintenance regimen. However, physicians need to be diligent in initiating such a regimen and monitoring patients as they progress. An awareness of the benefits and limitations of this setting will help physicians to utilize post-acute care to the best advantage of their diabetic patients.

LONG-TERM CARE FACILITIES
Introduction

Diabetes is a significant diagnosis in long-term care facilities. Studies estimate its prevalence anywhere from 14.5% to 26.7% (2–4) and its cost at around $6 billion annually (8). Diabetes has substantial comorbidity associated with it, and long-term care patients are disproportionately affected, with more than 90% having coronary artery disease or peripheral vascular disease (5), 50% having cognitive impairment (33% of which is at the moderate stage or greater) (3), and more than 50% having chronic pain (3). Despite the frailty of this population, diabetic patients in long-term care have been shown to have better glucose control than a healthier and younger ambulatory population (5). However, the associated comorbidities in this population may have progressed to such a degree that improved glucose control is "too little, too late," since the majority of long-term care diabetics have functional and cognitive impairment (4), 20% are underweight and at a risk of malnutrition (5), and a significant proportion have neuropathy, retinopathy, and nephropathy. Physicians need to take multiple factors into account when implementing a treatment plan for diabetes. It is clear that good glycemic control slows the progression of microvascular disease and cognitive impairment (12). However, quality of life, prognosis, and functional status issues also need to be taken into account. What is clear is that the guidelines for ambulatory patients may not be appropriate for every long-term care patient. Physicians need to find a balance between the rigidity of tight glycemic control and the pessimism of undertreatment based solely on age and institutionalization.

Goals of Treatment

The treatment goals for patients in long-term care facilities need to strike a balance between good glycemic control and maintenance of quality of life and include

1. Recognizing the diabetic patient on admission to the facility, and screening and diagnosing patients at risk for development of diabetes, both at the time of admission and at set intervals during the stay at the facility (see Chapter 4 for more information on screening and diagnosis of diabetes in the elderly).
2. Establishing, monitoring, adjusting, and maintaining a glycemic control regimen. See Table 4 for recommended frequency of monitoring in various clinical situations.
3. Modifying the glycemic control regimen in response to factors such as malnutrition, increased metabolic need secondary to medical illness, cognitive impairment, end-stage disease, patient preference, and the realities of long-term care facility capabilities.
4. Providing and overseeing diabetes-health maintenance care available onsite, such as foot care, podiatry evaluation, nutrition evaluation, oral care, screening for orthostasis, renal disease, cognitive impairment, and immunization.
5. Facilitating access to diabetes-health maintenance care available off site, such as ophthalmologic examination and dental and periodontal care. See Table 5 for recommended health maintenance.
6. Diagnosing and managing common comorbidities such as peripheral vascular disease, hypertension, coronary artery disease, peripheral neuropathy, chronic pain, depression, hyperlipidemia, infection, and renal disease.
7. Reviewing the medication regimen for polypharmacy, side effects, redundancy, and inappropriate, contradictory, or unnecessary medications.
8. Educating patients' families, caregivers, and staff about the goals of treatment, the course of disease, and sentinel signs of progression or inadequate treatment.
9. Providing input to facility management regarding policies and guidelines for care and issues relating to suboptimal care or resource availability.
10. Documenting goals of care, risks, and benefits of medications or procedures and patient and family preferences for various care options.
11. Communicating with caregivers and other health-care providers to prevent duplication of care or gaps in care delivery.

TABLE 4 Recommended Frequency of Blood Glucose Monitoring

Oral hypoglycemic regimen	HgA1C on admission HgA1c q6 mo if <8 HgA1c q3 mo if >8	Fingerstick blood glucose twice weekly if no regimen changes
		Fingerstick blood glucose b.i.d.. × 72 hr if increasing oral agent Fingerstick blood glucose q.i.d. × 72 hr if adding insulin (either sliding scale or longer acting prep)
Insulin regimen Short-acting agent (regular insulin, lispro) (not recommended for ongoing maintenance)	HgA1C on admission HgA1C q3 mo	Fingerstick blood glucose q.i.d. until patient is on intermediate or long-acting agent
Insulin regimen Intermediate agent (NPH, Lente®)	HgA1C on admission HgA1C q6 mo <8 HgA1C q3 mo >8	Fingerstick blood glucose b.i.d. if no regimen changes
		Fingerstick blood glucose q.i.d. if increasing insulin Fingerstick q.i.d. for status change including fever, infection, vomiting, inability to eat
Insulin regimen long-acting agent (Ultralente®, Lantus®)	HgA1C on admission HgA1C q6 mo <8 HgA1C q3 mo >8	Fingerstick blood glucose b.i.d. if no regimen change
		Fingerstick blood glucose q.i.d. if increasing insulin Fingerstick twice weekly for stable blood sugar >3 mo Fingerstick q.i.d. for status change including fever, infection, vomiting, inability to eat

Abbreviations: HgA1C, hemoglobin A1C; NPH, isophane insulin.

TABLE 5 Recommended Diabetes Health Maintenance

Blood pressure	Every shift × 72 hr after admission Every shift × 72 hr after medication increase Weekly if stable × 72 hr Monthly if stable >12 wk Every shift for status change including fever, infection, change in intake
Orthostatics	Every 6 mo if no signs or symptoms of neuropathy Every 3 mo if peripheral neuropathy present Every shift × 72 hr if initiating or changing medication Weekly if stable on medication × 72 hr Monthly if stable >12 wk
Eye exam	Yearly or q6 mo as per ophthalmology
Oral exam	Daily care by unlicensed staff or patient Yearly by dentist
Foot exam	Daily during A.M. or P.M. care by unlicensed staff or patient; Weekly by licensed staff; yearly by podiatrist if no signs/symptoms
Urine studies	Yearly if protein/Cr< 30 mcg/mg Every 6 mo if protein/Cr > 30 mcg/mg
Lipid studies	Yearly; 6–12 wk after initiating or changing therapy
Weight	Monthly if stable Weekly if has changed by >5%
Pain	Every shift assessment by licensed staff Every visit by physician
Cognition	On admission Yearly; 6 mo after initiation of drug therapy
Depression	On admission; qvisit by physician if on medication

Abbreviation: Cr, creatinine.

Barriers to Care
Underdiagnosis

Underdiagnosis of diabetes is a significant problem, both in the community and in the long-term care setting. Studies have estimated the prevalence of undiagnosed diabetes in the community to be 12% to 22%, a finding of concern when considering that the comorbidities of diabetes, especially retinopathy, may begin to develop years before the clinical diagnosis is made. Despite the increased access to physician and nursing care present in long-term care facilities, underdiagnosis has been shown to be prevalent, with studies finding 8.5% to 16.7% of patients with evidence of diabetes, either by oral glucose tolerance testing or by HgA1C above 7. An even larger percentage, that is, 30.2% to 38.7% had evidence of impaired glucose tolerance (18,39). Given the frailty, multiple diagnoses, polypharmacy, and high-risk status of the long-term care population, undetected diabetes may be contributing to substantial excess morbidity. Although studies have shown that approximately eight years of treatment are needed before the benefits of glycemic control can be shown (40), a time frame that may not be relevant to a long-term care patient with an average life expectancy of three years, undiagnosed diabetes may lead to episodes of hyperglycemia, which have more immediate consequences for frail elders. Hyperglycemia may contribute to dehydration, lethargy, falls, infections, incontinence, and delirium (41), conditions that are all associated with significant morbidity and mortality. Workup of these conditions frequently demonstrates elevated blood glucose. Often this is assumed to be a consequence of the dehydration, infection, etc., rather than a cause. Physicians should be aware that undiagnosed diabetes is very prevalent and plan for follow-up testing on these patients to rule it out, so as to avoid future morbidity from hyperglycemia.

Patient Frailty/Comorbidities

Frailty and the existence of significant comorbidities are the main reasons for undertreatment of diabetes in the long-term care setting. Diabetic patients in long-term care are much more impaired than their peers in the community, averaging 6.4 diagnoses and 6.1 medications at admission (5). Cognitive impairment and functional impairment are present in over 50% of patients, and the prevalence of comorbidities such as retinopathy, neuropathy, nephropathy, and late-stage vascular disease, is more common in long-term care diabetics than either community diabetics or long-term care nondiabetics (3,5). Important comorbidities in this setting that limit good glycemic control include the following:

Cognitive Impairment: Diabetics with cognitive impairment have multiple issues with glycemic treatment. They may be combative and less accepting of fingerstick glucose monitoring or phlebotomy, limiting staff's ability to appropriately gather data with which to adjust medications. They may be limited in their ability to verbalize symptoms or hypo-/hyperglycemia, raising clinician concern about aiming for tight glucose control. The cognitively impaired are at an increased risk of delirium, depression, falls, and weight loss, especially in the later stages of the illness. Additionally, they are dependent on staff monitoring and performance of oral care, foot care, skin care, and in the late stages, feeding and hydrating. Caregiver concerns about the performance of these essential activities also limit ability to appropriately manage diabetes. Cognitively impaired patients with behavioral problems may need treatment with antipsychotics, including those known to raise glucose levels. Lastly, family members of cognitively impaired patients may prefer to minimize treatment, so as to maintain comfort and avoid agitation and behavioral issues.

Depression: Patients with depression are prone to changes in weight (frequently weight loss, but weight gain is also well described), which may impair a previously stable regimen. Additionally, they may neglect or refuse to comply with oral and foot care, phlebotomy, and fingerstick monitoring.

Delirium: Patients in long-term care are at an increased risk of delirium as compared with those in the community. Delirium may go unrecognized or attributed to worsening cognitive impairment or psychiatric disease, delaying treatment of the underlying cause and put the patient at risk for hypo-/hyperglycemia. The fluctuating level of consciousness may impair oral intake, further putting the patient at risk.

Enteral Feeding: Patients requiring long-term enteral feeding may be difficult to manage without need for frequent fingerstick monitoring and use of multiple insulin products. If feedings can be changed to bolus-type three or four times daily, or nocturnal feedings only, improved glycemic control may be more easily achieved.

Quality-of-Life Issues

Physicians are often faced with decisions about treatment options for diabetes that must take into account the patient's quality of life. Of particular importance in the long-term care setting is dietary restriction or limitation. Studies have shown that a regular diet in a long-term care facility versus a calorie- and carbohydrate-limited ("diabetic") diet does not lead to poorer glycemic control (42), and the use of such diets is not recommended in general. However, physicians and staff may wish to limit dietary excesses that clearly exceed the patient's metabolic needs and are detrimental to glycemic control. Unfortunately, these may be the foods that most contribute to the patient's quality of life. Many social activities in long-term care facilities revolve around food, usually sweets, ethnic, and holiday foods. Additionally, many patients socialize with family members and friends in the community via sharing favorite community foods, and removing these sources of pleasure in the interest of glycemic control is resisted by many patients. Physicians may try incorporating these foods into the patient's glycemic regimen, with extra glycemic coverage, rather than limit patient socialization and risk an antagonistic relationship between patient and staff.

Frequent phlebotomy and fingerstick glucose monitoring can also impair the patient's quality of life, particularly if these measurements persist over a long period of time despite stability of patient status. Minimizing these measurements, especially in the cognitively impaired, promotes increased patient ability to participate in facility activities and trips and limits potential conflicts between patients and staff.

Agism and Pessimism

Physicians and staff may undertreat diabetes in elderly patients in long-term care because of personal beliefs about the efficacy of treatments in the elderly that do not have objective data to substantiate them. Also, many caregivers "put themselves in the patient's shoes" with respect to treatments that may prolong life and prevent complications. Although no specific studies have been done on diabetes with regard to this issue, studies looking at patient preferences for advance directives and intensive-care-unit care demonstrate that physicians and caregivers are not accurate at predicting patient preferences. Physicians need to avoid ageism, even in the very old, if functional status is good and patients perceive that they have a good quality of life.

Lack of Trained/Educated/Available Staff

Long-term care facilities are chronically understaffed, and, as in post-acute care, the majority of direct care is performed by unlicensed staff. Skill levels vary widely and staff may not have the education in diabetes management that they need to recognize hypo-/hyperglycemia and emerging complications of diabetes, such as orthostasis, infection, and foot ulceration. Additionally, facility staff itself is a limited resource, and physicians may be faced with decisions about how to allocate this scarce resource. For example, an order to check fingerstick glucose more frequently may be at the expense of oral and foot care, or orthostatic blood pressure. Realistically, staff may not physically be able to carry out all ordered monitoring, especially if the patients are cognitively impaired or noncompliant. Physician awareness of staff limitations will allow more judicious ordering of testing and care.

Lack of Physician Presence

Poor reimbursement and the demands of an ambulatory and hospital practice lead many physicians to place their long-term practice low on their list of priorities. Although practice patterns are changing and long-term care specialists are becoming more common, physician presence in the long-term care facility is still suboptimal. This may disproportionately affect diabetic patients, who require frequent monitoring and coordination of care. To combat this, facilities and physicians have turned to physician extenders, such as nurse practitioners; this has proved to be cost effective and to promote quality long-term primary care (38). However, many small physician groups and solo practitioners cannot afford a salaried midlevel practitioner, especially since they are reimbursed at only 80% of the (already low) physician rate. This often leaves coordination of diabetes care to nursing staff, which may not have the expertise to recognize when physician input and change of management strategy is necessary.

Lack of Clear Treatment Goals

Maintaining good glycemic control is clearly important for prevention of both the short-term effects of hyperglycemia and the long-term effects of microvascular disease. However, many factors may be present that modify the goals of therapy. If these are not clearly documented, patients may receive over-/undertreatment, especially if hospitalized or moved to another setting, such as a post-acute unit, where the previous course of treatment may not be known or communicated. Similarly, many facilities are covered at night by on-call physicians who know nothing about the patients in advance. Late-returning results may lead to changes in regimen that are not appropriate if the goals of treatment are not documented up front. Lastly, the long-term care industry is one of the most heavily regulated of health-care industries, and outside entities, including state and federal regulating agencies, third-party payers, private licensing agencies, and corporate compliance agencies are frequently onsite to review charts and evaluate ongoing treatment. If goals of care are not clearly documented, patients may be found to be undertreated with regard to evidence-based guidelines, and the facility, and even the physician, could be penalized. Documentation of patient comorbidities and patient and caregiver preferences is crucial to maintaining an effective and appropriate plan that will stand up to any fragmentation of care or review.

Strategies for Quality Improvement
Education and Policy Development

Several studies in the literature have shown that diabetes education for nursing home staff works to improve quality of care (43,44). Physicians should take a lead role in helping to implement educational programs in long-term care facilities. Also, guidelines for diabetes management in this setting, such as the American Medical Directors Association Clinical Practice Guideline, are available for reference and implementation. Physicians may also want to work with facility management to designate a licensed nurse to coordinate diabetes care for the facility and assist in educating and training such an individual to review glycemic regimens, facilitate appropriate screening, and educate and monitor unlicensed staff providing direct care.

Equitable Allocation of Resources

Many studies have documented the excess resources spent on the elderly during the end-stage portion of their lives. Reallocation of resources toward preventive care would improve quality of life for many of these patients. Organizations such as the Evercare program have documented improved quality of life and reduction in mortality when an resource are spent on facility-based care, even in acute illnesses, rather than hospital care (46). The keys to this strategy are empowerment of the facility staff through education and physician or physician extender availability and support, and communication with family and caregivers, stressing the benefits to patients of preventive and facility-based care. Enrolling family members or caregivers in the patient's diabetic care plan, including help with feeding, oral, and foot care may extend the capabilities of limited staff and allow complications of diabetes to be recognized and treated earlier, resulting in improved outcomes and increased patient satisfaction.

SUMMARY

Long-term care facilities are a challenging setting for care of the diabetic patient, since this population is frail and complex. However, if realistic, appropriate, individualized treatment goals are established, patients can thrive in this setting. Glycemic control in long-term care facilities has been shown to be better than in the community, and most physicians agree that the care of these patients is still not optimal. With some education and direction by physicians, staff in long-term care facilities can provide even better care for diabetic residents and promote life quality as well.

CONCLUSION

Diabetes management in chronic care settings has a unique set of challenges for physicians. The patient population in assisted-living facilities, post-acute facilities, and long-term care facilities is frail, medically complex, and often requires an individual approach to treatment rather than use of guidelines or standards developed for a younger, healthier population. However, for the physician familiar with each setting's benefits and challenges, managing diabetic patients in chronic-care settings can be successful and rewarding. The elderly population is increasing, and these settings will become even more utilized in the future. More physician involvement in research, education, and policy development is absolutely crucial if this vulnerable population is to age successfully.

REFERENCES

1. US Census Bureau. The Population 65 Years and Over. US Census Brief, October 2001.
2. National Center for Health Statistics. The National Nursing Home survey 1997–Summary for the United States. Vital and Health Statistics, Series 3 No: 143.
3. Travis SS, Buchanan RJ, Wang S, et al. Analyses of nursing home residents with diabetes at admission. J Am Med dir Assoc 2004; 5:320–327.
4. Benbow SJ, Walsh A, Gill GV. Diabetes in the institutionalized elderly: a forgotten population? BMJ 1997; 315:1868–1870.
5. Mooradian AD, Osterweil D, Petrawek D, Morley JE. Diabetes mellitus in elderly nursing home patients. A survey of clinical characteristics and management. J Am Geriatric Soc 1988; 37:391–396.
6. Russell LB, Valiyeva E, Roman SH, et al. Hospitalizations, nursing home admissions, and deaths attributable to diabetes. Diabetes Care 2005; 28(7):1611–1617.
7. Tsuji J, Whalen S, Finucane TE. Predictors of nursing home placement in community-based long-term care. J Am Geriatr Soc 1995; 43:761–766.
8. National Center for Health Statistics, US Centers For Disease Control and Prevention. http://www.cdc.gov/nchs/agirgact.htm
9. Taylor CD, Hendra TJ. The prevalence of diabetes mellitus and quality of diabetic care in residential and nursing homes. A postal survey. Age Ageing 2000; 29(5):447–450.
10. Reed RL, Mooradian AD. Management of diabetes mellitus in the nursing home. Ann Long-Term Care 1998; 6(2):102–108.
11. Spooner J, Lapane K, Hume, et al. Pharmacological treatment of diabetes in long-term care. J Clin Epidemiol 2001; 54:525–530.
12. Orchard TJ. From diagnosis and classification to complications and therapy. DCCT. Part II: diabetes control and complications trial. Diabet Care 1994; 17(4):326–338.
13. Kovner CT, Harrington C. Nursing care in assisted living facilities. Am J Nursing 2003; 103(1):97–98.
14. Chao S, Hagisava V, Mollica R, et al. Time for assessment of nutrition services in assisted living. J Nutr Elder 2003; 23(1):41–55.
15. Sloane PD, Gruber-Baldini AL, Zimmerman S, et al. Medication undertreatment in assisted living settings. Arch Intern Med 2004; 164(18):2031–2037.
16. Magsi H, Molloy T. Underrecognition of cognitive impairment in assisted living facilities. J Am Geriatr Soc 2005; 53(2):295–298.
17. Sung KW. Comparison of health conservation for elders in assisted living facilities and nursing homes. J Nutr Elder 2005; 35(7):1379–1389.
18. Sinclair AJ, Gadsby R, Penfold S, et al. Prevalence of diabetes in care home residents. Diabetes Care 2001; 24(6):1066–1068.
19. Grobin W. A longitudinal study of impaired glucose tolerance and diabetes mellitus in the aged. J Am Geriatr Soc 1989; 37(12):1127–1134.
20. Port CL, Zimmerman S, Williams CS, et al. Families filling the gap: comparing family involvement for assisted living and nursing home residents with dementia. Gerontologist 2005; 45 Spec No. 1(1): 87–95.
21. Hawes C, Phillips CD. High service or high privacy assisted living facilities, their residents and staff: results from a national survey. Washington, DC: U.S. Department of Health and Human Services, November 2000.
22. McPhee SD, Johnson TR, Dietrich MS. Comparing health status with healthy habits in elderly assisted living residents. Fam Community Health 2004; 27(2):158–169.
23. Reed PS, Zimmerman S, Sloane PD, et al. Characteristics associated with low food and fluid intake in long-term care residents with dementia. Gerontolgist 2005; 45 Spec No. (1):74–80.
24. http://www.medpac.gov/publications/congressional_reports/jun04_ch9.pdf
25. http://aspe.hhs.gov/daltcp/reports/mpacb.htm

26. Resnick B. Diabetes management: the hidden challenge of managing hyperglycemia in long-term care settings. Ann Long-term Care 2005; 13(8):26–32.
27. Coleman EA, Min SJ, Chomiak A, et al. Posthospital care transitions: patterns, complications and risk identification. Health Serv Res 2004; 39(5):1449–1465.
28. Inouye SK. Delirium in older persons. N Engl J Med 2006; 354(11):1157–1165.
29. Bellelli G, Trabucchi M. Outcomes of older people admitted to postacute facilities with delirium. J Am Geriatr Soc 2006; 54(2):380–381.
30. McAvey GJ, Van Ness PH, Bogardus ST, et al. Older adults discharged from the hospital with delirium: 1-year outcomes. J Am Geriatr Soc 2006; 54(8):1245–1250.
31. Levkoff SE, Evans DA, Liptzin B, et al. Delirium. The occurrence and persistence of symptoms among elderly hospitalized patients. Arch Intern Med 1992; 152(2):334–340.
32. Thomas DR, Zdrowski CD, Wilson MM, et al. Malnutrition in subacute care. Am J Clin Nutr 2002; 75(2):308–313.
33. Baldelli MV, Boiardi R, Ferrari P, et al. Evaluation of the nutritional status during stay in the subacute nursing home. Arch Gerontol Geriatr Suppl 2004; (9):39–43.
34. Sullivan DH, Patch GA, Walls RC, et al. Impact of nutrition status on morbidity and mortality in a select population of geriatric rehabilitation patients. Am J Clin Nutr 1990; 51(5):749–758.
35. Mayer GG, Buckley RF, White TL. Direct nursing care given to patients in a subacute rehabilitation center. Rehabil Nurs 1990; 15(2):86–88.
36. Manning EH, Jackson L. An evaluation of the timing between key insulin administration-related processes: the reasons why these processes happen when they do, and how to improve their timing. Aust Health Rev 2005; 29(1):61–67.
37. Weinberg AD, Lesesne AJ, Richards, CL, et al. Quality care indicators and staffing levels in a nursing facility subacute unit. J Am Med Dir Assoc 2002; 3(1):1–4.
38. Kane RL, Garrard J, Buchanan JL, et al. Improving primary care in nursing homes. J Am Geriatr Soc 1991; 39(4):359–367.
39. Hauner H, Kurnaz AA, Haastert B, et al. Undiagnosed diabetes mellitus and metabolic control assessed by HbA(1c) among residents of nursing homes. Exp Clin Endocrinol Diabetes 2001; 109(6):326–329.
40. United Kingdom Prospective Diabetes Study Group. Tight blood pressure control and risk of microvascular and macrovascular complications in type 2 diabetes. BMJ 1998; 7:703–713.
41. Resnick B. Diabetes management: the hidden challenge of managing hyperglycemia in long-term care settings. Ann Long-Term Care 2005; 13(8):26–32.
42. Coulson AM, Mandelbaum D, Reaven GM. Dietary management of nursing home residents with non-insulin-dependent diabetes mellitus. Am J clin Nutr 1990; 5(1):67–71.
43. Parker MT, Leggett-Frazier M, Vincent Pa, et al. The impact of an educational program on improving diabetes knowledge and changing behaviors in long-term care facilities. Diabet Educ 1995; 21(6):541–545.
44. Deakin TA, Littley MD. Diabetes care in residential homes: staff training makes a difference. J Hum Nutr diet 2001; 14(6):443–447.
45. The American Medical Directors Association Clinical Practice Guideline. Managing diabetes in the long-term care setting, 2002.
46. Kane RL, Flood S, Keckhafer G, et al. Nursing home residents covered by Medicare risk contracts: early findings from the EverCare evaluation project. J Am Geriatr Soc 2002; 50(4):719–727.

28 | Economic Considerations in the Management of Older Adults with Diabetes: Role of Patient Self-Management

James L. Rosenzweig
Joslin Diabetes Center, Harvard Medical School, Boston, Massachusetts, U.S.A.

PRESENT AND PROJECTED COST OF MANAGEMENT OF DIABETES IN THE ELDERLY POPULATION

Diabetes is largely a disease affecting those in middle and old age. The incidence and prevalence of diabetes in the United States, 95% of which represents type 2 diabetes, progressively increase after age 50 (1–3). The burden of diabetes care in the general population has dramatically increased in the United States, doubling in the past 20 years, with enormous projected further increases in the next 50 years in the United States and throughout the world, especially in South and East Asia and in South America. As individuals with type 2 diabetes age and have the disease for longer periods of time, the burden of care and treatment of the major complications increases. The major emphasis of care shifts from control of glucose to the surveillance and treatment of chronic complications including cardiovascular disease, retinopathy, chronic renal insufficiency, and the protean manifestations of neuropathy. In one study of elderly Medicare beneficiaries with type 2 diabetes, it was found that 96% of beneficiaries had a comorbidity, and 46% had five or more comorbidities. Among beneficiaries with type 2 diabetes, cardiovascular-related comorbidities were common and accounted for greatly increased odds of preventable hospitalization, controlling for other factors. It was estimated that nearly 7% of all hospitalizations could have been avoided (4,5). Medical care costs related to diabetes increase further, the longer one is affected with the disease.

Interestingly, in the elderly, it is not necessarily the number of complications that is the major indicator of health-care cost. The very nature of the disease, which requires time spent with the patient, extensive counseling, supervision, self-management training, and the use of complex medication strategies, predisposes to higher cost. In one study of vulnerable elderly patients in two senior managed care plans, patients with diabetes and those whose conditions required more history taking, counseling, and medication prescribing care processes received lower-than-expected quality of care (6). A greater number of comorbid conditions were associated with a higher-than-expected quality of care. This suggests that age, complexity of illness, and vulnerability do not necessarily predispose older persons to receive poorer-quality care. Since those older persons with conditions such as diabetes, whose care requires time-consuming processes such as history-taking and counseling, are at risk for worse quality of care; they should be major targets for intervention to improve care. Unfortunately, the current health-care system tends to undervalue the time spent on history taking and counseling in favor of high-cost procedures to remedy acute illness.

Prevalence rates of diabetes are especially high in minorities within the general population of Medicare patients. The Center for Disease Control and Prevention reports that 23% of black males and 23.5% of Hispanic males aged 65 to 74 have diabetes as compared to 16.4% of white males and 15.4% of all individuals in that age range. Black and Hispanic females have correspondingly increased prevalence rates of diabetes: 25.4% and 23.8%, respectively, compared to 12.8% for Caucasian females and 12.8% for all women in that age group (7). Levels of preventative care for diabetes-related problems are much lower in these ethnic minority groups than in whites (8).

In a survey by the American Diabetes Association of the economic burden of diabetes in the United States, total direct and indirect costs of diabetes were estimated nationwide at

132 billion dollars. Direct medical care payments alone totaled 91.8 billion dollars for diabetes care; this comprised 23.2 billion dollars for care of diabetes itself, 24.6 billion for chronic complications due to diabetes, and 44.1 billion dollars for excess prevalence of general medical conditions related to having diabetes. Inpatient days were by far the greatest determinant of expenditures, totaling 43.9%, with nursing home care representing 15.1% and office visits only 10.9% (9).

A disproportionate amount of the costs attributable to diabetes occurs in the population aged 65 years or older. Office-based physician encounters for the elderly were more than twice those in the 50- to 65-year age group, and the use of the emergency room, home health care, and hospice were substantially higher than for those individuals with diabetes, aged 45 to 64. The largest increase in costs in the elderly with diabetes was attributed to the worsening of their general medical condition, contributing to increased number and length of hospitalizations. It was predicted that costs for patient care would increase substantially in the next 18 years, but costs for those aged 65 and older would increase greater than for any other age group (9,10).

A summary of the effect of age on costs in the diabetic population is shown in Table 1. The greatest determinant of costs in this patient population is cardiovascular disease, especially hospitalizations related to problems associated with cardiovascular disease. A disproportionate amount of these costs were seen in the older age population, those 50 to 64 and 65 to 75 years of age.

The prevalence of diabetes in the United States Medicare population is increasing at a rapid rate. From 1980 to 2004, the number of people aged 65 or older with diagnosed diabetes increased from 2.3 to 5.8 million individuals. According to the Centers for Medicare and Medicaid Services (CMS), 32% of Medicare spending is attributed to the diabetes population. Since its inception, Medicare has expanded medical coverage of monitoring devices, screening tests and visits, educational efforts, and preventative medial services for its diabetic enrollees. However, oral antidiabetic agents and insulin were excluded from reimbursement (11). In 2003, Congress passed the Medicare Modernization Act, which includes a drug benefit to be administered either through Medicare Advantage drug plans or privately sponsored prescription drug plans for implementation in January 2006. However, studies of the estimated 3.2 million patients with diabetes over age 65 in the Medicare population in 2001 eligible for the standard drug benefit suggest that approximately 64% had medication expenditures in excess of the coverage limit of $2250 in 2006 adjusted dollars. The proportion exceeding the initial coverage limit varied by type of hypoglycemic agent used from 60% using traditional hypoglycemic agents to more than 75% of those using novel hypoglycemics. It is quite clear that having to pay out-of-pocket costs for medications can have a significantly adverse impact on elderly patients with diabetes. In a national survey of 875 older patients with diabetes, 19% reported cutting back on medications due to cost, and the cost of medications placed a significant burden on many of the respondents (12).

TABLE 1 Health-Care Expenditures for Patients with Diabetes in the United States in 2002, by Age and Type of Service (in Millions of Dollars)

Type of service	Age < 45	Age 45–64	Age ≥ 65	Total
Institutional care	—	—	—	—
Hospital inpatient	5,207	13,838	21,293	40,337
Nursing home days	2,552	5,528	5,798	13,878
Outpatient care	—	—	—	—
Office-based physician encounters	1,851	2,679	5,708	10,033
Emergency department encounters	151	439	1,572	2,162
Hospital outpatient and ambulatory surgery	26	1,345	1,944	3,315
Home health visits	133	524	3,273	3,930
Hospice care	5	46	492	543
Other expenditures	—	—	—	—
Ambulance services	28	40	77	146
Outpatient medication	756	1,991	2,769	5,516
Oral agents	533	2,318	2,157	5,009
Insulin and delivery supplies	1,355	2,891	2,745	6,991
Total	12,596	31,640	47,626	91,861

Source: From Ref. 9.

However, use of medications to control glucose is only one part of the puzzle in the care of older patients with diabetes. Approximately 80% of patients with type 2 diabetes in the elderly population have some degree of hypertension and need to be treated with antihypertensive medications. Patients with more comorbidities and poorer health status in the population of patients with diabetes are at greater risk of exceeding the initial coverage limit. As a result, a large proportion of older adults with diabetes mellitus exceed the initial coverage limit under the standard Medicare Part D drug benefit and incur significant out-of-pocket spending (13).

The major failings of management of patients with chronic diseases and the lack of provisions for effective chronic care and preventative care are a recognized problem throughout the United States. Studies have identified the challenges of assuring that patients with major chronic conditions such as diabetes receive adequate care (14). Many of these failings are due to problems with the health-care system rather than the lack of effort or intent by providers to deliver health care of high quality. The current health-care system is structured and financed largely to manage acute care episodes, not to manage and support individuals with progressive chronic diseases. Providers see patients in discrete locations such as hospital, physician offices, home health care, and long-term care facilities and they are usually paid for their services separately in those settings. Existing incentives for provider care tend to promote the focusing on each patient only while he or she is within the provider's care setting (15). Especially among the elderly, this can be an inefficient process, because optimal care of their chronic conditions requires proper coordination and integration of efforts over a variety of settings including the home and general and specialized care locations. Interventions to avoid the fragmentation of care often involve collecting data that can be shared in these different settings to minimize efforts that are redundant and internally conflicting. Making the optimal use of resources can best prevent complications and comorbidities. It is currently rare for seniors to receive support for managing their diabetes outside the physician office setting.

Fragmentation of care is a major problem for Medicare beneficiaries. The average beneficiary sees several different physicians and fills upward of 20 prescriptions per year (16). In a recent survey, 18% of people with chronic conditions reported having duplicate tests or procedures and 17% received conflicting information from providers (17). Providers reported feeling ill-prepared to manage chronically ill patients and reported that poor coordination of care led to poor outcomes (18).

In addition, studies have shown that there is a large gap between what we know is appropriate care for patients with chronic disease and the actual care they receive. A review of all of the currently accepted performance measures and indicators of quality of care for patients with diabetes shows that goals of care are not being met in the United States and in the world at large (19). Nevertheless, some studies have shown small but significant improvement in diabetes processes of care and intermediate outcomes (20).

In one U.S. study, only 56% of patients with chronic disease received recommended care based on well-established guidelines. Only 24% of diabetes patients in the study received three or more glycosylated hemoglobin tests over a two-year period (21). In another study of practice patterns under Medicare, researchers found that, across all states, an average of 66% of Medicare beneficiaries with heart failure received angiotensin converting enzyme inhibitors and only 16% with diabetes received a lipid test (22).

Beneficiaries of Medicare are affected by these problems disproportionately because they typically have multiple chronic health problems (23). Beneficiaries who have multiple progressive chronic diseases are a large and costly subgroup of the Medicare populations: Medicare beneficiaries with five or more chronic conditions represent 20% of the Medicare population but they consume 66% of program spending.

Diabetes is one of the five most common chronic diseases in the Medicare population. Beneficiaries with diabetes tend to have complex self-care regimens and medical care needs. Many of these beneficiaries have other chronic conditions that add to their self-care burdens and risks of developing comorbid conditions, complications, and acute care crises. Risks to health care for these patients are largely affected by how care can be coordinated and whether appropriate care can be delivered in the context of their daily lives. Proper management to prevent the development of complications and comorbidities may require ongoing guidance and support beyond individual provider settings.

As shown in the 1999 Medicare Current Beneficiary Survey, individuals with diabetes represent 18% of beneficiaries and 32% of fee-for-service (FFS) Medicare Expenditures (24). Each year, 10% of the Medicare population accounts for two-thirds of all Medicare FFS program payments (25). Many of these high-cost patients suffer from chronic progressive diseases such as diabetes, and most of their Medicare expenditures are for multiple and often preventable hospitalizations.

DISEASE MANAGEMENT ISSUES PERTAINING TO DIABETES AND THE ELDERLY

Disease management is a complete and comprehensive method of providing health care that focuses on management of care across the continuum for populations of patients with chronic diseases. When used properly, it can be a comprehensive integrated approach to care and reimbursement based fundamentally on the natural course of the disease, with treatment designed to address the illness with maximum effectiveness and efficiency (26). Disease management can be thought of as an approach to care that identifies the optimal processes for care of a patient with a specific condition and implements those processes while measuring the outcome to demonstrate improvement economically, humanistically, and clinically. Disease management is oriented toward wellness and prevention. The goals of disease management are to extend the periods of wellness that patients experience, to improve the overall quality of their lives, to prevent occurrence or exacerbation of complications or acute episodes, to direct utilization of services and resources appropriately, and to consistently measure outcomes. In practice, disease management is being implemented as a way to contain costs while maximizing the overall quality of care across an insurance company or employer's population. Therefore, disease management is being implemented most widely in patients with conditions for which cost savings are most substantial.

Whereas major disease management interventions have shown substantial beneficial effects in the process and outcomes of diabetes care in the commercial and Medicaid managed care sectors (27–29), there is less information available for the outcomes of disease management programs for the elderly in the Medicare population. Some studies in Medicare health maintenance organization among elderly patients with diabetes suggest that they represent a heterogeneous population with a wide range of medical interventions. It has been found that those patients with high comorbidity severity and numerous emergency room visits had reduced compliance with antidiabetic medications (30). Conversely, an increased antidiabetic medication possession ratio (the degree to which patients refilled their medications) was the strongest predictor of decreased annual health-care costs. There was an 8.6% to 28.9% decrease in annual costs with every 10% increase in medication possession ratio. Therefore, there is reason to believe that concrete disease management interventions to improve medication compliance can have a major impact in reducing medical care costs.

Avoiding polypharmacy is often considered an important goal in the elderly population, but elderly patients with diabetes almost always require multiple medications. It has been found that the use of multiple oral antidiabetic agents in the population of patients with diabetes can serve as a marker of poor glycemic control; in one study only 13% of patients receiving three or more oral agents were found to have optimal glycemic control (31). These might be an especially important group of patients, especially in the elderly, to be targeted for disease management interventions. However, another study has indicated that patients with diabetes often can adhere to appropriate regimens regardless of the number of medications prescribed (32).

Why Is Disease Management Necessary?

Diabetes is one of the most complex and significant chronic diseases requiring health care. Its emergence as a major cause of clinical morbidity and increasing health-care costs was discussed earlier in this chapter. Many people are diagnosed only upon developing serious and life-threatening complications related to the underlying diabetes. In evaluations of the impact of diabetes on the health-care system and the effect it has on a population, the facts give a convincing picture of diabetes as an appropriate target for disease management. According to the results of the diabetes control and complications trial (DCCT), maintaining blood glucose levels as close to normal as possible slows the onset and progression of eye, kidney, and nerve complications related to diabetes (33). The DCCT showed that sustained lowering of blood glucose levels had positive effects, even in those patients who had prior histories of poor control. Tighter control also contributed to a lower number of glycemic events leading to hospitalizations. Achieving and maintaining consistent blood glucose control is extremely challenging both for people with diabetes who are attempting to balance busy lives with management of this disease and for their care providers. Disease management offers an infrastructure for integrating all the key members of the health-care team with the patients and their significant others, in combination with proactive and comprehensive services to improve the quality and cost-effectiveness of diabetes care.

Notable challenges in the health-care system that affect the ability of clinicians to manage diabetes successfully and practice disease management include the following:

- The lack of standardized care throughout the continuum of care. This has contributed to high variability in physician practice and in resultant patient outcomes.
- The lack of accessible and immediately available screening, treatment, prevention, and pharmacologic utilization guidelines and protocols for clinicians in active practice settings.
- The lack of resources and systems that provide consistent education and reinforcement for professional care providers.
- Inappropriate utilization of services and resources including hospitalizations and emergency department visits secondary to often-preventable glycemic occurrences and events related to acute and/or chronic complications of diabetes.
- The lack of consistent systems that can assist clinicians to identify high-risk patients, to institute comprehensive preventive and education programs, and to coordinate appropriate utilization of services.
- Absence of systems, formats, and resources for performance and outcome measurement; data collection and analysis; trend analysis; patient identification and risk stratification; tracking and monitoring of patients; and reporting and feedback mechanisms that have strong potential to influence effective health-care delivery.
- Inadequate resources and systems to provide comprehensive patient education and support in long-term self-management.
- Inadequate systems for coordinating the care and priorities of multiple participants including the patient, the primary care physician, the specialists, case managers, nurses, and other care providers—in a focused concerted integrated team approach.

Diabetes is a disease with multiple stakeholders who have a vested interest in improved systems and outcomes, i.e., patients, providers, employers, community agencies, health plans, health facilities and agencies, and pharmaceutical and other vendors. As a disease state, diabetes presents a combination of high variability in practice and cost, high prevalence of work or school days lost, and significant difficulties in management. However, there is a realistic ability to alter the course of the disease across the continuum of care through implementation of a disease management program that provides a focused and specific set of goals and interventions, as well as a consistent evaluative process.

Recommended Elements for a Diabetes Disease Management Program

A diabetes disease management program should be designed to address the overall needs of the general patient population that has been identified, as well as to target specific activities for patients who have been identified as at high risk for complications. The core components of an effective diabetes disease management program include the following:

- Establishment of a collaborative work team
- Development of an assessment process
- Implementation of a risk management process
- Physician education programs and processes

- Implementation of clinical guidelines
- Educational programs and support mechanisms for professional and office staff
- Programs and tools for patient self-management
- Data management and technological support
- Integration into quality improvement
- Management of care coordination and utilization
- Ongoing support mechanisms

Risk Stratification

A diabetes disease management program is designed to improve the quality and cost-effectiveness for the entire patient population that has been identified. However, within that larger population, there is a group of patients who are considered to be high risk for complications and who account for a significant proportion of resource utilization and medical costs. This subset of patients represents candidates for intensified therapy and intervention. It does not matter that the entire population, by virtue of being elderly and having diabetes mellitus, would already be considered "high risk." Within that population, there is substantial variability of severity of illness, determined not only by level of glycemic control, but by incidence and severity of complications and the many problems of daily functioning that complicate diabetes care in the elderly.

Risk stratification is a critical process in disease management because it provides a detailed patient profile and identifies those patients who are at risk for developing severe chronic complications (34). The risk stratification information is used as a guide for care providers to enable them to achieve two objectives.

1. *The development of programs, systems, processes, and tools targeted at the high-risk patient group*: Patient educational tools and processes, care coordination, and case management activities, referrals to certified diabetes educators or specialists, and follow-up regimens are directed by the information that is provided by risk stratification.
2. *Individualization of care on the basis of scientific information that describes the patient's circumstances*: Predictive modeling systems that identify patients likely to have high costs in the future, based upon previous costs and characteristics, may be a part of the risk stratification process, but they are not essential to it.

The goals for integrating a risk stratification component into the diabetes disease management program include (*i*) prevention or delay of onset of chronic complications or acute events; (*ii*) decrease in the severity of complications that do occur; (*iii*) extension of the patient's life, (*iv*) improvement in the patient's quality of life; (*v*) decrease in costs by reduction of preventable hospitalizations, emergency department visits, or inappropriate utilization of resources; and (*vi*) improvement in patient and care-provider satisfaction.

Patient Self-Management

Education in self-management of diabetes is a critical element in providing patients with the mechanisms necessary for managing the disease and its subsequent effects on their lives. Empowering patients and helping them acquire the skills for effective self-management are the foundation of the educational process for the patient with diabetes.

For people with diabetes, management of their disease relies on continual treatment and constant balancing of the integral parts of their everyday lives. Effective management of diabetes requires vigilance and commitment on a 24-hour-a-day basis and significant lifestyle modifications. Education and self-management play vital roles in guiding the patient toward independent and competent management of diabetes. The goal of the patient educational component of disease management is to facilitate the patient's and the family's ability to increase their diabetes knowledge base for self-management, to increase their confidence in applying the knowledge to practical situations, and to share experiences with other people with diabetes. The effective diabetes disease management program incorporates multiple individual and group formats, with an emphasis on interactive participation. The health-care team is provided with standardized patient educational materials so that the patient is receiving consistent information. Technology has enabled care providers to present educational material to patients in a wide range of creative ways including and not limited to call centers, telemedicine communication devices in the home to improve compliance, videos, e-mail, interactive websites, and interactive software (35). Curricula can focus on meaningful topics ranging from survival skills, to meal planning, to intense monitoring of blood glucose, to more in-depth self-management techniques and information. Incentives for maintaining attendance and compliance with educational programs may be helpful tools for supporting the patient. It is important for the educational programs to address psychosocial needs and the enormous emotional and psychological toll exacted by living with diabetes. Engaging the patient and family as active partners in the health-care team and addressing educational needs across the continuum are important attributes for success.

Clinical Guidelines

Clinical guidelines provide a basis for screening, treatment, evaluation, and pharmacologic management in the delivery of care to patients with diabetes. Part of every disease management program entails the development, implementation, and evaluation of disease-specific clinical pathways, which can also encompass care algorithms or protocols (36–38). The guidelines must incorporate current knowledge and reference reliable resources. It is clear that general guidelines for patients with diabetes do not always apply to elderly patients with diabetes. In many cases, the goals for glucose and hemoglobin A1C may be higher in order to avoid hypoglycemia, and the anticipated benefit due to tight glycemic control may not be as great. There is a strong rationale for providing simpler insulin regimens, using premixed insulin combinations, which would be less likely to be used in younger patients.

Continuous review, updating, and modification contribute to the credibility of the guideline. Clinical guidelines that are evidence based and have been stringently and authoritatively tested receive much stronger positive response from physicians and integration into practice (35,39).

Easy accessibility and user-friendly formats that facilitate guideline use in a busy practice are a prerequisite to successful implementation. Tools that support the guidelines including documentation forms, physician order sheets, patient surveys, and data collection forms frequently are developed for use in conjunction with the guidelines. Increased efforts are being made to provide online and web-based applications. The objectives of the clinical guidelines are (*i*) to support optimal clinical practice, (*ii*) to influence clinical behavior to produce improved patient outcomes, and (*iii*) to ensure that patients' expectations are informed and reasonable.

Care Coordination, Utilization Management, and Case Management

Care coordination, utilization management, and case management are critical to the implementation of a successful diabetes disease management program. The population of patients with diabetes includes a significant number who are actively experiencing serious or life-threatening complications, have been identified as being in a high-risk category for development of complications, or demonstrate the potential for progression to a high-risk level. Also, because of the complexity of managing this difficult chronic disease on a daily basis, patients require the intensive support and coordination offered by disease management programs via care and case management. Elderly patients with diabetes need to have a supportive service that is geared to assist them toward better self-management and ultimately to an improved quality of life.

The role of the case or care manager has expanded beyond the original context of acute, inpatient care and extends into continued management of the patient's care throughout the outpatient/community experience and primary medical care. The case manager supports the disease management process from the perspective of both the individual patient and the population as a whole.

Quality Improvement

A major purpose of disease management programs is to support quality-improvement initiatives and to provide a system for outcomes analysis. Within the context of a diabetes disease management program, the evaluative process that contributes to effective quality improvement is reorganized to encompass entire populations. In this population-based concept, the ability to stratify for risk and identify high-risk patients; to develop and implement "best-practice" protocols, guidelines, interventions, and processes; and to measure patient and system responses and outcomes is increasingly important to the many stake-holders in health-care delivery.

Integration of valuable data on patient outcome into the quality-improvement program enables the care providers to respond to the physical, psychological, functional, and environmental needs of the patients in the population with diabetes. Consistent and reliable reporting structures provide a mechanism for utilizing the data in meaningful and productive ways. Including the perspectives of the patient and care provider in the evaluation of quality promotes a comprehensive viewpoint. Prompt response to the data through the development and implementation of plans for improvement or corrective action strengthens the program and increases its credibility.

Some of the indicators measured to evaluate quality and incorporated into the quality-improvement program are level of clinical quality; accessibility to care and services; the patient's quality of life and functional status; levels of satisfaction; and levels of utilization management.

Quality of life and functional status: Evaluation of quality of life and functional status includes monitoring for improvements in self-care ability, achievements in individual- and population-based goals for self-management and behavior change, treatment and follow-up compliance rates, and patient/family comprehension of self-management.

Satisfaction levels: To obtain a comprehensive view of how the quality and the effectiveness of the diabetes disease management is perceived, assessments need to consider satisfaction levels from the perspectives of multiple stake-holders in the care-delivery process: patients, families, care providers, payers, employers, and others. The indicators for such assessment include levels of satisfaction with the care provided, the accessibility to care and services, and the resultant outcomes of the care provided.

Data Management and Technology

Advanced technology is essential in the current complicated health-care industry, with its need for managing enormous amounts of detailed and complex patient information. The establishment of disease management has promoted the need for increasingly powerful and sophisticated technology that can support multiple demands.

Technology should not be used to substitute for the human interaction and personal relationships that exist between patients and care providers but should be integrated into the disease management program to facilitate and strengthen those components (40).

Physician Support for Disease Management

Disease management programs have a significant potential to improve outcomes and reduce costs; however, many physicians remain wary about participating (35). Physician resistance is one of the top three reasons why disease management programs are not implemented (35). If physicians perceive that the disease management program reduces their control over the management of patient care or dilutes their relationships with their patients, they will not accept the program.

Several success factors have been identified that influence physician participation. First, structuring the program on evidence-based medicine establishes credibility and a more positive response by physicians. Educating the physician about the program, its value to the patient, its support of the physician's role in the coordination of care, and its value to the physician is an important element (35). Maximizing the opportunities for physicians to have input in the development, implementation, and evaluation of the program helps them to become more comfortable with the concept of disease management. Modifying the program according to physician input or practices builds support. Demonstrated success of positive outcomes in previous activities encourages physicians to participate. Structuring the program so that the physician truly owns and champions the program is an element for success (35). The impetus of the program should be to support and strengthen the physician/patient relationship.

Lifestyle Modifications and Psychosocial Issues

Diabetes is a chronic disease that affects the patient physically, psychologically, socially, spiritually, cognitively, and economically. It requires a careful balance of activities, 24-hour-a-day management, and significant lifestyle changes. Living well with diabetes means combining a lifelong commitment to maintaining a lifestyle that balances sound nutrition, activity, and overall health habits with adherence to a strict medical management regimen. Patients with diabetes live with it all day, every day. The person's self-esteem, sense of independence, and self-image all experience enormous strain as his or her lifestyle undergoes significant modifications and alterations. Providing systems, processes, and supports that assist the patient to learn self-management of diabetes is an important factor in the health-care plan.

Education regarding self-management and lifestyle modification is important to help patients take control of diabetes and its impact on their lives. Education about managing diabetes is about mastering a wide range of new skills and activities as well as about adapting to life with a chronic disease (41). Patients are faced with learning self-management skills including monitoring blood glucose levels, planning meals, scheduling meals and medications, and maintaining exercise programs. They also are faced with the challenge of learning to prioritize commitment to a treatment plan over other activities, to manage unexpected events, to develop contingency plans, to know when to contact supportive resources, and to maintain eternal vigilance to stay well. Effective education in diabetes self-management and nutritional management is cost-effective (42). It is associated with many positive outcomes including improvement in patients' physical and emotional health, improvement in ability to achieve glycemic and metabolic control, a reduction in hospitalizations, a reduction in diabetes-related health-care costs, and fewer acute and chronic complications.

The Patient's Role in Diabetes Management

The patient plays the most important role in diabetes management. Patients with diabetes must perceive themselves as active, empowered members of the health-care team and be able to accept responsibility for self-management and for adhering to treatment plans (43). There must be a commitment to understanding the disease as well as possible and a willingness to continue to learn. The patient's active participation in decision-making and planning treatment as a member of the health-care team contributes substantially to successful self-management. The patient must be able to change behaviors and learn new skills to be able to feel better, be healthier, and, in some cases, survive. Working with the team to set goals for treatment and behavior allows the patient to have more immediate control over care that reflects his or her preferences and priorities. The patient needs to make appropriate decisions, multiple times, on a daily basis about self-management and to act on those decisions accordingly (43). The patient must have strong communication skills and a sense of assertiveness to be able to inform the health-care team when difficulties arise, when circumstances change that impact the treatment plan, or when the goals for glycemic control have not been met.

Issues that Affect Proficient Self-Management

Changes in behavior and adjustments of lifelong habits and choices are difficult processes. The difficulties for the patient of learning new skills, understanding how and why to control a chronic disease, and managing all the associated feelings often lead to frustration and discouragement. Associated dementia, reduced functional status, and depression are major complicating issues.

DISEASE MANAGEMENT IN MEDICARE

The Medicare Prescription Drug and Modernization Act of 2003 provided, for the first time, a comprehensive pharmaceutical benefit for Medicare beneficiaries (Medicare Part D). Section 1807 of this Act specified that the Secretary of Health and Human Services, through the CMS, would provide for the phased-in development, testing, evaluation and implementation of chronic care improvement programs. Each program was to be designed to improve quality of care and provider satisfaction and achieve spending targets related to expenditures for one or more threshold conditions.

The program has been implemented as a voluntary chronic care improvement program for FFS Medicare patients with complex diabetes and/or congestive heart failure, called Medicare Health Support. Following the enactment of the Act, CMS conducted a competitive contracting process and awarded nine contracts for Phase 1 pilot programs. Each program must be accomplished over a three-year period (44). The pilots are being implemented in eight regional areas including Chicago, Northwest Georgia, Western Pennsylvania, the District of Columbia and Maryland, Central and South Florida, Oklahoma, Mississippi, and Tennessee. The awardees were large payers or disease management companies.

Each of the pilots is designed to serve 20,000 Medicare patients in each of the regions listed above. They are offered to beneficiaries for free with an opt-out strategy. The 20,000 beneficiaries are to be compared with 10,000 control patients, assigned by Medicare to each group on a randomized basis.

The three-year pilots will enable each awardee to set up its own program, combining the classic elements of disease management programs designed for diabetes and congestive heart failure. These are currently including mixes of care management via call centers, home health-care support, provider support and quality improvement programs, including in certain cases pay-for-performance incentives, case management of high-risk patients, telemedicine initiatives, information systems and registries, and education and training for both patients and providers. Payments to the awardees will be based upon performance, and if each pilot fails to save at least 5% of health-care costs over the three-year period compared to the control group, they will be subject to up to a 100% refund of the performance-based revenue.

The goal of the program is to improve clinical outcomes, increase patient satisfaction, and meet the Medicare spending targets assigned for the population. As of yet, no outcome data are available. It is anticipated that this program will be able to provide a wealth of data on the success of disease management and quality improvement programs in the Medicare population.

REFERENCES

1. Harris MI, Flegal KM, Cowie CC, et al. Prevalence of diabetes, impaired fasting glucose, and impaired glucose tolerance in adults. Diabetes Care 1998; 21:518–524.
2. World Health Organization. Diabetes: diabetes estimates. Available at: http://www.who.int/ncd/dia/databases/htm.
3. Centers for Disease Control and Prevention. Diabetes Fact Sheet, 2005. Available at: http://www.cdc.gov/diabetes/pubs/estimates05.htm#prev4.
4. Niefeld MR, Braunstein JB, Wu AW, Saudek CD, Weller WE Anderson GF. Preventable hospitalization among elderly Medicare Beneficiaries with type 2 diabetes. Diabetes Care 2003; 26:1344–1349.
5. Harris MI, Eastman RC. Early detection of undiagnosed non-insulin–dependent diabetes mellitus. JAMA 1996; 276:1261–1262.
6. Min LC, Reuben DB, Maclean CH, et al. Predictors of overall quality of care provided to vulnerable older people. J Am Geriatr Soc 2005; 53:1705–1711.
7. Centers for Disease Control and Prevention, National Center for Chronic Disease Control and Prevention and Health Promotion, Disease Surveillance System. See www.cdc.gov/diabets.statistics/prev/nationa/f5dt2000.htm.
8. Kirk JK, Bell RA, Bertoni AG, et al. A qualitative review of studies of diabetes preventative care among minority patients in the United States, 1993–2003. Am J Manag Care 2005; 11:349–360.
9. Hogan P, Dall T, Nikolov P. Economic costs of diabetes in the US in 2002. Diabetes Care 2003; 26:917–932.
10. American Diabetes Association. Economic consequences of diabetes mellitus in the US in 1997. Diabetes Care 1998; 21:296–309.
11. Ashkenazy R, Abrahamson MJ. Medicare coverage for patients with diabetes. A national plan with individual consequences. J Gen Intern Med 2006; 21:286–292.
12. Piette JD, Heisler M, Wagner TH. Problems paying out-of-pocket medication costs among older adults with diabetes. Diabetes Care 2004; 27:384–391.
13. Tjia J, Schwartz JS. Will the Medicare prescription drug benefit eliminate dost barriers for older adults with diabetes mellitus? J Am Geriatr Soc 2006; 54:606–612.
14. Institute of Medicine. Crossing the Quality Chasm: A New Health System for the 21st Century. Washington, D.C: National Academy Press, 2001.

15. Todd W, Nash T, eds. Disease Management a Systems Approach to Patient Outcomes. Chicago: American Hospital Pub., 1997:1–357.
16. Anderson G. Chronic Conditions: Making the Case for Ongoing Care. Partnership for Solutions and the Robert Wood Johnson Foundation, 4.
17. Anderson G. Chronic Conditions: Making the Case for Ongoing Care. Partnership for Solutions and the Robert Wood Johnson Foundation, 32.
18. Anderson G. Chronic Conditions: Making the Case for Ongoing Care. Partnership for Solutions and the Robert Wood Johnson Foundation, 36.
19. Kenny SJ, Smith PJ, Goldschmid MG, et al. Survey of physician practice behaviors related to diabetes mellitus in the U.S.: physician adherence to consensus recommendations. Diabetes 1993; 16:1507–1510.
20. Saaddine JB, Cadwell B, Gregg EW, et al. Improvement in diabetes processes of care and intermediate outcomes: United States, 1988–2002. Ann Intern Med 2006; 144:465–474.
21. McGlynn E, Asch S, Adams J, et al. The quality of health care delivered to adults in the United States. N Engl J Med 2003; 348:2635–2645.
22. Jencks S, Huff E, Cuerdon T. Change in the quality of care delivered to medicare beneficiaries 1998–1999 to 2000–2001. J Am Med Assoc 2003; 289:305–312.
23. Anderson G. Testimony before the Subcommittee on Health of the House Ways and Means Committee, Hearing on Promoting Disease Management in Medicare, 16 April 2002. www.partnershipforsolutions. org/dms/files/4_16_o2_testimony.doc.
24. Foote S. Population-based disease management in fee-for-service medicare. Health Affairs, Web Exclusive, 30 July 2003 W3-350.
25. Centers for Medicare and Medicaid Services. CMS Chart Book June 2002 edition, Section III, Am, 29.
26. Moran M. Disease management spreading. Am Med News 1999; 42(16).
27. Shojania KG, Ranji SR, McDonald KM, et al. Effects of quality improvement strategies for type 2 diabetes on glycemic control: a meta-regression analysis. JAMA 2006; 269:427–440.
28. Clarke J, Crawford A, Nash DB. Evaluation of a comprehensive diabetes disease management program: progress in the struggle for sustained behavior change. Dis Manag 2002; 5:77–86.
29. Villagra VG, Ahmed T. Effectiveness of a disease management program for patients with diabetes. Health Aff 2004; 23:255–266.
30. Balkrishnan R, Rajagopalan R, Camacho FT, Huston SA, Murray FT, Anderson RT. Predictors of medication adherence and associated health care cost in an older population with type 2 diabetes mellitus: a longitudinal cohort study. Clin Ther 2003; 25:2958–2971.
31. Willey CJ, Andrade SE, Cohen J, Fuller JC, Gurwitz JH. Polypharmacy with oral antidiabetic agents: an indicator of poor glycemic control. Am J Manag Care 2006; 12:435–440.
32. Grant RW, Devita NG, Singer DE, Meigs JB. Polypharmacy and medication adherence in patients with type 2 diabetes. Diabetes Care 2003; 26:1408–1412.
33. Diabetes Control and Complications Trial Research Group. The effect of intensive treatment of diabetes on the development and progression of long-term complications in insulin-dependent diabetes mellitus. N Engl J Med 1994; 329:977–986.
34. Rosenzweig J, Weinger K, Poirier-Solomon L, Rushton M. Use of a disease severity index for evaluation of healthcare costs and management of comorbidities of patients with diabetes mellitus. Am J Manag Care 2002; 8:950–958.
35. Brown J. Physicians support disease management programs with right combination of incentives, education, medical evidence. Physicians Partnership Report. Washington, DC: Atlantic Information Services, 1999.
36. Durso SC. Using clinical guidelines designated for older adults with diabetes and complex health status. JAMA 2006; 295:1935–1940.
37. Brown AF, Mangione CM, Saliba D, Sarkisia CA. Guidelines for improving the care of the older person with diabetes mellitus. J Am Geriatr Soc 2003; 5(suppl):S265–S280.
38. Blaum CS. Management of diabetes in older adults; are national guidelines appropriate? J Am Geriatr Soc 2002; 50:581–583.
39. Special Supplement. Disease management: an industry emerges. Healthcare Business Roundtable 1999.
40. Zitter M. Disease management: a new approach to health care. Med Interface 1995; 7(8):70–72,75–76.
41. Clement S. Diabetes self management education. Diabetes Care 1999; 18:1204–1214.
42. Sheils JF, Rubin R, Stapleton DC. The estimated costs and saving of medical nutrition therapy: the medicare population. J Am Diet Assoc 1999; 99:428–435.
43. Poirier L, Maryniuk M, de Groot M. The Joslin Way; a Healthcare Professional's Guide to Diabetes Patient Care. Boston: Joslin Diabetes Center, 1999.
44. Boston Consulting Group. Realizing the promise of disease management. Payer trends and opportunities in the United States. BCG Report 2006; 3–27.

29 | Optimizing Diabetes Care in Older Adults—What Else Is Needed?

Alan J. Sinclair
Bedfordshire and Hertfordshire Postgraduate Medical School, University of Bedfordshire, Luton, U.K.

INTRODUCTION

In a comprehensive textbook on geriatric diabetes, there are rarely large omissions in diabetes care. This chapter will reflect on those aspects of care where little objective evidence exists and provide guidance designed to optimize clinical care and the attainment of goals. It will necessarily explore the relatively unresearched area of caregiver-related issues, importance of specialist approaches, and how best to implement the available evidence base. In this way, we can move closer to that ideal (optimal) platform in which we feel that everything possible is being done in not only the "medical" sense but also in the equally important areas of socioeconomic and psychological support, family and caregiver interaction with the patient, and specialist access.

CAREGIVER ISSUES

Many studies have testified to the considerable social, economic, and health burden of diabetes on the community, with the focus generally being the individual with diabetes (1). These studies lack details about the corresponding burden of informal (unpaid) caregivers who provide considerable, if not the majority of, community-based care in domestic settings and this need is likely to increase dramatically over the next 25 years (2). Part of this burden relates to lost earnings (as many caregivers are in the working-age category), which may be as high as $20,000 per year (3) and to an increased risk of depressive illness (4). In the United States, it has been estimated that the total cost of informal care is between three and six billion dollars per year (5).

Chronic diseases (which includes diabetes) or the presence of physical disability, falls and fractures, or dementia is likely to impose a particularly heavy burden, but this area remains understudied. We also have little knowledge of caring for older people with diabetes from other ethnic backgrounds but earlier reports suggest that a particularly heavy burden is borne by informal caregivers among black and minority ethnic groups (6). Their burden may be more unique and intense since issues such as greater lack of access to services, problems relating to living within poor, inner city environments including poverty and overcrowding, and difficulties in accessing nursing-home placements are more prominent. Indeed, some studies have focused on strategies to improve care-giving roles among minority ethnic populations, for example, in one study of African American women (7) with type 2 diabetes, who participated in several lifestyle behavior programs, family and care-giving roles were considered culturally meaningful strategies to improve diabetes self-care. Improvement in caregiver role may be one factor observed in a study of Mexican Americans with type 2 diabetes aged 35 to 70 years, where a culturally competent diabetes self-management program over three months (involving 52 contact hours over three months with a dietician, Mexican American nurses, and community workers comprising weekly instructional sessions on nutrition, self-monitoring of glucose, exercise and other self-care topics), which also involved a family member or friend (8) improved glycemia as measured by a 1.4% fall in HbA1c, and particular benefits were observed in those whose HbA1c was greater than 10%.

In a study of family members of American Indian Elders with diabetes (9) using a focus group approach, it is obvious that informal caregivers have a wide range of care responsibilities including skin and wound care, medication management, dietary provision, financial care, and even in-home dialysis where needed. Several anxieties were revealed by caregivers including anxiety about in-home care, coping with psychosocial issues, and decision-making and communication problems with other family members. The effect of care giving on health-related quality of life using the short form-36 questionnaire was recently studied in a group of primary caregivers of inpatients with stroke or diabetes (10). In each case, poorer mental well-being was observed compared with the population norm, but physical well-being was higher! Using a multivariate regression model and data in patients aged 70 years and over from the 1993 Asset and Health Dynamics Among the Oldest Old Study, Langa et al. (5) determined that patients with diabetes received between 10.1 and 14.4 hours of informal care per week (compared with 6.1 hours of those without diabetes). The presence of heart disease, stroke, or visual impairment was an important predictor of informal care.

In Box A, based on the available evidence we have in relation to care-giving roles in both Caucasian and ethnic minority populations, is a summary of the optimal content of informal caregiver "support packages," which should be of special importance in areas of high ethnic diabetes prevalence. These recommendations are taken from a comprehensive report provided to the British Diabetic Association by the author (11) following a descriptive analysis of the roles and the responsibilities of informal caregivers of older people with type 2 diabetes from several ethnic backgrounds.

Language difficulties remain an important issue since language barriers can hinder trust among patients and health professionals, increase the likelihood of staff failing to recognize complexity in a patient, and decrease adherence to therapy (12). It is important to ensure that the information and instruction provided in the "support package" has several important characteristics: firstly, it should be translatable into relevant languages; secondly, it should be simple and easy to read and illustrated where appropriate; thirdly, it should be sensitive to the cultural, educational, religious, and ethnic issues for each group of subjects; and lastly, it should be designed to empower individuals in diabetes and other healthcare issues.

It is clear that in future evaluations of the costs of diabetes, including the important issue of cost effectiveness of care, there should be an important consideration relating to the substantial informal care-giving costs associated with this metabolic disorder.

SPECIAL CASE OF FRAIL NURSING HOME RESIDENTS

A detailed account of this area has also been given in Chapter 27 but it is important to emphasize the deficiencies in diabetes care in these settings and to suggest possible ways to enhance care. More than one in four residents of nursing homes have diabetes (13) and the presence of diabetes imposes an increased risk of admission to a nursing home (14). Several factors are likely to affect this admission scenario and are summarized as (*i*) nature and severity of medical condition (s)/functional status; (*ii*) availability of family/caregiver support, and (*iii*) availability of community-based programs.

Despite their significant numbers, residents of nursing homes are a vulnerable and often neglected group of subjects with diabetes lacking comprehensive assessment, monitoring, and

BOX A   Informal Caregivers of Older Patients with Diabetes—Requirements of the "Support Package"

Information about the basic essentials of diabetes as a medical disorder
Practical guidance on the following
Monitoring of blood glucose and urinary glucose
Insulin administration where appropriate
Dietary instruction
Exercise and lifestyle "desirable" practices
Caregiver management of hypoglycemia, worsening glycemic control of patient index, and management of "sick days"
Information about local diabetes teams and other health professionals involved in diabetes care including contact persons and telephone numbers
Information about community and neighborhood services and social services that are available locally to support older adults with diabetes, from varying ethnic backgrounds, and their informal caregivers
Information about local ethnic diabetes support groups, which can provide further information advice on living with diabetes and the caring role and provide a forum and link for networking in any one district

Source: From Ref. 11.

BOX B Specific Interventions in Care Homes Likely to Bring About Change

Develop and implement care home diabetes clinical guidelines widely: pressure major professional diabetes organizations
(e.g., American Diabetes Association) to include care homes in their national strategies
Agree on a minimum data set for residents with diabetes
Examine feasibility of a cost-effective "domiciliary" photographic screening program for diabetic eye disease
Introduce an annual "protective sensory" test using a Semmes Weinstein monofilament or vibration test for each resident
Establish a hypoglycemic preventative program in each care home

specialist access (15). They are characterized by a high prevalence of vascular disease, repeated chest, urine, and skin infections and may be nutritionally impaired. In one recent study of Danish nursing homes, a third of residents had a body mass index of below 20 (16). Unfortunately, other issues compound the difficulties of maintaining functional well-being among residents, such as the dangerous and, often, inappropriate drug-prescribing patterns such as both excessive (e.g., neuroleptics) and deficient (e.g., β-blockers after acute myocardial infarction) use of medications (17).

There is a real need to rethink current approaches for treating diabetic residents within institutions. This involves both an evidenced-based and a realistic viewpoint, for example, emphasizing that in the prevention of vascular complications in older patients with type 2 diabetes, blood pressure control may be more important than glucose control or that detection and treatment of depression improves outcome more than controlling blood glucose and prevents more nursing-home admissions. Specific interventions that may bring about change are given in Box B.

These are not difficult interventions to implement but will require a culture change in diabetes care and a commitment from geriatricians and specialists in diabetes care to recognize the problem. National clinical guidelines on nursing homes diabetes are already published by the British Diabetic Association (18) as well as the American Medical Directors Association (19), but their implementation has been slow and uncoordinated. A great opportunity exists for cooperation across the Atlantic to come to a consensual approach in this area.

SPECIALIST DIABETES CARE FOR OLDER PEOPLE

Access to a specialist in diabetes care with a special expertise in older people is a mandatory requirement if high quality care is to be achieved. The rationale for this care and its associated grade of recommendation (A highest, D lowest) can be summarized as in Box C.

This care can be delivered via either secondary care (hospital) or community-based approach (or both). There has been conflicting evidence on whether hospital-based care is superior to routine primary care for patients with diabetes. One of the earliest studies in patients with type 2 diabetes (aged 40–80 years) (21) demonstrated that hospital care was superior in terms of HbA1c and lower mortality after a five-year follow-up review. This was in a relatively small number of patients and diabetes care by primary care providers in the community has moved on considerably since then. A recent meta-analysis of five randomized controlled trials in more than a 1000 patients (22), examining the same issue demonstrated no difference in glycemia and a suggestion of improved mortality in hospital care settings.

There are, of course, many factors that may influence the type of care provided: geographical location, access to hospital and community services across health-care boundaries

BOX C Rationale for High-Quality Diabetes Care for Older People with Type 2 Diabetes

Screening and early diagnosis may prevent progression of undetected vascular complications (C)
Improved metabolic control will reduce cardiovascular risk (B)
Improved screening for maculopathy and cataracts will reduce visual impairment and blind registrations (C)
An integrated approach to the management of peripheral vascular disease and foot disorders will reduce amputation rate (B)
Improved primary care and specialist followup will reduce hospital admission rate (D)

Note: B, C, and D are levels of recommendations.
Source: From Ref. 20.

BOX D   Criteria for Referral to Hospital-Based Specialists and Members of the Diabetes Care Team

Where diabetes care may be deficient
Newly diagnosed patients with treatable vascular complications or foot ulceration
Recurrent hypoglycemia
Patients with persistent poor metabolic control where HbA1c, blood pressure, or lipid level targets have not been achieved
Patients with increasing dependency and immobility, e.g., due to a previous stroke, neuropathy (geriatrician), and/or development of falls syndrome
Diabetic patients with suspected depressive symptoms or cognitive dysfunction/memory problems
Development of early heart failure or unstable angina (cardiologist)
Patients whose serum creatinine is 140–250 µmol/L (diabetologist) or 250 µmol/L (nephrologist)

as well as national drivers such as the increasing trend for integrated (shared) care, and policy formation from professional diabetes societies.

Where a strong community diabetes setup exists, there must be agreement on when to refer to the specialist physician and/or to the diabetes care team. These are outlined in Box D.

EVIDENCED-BASED MEDICINE APPROACHES

The evidenced-based medicine approach has become sacrosanct in health-care delivery, with health professionals signing up to it as disciples! Regrettably, in geriatric diabetes, there are few major examples of benefit seen from therapeutic interventions in major clinical trials, which have had older people as the focus. In addition, what evidence there is has been poorly interpreted or its impact unmeasured. The current situation, therefore, is reflected in Box E.

These issues, perhaps paradoxically because of lesser evidence available, provide a platform for the development of clinical guidelines based on an evidenced-based medicine approach.

CLINICAL GUIDELINES OF CARE—A EUROPEAN UNION APPROACH

Modern diabetes care systems for older people require integrated care that is characterized by a multidimensional approach, with an emphasis on prevention of diabetes and its complications, early detection and intervention for vascular disease, and assessment of functional status. Variations in clinical practice across the European Union for managing older people with diabetes are recognized (Box F) but it is not certain how much lack of resources are responsible and how much the "culture" of treating older people plays a part. What is clear, however, is that

BOX E   Evidence-Based Medicine—the Bottom Line Relating to Diabetes in Older People

No large scale intervention studies in older people with diabetes (subjects aged >75 yr)
No substantial evidence of benefit for glucose-lowering
Limited evidence for lipid lowering—PROSPER (2002) and ASCOT (2003)
No evidence to recommend a particular diabetes care model
No evidence to support metabolic or educational interventions in care home residents or those who are housebound

Abbreviations: ASCOT, Anglo-Scandinavian Cardiac Outcomes Trial; PROSPER, Prosepective Study of Pravastatin in the Elderly at Risk.

BOX F   Variations in Clinical Practice in Europe—Inequalities in Diabetes Care for Older People

Lack of access to local diabetes services
Inadequate specialist provision
Inadequate assessment of needs
Poorer clinical outcomes and premature mortality
Patient and family dissatisfaction
Lack of involvement in clinical research and intervention studies

BOX G Shortfalls Relating to Older People in Current Type 2 Diabetes Clinical Guidelines

Lack of recognition of older people as a special group with diverse and differing needs
Recommendations often do not apply to individuals older than 75 yr, those with frailty or multiple comorbidities, or those residing in institutions
Failure to consider the major role of caregivers or the support they require in delivering diabetes care
Failure to consider the ethical dimensions and dilemmas in diabetes care
No consideration to the nature/type of diabetes care model adopted

wide variations in clinical standards exist. Where is the evidence that this is not an issue for North America as well?

Apart from the excellent clinical guidelines by the American Geriatrics Society (AGS) (23), most other major clinical guidelines have not included special provision for this vulnerable group. Other shortfalls relating to older people in current clinical guidelines for type 2 diabetes are indicated in Box G.

The Clinical Guidelines of the European Diabetes Working Party for Older People are meant to fill this important gap and complement other published work (20). They are designed to provide an up-to-date, evidence-based approach to practical clinical decision making for older adults with type 2 diabetes aged 70 years and over and improve consistency of diabetes care across other countries. Other aims such as improving cost effectiveness and influencing national and international policy making requires further investment in research and greater lobbying by the government.

Following a strategic meeting of the European Working Party ("Paris Declaration") in December 2000, "Primary Areas of Concern and Targeted Areas for Concerted Action" were identified—Box H.

These were researched for guideline inclusion by using the Scottish Intercollegiate Guideline Network 50 guideline developer's handbook approach. Relevant studies were critically appraised and reviewers assigned a level of evidence and graded each recommendation made. All major clinical and health-related databases were examined including Embase, Medline/PubMed, Cochrane Trials register, Cinahl, and Science Citation. A rigorous guideline development plan was adopted with later external review endorsement. Seven sections have been included: aims of care (including education, screening/diagnosis, prevention, and ethics of care); framework and models of care; functional impairment/disability; cardiovascular disease and risk assessment; treatment strategies; nursing home diabetes; and specific problems: foot disease, visual loss, erectile dysfunction, and pain. Recommendations for care were made in each section, including key clinical messages, best practice points, and key research areas. These guidelines represent the most up-to-date and detailed evidence-based description of diabetes care for subjects of advanced age. They have been presented and well received in Italy, Spain, United Kingdom, United States, Costa Rica, and other parts of the European Union. A revision of the guidelines is due to take place in November 2006.

RESEARCH IN GERIATRIC DIABETES ARISING FROM CLINICAL GUIDELINE DEVELOPMENT

An analysis of both AGS and European Working Party guidelines suggests a number of important areas for future research. These have been summarized in Box I.

BOX H Paris Declaration 2000: Primary Areas of Concern—Targets for Concerted Action

Emphasizing the importance of functional and vascular assessment
Need to explore relationship between functional outcome and metabolic control
Management of diabetes in primary care
Routine screening for cognitive impairment and depressive illness
Care home diabetes
Management of specific problems: visual loss, pain, and foot disease
Ethical and moral aspects of treatment

BOX I   Areas of Future Clinical Research in Geriatric Diabetes

Evaluation study of educational interventions
Benefits of early and regular functional status assessment in the management of older people with type 2 diabetes mellitus
Benefits of lifestyle intervention and/or therapeutic approaches (e.g., ACE inhibitor, insulin sensitizer, etc.) in reducing the incidence of type 2 diabetes in older subjects (>70 yr) with hypertension or other cardiovascular risk factors
Outcome of intensive treatment with oral agents and/or insulin in older subjects with type 2 diabetes (>70 yr) to evaluate primary macrovascular and microvascular outcomes and mortality
Does lowering blood pressure reduce the risk of dementia in people with type 2 diabetes and hypertension?
Benefits (vascular/mortality outcome data; cost effectiveness) of statin and/or fibrate therapy in older subjects with type 2 diabetes and proven cardiovascular disease using an RCT approach

Abbreviations: ACE, angiotensin converting enzyme; RCT, randomized control trial.

These have been provided to complement the scientific research themes given in Chapter 30. National campaigns to increase funding for this research, collaborative working across health disciplines, and international cooperation to deliver large randomized clinical trials is essential.

CONCLUSION

A pressing need in geriatric diabetes is to develop effective interventions that target the multifaceted nature of this disabling condition in older people—Box J. This requires considerable energy on the part of the clinician but with the promise of improved outcomes, it can be professionally very satisfying.

Other major challenges remain and include developing a model of diabetes care for older people based on the recognition that the traditional metabolic model is insufficient to meet the complete needs of many patients and that an effective model requires elements relating to the vascular approach (focus on cardiovascular and cerebrovascular disease, limb vascular disease, and eyes) and rehabilitation (focus on prevention and management of disability) (24). This and other challenges continue to make geriatric diabetes an area for further development and should be emphasized in the training of all geriatricians, diabetes specialists, and primary care physicians.

KEY POINTS

- Informal caregivers are a neglected group in diabetes care, whose contributions are associated with considerable healthcare cost savings, improved support for older patients with diabetes, evidence of unmet needs as well as an urgent need for support for themselves.
- Diabetes care for residents of institutions needs a rethink! Specific interventions need to be adopted and evaluated. Quality standards need agreement and regular audit established.
- Specialist care for older people with diabetes is to be enhanced and not downgraded but research needs to establish where this care is best delivered.
- Further research in geriatric diabetes will strengthen the evidence base and increase the validity of clinical decision making; some key interventions can already be justified. Clinical guidelines have a place in clinical care but require local interpretation.

BOX J   Interventions in Geriatric Diabetes: A Realistic and Justified Approach

Preventative: targeting middle-aged, high-risk individuals with diet/lifestyle changes and antihypertensive medication (where appropriate) to reduce onset of diabetes
Where calculated life expectancy is greater than 5 yr, aiming for strict metabolic control to reduce vascular complications and cardiovascular risk
Early detection of disability may prevent/delay further functional deterioration, for example, mobility, ADL function, and falls rate
Active screening for evidence of cognitive dysfunction and/or depressive symptomatology to prevent functional decline, improve adherence to therapy, and delay the need for caregiver support
Early detection of diabetes in care home settings with the purpose of improving well-being, reducing vascular endpoints and metabolic decompensation, and delaying onset of disability

Abbreviation: ADL, activities of daily living.

REFERENCES

1. Sinclair AJ. Aging and diabetes. In: De Fronzo RA, Ferrannini E, Keen H, Zimmet P, eds. International Textbook of Diabetes Mellitus. 3rd ed. Chichester, England: John Wiley & Sons Ltd, 2004.
2. Karlsson M, Mayhew L, Plumb R, Rickayzen B. Future costs for long-term care: cost projections for long-term care for older people in the United Kingdom. Health Policy 2006; 75:187–213.
3. Holmes J, Gear E, Bottomley J, Gillam S, Murphy M, Williams R. Do people with type 2 diabetes and their caregivers lose income? (T2 Ardis-4). Health Policy 2003; 64:291–296.
4. Tsai PF, Jirovec MM. The relationship between depression and other outcomes of chronic illness caregiving. BMC Nurs 2005; 4(1):3.
5. Langa KM, Vijan S, Hayward RA, et al. Informal caregiving for diabetes and diabetic complications among elderly Americans. J Gerontol B Psychol Sci Soc Sci 2002; 57(3):S177–S186.
6. Askham J, Grundy E, Tucker A. Caring: The Importance of Third Age Caregivers. Research Paper No 6. London: Carnegie United Kingdom Trust, 1992.
7. Samuel-Hodge CD, Skelly AH, Headen S, Carter-Edwards L. Familial roles of older African-American women with type 2 diabetes: testing of a new multiple caregiving measure. Ethn Dis 2000; 15(3): 436–444.
8. Brown SA, Garcia AA, Kouzekanani K, Hanis CL. Culturally competent diabetes self-management education for Mexican-Americans: the Starr County Border Health Initiative. Diabetes Care 2002; 25(2):259–268.
9. Hennessy CH, John R, Anderson LA. Diabetes education needs of family members caring for American Indian elders. Diabetes Educ 1999; 25(5):747–754.
10. Li TC, Lee YD, Lin CC, Amidon RL. Quality of life of primary caregivers of elderly with cerebrovascular disease or diabetes hospitalised for acute care: assessment of well-being and functioning using the SF-36 health questionnaire. Qual Life Res 2004; 13(6):1081–1088.
11. Sinclair AJ, Bayer AJ. British Diabetic Association Report 1999: Informal Caregivers of Older Adults with Diabetes from Varying Ethnic Backgrounds. The European Diabets Working Party for Older People.
12. Rivadeneyra R, Elderkin-Thompson V, Silver RC, Waitzkin H. Patient centeredness in medical encounters requiring an interpreter. Am J Med 2000; 108:470–474.
13. Sinclair AJ, Gadsby R, Penfold S, Croxson SC, Bayer AJ. Prevalence of diabetes in care home residents. Diabetes Care 2001; 24(6):1066–1068.
14. Rockwood K, Stolee P, McDowell I. Factors associated with institutionalisation of older people in Canada: testing a multifactorial definition of frailty. JAGS 1996; 44(5):578–582.
15. Sinclair A, Allard I, Bayer A. Observations of diabetes care in long-term institutional settings with measures of cognitive function and dependency. Diabetes Care 1997; 20(5):778–784.
16. Beck AM, Ovesen L. Body mass index, weight loss and evening intake of old Danish nursing home residents and home-care clients. Scand J Caring Sci 2002; 16(1):86–90.
17. Fahey T, Montgomery AA, Barnes J, Protheroe J. Quality of care for elderly residents in nursing homes and elderly people living at home: controlled observational study. BMJ 2003; 326:580.
18. BDA (British Diabetic Association). Guidelines of Practice for Residents with Diabetes in Care Homes. London: BDA, 1999.
19. http://www.amda.com/tools/cpg/diabetes.cfm.
20. Clinical Guidelines for Type 2 Diabetes Mellitus. The European Diabetes Working Party for older people 2001–2004 (www.eugms.org).
21. Hayes TM, Harries J. Randomised controlled trial of routine hospital clinic care versus routine general practice care for type II diabetics. BMJ 1984; 289:728–730.
22. Griffin S. Diabetes care in general practice: meta-analysis of randomised control trials. BMJ 1998; 319:390–396.
23. Care California Healthcare Foundation/American Geriatrics Society Panel in improving care for elders with diabetes. Guidelines for improving the care of the older person with diabetes mellitus. JAGS 2003; 51:265–294.
24. Sinclair AJ. Diabetes in old age: changing concepts in the secondary care arena. J Roy Coll Phys 2000; 34:240–244.

30 Promising Research, New Pharmacotherapy and Technologies, and Their Relevance to Older Adults

William M. Sullivan
Joslin Diabetes Center, Beth Israel Deaconess Medical Center, and Department of Medicine, Harvard Medical School, Boston, Massachusetts, U.S.A.

INTRODUCTION

Over the past year, there have been a number of new medications available for the treatment of diabetes mellitus. These medications include the incretin mimetic agent exenatide, the amylin analog pramlintide, and the insulin analogs including glulisine and detemir insulin. These medications were covered in Chapter 21. This chapter will review newer medications not yet available, including the α cannabinoid-1 (CB-1) receptor antagonist rimonabant, the new DPP-4 inhibitors, the long-acting glucagon-like peptide 1 (GLP-1) analog liraglutide, and inhaled insulin, including recently approved Exubera (Table 1).

NEWER MEDICATIONS
Oral and Injectable Agents

Since the majority of patients with type 2 diabetes are overweight or obese, an effective weight loss medication would be an attractive option in improving glycemic control as well as other metabolic parameters. Fenfluramine and dexfenfluramine had been effective weight loss medications and were widely prescribed but were taken off the market in 1997 when their association with primary pulmonary hypertension and valvular heart disease became apparent (1). The currently available agents—sibutramine (a centrally active inhibitor of serotonin and noradrenaline uptake) and orlistat (a lipase inhibitor that decreases absorption of fat from the gut by 30%) are modestly effective in promoting weight loss and improving diabetes control (2). Rimonabant, a CB-1 receptor antagonist, has been shown to decrease appetite and reduce weight (3,4). By affecting CB-1 receptors in the brain, there is less desire to eat and thus subsequent weight loss. In a one-year study involving over 1500 subjects with obesity [body mass index (BMI) > 30] or BMI > 27 with risk factors including hypertension or hyperlipidemia, (Rimonabant in Obesity—Europe), rimonabant at 20 mg/day was associated with weight loss (6.6 kg), decreased waist circumference, decreased triglycerides, increased high-density lipoprotein, and improved glucose tolerance (3). In a similar one-year study on over 3000 subjects in North America, there was a 6.3 kg weight loss with reduction in waist circumference and improved lipid status with rimonabant 20 mg/day (5). Rimonabant was generally well tolerated in both studies with most common side effects being nausea, diarrhea, and dizziness—all of which tended to be mild and transient. In the Rimonabant in Obesity (RIO)–North America study, 4% of the subjects were over the age of 65 years. Both RIO–North America and RIO–Europe excluded patients with diabetes mellitus, but rimonabant is currently being studied in patients with diabetes mellitus. It is important to note that rimonabant has not been shown to reduce morbidity and mortality. Also, patients tend to regain the weight they lost after rimonabant withdrawal and possible long-tem adverse effects are not currently known.

A new class of agents called dipeptidyl peptidase-4 inhibitors (DPP-4) have recently become available for use. Sitaglipton was approved by the Food and Drug Administration (FDA) in the 2006 and vildagliptin is currently under review. These agents inhibit the DPP-4 enzyme that rapidly degrades GLP-1. Thus, increasing GLP-1 concentrations in the blood cause a number of metabolic effects including increased insulin secretion in a glucose-dependent

TABLE 1 Newer Medications in the Treatment of Diabetes Mellitus

Rimonabant—cannabinoid-1 receptor antagonist
Vildagliptin and sitagliptin—DPP-4 inhibitors
Liraglutide—long-acting subcutaneous glucagon-like peptide 1 analog
Exubera—rapid-acting inhaled insulin

Abbreviation: DPP-4, dipeptidyl peptidase-4.

mechanism, decreased glucagon secretion, and delayed gastric emptying. In a 12-week, double-blind, placebo-controlled trial (followed by a 40-week extension study), vildagliptin at 50 mg once daily given orally, added to metformin treatment in patients with type 2 diabetes, lowered A1c by 0.7% at 12 weeks and the effect was sustained for the 52 weeks of the study (6). In a study of 521 patients aged 27 to 76 years, with a baseline A1c of 8.1%, sitagliptin in a dose of 100 mg/day lowered A1c by 0.6% (7). Patients with higher baseline A1c (>9%) experienced a greater placebo-subtracted A1c reduction (−1.2%) than those with A1c below 8% (−0.44%). In general, DPP-4 inhibitors tend to be well tolerated with no serious side effects reported to date (6,7). In contrast to exenatide, DPP-4 inhibitors (such as vildagliptin and sitagliptin) do not affect satiety and are not associated with weight loss.

Another new GLP-1–based therapy is liraglutide, which is a long-acting GLP-1 analog that has been made resistant to DPP-4 degradation (8). Liraglutide is a once-daily injection. In a 12-week study in 193 patients with type 2 diabetes (over the age of 30 years), A1c decreased from 7.6% to 6.8% in the liraglutide 0.75 mg/day group, which was similar to the A1c lowering in the comparison glimepiride group (mean dose of 2.7 mg/day of glimepiride) (8). There were rare reports (1 in 135 patients) of mild hypoglycemia (blood sugar less than 2.8 mmol/L) in the liraglutide group. Other side effects attributable to liraglutide were mild and transient, including headache, nausea, vomiting, and diarrhea. There was a 0.5- to 1.0-kg weight gain in the glimepiride group versus no weight gain and up to 1.2 kg weight loss in the liraglutide group (depending on dose given). Thus, liraglutide in early studies shows promise for lowering blood glucose without weight gain or increased risk of hypoglycemia. The low risk of hypoglycemia with both DPP-4 inhibitors and liraglutide would make them attractive agents for the elderly where hypoglycemia is avoided whenever possible.

Newer Insulin

Inhaled insulin is another novel approach to delivering insulin into the blood stream. The first available inhaled insulin will be Exubera, which was approved by the FDA in January 2006 for the treatment of both type 1 and type 2 diabetes in adults. Exubera is a rapid-acting, dry powder insulin delivery system developed by Pfizer (New York, U.S.A) and Sanofi-Aventis group (Bridgewater, New Jersey, U.S.A) in conjunction with Nektar Therapeutics (San Carlos, California, U.S.A) (9). Clinical studies indicate that it is comparable to other bolus insulins in controlling postprandial excursions (10). Exubera has been shown to be effective in patients with inadequate control on diet and exercise alone (11) and with multiple oral agents (12–14). Adverse effects have included a mild cough and hypoglycemia (with similar rates as subcutaneous insulin). In studies to date, there have been no significant changes in pulmonary function tests over time. Exubera in not recommended if there is any underlying lung disease such as emphysema or asthma. It is also not recommended in current smokers or if there is any history of smoking in the preceding six months. Pulmonary function tests are recommended at baseline, six months after initiating Exubera, and then annually. The issue of long-term pulmonary safety is still a major concern. In clinical studies with Exubera, the age range was typically 30 years to 80 years—so there have been studies in the elderly population. Potentially, Exubera (as well as other pulmonary insulin preparations that may become available in the future) will especially be helpful in the elderly patients with type 2 diabetes, who are very reluctant to start subcutaneous insulin therapy.

NEW METERS AND MONITORING SYSTEMS

Since home blood glucose monitoring became available in 1963, there has been considerable improvement in this technology. The initial Dextrostix was a paper strip to which blood was added. This was then timed for one minute and the blood was wiped off. A blue color then developed and was compared to a color chart for an approximate blood glucose reading. Later, meters were developed that gave a digital readout of the blood glucose level. These early meters were relatively cumbersome and difficult to use. Newer glucose monitoring meters are smaller, easier to use, and more accurate than the earlier versions. Also, the current models require only a minimal amount of blood and blood glucose results are available within seconds. In addition, many newer meters can check finger stick blood specimens as well as blood from alternate sites such as palm or forearm. Some elderly patients also prefer the meters that do not require handling of the small glucose strips, but rather use multiuse drums, such as the Accuchek Compact meter. Also, meters that do not require coding (such as the Accuchek Compact or Ascensia Contour) may be preferable in the elderly population.

Despite these advances in glucose meter technology, the ultimate goal is for truly noninvasive glucose testing. Many patients still find finger stick glucose testing painful and obtrusive. Less invasive devices are currently being developed and hopefully will be available in the near future.

A relatively new technology is continuous glucose monitoring systems (CGMS) (15). Using an inserted catheter (similar to that which delivers insulin as part of an insulin pump), these devices measure glucose levels multiple times every hour. They can be attached for 72 hours and are particularly helpful with glucose pattern analysis. The two recently approved devices are the Medtronic MiniMed CGMS and the DexCom system. The FDA has not yet approved a third system called the Abbott Navigator. These three devices are particularly designed for individuals with type 1 diabetes on intensive insulin therapy—in particular, patients on insulin pump therapy. These devices are not meant to replace finger stick testing but are meant to be supplemental. In fact, finger stick testing is still needed to calibrate the CGMS. Now, a major barrier to use of CGMS is the lack of third-party insurance coverage. CGMS can be helpful, in particular, with analysis of blood glucose patterns over a three-day period. Although there are no specific studies of CGMS in the elderly, one would expect that it could be especially useful in elderly patients with erratic diabetes control or recurrent hypoglycemia, on intensive insulin regimens.

INSULIN PUMPS

Although insulin pumps have been available since 1963, there has been significant improvement in both size and programmability since that time. The current pump models are much more compact and user friendly. The advantages of insulin pump therapy are greater lifestyle flexibility, less hypoglycemia, improved weight control, better control with exercise, and better insulin coverage for the dawn phenomenon. On the other hand, the demands of insulin pump therapy include frequent blood sugar testing (at least four times/day), inconvenience of wearing the pump and taking care of catheter sites and pump, need for trouble-shooting skills, potential increased risk of diabetic ketoacidosis, and extra cost (16).

A number of new features of the so-called smart pumps make the use of insulin pumps more user friendly. These features include alerts for blood glucose reminders as well as reminders for bolus and set change. Insulin-to-carbohydrate ratios and correction factors can be customized with different settings throughout the day. In addition, a bolus calculator within the pump can suggest a meal coverage dose based on carbohydrate intake and the measured blood sugar.

There are limited studies in the elderly population using insulin pump therapy. Rizvi et al. (17) report on five older subjects who were converted from insulin injections to pump therapy. There was a significant improvement in the glycohemoglobin level and less hypoglycemia after being changed over to pump therapy. Studies by Raskin et al. (18) and Wainstein et al. (19) have shown benefit with the use of insulin pump therapy in patients with type 2 diabetes, but there were limited number of patients over the age of 65. Herman et al. (20) compared pump therapy versus multiple daily injections in older adults (mean age 66) with insulin-treated type 2 diabetes. Both treatments achieved excellent glycemic control and good patient satisfaction. Weight gain and hypoglycemic events were similar in both groups. The study supported the use of multiple daily injections in difficult-to-control patients with insulin-treated type 2 diabetes before considering insulin pump therapy. As life expectancy of patients with

TABLE 2 Medicare Insulin Pump Coverage—Revised 2/05

Criterion A—new pump patient
  Completion of a comprehensive diabetes education program
  Requiring of at least 3 insulin injections per day
  Frequent self-adjustments of insulin for 6 mo prior to starting pump therapy
  Documented blood sugar testing at least four times/day for 2 mo prior to starting pump therapy
  Meeting of one or more of the following criteria—A1c > 7%, history of recurrent hypoglycemia,
    wide variation of premeal glucose levels, dawn phenomenon with fasting sugars over
    200 mg%, or history of severe glycemic excursions
Criterion B—patient previously on pump therapy prior to Medicare enrollment
  Documented testing of at least 4 times/day—for 1 mo prior to Medicare enrollment

type 1 diabetes increases, we may see more older patients using the insulin pump. In elderly patients with other medical comorbidities, especially cognitive dysfunction, patients' ability to use pump safely should be frequently assessed.

In the care of older individuals with diabetes on insulin pump therapy, one needs to be aware of recent Medicare revisions concerning pump coverage (21,22). Implemented in February 2005, insulin pumps are covered as medically necessary if (*i*) they satisfy criteria A or B (Table 2) and (*ii*) meet the fasting C-peptide requirement or are β-cell antibody positive (Table 3).

PANCREAS AND ISLET-CELL TRANSPLANTATION

Both pancreas and islet-cell transplantation have been used in selected cases to treat insulin deficiency in diabetes. Pancreas transplantation was first performed on an experimental basis in the 1960s and then became more widely available in the 1980s. Benefits of pancreas transplantation include stabilization of both diabetic neuropathy and retinopathy (23,24). With regard to nephropathy, studies have shown reversal of histological changes toward normal after 10 years of a pancreas transplant (but there were no histological changes five years after pancreas transplant) (25). There has also been improved quality of life with no further need for insulin injections and food restrictions. With pancreas transplantation, there has been an 85% one-year survival and a 70% five-year graft survival—with better outcomes with simultaneous pancreas and kidney transplantation (SPK) when compared with pancreas transplant alone or pancreas transplant after kidney transplant (26). On the other hand, pancreas transplantation is a major abdominal surgery requiring extended hospitalization with a cost of approximately $100,000 per patient (27). Also, there is a need for long-term immunosuppression with its attendant side effects. Now, the most common procedure is the simultaneous pancreas and kidney transplant given to patients with type 1 diabetes and advanced renal disease. As of registry data from 2002, the number of potential recipients on the kidney–pancreas (SPK) transplant waiting list is mostly in the 35- to 49-year age group (60%) with less than 10% in the 65-year and older group (26).

Islet-cell transplantation is an experimental procedure of infusing insulin-secreting β-cells via a transhepatic approach to selected patients with type 1 diabetes. Prior to 2000, the results of islet-cell transplantation were disappointing. In 2000, Shapiro et al. (28) reported initial findings in seven patients who achieved insulin independence after islet-cell transplantation with up to a year of followup. They used a different immunosuppressive regimen including rapamycin (sirolimus) and tacrolimus (FK-506) without the use of glucocorticoids. For induction, daclizumab (antibody to the interleukin-2 receptor) was added. In addition, islets from

TABLE 3 Patient Eligibility for Medicare Coverage of Insulin Pump

Having a positive β-cell antibody test or
C-peptide being less than 110% of lower limit of normal concurrently with fasting glucose less
  than 225 mg%
Renal insufficiency being present with a glomerular filtration rate < 50 mL/min, then the C-peptide
  criteria is less than 200% of laboratory's lower limit of normal concurrently with a fasting
  glucose <225 mg%

more than one cadaver donor were required and the islets were used immediately after their isolation. The Edmonton group was treating a subgroup of patients with type 1 diabetes, who had been disabled by recurrent severe hypoglycemia—thus justifying the use of potentially harmful immunosuppressive medications. More recently, an international trial of the Edmonton protocol for islet transplantation was published (28). There were 36 subjects with type 1 diabetes, who underwent islet transplantation at nine international sites. The primary endpoint was defined as insulin independence with adequate glycemic control (A1c less than 6.5%) one year after the final transplantation. Although a majority (58%) attained insulin independence with good glycemic control at any point during the trial, approximately three-quarters of those patients required insulin again by two years. Thus, insulin independence was not usually sustainable, although persistent islet function did provide protection from severe hypoglycemia and improved levels of glycohemoglobin. In the international trial of the Edmonton protocol, the age range for subjects was 23 to 59 years (mean age of 41); thus, this study did not involve a geriatric population. In general, pancreas and islet-cell transplantation are being done in selected individuals with diabetes—and usually in younger age groups rather than the elderly population.

STEM-CELL RESEARCH

Currently, the main source of insulin-producing cells for transplantation is cadaver pancreata. Since the incidence of type 1 diabetes is approximately 30,000 new cases per year and there are less than 3000 cadaver pancreata available each year, there is a significant imbalance of supply and demand. Thus, one new avenue of research is the potential of stimulating stem cells into functional insulin-secreting β cells (29). Different types of stem cells include hematopoietic or intestinal cells; embryonic stem cells found in blastocytes or pancreatic duct cells—all cells that might be able to be stimulated to form new islet cells. However, major issues for the process of converting stem cells into functional β cells include the need for a large number of replacement β cells (islet-cell transplants use up to two to four times 10^9 β cells per recipient), the need to control the proliferative capacity of the replacement cells in vivo to avoid the development of hyperinsulinemic hypoglycemia, and then the need to avoid destruction by the recipient's immune system (29). Although stem-cell therapy offers the potential for an unlimited supply of β cells, we are still in the early stages of research and there are a number of unresolved ethical and scientific issues that are being confronted.

SUMMARY

1. Newer medications may offer significant benefit to the elderly patient with diabetes. Rimonabant may be helpful in promoting weight loss, but more long-term data is needed due to prior experience with rare side effects with fenfluramine and dexfenfluramine. The new DPP-4 inhibitors and liraglutide may improve glycemic control without risk of hypoglycemia or weight gain. Inhaled insulin may be helpful especially in the elderly patient who is anxious and reluctant to accept subcutaneous insulin therapy.
2. Newer meters that use a multiuse drum (rather than handling individual strips) and do not require coding may be easier to use in the elderly population.
3. Although published data is limited, insulin pump therapy can be successfully used in the elderly patient with erratic diabetes control and recurrent hypoglycemia.
4. Pancreas and islet-cell transplantation have, at the present time, a limited role in the care of elderly patients with diabetes.
5. Stem-cell research is in its early stages but offers the potential to improve the supply of insulin-producing cells.

REFERENCES

1. Yanovski SZ. Pharmacotherapy for obesity—promise and uncertainty. N Engl J Med 2005; 353: 2187–2189.
2. Kennedy RL, Khoo EYH. New options for the drug treatment of obesity in patients with Type 2 diabetes. Diabet med 2005; 22:23–26.

3. Van Gaal LF, Rissanen AM, Scheen AJ, et al. Effects of the cannibinoid—receptor blocker rimonabant on weight reduction and cardiovascular risk facts in overweight patients: 1 year experience from the RIO-Europe study. Lancet 2005; 365:1389–1397.
4. Pagotto U, Pasquali R. Fighting obesity and associated risk factors by antagonising cannbinoid type 1 receptors. Lancet 2005; 365:1363–1364.
5. Pi-Sunyer FX, Aronne LJ, Heshmati HM, et al. Effect of rimonabant, a cannabinoid-1 receptor blocker, on weight and cardiometabolic risk factors in overweight or obese patients—RIO-North America: a randomized controlled trial. JAMA 2006; 295:761–775.
6. Ahren B, Gomis R, Standl E, et al. Twelve and 52-week efficacy of the dipeptidyl peptidase IV inhibitor LAF237 in metformin-treated patients with Type 2 diabetes. Diabetes Care 2004; 27:2874–2880.
7. Raz I, Hanefeld M, Xu L, et al. Efficacy and safety of the dipeptidyl peptidase-inhibitor sitagliptin as monotherapy in patients with type 2 diabetes mellitus. Diabetologia 2006; 49(11):2564–2571.
8. Masbad S, Schmitz O, Ranstam J, et al. Improved glycemic control with no weight increase in patients with type 2 diabetes after once-daily treatment with the long-acting glucagon –like peptide 1 analog liraglutide (NN2211). Diabetes Care 2004; 27:1335–1342.
9. Barnett AH. Exubera inhaled insulin: a review. Int J Clin Pract 2004; 58:394–401.
10. Hollander PA, Blonde L, Rowe R, et al. Efficacy and safety of inhaled insulin (Exubera) compared with subcutaneous insulin therapy in patients with type 2 diabetes: results of a 6 month randomized controlled trial. Diabetes Care 2004; 27:2356–2362.
11. DeFronzo RA, Bergenstal RM, Cefalu WT, et al. The Exubera Phase III Study Group. Efficacy of inhaled insulin in patients with type 2 diabetes not controlled on diet and exercise. Diabetes Care 2005; 28:1922–1928.
12. Weiss SR, Cheng SL, Kourides IA, et al. The inhaled insulin phase II study group: inhaled insulin provides improved glycemic control in patients with type 2 diabetes mellitus inadequately controlled with oral agents: a randomized controlled trial. Arch Intern Med 2003; 163:2277–2282.
13. Rosenstock J, Zinman B, Murphy LJ, et al. Mealtime inhaled insulin improves glycemic control in patients with type 2 diabetes failing two oral agents. Ann Intern Med 2005; 143:549–558.
14. Barnett AH, Dreyer M, Lange P, et al. An open, randomized, parallel-group study to compare the efficacy and safety profile of inhaled human insulin (Exubera) with glibenclamide as adjunctive therapy in patients with type 2 diabetes poorly controlled on metformin. Diabetes Care 2006; 29:1818–1825.
15. Kowalski A. Continuous glucose monitors and the new era of diabetes management. Endocr News 2006; 14–15.
16. Wolpert H. The pump advantage. In: Smart Pumping for People with Diabetes. Alexandria, Virginia: American Diabetes Association, 2002:8–16.
17. Rizvi AA, Arnold MB, Chakraborty M. Beneficial effects of continuous subcutaneous insulin infusion in older patients with long-standing type 1 diabetes. Endocr Pract 2001; 5(7):364–369.
18. Raskin P, Bode BW, Marck JB, et al. Continuous subcutaneous infusion and multiple daily injection therapy are equally effective in type 2 diabetes: a randomized, parallel group, 24-week study. Diabetes Care 2003; 26:2598–2603.
19. Wainstein J, Metzger M, Boaz M, et al. Insulin pump therapy vs. multiple daily injections in obese type 2 diabetic patients. Diabet Med 2005; 22:1037–1046.
20. Herman WH, Iiag LL, Johnson SL, et al. A clinical trial of continuous subcutaneous insulin infusion versus multiple daily injections in older adults with type 2 diabetes. Diabetes Care 2005; 28:1568–1573.
21. Wittlin SD. Treating the spectrum of type 2 diabetes—emphasis on insulin pump therapy. Diabetes Educ 2006; 32:39S–46S.
22. Hainer TA. Managing older adults with diabetes. J Am Acad Nurse Pract 2006; 18:309–317.
23. Ramsay RC, Goetz FC, Sutherland DE, et al. Progression of diabetic retinopathy after pancreas transplantation for insulin-dependent diabetes mellitus. N Engl J Med 1988; 318:208–214.
24. Landgraf R. Impact of pancreas transplantation on diabetic secondary complications and quality of life. Diabetologia 1996; 39:1415–1424.
25. Fioretto P, Steffes MW, Sutherland DER, et al. Reversal of lesions of diabetic nephropathy after pancreas transplantation. N Engl J Med 1998; 339:69–75.
26. Wynn JJ, Distant DA, Pirsch JD, et al. Kidney and pancreas transplantation. Am J Transplant 2004; 4(suppl 9):72–80.
27. Robertson RP, Holohan TV, Genuth S. Therapeutic controversy: pancreas transplantation for type 1 diabetes. J Clin Endocrinol Metab 1998; 83:1868–1874.
28. Shapiro AMJ, Ricordi C, Hering BJ, et al. International trial of the Edmondton Protocol for islet transplantation. N Engl J Med 2006; 355:1318–1330.
29. Burns CJ, Persaud SJ, Jones PM. Stem cell therapy for diabetes: do we need to make β cells? J Endocrinol 2004; 183:437–443.

Index